Essentials of
Anesthesia
for
Neurotrauma

Essentials of Anesthesia for Neurotrauma

Edited by
Hemanshu Prabhakar
Charu Mahajan
Indu Kapoor

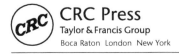

CRC Press
Taylor & Francis Group
Boca Raton London New York

CRC Press is an imprint of the
Taylor & Francis Group, an **informa** business

CRC Press
Taylor & Francis Group
6000 Broken Sound Parkway NW, Suite 300
Boca Raton, FL 33487-2742

First issued in paperback 2020

ISBN-13: 978-0-367-57144-3 (pbk)
ISBN-13: 978-1-138-89507-2 (hbk)

Library of Congress Cataloging-in-Publication Data
Names: Prabhakar, Hemanshu, editor. | Mahajan, Charu, editor. | Kapoor, Indu, editor.
Title: Essentials of anesthesia for neurotrauma / [edited by] Hemanshu Prabhakar, Charu Mahajan and Indu Kapoor.
Description: Boca Raton : Taylor & Francis, 2018. | Includes bibliographical references and index.
Identifiers: LCCN 2017053033| ISBN 9781138895072 (hardback : alk. paper) | ISBN 9781315166742 (ebook)
Subjects: | MESH: Trauma, Nervous System--surgery | Anesthesia--methods
Classification: LCC RD81 | NLM WL 140 | DDC 617.9/6--dc23
LC record available at https://lccn.loc.gov/2017053033

Visit the Taylor & Francis website at
http://www.taylorandfrancis.com

and the CRC Press website at
http://www.crcpress.com

To our parents, teachers, and the greatest gifts my parents gave to me, with whom I share my childhood memories, Kavita and Hemant.

Hemanshu Prabhakar

To our parents, teachers, and the greatest gifts my parents gave to me, with whom I share my childhood memories, Shelly, Shruti, and Aman.

Charu Mahajan

To our parents, teachers, and the greatest gifts my parents gave to me, with whom I share my childhood memories, Sunita, Poonam, and Tanzin.

Indu Kapoor

Contents

PART V NEUROSURGERY

PART VI NEUROMONITORING

PART VII NEURORADIOLOGY

PART VIII NEUROINTENSIVE CARE

PART XVI   WEBLIOGRAPHY

Index

Foreword

ESSENTIALS OF ANESTHESIA FOR NEUROTRAUMA

Globally, neurotrauma represents one of the most important causes of neurodisability. Despite the likely increase in neurodegenerative and cerebrovascular disease over the decades to come, the World Health Organization (WHO) estimates that traumatic brain injury (TBI) and spinal cord injury (SCI) will continue to be important drivers of disability and, hence, will represent important public health targets. This is particularly the case in low- and middle-income countries, where motor vehicle use is increasing at a rate far greater than the population's rate, with a consequent escalation in the burden of death and disability caused by neurotrauma.

Optimization of outcome from neurotrauma not only depends on definitive neurosurgical interventions but also requires skillful and well-informed anesthetic and critical care practice. Such practice can facilitate surgery when required and optimize the physiologic context for recovery from injury.

However, none of the interventions that we use in this context are risk free, and both knowledge and procedural expertise are required to ensure the best balance between the benefits and risks of individual interventions. Furthermore, these interventions need to be embedded in a clinical framework that delivers appropriate and timely care.

Given this context, this textbook, edited by a clinician with substantial expertise and experience in this area, is a welcome development. The contents of this textbook, which represent the output of an expert group of international authors, will help both trainees and specialists to make judgments that maximize benefit and minimize risk, with the result that we not only increase survival from neurotrauma but also improve the quality of this survival.

David K. Menon
Cambridge, UK

Preface

Neurotrauma is a preventable public health issue, yet it can have devastating consequences amounting to huge community and economic losses. The timely, proficient anesthetic and surgical management is impetus for improving the outcomes. Yet, there has never been a dedicated book covering all of the aspects of neurotrauma along with the various complications in the past. This book is simple to read and understand and highlights all of the practical aspects of anesthesia for patients with neurotrauma. This book aims to provide an overview of the basics of anesthesia for neurotrauma. Its target audience are trainees and fellows in neuroanesthesia and anesthesia, including physicians associated with neurosurgical and allied branches, such as neurology and neuroradiology. It will be very helpful, especially to those medical practitioners who are providing anesthesia for neurotrauma cases but who have not been formally trained in the subject.

The purpose of this book is to provide basic information on anesthesia for neurotrauma and to explain how the management of different neurotrauma cases may differ, especially those involving the head, spine, and/or polytrauma.

Straightforward issues, such as neurologic examination of such patients and understanding their CT and MRI scans, have been discussed in a simple, easy-to-understand manner. Starting with the prehospital management and resuscitation of these patients, the book covers perioperative management in great detail, including their care. Special considerations, such as pediatric, obstetric, and geriatric patients suffering neurotrauma have been dealt with separately. The less-often discussed issues, such as palliative care and rehabilitation, have also been included to make the readers aware of their importance and necessity. Another highlight is the clinical procedures section, which provides quick and easy access and can be quite helpful for all practical purposes. Thus, this book provides insight into all possible aspects of the anesthetic management of neurotrauma patients. The authors of this book are experts in their fields and we are grateful to all of the contributors who have made this work possible.

Hemanshu Prabhakar
Charu Mahajan
Indu Kapoor

Acknowledgments

We wish to acknowledge the support of the administration of the All India Institute of Medical Sciences (AIIMS), New Delhi, India, for allowing us to conduct this academic task.

We thank the faculty and staff of the Department of Neuroanesthesiology and Critical Care at AIIMS for their support.

Special thanks are due to the production team at CRC Press/Taylor & Francis: Shivangi, Mouli, Ritesh, Rajani, and Sunaina.

Editors

Hemanshu Prabhakar is a Professor in the Department of Neuroanesthesiology and Critical Care at All India Institute of Medical Sciences (AIIMS), New Delhi, India. He received his training in neuroanesthesia at the same institute. Recently, he completed a PhD and now has the honor of being the first PhD (in neuroanesthesia) in India. He is the recipient of the AIIMS Excellence Award for notable contributions in academics. He has more than 250 publications to his credit. He is a reviewer for various national and international journals. He is also a review author for the Cochrane Collaboration and has a special interest in evidence-based practice in neuroanesthesia. Dr. Prabhakar is a member of various neuroanesthesia societies and is a past secretary of the Indian Society of Neuroanesthesia and Critical Care. He is an invited faculty member of numerous conferences, is on the editorial board of the *Indian Journal of Palliative Care*, and is the executive editor of the *Journal of Neuroanaesthesiology and Critical Care*. Dr. Prabhakar has written many book chapters in his area of expertise. He is the editor of *Complications in Neuroanesthesia* (2016) and *Essentials of Neuroanesthesia* (2017), which were published by Elsevier. He is also the editor of the *Manual of Neuroanesthesia* (2017), which has been published by CRC Press/Taylor & Francis.

Charu Mahajan is an Assistant Professor in the Department of Neuroanesthesiology and Critical Care at AIIMS, New Delhi, India. After completing a MD in anesthesia, she was awarded a DM in neuroanesthesia at AIIMS and later joined as a faculty member. She has authored over 60 publications in various national and international journals. She is a reviewer for the Cochrane Collaboration. She also co-edited the book, *Manual of Neuroanaesthesia* (2017), which has been published by CRC Press/Taylor & Francis. She has authored chapters in many books and has received numerous awards for scientific presentations. Dr. Mahajan is a member of various scientific societies and is a reviewer for several reputable scientific journals.

Indu Kapoor is an Assistant Professor in the Department of Neuroanesthesiology and Critical Care at AIIMS, New Delhi, India. She received her training in neuroanesthesia at the same institute. She is the recipient of the Dr. T N JHA Memorial Award in 2009, which was awarded by the Indian Society of Anesthesiologists (ISA) in Chennai. She has also received the SMT Chandra and SH Narayan Wadhwani Memorial Award for best outgoing postgraduate in anesthesia at the University College of Medical Sciences, Delhi, in 2010. She has over 35 publications in national and international journals to her credit. She is also a reviewer of national journals and a review author for the Cochrane Collaboration. Dr. Kapoor has a special interest in evidence-based practice in neuroanesthesia. Additionally, she is a member of various national societies and has been an invited faculty member at various national conferences. Dr. Kapoor has written numerous chapters for various national and international books.

Contributors

Mohamed Samy Abdel Raheem
Department of Anesthesiology and Intensive
  Care
Asyut University Hospitals
Asyut University School of Medicine
Asyut, Egypt

Richa Aggarwal
Division of Trauma Surgery and Critical Care
JPNA Trauma Centre
AIIMS
New Delhi, India

Morfaizan Ahmad
Department of Anesthesia
Sheffield Teaching Hospitals
Sheffield, United Kingdom

Gocke Yilmaz
Department of Anesthesiology
Bahcelievler State Hospital
Istanbul, Turkey

Onat Akyol
Department of Anesthesiology
University of Health Sciences,
Istanbul Bagcilar Training and Research Hospital
Istanbul, Turkey

Zulfiqar Ali
Division of Neuroanesthesiology
  and Neurocritical Care
Sheri Kashmir Institute of Medical Sciences Soura
Jammu and Kashmir, India

Richard Applegate II
Department of Anesthesiology and Pain Medicine
University of California
Davis, California

Lauren Berkow
Department of Anesthesiology
Division of Neuroanesthesia
University of Florida College of Medicine
Gainesville, Florida

Suparna Bharadwaj
Department of Neuroanesthesia and
  Neurocritical Care
National Institute of Mental Health and
  Neurosciences
Bangalore, India

Prasanna Udupi Bidkar
Department of Anesthesiology and Critical Care
JIPMER
Puducherry, India

Barbara Cambiaghi
School of Medicine and Surgery
University of Milan–Bicocca
Milan, Italy

Maria Chiara Casadio
School of Medicine and Surgery
University of Milan–Bicocca
Milan, Italy

Matthew T.V. Chan
Department of Anesthesia and Intensive Care
The Chinese University of Hong Kong
Hong Kong Special Administrative Region, China

Dinu Chandran
Department of Physiology
All India Institute of Medical Sciences
New Delhi, India

Sheng Chen
Department of Neurosurgery
Second Affiliated Hospital
School of Medicine
Zhejiang University
Hangzhou, Zhejiang, China

Mandy H.M. Chu
Department of Anesthesia
Pamela Youde Nethersole Eastern Hospital
Chai Wan, Hong Kong Special Administrative
    Region, China

Giuseppe Citerio
School of Medicine and Surgery
University of Milan–Bicocca
Milan, Italy
and
Neurointensive Care
Department of Emergency and Intensive Care
San Gerardo Hospital
ASST Monza, Italy

Maria J. Colomina
Department of Anesthesiology, Reanimation
    and Pain Clinic
Hospital Universitari de Bellvitge–Hospitalet
Universitat de Barcelona
Barcelona, Spain

Marek Czosnyka
Section of Brain Physics
Division of Neurosurgery
Addenbrooke's Hospital
University of Cambridge
Cambridge, United Kingdom
and
Institute of Electronic Systems
Warsaw University of Technology
Warsaw, Poland

Eunice Y.L. Dai
Department of Imaging and Interventional
    Radiology
Prince of Wales Hospital
Hong Kong Special Administrative Region, China

Raffaele Di Fenza
School of Medicine and Surgery
University of Milan–Bicocca
Milan, Italy

Marco Echeverria
Department of Anesthesiology
Clinical Research
Wexner Medical Center
Ohio State University
Columbus, Ohio

Hossam El Beheiry
Department of Anesthesia
University of Toronto
Toronto, Ontario, Canada
and
Trillium Health Partners
Mississauga Hospital
Mississauga, Ontario, Canada

Neus Fàbregas
Anesthesiology Department
Hospital Clínic de Barcelona
University of Barcelona
Barcelona, Spain

Salia Farrokh
Department of Pharmacy
The Johns Hopkins Hospital
Department of Anesthesiology and Critical Care
    Medicine
The Johns Hopkins School of Medicine
Baltimore, Maryland

Magni Federico
Department of Emergency and Intensive Care
San Gerardo Hospital
ASST Monza, Italy

Daniela Ferlicca
Department of Emergency and Intensive Care
San Gerardo Hospital
ASST Monza, Italy

Alana M. Flexman
Department of Anesthesiology, Pharmacology
    and Therapeutics
University of British Columbia
Vancouver General Hospital
Vancouver, British Columbia, Canada

Vadim Gospodarev
Department of Physiology and Pharmacology
Loma Linda University School of Medicine
Loma Linda, California

Nidhi Gupta
Department of Neuroanesthesia
Indraprastha Apollo Hospital
New Delhi, India

Mohan Gurjar
Department of Critical Care Medicine
Sanjay Gandhi Postgraduate Institute
    of Medical Sciences
Lucknow, India

Zakir Hajat
Department of Anesthesia and Critical Care
Royal Hallamshire Hospital
Sheffield Teaching Hospitals NHS FT
Sheffield, United Kingdom

Shumaila Hasan
The Royal London Hospital
Barts Health NHS Trust
London, United Kingdom

Kiran Jangra
Department of Anesthesia and Intensive Care
Postgraduate Institute of Medical Education
    and Research
Chandigarh, India

Patricia K.Y. Kan
Department of Anesthesia and Intensive Care
Prince of Wales Hospital
Hong Kong Special Administrative Region, China

Indu Kapoor
Department of Neuroanesthesiology
    and Critical Care
Neurosciences Center
All India Institute of Medical Sciences
New Delhi, India

Manpreet Kaur
Department of Physiology
Vardhaman Mahavir Medical College
    and Safdarjung Hospital
New Delhi, India

Ankur Khandelwal
Department of Neuroanesthesiology and Critical
    Care
Neurosciences Centre
All India Institute of Medical Sciences
New Delhi, India

Priyanka Khurana
GB Pant Institute of Post Graduate Medical
    Education and Research
New Delhi, India

Matthew A. Kirkman
The National Hospital for Neurology
    and Neurosurgery
UCL Hospitals NHS Foundation Trust
Queen Square, London, United Kingdom

Alexandra Kisilevsky
Department of Anesthesiology, Pharmacology
    and Therapeutics
University of British Columbia
Vancouver General Hospital
Vancouver, British Columbia, Canada

Andrew W. Kofke
Department of Anesthesiology and Critical Care
and
Department of Neurosurgery
University of Pennsylvania
Philadelphia, Pennsylvania

Emily G.Y. Koo
Department of Anesthesiology, Intensive Care
    and Pain Medicine
Tan Tock Seng Hospital
Singapore, Singapore

Maylin Koo
Department of Anesthesiology, Reanimation
    and Pain Clinic
Hospital Universitari de Bellvitge–Hospitalet
Universitat de Barcelona
Barcelona, Spain

Sara Laxe
Brain Injury Department
Institut Guttmann
Hospital for Neurorehabilitation
Barcelona, Spain

Bastia Luca
School of Medicine and Surgery
University of Milan–Bicocca
Monza, Italy

Ankur Luthra
Department of Anesthesia and Intensive Care
Postgraduate Institute of Medical Education
    and Research
Chandigarh, India

Marta Magaldi
Department of Anesthesiology
Hospital Clínic de Barcelona
University of Barcelona
Barcelona, Spain

Charu Mahajan
Department of Neuroanesthesiology
    and Critical Care
Neurosciences Center
All India Institute of Medical Sciences
New Delhi, India

Vibha Mahendra
Department of Anesthesiology
Baylor College of Medicine
Houston, Texas

Panumart Manatpon
Division of Neurocritical Care
Department of Anesthesiology
University of Pennsylvania
Philadelphia, Pennsylvania

Basil Matta
Neurosciences Critical Care Unit
Addenbrooke's Hospital
University of Cambridge
Cambridge, United Kingdom

Pozzi Matteo
Department of Emergency and Intensive Care
San Gerardo Hospital
ASST Monza, Italy

Rajeeb K. Mishra
Department of Neuroanesthesiology
    and Critical Care
All India Institute of Medical Sciences
New Delhi, India

Manju Mohanty
Department of Neurosurgery
Post Graduate Institute of Medical Education
    and Research
Chandigarh, India

Srilata Moningi
Department of Anesthesia and Intensive Care
Nizam's Institute of Medical Sciences
Hyderabad, India

Athir Morad
Division of Neurocritical Care
Department of Anesthesiology
    and Critical Care Medicine
The Johns Hopkins School of Medicine
Baltimore, Maryland

Asha Nandakumar
Department of Anesthesia
Royal Hallamshire Hospital
Sheffield Teaching Hospitals
NHS Foundation Trust
Sheffield, United Kingdom

K. Narmadhalakshmi
Department of Anesthesiology
    and Critical Care
JIPMER
Puducherry, India

Jovany Cruz Navarro
Department of Neurology, Division of
    Neurocritical Care
Department of Anesthesiology and Critical Care
University of Pennsylvania
Philadelphia, Pennsylvania

Lamia Nayeb
London Postgraduate Medical and Dental
    Education
London, United Kingdom

Ashima Nehra
Clinical Neuropsychology at Neurosciences Centre
and
Division of Clinical Psychology
Department of Psychiatry
All India Institute of Medical Sciences
New Delhi, India

Julia Martinez Ocón
Department of Anesthesiology
Hospital Clínic de Barcelona
University of Barcelona
Barcelona, Spain

Valentina Ormas
School of Medicine and Surgery
University of Milan–Bicocca
Milan, Italy

Martina Ornaghi
School of Medicine and Surgery
University of Milan–Bicocca
Milan, Italy

Ana Ruiz Pardos
Department of Anesthesiology
Hospital Clínic de Barcelona
University of Barcelona
Barcelona, Spain

Hemanshu Prabhakar
Department of Neuroanaesthesiology
    and Critical Care
All India Institute of Medical Sciences
New Delhi, India

Ferenc Rabai
Department of Anesthesiology
Division of Neuroanesthesia
University of Florida
College of Medicine
Gainesville, Florida

Cesar Reis
Department of Physiology and Pharmacology
Loma Linda University School of Medicine
Loma Linda, California

Haley Reis
Department of Physiology and Pharmacology
Loma Linda University School of Medicine
Loma Linda, California

Luis Reyes
Department of Neurosurgery
Hospital Clínic de Barcelona
University of Barcelona
Barcelona, Spain

Chiara Robba
Neurosciences Critical Care Unit
Addenbrooke's Hospital
University of Cambridge
Cambridge, United Kingdom

Shivani Sharma
Department of Laboratory Medicine
Clinical Neuropsychology
Neurosciences Centre
All India Institute of Medical Sciences
New Delhi, India

Sarabpreet Singh
Department of Anaesthesia
Sheffield Teaching Hospitals
Sheffield, United Kingdom

Vasudha Singhal
Medanta
The Medicity
Gurgaon, India

José María Soto-Ejarque
Cap Territorial RSCC
Emergències Mèdiques–Departament de Salut
Generalitat de Catalunya, Spain
and
Serveid'Anestesiologia i Medicina Crítica
Hospital d'Igualada
and
University of Barcelona
Barcelona, Spain

Monica S. Tandon
G.B Pant Institute of Post Graduate Medical
    Education and Research
New Delhi, India

Emma Temple
Department of Anesthesia
Royal Hallamshire Hospital
Sheffield Teaching Hospitals
NHS Foundation Trust
Sheffield, United Kingdom

Shanali Thirunavukkarasu
Department of Anesthesia
Sheffield Teaching Hospitals
Sheffield, United Kingdom

Swagata Tripathy
Department of Anesthesia and Intensive Care
All India Institute of Medical Sciences
Bhubaneswar, Odisha, India

Ricard Valero
Department of Anesthesiology
Hospital Clínic de Barcelona
University of Barcelona
Barcelona, Spain

Marina Vendrell
Department of Anesthesiology
Hospital Clínic de Barcelona
University of Barcelona
Barcelona, Spain

Lashmi Venkatraghavan
University of Toronto
and
Department of Anesthesia and Pain Medicine
Toronto Western Hospital
Toronto, Ontario, Canada

Paola Cristina Volpi
School of Medicine and Surgery
University of Milan–Bicocca
Milan, Italy

Frederick A. Zeiler
Division of Anesthesia
Addenbrooke's Hospital
University of Cambridge
Cambridge, United Kingdom
and
Section of Neurosurgery
Department of Surgery
and
Clinician Investigator Program
University of Manitoba
Winnipeg, Canada

John Zhang
Department of Physiology and Pharmacology
and
Department of Neurosurgery
Loma Linda University School of Medicine
Loma Linda, California

PART I

Introduction to neurotrauma

Introduction

INDU KAPOOR, CHARU MAHAJAN, AND HEMANSHU PRABHAKAR

Trauma continues to be a major cause of morbidity and mortality in developed and developing countries worldwide. According to the Global Burden of Disease study report (2010), 89% of trauma-related deaths occur in low- and middle-income countries. Nearly 6 million people die every year as a result of trauma, accounting for 10% of the world's deaths, which is 32% more than deaths from infectious diseases.[1] Although almost all types of injuries have declined in recent years, neurotrauma has not, leading to major deficits, long-term morbidity, and deaths. Traumatic brain injury (TBI) and spinal cord injury (SCI) are the largest causes of death and disability, causing suffering and financial difficulties for the individual, his or her family, and society as a whole. The incidence of neurotrauma ranges from 200 to 600 injuries per 100,000 people. However, these data are scattered and the real incidences of central nervous system (CNS) injury are underestimated considerably.[2] The data from developed countries indicate that approximately 7.7 million people in Europe and 5.3 million people in the United States are having TBI-related disabilities. The major cause of CNS injuries in developed countries is motor vehicle accidents, whereas in developing countries, it is mainly motorcyclists, bicyclists, and pedestrians.[3] Also, there are differences in the age groups that are affected by neurotrauma disability: the older population in developed countries and the younger population in developing countries.[3] Common deficits that are associated with TBI, including depression, aggressive behavior, poor decision making, impulsivity,

and impaired attention have negative social consequences for individuals and for society as a whole.[4] Similar to TBI, data on SCI are also limited. In developed countries, the incidence of SCI is estimated to be approximately 250,000 to 500,000 per year.[5,6] However, because there is no SCI registry in developing countries, information on incidence of SCI is lacking. The most common causes of SCI globally are traffic accidents, falls, and violence.[7] As is the case with TBIs, most of the research on SCI is conducted in developed countries; the research focuses on the basic science of the disease's biologic process, which helps to develop treatment guidelines, as well as applying advanced technology to nerve reconstruction, sophisticated prostheses, and advanced rehabilitation.[7]

Approximately 85% to 90% of TBIs are mild and are described as acute brain injuries, resulting from motion and position of the head as a result of external forces with loss of consciousness of fewer than 30 minutes, post-traumatic amnesia of less than 24 hours, and a Glasgow Coma Scale (GCS) score of 13 to 15, observed at 30 minutes post injury or upon examination by a healthcare professional.[8] Recent research on brain injury has focused mainly on evaluating patients with concussions (mild TBIs). Only 1% of all patients with mild TBIs with a GCS score of 13 to 15 will have data on head computerized tomography (CT), which requires neurosurgical intervention.[9] In patients with a GCS score of 15, only 5% will have findings of hemorrhage on head CT; while this percentage rises to 30% in patients with a GCS score of 13. Moreover, a CT scan has very little ability to rule out the presence of diffuse axonal injury (DAI) and causes unnecessary exposure to radiation. Magnetic resonance imaging (MRI) has more sensitivity to DAI; its availability is limited. For this reason, there has been growing interest in serum biomarkers as a diagnostic tool in TBI. The most widely used biomarker is S100β. Others include neuron-specific enolase, creatine kinase isoenzyme, myelin basic protein, glial fibrillary acidic protein, fatty acid-binding proteins, ubiquitin C-terminal hydrolase-L1, and alpha II-spectrin breakdown products. The goal of managing anesthesia in patients with TBI is to avoid secondary brain injury by preventing hypotension, hypoxemia, too much or too little carbon dioxide in the blood, fever, hypoglycemia or hyperglycemia, and/or increased intracranial pressure (ICP). The perioperative period is very important in TBI management. While it may make the patient more vulnerable to new secondary injuries, which may contribute negatively to outcomes, it is also an opportunity to detect and correct undiagnosed preexisting secondary causes. It may also be a potential opportunity to initiate interventions that may improve the severity of TBI. While waiting for the results of research that is focused specifically on intraoperative and perioperative TBI management, clinical management will continue to be based on physiologic development. A large number of patients with spinal cord injury (SCI) require operative intervention. It should be assumed that all patients with multiple traumas have an SCI until proven otherwise. The majority of SCI (55%) involves the cervical spinal column and 15% involves the thoracolumbar junction.[10] When it comes to anesthetic management, the most important approach in the treatment of spine trauma is a high probability for early detection and prevention of secondary injury through adequate oxygenation, blood pressure support through volume replacement, and immobilization. It is important to use different strategies to minimize blood loss during surgery. Multimodality neuromonitoring is sensitive and specific enough to detect neurologic injury during spine surgery and the anesthetic that is used has an impact on the quality of the multimodality neuromonitoring.

Currently, there is no definitive therapy; neurotrauma patients are treated with a combination of pharmacotherapy, surgery, rehabilitation, and managing post-trauma conditions, such as post-traumatic stress and depression. However, there are interventions that can effectively limit the impact, which include primary prevention, early management, and targeted early treatment. Evidence-based guidelines and management protocols help to guide care and are associated with better outcomes. Researchers around the world are continually striving to discover the best possible treatment; however, an effective treatment method is not yet available. Researchers are constantly working on preventing neurotrauma and improving treatment. Target-oriented treatment and prevention require a deep understanding of incidence, causes of injury, treatment approaches, and outcome results. The chapters in this book address, in detail, a scientific and evidence-based understanding of the conditions in its various dimensions, controversies regarding diagnostic and therapeutic approaches, outcome and impact of neurotrauma on an individual and rapidly transforming societies, challenges and opportunities in research, and recent advances and future trends to practice.

REFERENCES

1. Norton R, Kobusingye O. Injuries. *N Engl J Med.* 2013;368(18):1723-1730.
2. Reilly, P. The impact of neurotrauma on society: An international perspective. *Prog. Brain Res.* 2007;161:3-9.
3. Horton, R. GBD 2010: Understanding disease, injury, and risk. *Lancet.* 2012;380(9859):2053-2054.
4. Hofman K, Primack A, Keusch G, Hrynkow S. Addressing the growing burden of trauma and injury in low- and middle-income countries. *Am J Public Health.* 2005;95(1):13-17.
5. Furlan JC. Databases and registries on traumatic spinal cord injury in Canada. *Can J Neurol Sci.* 2013;40(4):454-455.
6. National Spinal Cord Injury Statistical Center. The 2013 Annual Statistical Report for the Spinal Cord Injury Model Systems (University of Alabama at Birmingham, 2013).
7. Rubiano AM, Carney N, Chesnut R, Puyana JC. Global neurotrauma research challenges and opportunities. *Nature.* 2015;527(7578): 193-197.
8. Carroll LJ, Cassidy JD, Peloso PM et al. Prognosis for mild traumatic brain injury:

Results of the WHO Collaborating Centre Task Force on Mild Traumatic Brain Injury. *J Rehabil Med.* 2004;43(suppl):84-105.

9. Borg J, Holm L, Cassidy JD et al. Diagnostic procedures in mild traumatic brain injury: Results of the WHO Collaborating Centre Task Force on Mild Traumatic Brain Injury. *J Rehabil Med.* 2004;43(suppl):61-75.

10. Goldberg W, Mueller C, Panacek E. Distribution and patterns of blunt traumatic cervical spine injury. *Ann Emerg Med.* 2001;38 (1):17-21.

PART II

Neuroanatomy

2

Anatomy for neurotrauma

VASUDHA SINGHAL AND SARABPREET SINGH

INTRODUCTION

Neurotrauma, either to the brain or spinal cord, is one of the most disabling forms of traumatic injury to humans, associated with a very high rate of mortality and morbidity. In order to understand the physiology, impact, and treatment of neurotrauma better, it is imperative to have an in-depth knowledge of the anatomical features that we are dealing with.

OVERVIEW OF THE NERVOUS SYSTEM

The nervous system is divided into the *central nervous system* (CNS) and the *peripheral nervous system* (PNS). The CNS comprises of the brain and the spinal cord, the main centers for integration and processing of all information. They consist of the gray matter, which contains the neuronal cell bodies, their dendrites and synaptic interactions; and the white matter, which is formed by the myelinated axons. The PNS comprises of the cranial and spinal nerves, and their associated ganglia. These conduct information to and from the CNS, via afferent fibers carrying information from sensory receptors and efferent fibers running to effector organs. These peripheral nerves are relatively unprotected as they are covered with fibrous nerve sheaths only, and so are prone to damage by trauma. There are 12 pairs of cranial nerves, and 31 pairs of spinal nerves—8 cervical, 12 thoracic, 5 lumbar, 5 sacral, and 1 coccygeal.

Another classification divides the nervous system into *somatic* and *autonomic* components, the fibers of each are distributed through both the CNS and the PNS. The autonomic nervous system, comprising of the sympathetic and the parasympathetic system, controls the internal environment by innervation of the secretory glands, and the cardiac and smooth muscles.

ANATOMY FOR HEAD INJURIES

Head injury is any form of injury to the brain, skull, or scalp—common injuries include scalp lacerations, skull fractures, brain concussions, and diffuse axonal injury. A brief discussion on the pertinent anatomy of the scalp, skull, and the brain thus helps to appreciate the pathophysiology of head trauma more effectively.

Scalp

The scalp is the soft tissue cover over the cranial vault. It consists of five layers—*skin, connective tissue, aponeurosis (galea aponeurotica), loose areolar tissue,* and *pericranium*. The first three layers are bound together as a single unit, which can move along the areolar tissue over the pericranium. The pericranium becomes continuous with the endosteum along the suture lines, and therefore, a hematoma beneath this layer outlines the affected skull bone.

Blood vessels in the scalp are attached to the fibrous connective tissue layer, and this attachment prevents vasoconstriction if the vessels are cut, causing profuse bleeding after scalp injury. Scalp lacerations, in fact, may be an occult cause of hypovolemic shock and acute anemia in blunt trauma victims (1). The aponeurosis provides attachment to the occipitofrontalis muscle. Anteriorly, the subaponeurotic space extends to the upper eyelids due to the lack of a bony insertion, accounting for the occurrence of orbital hematomas after head injuries. The loose areolar tissue contains numerous blood vessels, including the valveless emissary veins, which connect the veins of the scalp to the diploic veins and intracranial venous sinuses. This layer is sometimes referred to as the "danger zone," as infections may spread from the scalp to the brain through these emissary veins. Also, scalp lacerations through this layer would mean that the anchoring of the superficial layers is lost, and gaping of the wound occurs, necessitating suturing.

Blood supply: The scalp has a rich blood supply derived from the external and internal carotid arteries. The supratrochlear and supraorbital arteries are derived from the ophthalmic division of the internal carotid artery. The superficial temporal artery, the occipital artery, and the posterior auricular artery are branches of the external carotid artery. The scalp veins accompany the arteries with similar names. All the blood vessels anastomose freely in the scalp. Hence, the viability of the scalp is retained even in cases of major scalp avulsions.

Nerve supply: The sensory innervation of the scalp is derived from the trigeminal nerve (supratrochlear, supraorbital, zygomaticotemporal, and auriculotemporal branches) and the cervical nerve (greater and lesser occipital nerves). The motor supply is through the frontal and auricular branches of the facial nerve.

Skull

The skull is the bony skeleton of the head, which consists of the cranium, facial skeleton and mandible. It may be subdivided into—the neurocranium and viscerocranium.

The *neurocranium* houses the brain, meninges, blood supply, cranial nerves, and cerebrospinal fluid (CSF) within the cranial cavity. It has eight cranial bones—frontal, ethmoid, sphenoid, 2 parietal, 2 temporal, and an occipital bone. It is subdivided into the cranial vault or calvaria, and the basicranium or skull base. The base of the skull is further divided into three regions, corresponding to the floor of the anterior, middle, and posterior cranial fossae.

The *viscerocranium* or the facial skeleton consists of 14 bones. These include: a vomer, 2 nasal chonchae, 2 nasal bones, 2 lacrimal bones, 2 palatine bones, 2 zygomatic bones, 2 maxilla, and a mandible.

Most of the bones in the neurocranium are flat or *diploic bones* consisting of two tables enclosing a medullary cavity with red bone marrow. The inner table is thin and brittle, while the outer table is thick and resilient. The diploe do not form where the skull is covered with muscles, leaving the vault thin and prone to fracture. The skull bones vary in thickness in different regions—it is thickened at the glabella, occipital protuberance, mastoid processes, and external angular process of the frontal bone. The thinnest part of the cranium, particularly prone to fractures, is the *pterion*, an H-shaped junction between the frontal, temporal, parietal, and sphenoid bones. A fracture here can lacerate the underlying middle meningeal artery, resulting in an extradural hematoma. The bones in the viscerocranium are rather delicate and hence susceptible to fracture.

The bones in the skull articulate via fibrous joints, which are immovable, called *sutures*. The main sutures in the adult brain are: the *coronal* suture (fusing the frontal bone with the two parietal bones), the *sagittal* suture (fusing the two parietal bones), and the *lambdoid* suture (fusing the occipital bone with the two parietal bones). These are points of potential weakness, and fractures along suture lines are common in pediatric population, causing *diastasis* or widening of sutures.

SKULL BASE: The base of the skull is a complex anatomical region, as it allows entry and exit of many important neurological and vascular structures, including the spinal cord, which might be at risk of damage following skull base fractures.

The **external surface of the skull base** consists of the *hard palate*; posterior nasal apertures or *choanae*, separated from each other by the *vomer*; the *sphenoid* bone, with its greater and lesser wings, and the pterygoid processes; *temporal* bone, with the auditory groove and the mandibular fossa; and the *occipital* bone arranged around the *foramen magnum*. The major structures passing through the foramen magnum are the spinal cord, meninges, anterior and posterior spinal arteries, vertebral arteries, and spinal accessory nerve. The cranium articulates with the vertebral column by means of *occipital condyles*, located on the lateral parts of the occipital bone. The *jugular foramen* is located between the occipital bone and the petrous temporal

bone—the internal jugular vein and cranial nerves IX-XI emerge through this foramen. The internal carotid artery enters the cranium through the *carotid canal* just anterior to the jugular foramen.

The **internal surface of the skull base** forms a concave, bowl-shaped floor of the cranial cavity. It has three large depressions, namely the *anterior, middle, and posterior cranial fossae*, with the anterior cranial fossa at the highest level, and the posterior at the lowest.

The ***anterior cranial fossa*** supports the frontal lobes of the cerebral hemispheres. Its floor is formed by the orbital plate of the frontal bone; the cribriform plate (for passage of the olfactory nerve) and crista galli (for attachment of falx cerebri) of the ethmoid bone; and the lesser wings, planum sphenoidale, and prechiasmatic sulcus of the sphenoid bone. The olfactory tracts lie above the planum sphenoidale, while the optic chiasma usually lies above the prechiasmatic sulcus. Skull base fractures (Figure 2.1) in the region of the anterior cranial fossa may cause CSF rhinorrhoea, pneumocephalus, olfactory nerve damage leading to anosmia (due to damage to the cribriform plate), bilateral periorbital ecchymosis (*Raccoon's eyes*), and damage to optic nerve

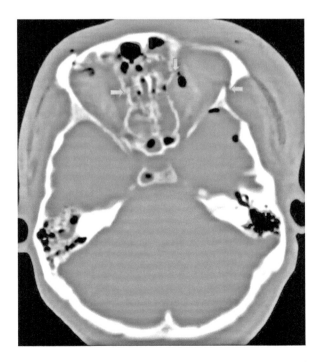

Figure 2.1 Computed tomography (CT image) depicting skull base fractures (shown by blue arrows) in a blast victim. The patient presented with pneumocephalus and CSF rhinorrhoea, along with basifrontal contusions following fracture of the anterior cranial fossa.

and orbital contents. Frontal lobe injury leading to personality and behavioral changes may also occur in such fractures.

The **middle cranial fossa** is a butterfly-shaped structure, with *sella turcica* on the body of the sphenoid centrally, and large depressions formed by greater wings of sphenoid and squamous temporal bones, supporting the temporal lobes of the brain, laterally. The sharp sphenoidal crests, along with the anterior clinoid processes, formed by the lesser wings of sphenoid, separate it from the anterior cranial fossa. The petrous temporal bone and the dorsum sella of the sphenoid forms a boundary between the middle and the posterior cranial fossae.

The *sella turcica* is a saddle-shaped bony formation on the upper surface of the body of sphenoid, surrounded by the anterior and posterior clinoid processes. Its anterior edge is formed by a bony prominence known as the *tuberculum sellae*, which continues with the prechiasmatic sulcus. The median depression housing the pituitary gland is the *hypophysial fossa*. The posterior boundary of the sella presents a vertical pillar of bone called the *dorsum sellae*. The sigmoid groove for the internal carotid artery lies in this region, as it traverses the petrous apex through the cavernous sinus. A fold of dura attached to the anterior and posterior clinoid processes, forming a roof over the pituitary fossa, is the *diaphragma sellae*. The cavernous sinus lies lateral to the pituitary fossa.

The greater wing of sphenoid presents four prominent foramina on each side of the body of sphenoid, in a posterolateral plane—the *superior orbital fissure* (transmitting the cranial nerves III, IV, V_1, VI, along with the ophthalmic vein); the *foramen rotundum* (transmitting the cranial nerve V_2); the *foramen ovale* (cranial nerve V_3 and accessory meningeal artery); and the *foramen spinosum* (meningeal branch of cranial nerve V_3, middle meningeal artery and vein).

The trigeminal impression is present on the anterior surface of the petrous temporal bone near its apex, which accommodates the trigeminal ganglion. Lateral to the trigeminal impression, lies a narrow groove for the greater petrosal nerve, and another small groove for the lesser petrosal nerve further laterally.

The *temporal bone* is divided into three parts in the middle cranial fossa—the petrous part, the squamous part, and the mastoid part. The *petrous part* contains the auditory tube, the carotid foramen (for passage of internal carotid artery), and the jugular foramen (for internal jugular vein, CN IX, X, XI). The *squamous part* includes the zygomatic process and the temporo-mandibular joint. The *mastoid part* contains the mastoid air cells, the internal auditory meatus (for passage of CN VII, VIII), and the stylomastoid foramen (for CN VII, stylomastoid artery).

Fractures of the middle cranial fossa may be associated with pituitary dysfunction, if the sella turcica is damaged. Skull base fractures in the temporal region may lead to deafness due to injury to the middle ear cavity or the eighth cranial nerve. Patients with fractures of the petrous temporal bone present with CSF otorrhoea and bruising over the mastoid (Battle's sign).

The **posterior cranial fossa** is the largest and deepest fossa formed mostly by the occipital bone, and accommodates the cerebellum, pons, and medulla oblongata. The anterior boundary of the fossa is formed by the dorsum sella of sphenoid centrally, while the occipital bone (with grooves for the transverse and sigmoid sinuses) forms the rest of the fossa. The anterolateral walls of the posterior fossa are marked by the petrous and mastoid parts of the temporal bone. At the base of the petrous ridge is the jugular foramen, transmitting the cranial nerves and internal jugular vein. The internal acoustic meatus lies anterosuperior to the jugular foramen, and transmits CN VII, VIII, and the labyrinthine artery. Superior to the foramen magnum anterolaterally, lies the hypoglossal canal for CN XII.

The medulla exits the cranial cavity through the foramen magnum to continue as the spinal cord. When the lower part of the cerebellum (the cerebellar tonsils) descend abnormally through the foramen magnum (due to increased intracranial pressure during head trauma), they may cause medullary compression, which is an ominous event leading to brain death.

FRACTURES OF THE SKULL: Cranial fractures may be linear, depressed or comminuted. *Linear fractures* (Figure 2.2a) are the most common fractures—there is a simple break in the entire thickness of the bone, with fracture lines radiating away from the point of impact. They are managed conservatively. *Depressed fractures* (Figure 2.2b) are caused as a result of a direct, hard blow, causing skull indentation, compressing and injuring the underlying brain. A depressed bone segment >5 mm below the inner table of the adjacent bone usually needs a surgical

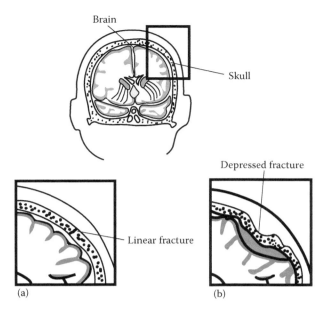

Figure 2.2 Diagrammatic representation of skull fractures: (a) Linear fracture. (b) Depressed fracture.

intervention. Elevation of the depressed fracture is particularly indicated if there is a gross contamination, or a dural tear with pneumocephalus, or an underlying hematoma. Frontal bone fractures are more likely to necessitate repair (2). In *comminuted fractures*, the bone is broken into several pieces.

THE CRANIUM

The cranium consists of the meninges, the blood vessels, the brain, and cerebrospinal fluid (CSF).

Meninges

The brain and spinal cord are covered by three connective tissue membranes or meninges: the dura mater, the arachnoid mater, and the pia mater, which protect these structures and form a supporting framework for the blood vessels and CSF.

Dura mater, or pachymeninx, is a thick, bilaminar membrane that incompletely divides the cranial cavity into compartments (by means of infoldings) and accommodates the dural venous sinuses. The two layers of the dura are: an *external periosteal layer*, formed by the inner periosteum of the skull bones; and an *inner meningeal layer*, which forms four inward processes or folds in the cranium—falx cerebri, tentorium cerebelli, falx cerebelli and

diaphragma sellae. The meningeal layer provides tubular sheath for the cranial nerves during their exit from the cranial foramina, finally blending into their epineurium. The optic nerve, however, is an exception. The meningeal dura, along with the arachnoid and pia, envelop the entire course of the optic nerve up to the eyeball. Hence, an increased intracranial pressure is reflected as a raised optic nerve sheath diameter on ultrasonographic studies and is used as a noninvasive method of monitoring raised ICP. On the other hand, in sella turcica, all the three meninges blend intimately with one another and with the fibrous capsule of the pituitary. Therefore, the hypophysis cerebri is not affected by changes in intracranial pressure. The spinal dura presents the meningeal layer only. The collection of blood between the periosteum and the meningeal layer due to high pressure arterial bleeding caused by trauma, results in an extradural hematoma, which is a medical emergency.

Dural partitions—*Falx cerebri* is a sickle-shaped structure that projects mid-sagitally into the median longitudinal fissure, separating the right and the left cerebral hemispheres. It is attached in the median plane from the crista galli of the ethmoid bone anteriorly to the internal occipital protuberance posteriorly and blends with the tentorium cerebelli.

The *tentorium cerebelli* separates the occipital lobes of the cerebral hemispheres from the cerebellum. It is attached anteriorly to the posterior clinoid process of sphenoid, laterally to the petrous temporal bone, and posteriorly to the transverse sulci of the occipital bone. The falx cerebri attaches to the tentorium in the midline, pulling it upwards, giving it a tent-like appearance. The tentorium cerebelli divides the cranial cavity into supratentorial and infratentorial compartments. The free concave anteromedial border forms a U-shaped gap called the tentorial notch, filled by the midbrain and the anterior part of the superior aspect of the cerebellar vermis.

The *falx cerebelli* is a small, sickle-shaped infolding of dura below the tentorium, partially separating the cerebellar hemispheres. It extends forwards from the internal occipital crest to the posterior cerebellar notch.

The *diaphragma sellae* is a circular sheet of dura forming the roof of the sella turcica. It is perforated in the center by the infundibular stalk and the hypophyseal veins.

In the event of a large intracerebral hematoma, or diffuse axonal injury with gross cerebral edema following head injuries, the raised ICP may cause the brain to herniate under the falx cerebri (*subfalcine herniation*), or through the tentorial notch (*uncal herniation*, with the uncus or medial temporal lobe compressing the oculomotor nerve, midbrain and posterior cerebral arteries). A space occupying lesion in the infratentorial compartment may lead to *downward transtentorial tonsillar herniation* through the foramen magnum, or an *upward transtentorial herniation of the cerebellar vermis* (Figure 2.3). Brain herniation is a neurosurgical emergency, warranting urgent decompression.

The **arachnoid mater** (thin, avascular intermediate layer) and the **pia mater** (delicate, highly vascular internal meningeal layer) collectively make up the *leptomeninges*. Numerous spider like trabeculae extend between the arachnoid and pia. The arachnoid is separated from the pia by the *subarachnoid space*, containing the cerebrospinal fluid, which nourishes and cushions the brain. The pia adheres to the surface of the brain and follows its contours.

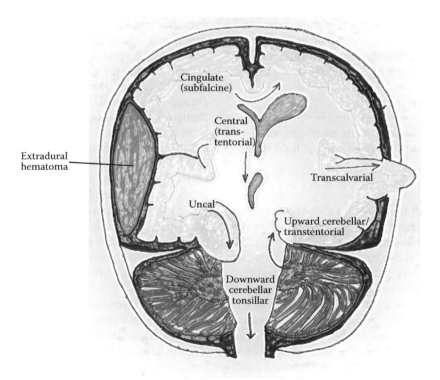

Figure 2.3 Image depicting the various types of brain herniations that may occur as a result of increased intracranial pressure (due to an extradural hematoma in this case).

The cranial meninges receive the blood supply primarily from the middle meningeal branches of the maxillary artery. Sensory innervation is from the meningeal branches of all three divisions of the trigeminal nerve and fibers from the C2 spinal ganglion.

Damage to small bridging veins in the subdural space due to sudden deceleration injuries may lead to a *subdural hematoma. Subarachnoid hemorrhage* is the collection of blood between the arachnoid and dura, occurring as a result of arterial rupture in the subarachnoid space.

THE BRAIN

The brain is contained within the cranium, and broadly consists of the cerebrum, cerebellum, and brainstem (midbrain, pons, medulla). In the cerebrum and cerebellum, the gray matter appears at the surface, and the white matter lies in the interior. On the other hand, in the brainstem and spinal cord, the reverse is true—the gray matter lies within and the white matter outside. The adult brain weighs only 2% of the total body weight but receives a blood flow that is approximately one-sixth of the total cardiac output. The total number of neurons in the human cortex average around 10–15 billion.

Embryologically, the brain is subdivided into three parts: the forebrain (prosencephalon), midbrain (mesencephalon), and hindbrain (rhombencephalon). The *forebrain* consists of the telencephalon (two cerebral hemispheres and the lateral ventricle), and the diencephalon (thalamus, hypothalamus, and the third ventricle). The *midbrain* consists of the cerebral peduncles and the aqueduct, while the *hindbrain* consists of the pons and medulla ventrally, and the cerebellum dorsally, separated by the fourth ventricle.

Cerebrum

The cerebrum consists of two cerebral hemispheres, incompletely separated from each other by a median longitudinal fissure, which is occupied by the falx cerebri. The two hemispheres are partially connected in the midline by a band of commissural fibers, called the corpus callosum.

The cerebral cortex is folded into numerous convolutions called gyri, separated by fissures or sulci, for accommodation in a limited space within the skull, rendering the cortex a massive surface area of around 2200 square centimeters. The lateral

sulcus (Sylvian fissure), and the central sulcus (Rolandic fissure), along with an imaginary line connecting the parieto-occipital sulcus to the preoccipital notch, divide the cerebral hemisphere into four lobes—the frontal, parietal, temporal, and occipital. The frontal lobe lies anterior to the central sulcus and above the lateral sulcus; the parietal lobe lies behind the central sulcus and above the lateral sulcus; the temporal lobe is below the lateral sulcus; and the occipital lobe lies below and behind the imaginary line from the parieto-occipital sulcus to the preoccipital notch.

Insula is a pyramidal-shaped portion of the cortex lying at the bottom of the stem and posterior ramus of the lateral sulcus. The insula integrates sensory and autonomic information from the viscera and is considered a cornerstone for conscious awareness.

One hemisphere, usually the left in right-handed people, is slightly larger than the other and constitutes the dominant hemisphere. The dominant hemisphere is concerned with handedness and speech—language related activities such as reading, writing and speaking, and complex intellectual functions such as analytical and computational skills are localized to the dominant hemisphere. The non-dominant hemisphere preserves functions like spatial and pictorial concepts, and the recognition of faces and music.

FUNCTIONAL AREAS OF THE BRAIN: Different areas of the cerebral cortex have specific functions, often described as **Brodmann's areas**. The *frontal lobe* is involved in cognitive functions like reasoning and judgment, and in speech and language. The control of voluntary movement of skeletal muscles lies in the precentral gyrus (*Brodmann's area 4*), also called the primary motor area or motor strip, immediately anterior to the central sulcus. It contains the cell bodies of the pyramidal tract. The area of the cortex representing a part of the body is proportional to the amount of motor control needed by that area, not just its size. Large areas of the cortex are, therefore, dedicated to the lips and hands (**motor homunculus**). The premotor area (*Brodmann's area 6*), immediately anterior to the motor strip, is responsible for programming of motor movements. The frontal eye field in the middle frontal gyrus just anterior to the precentral gyrus (*Brodmann's area 8*) controls the conjugate eye movements, visual reflexes, and pupillary constriction and dilatation. The motor commands for speech are programmed in the Broca's area (*Brodmann's area 44,45*), located in the inferior frontal gyrus of the dominant hemisphere. Biological intelligence, or executive functions such as reasoning and judgement, are controlled in the most anterior part of the frontal lobe (*Brodmann's area 9,10,11*).

The *parietal lobe* is involved in somatosensory processing. Immediately posterior the central sulcus is the postcentral gyrus (*Brodmann's area 1,2,3*) involved in sensory reception from various parts of the body. Similar to the motor strip, this area is represented upside down, and the area represented by a particular body part is proportional to the complexity of sensations received from it (**sensory homunculus**). Posterior to the primary sensory strip lie the presensory association areas, involved in somatosensory processing (*Brodmann's area 5,7,40*). The angular gyrus (*Brodmann's area 39*), in the anterolateral region of the parietal lobe, is responsible for transferring visual information to Wernicke's area, in order to derive meaning from visually perceived words.

The *temporal lobe* controls memory, auditory processing, receptive component of speech and emotion. Wernicke's area (*Brodmann's area 39,40*), responsible for producing meaningful speech, is located on the posterior portion of the superior temporal gyrus in the dominant hemisphere. The primary auditory area lies in the anterior transverse temporal gyrus (*Brodmann's area 41,42*). The auditory association areas (*Brodmann's area 21,22*) make important contributions to the comprehension of speech.

The *occipital lobe* is responsible for visual processing. The primary visual area (*Brodmann's area 17*) receives input from the optic tract via thalamus. The secondary visual areas (*Brodmann's area 18,19*) integrate visual information.

Injury to specific parts of the cerebral cortex result in loss of function subserved by the particular area.

Coup and contrecoup injuries: These are brain injuries, most often cerebral contusions, where the damage is located both at the site of impact (*coup*), as well as on the side opposite to it (*contrecoup*) (Figure 2.4). They are a type of closed head injuries and occur due to a strong blow on the head, which causes a contusion not only at the site of trauma, but also accelerates the skull and causes the brain to slam against it on the opposite side, causing an additional contusion. Damage from contrecoup injuries frequently surpass that caused by the coup injuries. Areas affected most commonly are the inferior surface of frontal bones (behind the forehead) and the temporal poles (underneath the

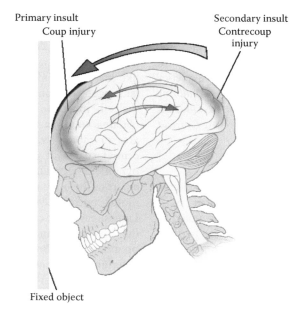

Figure 2.4 Coup and contrecoup injuries. (Creative credits: Patrick J. Lynch, medical illustrator; C. Carl Jaffe, MD, cardiologist. http://creativecommons.org/licenses/by/2.5/.)

temples), characteristically leading to memory impairment and personality changes.

DIENCEPHALON

The diencephalon consists of masses of gray matter surrounding the slot-like third ventricle, superior to the midbrain. The main structures of the diencephalon include the thalamus, hypothalamus, epithalamus (including the pineal gland), and subthalamus.

The *thalamus* is located on each side of the third ventricle, interconnected by the interthalamic connection. It is referred to as the "*gateway to the cortex*," as it relays and processes sensory and motor information to the cerebral cortex.

It receives sensory input via the *spinothalamic tracts*—the *lateral spinothalamic tract* transmits pain and temperature, while the *ventral spinothalamic tract* transmits crude pain and pressure. All sensory pathways (except olfactory), including visual, tactile, auditory and gustatory, relay in the thalamus, where the information is processed and integrated with cerebral activity. It is functionally connected to the hippocampus of the limbic system via anterior thalamic nuclei, playing a role in spatial memory. Through its connections to the prefrontal cortex, it provides the "mood or feeling tone" to the emotional aspect of behavior. It receives fibers from the cerebellum and basal ganglia (corpus striatum and substantia nigra), and conveys information to the motor areas of the frontal lobe, thereby regulating motor activity. The thalamus also plays a significant role in the ascending reticular activating system for arousal and alertness. Damage to the thalamus may lead to permanent coma.

The *hypothalamus* is located below the thalamus and forms the ventral part of the diencephalon. Though small in size (~4 g), it is an integral part of the brain, as it controls the autonomic nervous system, as well as the endocrine system through its complex interaction with the pituitary gland (hypothalamic-hypophyseal axis), thereby maintaining homeostasis.

Anatomically, the hypothalamus is divided anteroposteriorly into four regions: *preoptic* region (adjoining the lamina terminalis), *supraoptic* region (above the optic chiasma), *tuberal* region (above the tuber cinereum), and the *mammillary* or posterior region.

The supraoptic and paraventricular nuclei in the supraoptic region, form the *hypothalamo-hypophyseal tract*. These nuclei are surrounded by a dense capillary plexus. Their axons pass down through the infundibulum to reach the neurohypophysis or posterior pituitary, where they branch profusely to end in relation to the capillaries, around which they release the neurohormones—vasopressin (ADH or antidiuretic hormone) and oxytocin.

The arcuate nuclei of the tuberal region produce various releasing and inhibitory hormones that control the secretion of hormones by the adenohypophysis or anterior pituitary. The axons of these nuclei give rise to the *tuberohypophyseal tract*, which terminates in the *hypophyseal portal system* of the median eminence and infundibulum.

The hypothalamus also modulates the autonomic nervous system—its anterior and medial parts (preoptic and supraoptic nuclei) control the parasympathetic activity, while the posterior and lateral parts regulate the sympathetic activity.

Other important functions under the control of the hypothalamus include—temperature regulation, food and water intake, sexual activity and reproduction, emotional behavior, and maintenance of circadian rhythm.

There is a high incidence of pituitary and hypothalamic dysfunction following moderate to severe traumatic brain injury (3). Basal skull fractures and subsequent fracture of the sella may result in a direct damage to the pituitary, infundibulum, or hypothalamus through axon shearing stress. Secondary brain injury in the form of hypoxia, hypotension, raised ICP, and hypoperfusion may cause ischemic damage to the pituitary, resulting in pituitary dysfunction. The most common endocrine complication following traumatic brain injury is a syndrome of inappropriate antidiuretic hormone (SIADH) by the hypothalamus, usually transient, causing dilutional hyponatremia and brain edema.

The *epithalamus* comprises the pineal body, along with the habenular nuclei and posterior commissure. The pineal body is an endocrine gland that produces melatonin, which controls the sleep patterns in both circadian and seasonal cycles.

The *subthalamus* contains the subthalamic nuclei, which exert excitatory effects on the globus pallidus through its glutaminergic neurons.

BASAL GANGLIA

The basal ganglia include clusters of neurons located deep beneath the cerebral cortex, associated with the modulation of motor activities in the brain. It comprises of the **corpus striatum**, divided by the fibers of the internal capsule into a medial *caudate nucleus*, and a lateral *lentiform nucleus*; the **claustrum**; and the **amygdaloid body**. The lentiform nucleus is further subdivided into *putamen* and *globus pallidus*. The caudate nucleus and the putamen are together referred to as the *striatum*, while the globus pallidus is called the *pallidum*. Recent researches indicate the **subthalamic nucleus** (part of the diencephalon) and the **substantia nigra** (part of the midbrain) to be functionally related to the basal ganglia.

The striatal neurons receive *excitatory glutaminergic* fibers from the cortex and the thalamus, and *inhibitory dopaminergic* fibers from the substantia nigra. The balanced interaction of these neurotransmitters help in regulating muscle tone and suppressing involuntary movements during execution of purposeful motor activity.

LIMBIC SYSTEM

Classically termed as the "feeling and reacting brain," the limbic system is situated just beneath the cerebrum on both sides of the thalamus (limbic means border or edge). It is considered the epicenter of memory, emotion and behavioral expression, and operates by influencing the endocrine and autonomic systems of the brain. The brain centers constituting the limbic system are (4):

1. Limbic cortex—situated at the inferomedial aspect of the cerebral hemisphere
   i. Cingulate gyrus—lies dorsal to the corpus callosum, and is interconnected with the association areas of cerebral cortex. It functions to regulate the heart rate and blood pressure and is also involved in cognitive and emotional processing.
   ii. Parahippocampal gyrus is located in the medial temporal lobe and plays a major role in spatial memory. It contains the entorhinal cortex, which is concerned with olfactory memories.
2. Hippocampal formation—extends for around 5 cm from the amygdala anteriorly to the splenium of the corpus callosum posteriorly, in the medial temporal lobe. It consists of three distinct zones:
   i. The dentate gyrus
   ii. Hippocampus (means "sea horse" in Greek)—is present as an elongated prominence along the floor of the inferior horn of the lateral ventricle. It is involved in long term memory.
   iii. Subicular complex
3. Amygdala—an almond-shaped structure lying deep beneath the uncus. It controls anxiety, aggression, and fear conditioning, and also plays a role in social cognition and emotional memory.
4. Septal area—lies immediately above the anterior commissure, and has extensive connections with the hippocampus via the fornix. It is believed to inhibit aggressiveness and produce pleasure reaction.
5. Hypothalamus—is the primary output node for the limbic system and regulates autonomic, endocrine, sexual, and emotional behavior.

The limbic system also includes the anterior nuclei of thalamus, which helps in memory processing; and the nucleus accumbens, involved in reward and addiction.

Limbic system is of particular importance in rehabilitation and recovery post trauma, as it is responsible for emotional control, memory, and learning.

WHITE MATTER OF THE CEREBRAL HEMISPHERES

The greater part of the cerebral hemisphere deep to the cortex is occupied by nerve fibers constituting the white matter. The white matter in the cerebral hemispheres may be:

a. Association fibers—interconnecting areas within the same hemisphere
b. Projection fibers—connecting cerebral cortex with other masses of gray matter in the brain and spinal cord
c. Commissural fibers—interconnecting identical areas in the two hemispheres.

ASSOCIATION FIBERS include the *superior longitudinal fasciculus* (connecting the frontal and occipital lobes); the *inferior longitudinal fasciculus* (that connect the temporal with the occipital lobe); the *arcuate fasciculus* (connecting the frontal lobe with the occipito-frontal cortex); the *uncinate fasciculus* (that connect the frontal and anterior temporal lobes); and the cingulum (underlying the cortex of the cingulate gyrus).

PROJECTION FIBERS connect the cortex to centers in the brainstem and spinal cord, in both directions (corticopetal/corticofugal). They also connect the cortex with the thalamus, basal ganglia, and hypothalamus. They are represented by the fimbria and fornix in the hippocampal formation, and the corona radiata and internal capsule in the neocortex.

The **corona radiata** is a fan-shaped arrangement of projection fibers, extending from the cerebral cortex above, to the internal capsule below. It consists of motor fibers, which are somatotopically arranged anterolateral to posteromedially (5).

Internal capsule is a dog-leg-shaped compact band of projection fibers, forming the main highway for the afferent and efferent fibers from the cerebral cortex. It can be divided into five parts, from before backwards –

a. *Anterior limb*—between the head of the caudate nucleus and the lentiform nucleus—consists of the corticopontine fibers and the anterior thalamic radiation
b. *Genu*—forms an angulation between the anterior and the posterior limb, and contains the corticobulbar fibers and the superior thalamic radiation
c. *Posterior limb*—lies between the thalamus medially and the lentiform nucleus laterally—consists of the corticospinal tract in its anterior two-third, and the afferent projection fibers in the posterior one-third
d. *Sublentiform part*—extends below the lentiform nucleus and consists of fibers of the auditory radiation arising from the medial geniculate body
e. *Retrolentiform part*—extends backwards behind the lentiform nucleus as a continuation of the posterior limb, and contains fibers of the optic radiation arising from the lateral geniculate body

COMMISSURAL FIBERS connect wide areas of cerebral cortex of the two hemispheres across the midline and are mostly derived from the axons of the pyramidal cells. There are five sets of commissural fibers: corpus callosum, anterior commissure, hippocampal, habenular, and posterior commissure.

The **corpus callosum** is the largest band of commissural fibers connecting the two hemispheres, thereby keeping them working together. It transfers memory and speech function from the trained hemisphere (dominant hemisphere, usually the left) to the uneducated hemisphere. The corpus callosum is an arched structure, with an anterior end or genu, a central part or trunk, and a posterior end or splenium. The rostrum projects posteriorly and inferiorly from the genu, connecting it to the anterior commissure.

White matter disruption during traumatic brain injury may result in severe impairment of cognition, including loss of associative learning, memory and executive functions (6). Conventional CT and standard MRI may underestimate the extent of white matter damage, and a diffusion tensor imaging may be indicated.

BRAINSTEM

The brainstem extends from the caudal part of the diencephalon to the cranial end of the spinal cord, and consists of the midbrain, pons, and medulla, from above downwards. The pons and medulla are posteriorly separated from the cerebellum by the fourth ventricle. The cerebellum is connected to the brainstem by the superior, middle, and inferior peduncles, for the midbrain, pons, and medulla, respectively. The brainstem provides attachment to most cranial nerves—cranial nerves (CN) III and IV emerge from the midbrain; CN V from the pons; CN VI, VII, VIII from the junction of pons and medulla; and CN IX, X, XI, XII, from the medulla.

Damage to the brainstem during trauma is often devastating and life threatening, as it contains vital cardiac and respiratory centers, and is the highway for most ascending and descending pathways, including all motor and sensory tracts.

Midbrain

Midbrain is the shortest brainstem segment that traverses the hiatus in the tentorium cerebelli. It consists of a tectum dorsally, and two cerebral peduncles—right and left, ventrally.

The tectum consists of a pretectal area, and the paired superior and inferior colliculi. The *superior colliculi* process visual information, while the *inferior colliculi* process auditory information. The *trochlear nerve (IV)* emerges below the inferior colliculus on each side.

The peduncles are further divided by a pigmented lamina called substantia nigra into a dorsal tegmentum and ventral crus cerebri. The tegmenti are continuous across the midline, but the crura are separate. The cerebral aqueduct lies between the tectum and tegmentum, and connects the third and the fourth ventricles. The optic tracts wind around the midbrain at its junction with the diencephalon. The *oculomotor nerve (III)* emerges from the medial surface of the peduncle. Lateral to the midbrain is the uncus of the temporal lobe.

Each crus cerebri consists of corticospinal, corticopontine, and corticobulbar fibers. The two crura are separated by a notch on the anterior aspect of the midbrain. The tegmentum contains the red nucleus (involved in motor coordination), medial longitudinal fasciculus, CN III nucleus, lateral spinothalamic tract, the reticular formation (continuous below with that of the pons and medulla), and the medial lemniscus.

Trauma to the midbrain may result in contralateral weakness (corticospinal tract), contralateral loss of proprioception and vibration (medial lemniscus), involuntary movements (corticobulbar tract), upward gaze palsy and ipsilateral ophthalmoplegia (medial longitudinal fasciculus), and loss of pupillary light reflex (CN III). Impairment of reticular activating system may lead to progressive loss of consciousness. *Raised ICP* in the setting of an intracranial hematoma or cerebral edema due to diffuse axonal injury, may lead to uncal herniation through the tentorial notch, leading to direct *midbrain compression* leading to a progressive oculomotor palsy (ophthalmoplegia, pupillary dilatation, and ptosis), contralateral limb weakness and falling level of consciousness.

Pons

The pons lies caudal to the midbrain, separated ventrally from the clivus by the cisterna pontis, and dorsally from the cerebellum by the upper part of the rhomboid fossa of fourth ventricle. The *cerebellopontine angle*, which lies lateral in relation to the pons, contains the roots of CN VII, VIII and IX, and the nervus intermedius, overlying the choroid plexus of the fourth ventricle. The ventral surface of the pons is convex and lodges the basilar artery in a vertical median sulcus. On each side, the ventral surface is continuous with the middle cerebellar peduncle. The motor and sensory roots of the CN V emerge at the junction of the pons and the middle cerebellar peduncle. Bundles of transverse cerebellopontine fibers produce faint ridges or grooves on the ventral surface. The dorsal surface of the pons is formed by the rostral part of the floor of the fourth ventricle. A rounded elevation, called the *facial colliculus*, on the dorsal surface, is produced by the underlying CN VI nucleus and the internal genu of motor fibers of CN VII.

Internally, the pons is divided into a ventral, basilar part and a dorsal, tegmental part. The *basilar part* is a continuation of the pyramids, which contains longitudinal fibers of the corticopontine, corticonuclear and corticospinal tracts descending from the crus cerebri of the midbrain. The *dorsal tegmentum* of the pons contains the motor nuclei of CN V, VI, VII, and VIII. The medial and lateral lemniscus and the pontine part of the reticular formation also lie in the tegmentum.

Pontine involvement during trauma may, therefore, present with loss of facial sensation and weakness of masticatory muscles (CN V), eye abduction weakness (CN VI), facial weakness (CN VII), or deafness and vertigo (CN VIII), along with contralateral hemiparesis (corticospinal tracts) and impairment of level of consciousness (reticular activating system).

Locked-in syndrome may occur due to trauma to the base of pons, involving bilateral corticospinal and corticobulbar tracts. The patient is typically quadriparetic, but conscious and intact cognitively. The oculomotor and trochlear nerves are preserved, and hence the patient can communicate through blinking and vertical eye movements.

Medulla

The medulla oblongata extends from the pons above to the spinal cord below. It is somewhat piriform in shape (~3 cm long, 2 cm wide), with the upper part being open and forming the caudal part of the floor of the fourth ventricle, and the lower part being closed and containing the central canal. The ventral surface of medulla rests on the basilar part of occipital bone, while the dorsal surface lodges in the inferior cerebellar notch, separated from the vermis by the cavity of the fourth ventricle. The caudal end of the medulla corresponds with the upper border of the atlas behind, and the middle of the odontoid process of the axis in front, making it prone to injury in upper cervical trauma.

The medulla is divided incompletely into two symmetrical halves by an anterior median fissure and a posterior median sulcus. Each half is further subdivided by the antero-lateral and postero-lateral sulci into anterior, lateral and posterior areas.

Immediately lateral to the anterior median fissure is a prominent elongated ridge, the *pyramid*, which contains the descending corticospinal and corticobulbar fibers. The shallow anterolateral sulcus, lateral to the pyramid, provides attachment to the rootlets of the CN XII, in line with the ventral spinal roots. Lateral to the anterolateral sulcus and the pyramid, is an oval prominence, called the *olive*, containing the inferior olivary nucleus. The posterolateral sulcus lies lateral to the olive, and provide attachment to the CN IX, X, and XI, in line with the dorsal spinal nerve roots. Between the posterolateral sulcus and the posterior median sulcus, are located the ascending dorsal columns—*fasciculus cuneatus* laterally and *fasciculus gracilis* medially. These end into elongated swellings called cuneate and gracilis *tubercles*, produced by the corresponding *nucleus cuneatus* and the *nucleus gracilis*. At the nucleus cuneatus and gracilis, these sensory fibers, which are responsible for fine touch, proprioception and two point discrimination, decussate to the opposite side (**sensory decussation**) to continue as the internal arcuate fibers in the ascending bundle, termed *medial lemniscus*. Lateral to the fasciculus cuneatus is a low elevated area, called the *tuberculum cinereum*, beneath which lies the nucleus and spinal tract of the CN V.

At the most caudal end of the pyramids, the corticospinal fibers cross over the midline or decussate to continue down in the spinal cord as the lateral corticospinal tract on the contralateral side (**decussation of pyramids**). Around 90% fibers decussate to continue in the lateral corticospinal tract, while the remaining 10% continue down in the anterior corticospinal tract without crossing over.

It is important to note that the medulla controls several major autonomic functions of the body, including respiration (via dorsal and ventral respiratory groups), heart rate, blood pressure, reflex arcs, vomiting, swallowing, defecation and so on.

Whiplash, or sudden cervical acceleration-deceleration injuries can cause a dislocation at the occiput or C1 level, leading to injury at the level of medullary pyramids, causing quadriplegia. Isolated lesions of medulla may lead to contralateral sensory and motor weakness along with ipsilateral tongue deviation, if the lesion occurs medially in the medulla; and ataxia, sensory deficits, dysphagia, Horner's syndrome, facial pain, diplopia, and so on, if the lesion occurs laterally (due to vertebral artery dissection or posterior inferior cerebellar artery damage).

Bilateral lesions of the brainstem are fatal if untreated, due to damage to the vital medullary centers that control heart rate, respiration and blood pressure, and to the reticular activating system, which controls the level of consciousness. The patients are termed brain-dead, with absent brainstem reflexes, on artificial support.

CRANIAL NERVES

Cranial nerves are the conduits that relay information to and from the brain to other body parts, primarily the head and neck. There are 12 pairs of cranial nerves, most of which (except CN I and II, which arise from the cerebrum) originate from the brainstem. Cranial nerves are numbered according to their structure or function, using roman numerals, in a rostro-caudal sequence as they occur in the brain.

CN I (*olfactory nerve*) conveys the sense of smell and is functionally associated with the limbic system. It directly terminates in the cortical and subcortical areas of the fronto-temporal lobes. **CN II** (*optic nerve*) transmits visual information. Its fibers emerge in the optic tract after traversing through the optic chiasma, and terminate into the lateral geniculate nucleus of the thalamus. **CN III** (*oculomotor nerve*), **IV** (*trochlear nerve*) and **VI** (*abducens nerve*) coordinate eye movement. **CN V** (*trigeminal nerve*) consists of three distinct parts – *ophthalmic* (V1), *maxillary* (V2) and *mandibular* (V3) nerves. Together, these nerves provide sensation to the skin of face, and control the muscles of mastication. **CN VII** (*facial nerve*) provides motor innervation to the face, and damage to this nerve results in facial palsy. **CN VIII** (*vestibulocochlear nerve*) is responsible for hearing (*cochlear nerve*) and balance (*vestibular nerve*). **CN IX** (*glossopharyngeal nerve*) provides sensory innervation to the oropharynx and back of the tongue. **CN X** (*vagus nerve*) is responsible for parasympathetic innervation to a number of organs, and also innervates the larynx—damage to the vagus may cause an increase in heart rate and blood pressure, hoarseness of voice, and difficulty in swallowing. **CN XI** (*accessory nerve*) helps in shoulder elevation and head turning by innervating the trapezius and sternocleidomastoid muscle. **CN XII** (*hypoglossal nerve*) helps in tongue movement.

The cell bodies of the neurons of most cranial nerves lie in various nuclei in the brainstem—the nuclei of CN III, IV lie in the midbrain; nuclei of CN V, VI, VII and VIII are present in the pons; and those of CN IX, X, XI, and XII are contained in the medulla. Damage to these nuclei due to trauma may lead to the associated cranial nerve dysfunction. The cranial nerves may also get compressed due to raised intracranial pressure or mass effect of an intracerebral hematoma.

CEREBELLUM

Literally meaning "the little brain," the cerebellum is located behind the fourth ventricle, pons, and medulla, separated from the occipital and temporal lobes of the cerebral hemispheres by the tentorium cerebelli. It plays an important role in motor control and coordination, maintenance of balance and posture, and cognition.

The cerebellum is divided into two cerebellar *hemispheres* connected by a narrow midline *vermis*. The surface is divided by numerous curved transverse fissures or *folia*, giving it a laminated appearance. Although being only 10% of the total weight of the total brain volume, it contains 3.6 times as many neurons as in the cortex due to the folded pattern in the cerebellar gray matter. The white matter of the cerebellum is largely made of myelinated nerve fibers to and from the cortex, and is referred to as *arbor vitae*, due to its branched, tree-like appearance in cross-section. Embedded within the white matter, are four deep gray matter nuclei—*dentate, globose, emboliform*, and *fastigial*, which are the main sources of output from the cerebellum.

The cerebellum is connected with the other parts of the nervous system by three paired cerebellar peduncles—superior, middle, and inferior. The *superior cerebellar peduncle* carries efferent fibers to the upper motor neurons in the cerebral cortex via thalamic nuclei. The *middle cerebellar peduncle* receives its input from the pontine nuclei via transverse pontine fibers. The *inferior cerebellar peduncle* receives afferent fibers from the vestibular nuclei, tegmentum, and the spinal cord.

The surface of the cerebellum is distinguished into three lobes—*anterior, posterior* and *flocculonodular* lobes. The flocculo-nodular lobe is the smallest region, involved mainly in spatial orientation and balance. Functionally, the cerebellum is divided into a medial sector, called the *spinocerebellum*, involved in limb movements and fine-tuning of the body; and a larger lateral sector, called the *cerebrocerebellum*, involved in planning and cognition.

The cerebellum is relatively well protected from trauma in comparison to the frontal and temporal lobes and the brainstem, due to its location on the skull base behind the brainstem. However, injury to the cerebellum may occur by indirect as well as direct trauma, leading to cerebellar symptoms like ataxia, hypotonia, dysarthria, imbalance, intention tremors, and nystagmus.

VENTRICULAR SYSTEM

The ventricular system consists of a series of interconnected cavities or ventricles within the brain, which contain the cerebrospinal fluid (CSF) secreted by a network of ependymal cells, called choroid plexus, located within. The ventricular system is continuous with the central canal of the spinal cord, allowing the CSF to circulate.

The system comprises of four ventricles—*lateral ventricles* (right and left), *third ventricle*, and *fourth ventricle*. The interventricular *foramina of Monro* connect each lateral ventricle to the third ventricle, located between the right and left thalamus. The third ventricle opens into the fourth ventricle located behind the pons and upper half of medulla, via the *aqueduct of Sylvius*. The fourth ventricle then communicates with the subarachnoid space via the median *aperture of Magendie*, and two *lateral apertures of Luschka*. The CSF then flows around the cerebral hemispheres, and are reabsorbed by the arachnoid villi into the venous sinuses, finally draining into the internal jugular vein. CSF provides buoyancy and support to the brain against gravity, protecting it from concussive, injury to a great extent.

Post-traumatic hydrocephalus is a frequent complication following traumatic brain injury. It occurs either due to overproduction of CSF, blockage of normal CSF outflow, or impaired absorption. Four main factors associated with post-traumatic hydrocephalus are intraventricular hemorrhage, subarachnoid hamorrhage, base of skull fracture, and interhemispheric subdural hygroma (7). These patients typically need a venticulo-peritoneal shunt for CSF diversion.

Blood supply of the brain

Despite being only 2% of the total body weight, the brain receives 15% of the total cardiac output, and utilizes 20% of the total body oxygen. The cerebral blood flow averages ~75 ml/min, and therefore, the brain has a rich blood supply.

ARTERIAL SUPPLY

Blood supply to the brain is mainly derived from two main arteries—the **internal carotid artery** that supplies the anterior brain (frontal, parietal, and part of the temporal lobes), and the **vertebral artery** that supplies the posterior brain (occipital and part of temporal lobes, brainstem, and cerebellum). The connection between the anterior and posterior cerebral circulation is via bilateral posterior communicating arteries, thereby completing a circle, commonly referred to as the circulus arteriosus, or the circle of Willis.

Circle of Willis: Each internal carotid artery gives off the anterior and the middle cerebral arteries to form the anterior circulation. The two vertebral arteries from each side unite to form the basilar artery, which then bifurcates into two posterior cerebral arteries, forming the posterior circulation. The internal carotid and the vertebrobasilar systems are connected by the posterior communicating arteries. The two anterior cerebral arteries are connected by the anterior communicating artery, thereby completing the arterial anastomotic ring at the base of the brain and providing backup circulation. If one of the arteries supplying the circle is occluded, the interconnections between the anterior and posterior circulation prevent tissue ischemia.

The **internal carotid artery**, in its cranial part beyond the cavernous sinus, gives off the ophthalmic artery, the posterior communicating artery, the anterior choroidal artery, and the two terminal branches—anterior and middle cerebral arteries.

The *anterior choroidal artery* is often referred to as the **artery of thrombosis**, as it has a narrow lumen and a long subarachnoid course, making it vulnerable to thrombosis.

Above the optic chiasma, the **anterior cerebral artery** connects its corresponding artery from the opposite side via the *anterior communicating artery*. Just proximal to the anterior communicating artery, the *recurrent artery of Heubner* arises, which recurs backward to supply the internal capsule and head of the caudate nucleus.

The anterior cerebral artery supplies the corpus callosum, medial parts of the frontal and parietal lobes (up to the parieto-occipital sulcus), including the sensorimotor cortex of the paracentral lobule, basal ganglia, and medial part of orbital surface. Motor weakness and sensory loss of the contralateral lower extremity is the commonest symptom of anterior cerebral artery occlusion.

The **middle cerebral artery** gives off the *lenticulostriate arteries*, which are end arteries and supply the internal capsule. These arteries are sometimes referred to as the "**Charcot's artery of hemorrhage**" as these are particularly prone to rupture during accelerated hypertension.

The middle cerebral artery supplies the bulk of the supero-lateral surface of the cerebral hemisphere, including the sensori-motor areas around the central sulcus, and the Broca's and Wernicke's area. Occlusion of this artery, therefore, results in contralateral paresis affecting mostly the face and upper extremity, along with aphasia.

Vertebral arteries form the posterior circulation in the brain. Each vertebral artery arises from the subclavian artery, enters the cranium through the foramen magnum, and unites with the corresponding artery from the opposite side, at the base of the pons, to form the *basilar artery*, between the two sixth cranial nerves. As the *vertebrobasilar system*, they supply the posterior part of the brain, cerebellum, brainstem and the spinal cord. The basilar artery ascends ventral to the pons and divides into a pair of *posterior cerebral arteries* at the cephalic border of the pons, close to the pituitary stalk.

The vertebral artery gives off the *posterior inferior cerebellar artery*, which is its largest branch and supplies the cerebellum. The *anterior and posterior spinal arteries* also arise from the vertebral artery and supply the medulla in addition to the spinal cord.

The **basilar artery** gives off the pontine arteries, the superior cerebellar artery, and the anterior inferior cerebellar artery to the cerebellum.

The **posterior cerebral artery** gives off *cortical branches* supplying the inferior surface of the temporal lobe and occipital lobe; *posterolateral striate branches* supplying the caudal part of thalamus; and the *posterior choroidal artery*, supplying the choroid plexus, posterior part of the thalamus and midbrain.

In the central nervous system, the capillary endothelium and the perivascular feet of the astrocytes of neurons, form a highly selective semipermeable membrane barrier, termed the **blood–brain barrier**, which helps in maintaining a chemically optimal environment for neuronal function. This blood–brain barrier controls movements of ions and metabolites, most importantly glucose, across the brain, and also prevents entry of harmful substances or toxins into the central nervous system. The blood–brain barrier may break down following infection or ischemia, leading to cytotoxic edema. Some areas of the brain, such as the pineal body, posterior pituitary, area postrema, median eminence of hypothalamus and so on, are devoid of the blood–brain barrier, and are termed circumventricular organs.

VENOUS DRAINAGE

The venous drainage of the brain is through a complex system of superficial and deep veins, which are thin-walled and valveless and pierce the arachnoid and meningeal layer of duramater obliquely, to open into the dural venous sinuses. The oblique drainage of veins into the sinuses, against the current of blood, prevents their collapse during increased intracranial pressure.

DURAL VENOUS SINUSES: The dural venous sinuses lie between the periosteal and meningeal layers of duramater and drain venous blood from the central nervous system, face, and scalp, to drain into the internal jugular vein. They also drain CSF from the subarachnoid space via arachnoid granulations.

There are, in all, 11 venous sinuses. The *straight, superior, and inferior sagittal sinuses* run in the midline in the falx cerebri and converge at the *confluence of sinuses* over the internal occipital protuberance. From the confluence, the *transverse sinus* continues laterally on each side and curves into the *sigmoid sinus*, finally opening into the internal jugular vein. The *cavernous sinus* drains the ophthalmic veins on either side of the sella and drains blood into the internal jugular vein via the *superior and inferior petrosal sinuses.*

The **SUPERFICIAL VEINS** drain the cortex and the subcortical white matter, and include the superior cerebral, superficial middle cerebral, and inferior cerebral veins.

The *superior cerebral veins* (~8–12 in number) drain the superolateral and medial surfaces of each hemisphere. They mainly follow the sulci and drain into the superior sagittal sinus.

The *superficial middle cerebral vein* drains the lateral surface of the brain and ends in the cavernous sinus. A superior anastomotic vein connects the superficial middle cerebral vein to the superior sagittal sinus, and an inferior anastomotic vein connects it to the transverse sinus.

The *inferior cerebral veins* drain the inferior surface and ventral part of the lateral surface of the hemisphere. Inferior cerebral veins on the orbital surface of the frontal lobe drain into the superior sagittal sinus, and those on the temporal lobe drain into the superior petrosal, cavernous, and transverse sinuses.

The **DEEP VEINS** drain the diencephalon and the basal ganglia. They include the internal cerebral veins, basal veins, and the great cerebral vein of Galen.

The *internal cerebral vein* is formed by the union of the thalamostriate veins (draining the caudate nucleus and the thalamus) and the choroidal veins (draining the choroid plexus of the third and fourth ventricles, along with the hippocampus, fornix, and corpus callosum).

The *basal vein (of Rosenthal)* is formed by the union of the anterior and deep middle cerebral veins, beneath the anterior perforated substance. It also receives tributaries from the interpeduncular fossa, inferior horn of the lateral ventricle, parahippocampal gyrus, and midbrain.

The *great cerebral vein (of Galen)* is a short median vessel formed by the union of the two internal cerebral veins, which opens into the anterior end of the straight sinus. It also receives the basal veins, occipital veins, and the posterior callosal vein.

Venous drainage of brainstem: Veins of the midbrain drain into the great cerebral or basal vein.

Veins of the pons and medulla drain into the adjacent dural venous sinuses, mainly the superior and inferior petrosal sinuses, the transverse sinus, and the occipital sinus. Inferiorly, these veins are continuous with the veins of the spinal cord.

Veins of the cerebellum: The cerebellar veins constitute the superior and inferior cerebellar veins. The superior group of veins drain into the straight, transverse, and superior petrosal venous sinuses. The inferior cerebellar veins drain into the straight or sigmoid sinus (median vessels), or the inferior petrosal and occipital sinuses (lateral vessels).

ANATOMY FOR SPINAL INJURIES

Trauma to the spine may cause vertebral fractures, leading to spinal cord injury, which may be complete (no function below the site of injury), or incomplete. Injuries at the level of cervical spine are particularly dangerous, as they may affect the chest muscles (above C4), leading to ventilator dependence.

The spine

The spine or the vertebral column is a part of the axial skeleton, which houses the spinal canal, within which the spinal cord is enclosed and protected. The adult vertebral column consists of 33 vertebral segments—the upper 24 are articulating, separated from each other by an intervertebral disc; while the lower 9 (sacral and coccygeal) are fused. There are 7 cervical, 12 thoracic, 5 lumbar, 5 sacral, and 4 coccygeal vertebrae. The first two cervical vertebrae—atlas and axis—are specialized to allow for movement of the head.

Each vertebra consists of a vertebral body anteriorly and a vertebral arch posteriorly. The **vertebral body** is the weight-bearing component of the spine, and its size increases as the vertebral column descends. Adjacent vertebral bodies are separated by a fibrocartilaginous *intervertebral disc*, consisting of an *annulus fibrosus*, surrounding the *nucleus pulposus*. The *anterior and posterior longitudinal ligaments* strengthen the intervertebral joints. The vertebral body, along with the vertebral arch, encloses a hole called a *vertebral foramen*. The foramina of all the vertebrae line up to form the *vertebral canal*, which contains the spinal cord.

The **vertebral arch** is formed by a pair of *pedicles*, and a pair of *laminae*, along with two *transverse*

processes pointing laterally, and a *spinous process* pointing posteriorly. *Articular processes*—two superior and two inferior—are located at the junction of lamina and pedicles, and articulate with their counterparts on the vertebrae above and below. The part of the vertebra located between the superior and inferior articular processes of the facet joint is called the *pars interarticularis*. The *facet joints* between the articular facets of the adjacent vertebrae are strengthened by various ligaments— *ligamentum flavum* (between adjacent laminae), *interspinous* and *supraspinous ligaments* (between the spinous processes), and *intertransverse ligaments* (between the transverse processes). In between each pair of vertebrae, there are the *intervertebral foramina* on each side, which allow for the exit of spinal nerves.

The cervical and lumbar spines normally have a lordotic curve (convex forward), while the thoracic spine has a kyphotic curve (convex dorsally).

Spinal or vertebral fractures

Minor vertebral fractures (e.g., fracture of the transverse processes, or spinous processes etc.) are mechanically stable and do not result in a neurological sequelae. However, associated injuries in the thorax and abdomen should always be looked for in such cases, as the force causing these fractures is usually large.

The **major spinal fractures**, in increasing order of severity, include:

1. *Wedge fracture*—single column anterior vertebral fracture caused by a flexion compression mechanism.
2. *Burst fracture*—axial compression injury causing failure of both anterior and posterior columns, resulting in loss of height of the vertebral body. These are usually unstable fractures, and the possibility of cord impingement, nerve root compression, or vascular injury needs to be excluded, which may warrant a decompressive surgery.
3. *Chance (or seat-belt) fracture*—flexion distraction injury involving a failure of the posterior column, along with an injury to the ligamentous and bony components.
4. *Rotational fracture dislocations*—resulting in failure of posterior and middle columns, with varying degrees of insult to the anterior column.

These are usually unstable fractures, with neurological sequelae.

Apart from the mechanism of injury causing the fracture, there are other types of fractures, depending on the vertebra fractured—these are usually the cervical vertebral fractures.

- *Jefferson's fracture*—fracture of the anterior and posterior arches of the first cervical vertebra—caused by an impact on the back of the head.
- *Hangman's fracture*—fracture of both pedicles or pars interarticularis of the second cervical vertebra—caused by a forcible hyperextension of the head with distraction (commonly seen in car crashes when the driver is without a seat belt and slams his chin against the steering wheel or windshield).
- *Teardrop fracture*—fracture of the anteroinferior aspect of a cervical body—caused by flexion and vertical axial compression of the vertebral body—usually associated with a spinal cord injury.
- *Clay-shoveler fracture*—fracture through the spinous process of a vertebra, mostly the lower cervical or upper thoracic (C6, C7 being the commonest)—an avulsion fracture—usually stable.

SPINAL CORD

The spinal cord extends from the medulla oblongata above to the lower border of the first lumbar vertebrae below, and transmits nerve signals to and from the cortex to control the muscles of the body. It is anchored to the dura by the denticulate ligaments. The lower part of the spinal cord is known as the *conus medullaris*, which is continuous with a neuroglial thread-like structure known as *filum terminale*, which attaches it to the coccyx. The length of the spinal cord is approximately 45 cm in males, and 43 cm in females.

The spinal cord gives attachment to a series of *spinal nerves*, one on each side, via a *ventral (motor) root* and a *posterior (sensory) root*. Through them, it provides innervation for the trunk and limbs, both afferent as well as efferent. Just proximal to its junction with the ventral root, outside the spinal cord, the dorsal root has an oval enlargement consisting of sensory neurons, known as the *dorsal root ganglion*. The length of the spinal cord giving

origin to the roots of one spinal nerve constitutes a *spinal segment*. The spinal cord thus forms 31 segments—8 cervical, 12 thoracic, 5 lumbar, 5 sacral, and 1 coccygeal. These segments, however, do not lie opposite to the corresponding vertebrae, nor do they exit their corresponding intervertebral foramina. This is largely due to the upward recession of the spinal cord during growth. In early fetal life, the spinal cord is as long as the vertebral canal, but subsequently, the differential growth of the spinal cord as compared to the vertebral canal makes it end at the level of the third lumbar vertebra at birth, and lower border of the first lumbar vertebra in adulthood. As a result, the spinal nerve roots have to follow an oblique course to reach their corresponding foramen. Many of these roots occupy the vertebral canal below the level of the spinal cord, constituting the *cauda equina*.

The spinal cord is covered by three membranes or meninges—dura, arachnoid, and pia mater. The outermost dura mater forms a tough protective coating for the cord. The epidural space separates dura from the vertebral canal and contains a layer of fat, along with a network of epidural veins, called the Batson's plexus. The subarachnoid space between the pia and arachnoid is a relatively wide space filled with cerebrospinal fluid.

The spinal cord is divided roughly into two halves by a deep anterior median fissure, and a shallow posterior median sulcus. The anterolateral sulcus, lateral to the anterior median fissure, marks the exit of the ventral roots; while the posterolateral sulcus, lateral to the posterior median sulcus, is the site of entry of the dorsal nerve roots.

The spinal cord consists of butterfly-shaped gray matter, surrounded by three columns or *funiculi* of white matter—the ventral, lateral, and dorsal funiculi. The corticospinal tract descends the spinal cord in the lateral funiculus, while the dorsal column medial lemniscus pathway (represented by gracile and cuneate fasciculi), is contained in the posterior funiculus. An imaginary coronal line through the central canal divides the gray matter into *anterior and posterior horns or columns*. Ventral nerve roots emerge from the ventral gray horns, while the dorsal nerve roots enter the dorsal gray horns. In the thoracic region, the posterolateral part of the anterior column is termed the *intermediolateral column*, which contains the preganglionic cells of the autonomic nervous system. The intermediolateral column from T1 to L2 spinal segments gives rise to sympathetic axons, while that from the S2, S3, and S4 spinal segments give rise to parasympathetic preganglionic neurons.

Blood supply of the spinal cord: The spinal cord is supplied by one *anterior* (supplying anterior two-thirds of the cord) and two *posterior spinal arteries* (supplying posterior one-third of the cord), which are branches of the vertebral artery; and from the *radicular arteries* that arise from the spinal branches of ascending cervical, deep cervical, intercostal, lumbar, and sacral arteries. These branches form three longitudinal trunks (one anterior and two posterior), which communicate around the cord, forming a pial plexus, called the vasa corona.

Artery of Adamkiewicz or the arteria radicularis magna is the largest of the great radicular arteries, arising from the lower thoracic or upper lumbar branches of the aorta, which supplies nutrition to most of the lower two-thirds of the spinal cord.

The veins draining the spinal cord are arranged in the form of six longitudinal channels— *anteromedian* and *posteromedian* channels that lie in the midline; and *anterolateral* and *posterolateral* channels that are paired and lie laterally. These channels are interconnected by a plexus of veins forming a **venous vasocorona**. The longitudinal veins communicate with the internal vertebral or epidural venous plexus, and drain into the vena caval and azygos veins and into the basilar venous plexus.

Trauma to the spinal cord may result in tetraplegia (injury at the cervical region) or paraplegia (injury in the thoracic, lumbar, or sacral segments, including the cauda equina). It may be a partial or complete injury. Complete spinal cord injuries may result in spinal shock, which results in complete loss of all neurologic function below a specific level, including all reflexes, that is associated with autonomic dysfunction.

REFERENCES

1. Turnage B, Maull KI. Scalp laceration: An obvious 'occult' cause of shock. *South Med J.* 2000 Mar; 93(3):265-6.
2. Bonfield CM, Naran S, Adetayo OA, Pollack IF, Losee JE. Pediatric skull fractures: The need for surgical intervention, characteristics, complications, and outcomes. *J Neurosurg Pediatr.* 2014 Aug. 14(2):205-11.
3. Javed Z, Qamar U, Sathyapalan T. Pituitary and/or hypothalamic dysfunction following moderate to severe traumatic brain injury: Current perspectives. *Indian J Endocrinol Metab.* 2015 Nov-Dec;19(6):753-63.
4. Rajmohan V, Mohandas E. The limbic system. *Indian J Psychiatry.* 2007 Apr;49(2):132-9.
5. Song YM. Somatotopic Organization of Motor Fibers in the Corona Radiata in Monoparetic Patients With Small Subcortical Infarct. *Stroke.* 2007;38: 2353-2355.
6. Kinnunen KM, Greenwood R, Powell JH, Leech R, Hawkins PC, Bonnelle V, Patel MC, Counsell SJ, Sharp DJ. White matter damage and cognitive impairment after traumatic brain injury. *Brain.* 2011 Feb;134 (Pt 2):449-63.
7. Mohd Nor MA, Abdul Rahman NA, Adnan JS. Post-traumatic hydrocephalus. *Malays J Med Sci.* 2013 Jan;20(1):95-6.

PART III

Neurophysiology

3

Neurophysiology in neurotrauma

DINU CHANDRAN AND MANPREET KAUR

INTRODUCTION

The pathophysiology (functional changes that accompany a particular syndrome or disease) of traumatic brain injury (TBI) is intricately linked to alterations and dysregulation of cerebral metabolism and homeostatic mechanisms that regulate vital neurophysiologic variables, including intracranial (brain) blood flow, intracranial volumes, and intracranial pressures. The initial section of this chapter will lay the groundwork to understand the fundamental physiologic mechanisms that regulate these variables. The subsequent section will explain the pathophysiology of TBI in light of current literature and evidence from both animal models and human studies.

INTRACRANIAL COMPONENTS AND THE MONRO-KELLIE DOCTRINE

The skull is a nonexpandable, rigid, semiclosed compartment housing three intracranial components; namely, (1) brain parenchyma (the essential and distinctive tissue of an organ), including interstitial fluid; (2) blood; and (3) CSF (cerebrospinal fluid). Quantitatively, brain parenchyma occupies 80% of the available intracranial volume, along with interstitial fluid, while CSF and blood occupy 10% each of the total intracranial volume. The influence of the change in volume of one of these components on the volumes of the remaining components is explained clearly in the Monro-Kellie Doctrine.[1] The introduction of this doctrine by Alexander Monro in 1783 didn't take into consideration the presence of CSF as an important intracranial component. Subsequent observations and evidence that led to the doctrine being revised to its current form stated, "with an intact skull, the sum of the volumes of brain, blood, and CSF is constant." Therefore, an increase in volume of one of the components will be associated with a decrease in the volume of one or both other components.[1,2] To understand the physiologic implications of this doctrine, it is important to understand the quantitative relationship between the volumes of each component and the potential for compressibility of each (Figure 3.1). Brain parenchyma (tissue) cannot be compressed; a volume increase of any intracranial component is accompanied by changes in CSF and/or blood

volumes in compliance with the Monro-Kellie Doctrine.

CSF is produced by specific capillary networks in cerebral ventricles known as choroid plexus at a relatively constant rate of 0.35 mL/min in adults and approximately 0.40 mL/min in children.[3] The total CSF volume equals 100 to 150 mL in adults; the majority of that volume remains in the cerebral subarachnoid space and major cisterns of the brain. A relatively minor volume of CSF occupies cerebral ventricles and the spinal subarachnoid space and spinal canal.[4] CSF formation is constant when continuous absorption occurs through specialized structures called arachnoid villi (small protrusions of the thin, second layer covering the brain) and granulations. Arachnoid granulations are herniations of arachnoid membrane through the dura mater into cerebral venous sinuses. Arachnoid granulations function as one-way valves permitting all CSF components to flow in the same direction into the cerebral venous blood.[4]

The brain receives approximately 700 mL of blood every minute, which is equivalent to double

Schematic model depicting cranium and intracranial components

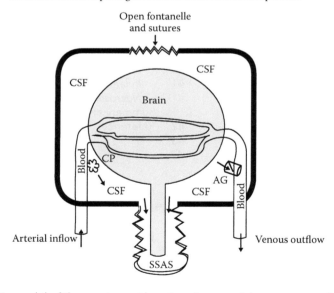

Figure 3.1 A schematic model of the cranium with various intracranial components. In steady state, arterial inflow is constantly balanced by venous outflow, keeping the total intracranial blood volume relatively constant. CSF is secreted from the choroid plexus (CP) and absorbed through the arachnoid granulations (AG), which act as one-way valves to the venous compartment. The spinal subarachnoid space (SSAS) acts as a high compliant space that can accommodate CSF translocated from the cranial compartment in response to a rise in volume of any other intracranial component. The presence of open sutures and fontanelles increases the compliance of the cranial compartment in infants and young children up to 2 years of age.

the total intracranial volume. In a steady state, the appropriate amount of arterial inflow is constantly balanced by an equal amount of venous outflow, negating any significant change in total intracranial blood (ICB) volume. ICB volume amounts to approximately 150 mL in adults. Forty-five percent of the blood volume stays in the microcirculation and the remaining percent stays in the venous (40%) and arterial compartments (15%).[2] Cerebral blood flow (CBF) is determined by cerebral perfusion pressure (CPP) and cerebrovascular resistance (CVR) by the relationship:

$$CBF = CPP/CVR,$$

where, $CPP = MAP - ICP$
MAP is mean arterial pressure, ICP is intracranial pressure, and,

$$CVR = 8\eta l/\pi r4,$$

where "l" is the length of the vessel, "η" is viscosity of blood, and "r" is the radius of the vessel.

Volume-buffering mechanisms and their decompensation

Change in volume of any intracranial component is often accompanied by compensatory changes in the volume of CSF and venous blood volume thereby buffering any change in total volume of the intracranial components. Intracranial CSF volume is displaced to the more compliant spinal subarachnoid space and spinal canal to make room for the increase in volume of intracranial components. A small increase in intracranial pressure also increases the reabsorption of CSF through arachnoid granulations[5] because the absorptive process is pressure dependent. These changes in CSF volume and flow dynamics are often accompanied by reduction in Intracerbral volume (ICV) blood volume as an additional mechanism of volume buffering.[5] Once the physiologic limit of these mechanisms is reached, any additional increase in volume of intracranial components will be accompanied by a rise in ICP. A progressive increase in volume or mass of the intracranial lesion can subsequently distort and block the subarachnoid pathways and cisterns there by preventing CSF translocation mechanisms from being able to buffer the volume change. Additionally, collapse of venous

outflow tracts due to rising ICP can cause back pressure on the cerebral microvascular bed, which will increase the capillary hydrostatic pressure (the force that is exerted by fluid against the capillary wall). A decrease in CPP in the wake of rising ICP can cause upstream resistance vessels to dilate due to autoregulatory mechanisms (mechanisms that automatically adjust [discussed below in the section of cerebral autoregulation]), leading to an increase in cerebral blood volume. Resulting arterial hypertension can augment the capillary hydrostatic pressure further and produce fatal cerebral edema.[5]

INTRACRANIAL PRESSURE

Intracranial pressure drives cerebral perfusion pressure and cerebral blood flow, making its monitoring essential for assessment and management of various clinical neurosurgical and neurologic conditions. At steady state, ICP is determined by input from CSF and vascular components as demonstrated by the relationship:

$$ICP = CSF\ component + vascular\ component$$

$$ICP = (If \times Ro) + Pv$$

where If is the CSF formation rate, Ro is CSF outflow resistance, and Pv is the vascular contribution to ICP.

It is understood from this mathematical relationship that any physiologic or pathologic factor that increases the CSF production rate or outflow resistance will increase ICP. The contribution of the vascular component to ICP is more complex and has not been modeled and expressed mathematically in a quantifiable manner.

Physiologic factors affecting ICP

ICP is lower in preterm infants compared with full-term infants. The normal range of ICP[6] progressively increases during childhood to adulthood (Table 3.1). Besides age, posture is another

Table 3.1 Normal intracranial pressure (ICP) values in children and adults

Age group	ICP value in mmHg
Term infants	1.5–6
Children	3–7
Adults	<10–15

important physiologic factor that affects ICP.[7] ICP is negative in the standing posture with mean ICP in adults falling to −10 mmHg in this posture.

MONITORING ICP

Clinically, ICP is monitored mostly by invasive methods. The methods can be classified based on the location of the catheter or pressure transducer into (1) intraventricular, (2) subdural/epidural, and (3) intra-parenchymal.[1,7,8] The gold standard technique for measuring ICP involves placing an intraventricular catheter in the lateral (sideways) ventricle connected to an external pressure transducer for continuous recording. Recording through ventricular catheters also allows therapeutic manipulation of the CSF pressure and prevents zero drifting of the pressure recording. Now that microtransducers exist, they can be placed in any of the recording locations; the infection rates associated with the procedure have been reported to decrease.[7] The prominent disadvantages of intra-parenchymal recording has been reported to be: zero drifting, which contributes to inaccuracy in ICP time estimation with and a limitation in deriving an estimate of real ICP based on the compartmentalized recording from a single parenchymal (tissue) site. Noninvasive methods to measure ICP based on various imaging methods, trans-cranial Doppler, and visual, evoked potentials (electric recordings of the nervous system) have been developed and tested with limited success and accuracy. A noninvasive estimation of ICP has been tried in infants by placing a pressure transduction system over the anterior fontanelle (the meeting point of coronal and sagittal sutures)[6] and also by assessment of hemodynamic response to anterior fontanelle compression using Doppler ultrasonography.[8]

FLUCTUATIONS IN MEAN ICP

Continuous ICP monitoring using an intraventricular catheter was pioneered by Lundberg et al., in the 1960s. Based on systematic analyses of pressure recordings from a series of patients, Lundberg reported three characteristic fluctuations in mean ICP.[1,6,8,9]

- **A waves or plateau waves:** These waves have a pathologic origin and indicate significant reduction in the intracranial compliance (see below). A waves are characterized by a sudden and steep increase in ICP to 50 mmHg or more from near normal values. These fluctuations usually last for 5 to 20 minutes followed by a sharp decline to the baseline values.

- **B waves:** B waves are also of pathologic significance and are associated with failing intracranial compensation to volume changes. B waves show rhythmic (0.5 to 2 Hz) oscillations in ICP rising steeply to 20 to 30 mmHg above baseline followed by a sudden decline to baseline values. Unlike A waves, B waves do not show sustained periods of intracranial hypertension. B waves most likely came about because of changes in cerebrovascular tone and cerebral blood volume.

- **C waves:** C waves are of limited pathologic significance. They are rhythmic oscillations in ICP with frequencies ranging from 4 to 8 per minute; they are synchronous with the spontaneously occurring Traube-Hering-Mayer wave oscillations in arterial blood pressure. C waves have lower amplitude than A and B waves.

INTRACRANIAL PRESSURE VOLUME RELATIONSHIP

Intracranial pressure volume curves graphically depict the changes in intracranial pressure in response to changes in intracranial volume (ICV). These graphic descriptions demonstrate the role of compensatory intracranial volume-buffering mechanisms and provide additional insights and quantifiable measures to predict the risk of intracranial hypertension with a steady increase in intracranial volume. The intracranial pressure volume curve (Figure 3.2) shows an initial compensated phase, the earlier half of which[1] shows a minimal increase in ICP with an increase in ICV. The volume-buffering mechanisms described above operate effectively during this phase, eliminating any change in ICP. The latter half[2] of the compensated phase shows a marginal increase in ICP with an increase in ICV, although ICP is still within the normal limits. More characteristic during this second half of the compensated phase is the change in slope of the intracranial pressure volume curve. The slope of the pressure volume curve that denotes a change in ICP for the unit change in ICV is defined as intracranial elastance ($\Delta P/\Delta V$). This slope has been widely expressed incorrectly as compliance in literature whereas in actual scientific terms, compliance denotes the change in volume

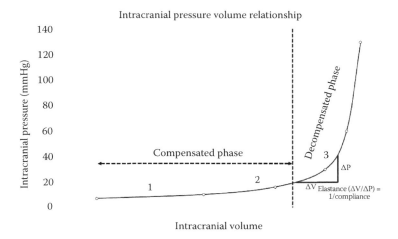

Figure 3.2 Shows the intracranial pressure volume relationship with intracranial volume (ICV) in the x-axis and intracranial pressure (ICP) in the y-axis. Phase 1 is characterized by a negligible rise in ICP with a rise in ICV, indicating a phase of complete compensation. Phase 2 is characterized by a minimal rise in ICP (still within normal limits) and a more prominent rise in cranial elastance (fall in compliance), as indicated by the changing slope of the pressure/volume curve. Phase 3 shows the decompensated phase where a marked rise in ICP is observed with any further rise in ICV.

for unit change in pressure ($\Delta V/\Delta P$). Thus, compliance bears an inverse relationship with intracranial elastance. The second half of the compensated phase shows an increase in intracranial elastance (fall in compliance) steeper than the rise in ICP per se. The decreasing intracranial compliance is indicative of the impending failure of volume-buffering mechanisms, which are already operating at their physiologic limits. Any increase in intracranial volume beyond this point produces a sharp decline in intracranial compliance and a large increase in ICP, which characterizes the decompensated phase of the intracranial pressure volume curve.

INTRACRANIAL COMPLIANCE AND ITS ESTIMATION

The recording of ICP responses to manipulation of ICV is necessary for the experimental or clinical estimation of intracranial compliance in order to generate the pressure-volume relationship. The procedure involves cannulation (inserting a tube) of the lateral ventricle, cisterna magna, or lumbar subarachnoid space to record neuraxis CSF pressure and produce increments or decrements in CSF volume by saline injection or CSF aspiration, respectively.[10] The cannula at the external end is connected to a pressure transducer to record the

changes in ICP. The volume manipulations are done using a syringe filled with sterile saline interposed between the cannula and transducer. After recording the steady state ICP after cannulation, volume manipulation is done initially by removing a specific volume of CSF ($-\Delta V$) by aspiration. Removal of volume will lead to an immediate fall in ICP ($-\Delta P$) followed by a gradual recovery to the steady state ICP values in 2 to 3 minutes. Similarly, a bolus (small) injection of sterile saline will increase the CSF volume by ΔV and a consequent immediate rise in ICP(ΔP) followed by recovery to steady state values in 2 to 3 minutes. Thus, a pressure volume curve is plotted with volume increments or decrements in the x-axis and ICP values are recorded immediately postvolume manipulation on the y-axis (Figure 3.3a). It can be inferred from the pressure volume curve that intracranial compliance (the inverse of the slope) changes as a function of ICV. Intracranial compliance is higher on the horizontal portion of the pressure volume curve than its vertical limb. Plotting the ICP changes of pressure volume curve on a logarithmic scale (base 10) can transform the curve to a linear plot (Figure 3.3b). The slope of this line has been used as an estimate of craniospinal compliance, indicated as pressure volume index (PVI). PVI is defined as the estimated volume in (mL) that is required to raise the ICP by a factor of 10.

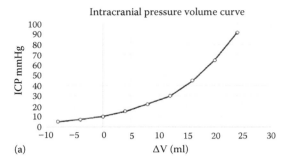

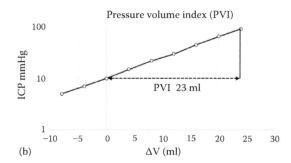

Figure 3.3 Shows the pressure volume curve derived by recording the ICP changes (y-axis) to bolus volume manipulation (ΔV) of intracranial volume as represented in the x-axis (a). A logarithmic plotting of the ICP data transforms the curve into a linear plot (b) and can be used to derive the pressure volume index (PVI).

In addition to the estimation of craniospinal compliance, the technique of bolus manipulation of ICV can also be used to estimate two important variables that determine the CSF pressure. CSF pressure is determined by the CSF production rate (If) and resistance to CSF outflow (Ro). Following the removal of a CSF bolus, ICP shows an immediate decrease followed by gradual recovery toward baseline steady-state values. The rate of this pressure recovery is proportional to the CSF production rate. Similarly, CSF outflow resistance can be estimated from the rate of pressure recovery observed after the immediate increase in ICP that is induced by the bolus volume increment.

The use of PVI in clinical practice to estimate craniospinal compliance has been limited by the need for bolus injections and removal of CSF. Another approach, which is based on ICP waveform analysis, was proposed by Aveezat et al.[1,11] in 1979 to determine craniospinal compliance. The ICP waveform shows changes in pulse that are synchronized with arterial pressure waveform. During each cardiac cycle, there is a pulsatile change in intracranial blood volume (ΔV), which might be equated with artificially induced volume increments, which are used to determine PVI. The pulse amplitude (the maximum extent of a vibration or oscillation) of ICP waveform (ΔP) thus represents the immediate pressure response to intracranial volume increments that are synchronized with each cardiac cycle. The synchronous cardiac volume increments remain largely constant in a stable hemodynamic state, which is not influenced by any changes in craniospinal elastance (a measure of the tendency of a hollow organ to recoil toward its

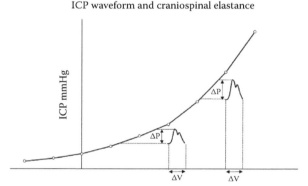

Figure 3.4 Depicts the changes in amplitude of ICP waveform with a rise in ICV. ICP waveform amplitude increases with the fall in intracranial compliance (rise in slope of the pressure volume curve).

original dimensions after removing a compressing or distending force). The pulsatile change in the ICP waveform due to these volume increments is plotted against the conventional pressure volume curve in Figure 3.4. Based on the graph, it can be inferred that the pulse amplitude of ICP waveform has an inverse relationship with the craniospinal compliance and thus can be used as a standard by which to measure.

CEREBRAL BLOOD FLOW

Adult healthy human brain, on average, receives 14% of the cardiac output every minute, which translates to approximately 50 mL/100 g/min. Because of its higher metabolic demands, gray matter receives approximately four times higher blood flow (80 mL/100 g/min) than white matter (20 mL/100 g/min) in adults.[12] There is paucity (scarcity) of data on cerebral blood flow measurements in healthy normal children. Based on available evidence, CBF has been reported to be significantly higher in healthy children (100 mL/100 g/min) than adults.[13,14] The age-dependent changes in CBF in children have been associated with similar changes in cerebral metabolic rate, as explained below.

CBF is influenced by the interaction of local and systemic factors exerted through humoral (relating to body fluids) and neural (relating to a nerve or the nervous system) mechanisms that include: (1) cerebral metabolic rate, (2) arterial partial pressure of CO_2, (3) Arterial partial pressure of O_2, (4) Hematocrit (the ratio of the volume of red blood cells to the total volume of blood), and (5) Cerebral autoregulation (the physiologic mechanisms that maintain blood flow at an appropriate level during changes in blood pressure).

Cerebral blood flow and metabolic rate and flow metabolism coupling

Cerebral metabolic rate is a measure of the energy used in the brain, which is calculated from the amount of oxygen used by the brain (cerebral metabolic rate for oxygen—$CMRo_2$) or amount of glucose metabolized by the brain (cerebral metabolic rate for glucose—CMRGlu) in unit time. The amounts of oxygen used and glucose metabolized are quantified by measuring the arterio-venous concentration difference of the substance of interest and CBF. Cerebral metabolism saves the energy expended by the brain during the resting state to maintain the ionic gradients (a gradient of electrochemical potential), biosynthetic (the formation of chemical compounds by a living organism) and other cellular housekeeping functions (basal need), and the additional energy used for neural (nerve) functioning and generation of electrical activity (functional need). Glucose is the metabolic fuel of choice for the brain, which derives 92% of its energy requirement through oxidative metabolism of glucose (the chemical process in which oxygen is used to make energy from carbohydrates).[12]

Flow metabolism coupling (a proportional increase in CBF) is the phenomenon by which CBF is tightly coupled to the metabolic demands of the brain, both regionally and globally.[13] An increase in

metabolic rate because of synaptic transmission (the passage of a neural impulse across a *synapse* from one nerve fiber to another by *means* of a neurotransmitter) temporally (with regard to time) and spatially (with regard to space, position, area, and size) coupled to increase in blood flow to meet the enhanced demands for oxygen and glucose. Flow metabolism coupling being a dominant controller of CBF is preserved during both sleep[15] and general anesthesia.[16] Adenosine and nitric oxide (NO), two potent vasodilatory (the widening of blood vessels) molecules, are believed to be the the the chief molecular mediators of flow metabolism coupling. An increase in cerebral metabolism due to neuronal activation has been linked to an increase in the concentration of these mediators in the surrounding area, resulting in vasodilatation (the dilatation of blood vessels, which decreases blood pressure) and an increase in blood flow to the metabolically active region.

Hypothermia reduces $CMRo_2$ and consequently reduces CBF through flow metabolism coupling. A low temperature reduces energy used by neurons for both basal and functional needs, producing a significant decrease in $CMRo_2$ to 10% of normothermic (normal body temperature) values at temperatures as low as 15°C.[13]

CO₂-MEDIATED VASOREACTIVITY

Carbon dioxide is one of the most potent known physiologic vasodilators of cerebral circulation. CO_2-mediated vasoreactivity is quantified as the change in cerebral blood flow or blood flow velocities to spontaneous or imposed changes in arterial or end-tidal (at the end of normal exhalation) CO_2 concentrations. An increase in arterial or end-tidal CO_2 concentrations is accompanied by an increase in CBF or flow velocities and vice versa. The reported values of CO_2-mediated vasoreactivity in healthy adults averages to 10.3% change in mean CBF velocity with each millimeters of mercury change in end-tidal CO_2.[17] Carbon dioxide quickly diffuses across the blood–brain barrier and changes the pH of cerebral perivascular (related to the tissues surrounding a blood vessel) milieu, which produces vasodilatation and an increase in blood flow. The vasodilatory action of CO_2 on pial arterioles in anesthetized cats has been mediated through changes in extracellular pH with CO_2 having no direct influence on vessel caliber.[18] Similarly, in chronic hypocapnia and hypercapnia, cerebral blood flow changes follow the adaptive changes in CSF pH rather than CO_2 concentrations.[12] Nitric oxide and prostaglandin E2 are considered to be the accepted molecular mediators of CO_2-mediated vasoreactivity, even though the exact mechanisms of action are unknown.[19,20]

CEREBRAL BLOOD FLOW RESPONSES TO CHANGES IN PO_2

Unlike CO_2-mediated vasoreactivity, the influence of changes in arterial/tissue partial pressure of O_2 on CBF is modest and of limited clinical significance. Hypoxemia (inadequate oxygen to the blood) below 50 mmHg produces a considerable increase in CBF, which compensates for the reduced oxygen delivery to neurons produced by a decrease in arterial PO_2 (partial pressure of oxygen). CBF responses to hypoxemia have a slower onset and a longer response time (approximately 6 minutes) to reach steady-state values compared with CO_2-mediated vasoreactivity.[12] The cerebral vasodilatory response to hypoxemia is thought to be the cause of the metabolic shift to anaerobic glycolysis (the transformation of glucose to lactate when limited amounts of O_2 are available) and consequent decrease in extracellular pH due to the accumulation of lactic acid. Additionally, it is believed that adenosine is a mediator of hypoxemia-induced vasodilatation[21] by way of its action through an opening of large-conductance, calcium-activated potassium channels, which lead to vascular smooth muscle relaxation. Nitric oxide that is released by neuronal nitric oxide synthase also plays an important role in mediating the cerebrovascular response to hypoxemia.[22,23] Unlike cerebral vasodilatation to hypoxemia, cerebrovascular response to hyperoxia is controversial and is not well defined.

VISCOSITY AND CEREBRAL BLOOD FLOW

Blood flow in any vascular bed (vascular system) is inversely related to viscosity of blood as given by Poiseuille's formula for calculating vascular resistance − $R = 8\eta l/\pi r4$, where "l" is the length of the vessel, "η" is viscosity of blood, and "r" is the radius of the vessel. The viscosity of blood is primarily a function of the hematocrit (the hematocrit measures how much space in the blood is occupied by the red blood cells). Hemodilution (decreased concentration of cells and solids in the blood as a result of gaining fluid) increases cerebral blood flow because of a decrease in viscosity and consequent reduction in resistance to blood flow as depicted

above. CBF increases in anemia because of both reduction in viscosity and metabolically induced vasodilation, which is produced by decreased oxygen delivery to neuronal tissue.[12]

CEREBRAL AUTOREGULATION

Autoregulation is a physiologic regulatory phenomenon that ensures a constant flow of blood to a vascular bed during changes in arterial blood pressure.[24] Autoregulation exists in most vascular beds but is particularly well developed in the brain.

Definition

Cerebral autoregulation is a homeostatic mechanism (a mechanism that maintains balance and equilibrium) to regulate and maintain a fairly constant brain blood flow over wide ranges of arterial blood pressures, or better, perfusion pressure.[25] The perfusion pressure of the brain is the difference between mean arterial pressure and intracranial pressure. The autoregulatory curve that depicts the relationship between CBF and MAP is shown in Figure 3.5. The quantitative relationship between CPP, CBF, and CVR is given as:

$$CBF = CPP/CVR,$$

and, therefore, $CVR = CPP/CBF$
where, $CPP = MAP - ICP$
MAP is mean arterial pressure, ICP is intracranial pressure.

Another approach to defining autoregulation is based on responses in the caliber (the diameter of a hollow, tubular structure) of *resistance vessels* as occurrence of vasodilatation in response to a decrease in cerebral perfusion pressure and vasoconstriction in response to an increase in cerebral perfusion pressure (Figure 3.5).[26] Third, autoregulation can be defined as changes observed in *CVR*. Autoregulation implies that CBF remains constant and that the CVR changes proportionally to changes in CPP. The definition of choice depends on the experimental model and the parameters of interest. CBF responses may be more effective in describing autoregulation during in vivo studies whereas the caliber changes properly define autoregulation in studies of isolated vessels. CVR seems to be a better parameter to understand the flow changes beyond the limits of autoregulation. CVR reaches a minimum somewhat below the lower limit of autoregulation (LLA) (Figure 3.5). At even

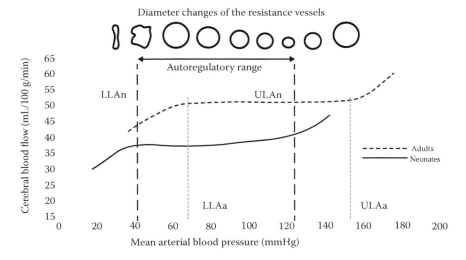

Figure 3.5 Shows the autoregulatory curve of cerebral circulation with mean arterial pressure (MAP) plotted in the x-axis and cerebral blood flow in the y-axis. Black vertical dashed lines indicate the lower (LLAn) and upper limits (ULAn) of autoregulation in neonates and gray dotted vertical lines indicate the lower (LLAa) and upper limits (ULAa) of autoregulation in adults. The top panel graphically depicts the diameter changes of resistance vessels with changes in mean arterial pressure. Below, LLAn vessels collapse, while with autoregulatory change, progressive decrease in diameter is observed with a rise in MAP. Vessels passively dilate beyond the ULAn.

lower pressures, there is a sharp increase in CVR due to the collapse of vessels. At the other end, beyond the upper limit of autoregulation (ULA), passive vasodilatation to high intravascular pressure results in a decrease in CVR and a corresponding increase in CBF (Figure 3.5).

Importance

The brain has a high metabolic demand, accounting for 20% of the body's resting energy used despite weighing only 2% of the total body mass.[26] Therefore, it requires adequate nutritional flow. This high perfusion demand means that the brain is highly susceptible to ischemic injury. On the other hand, disproportionately high CBF relative to the metabolic need is also problematic, because it can result in blood–brain barrier dysfunction with plasma protein extravasation (leakage) and transudation (the passage of fluid or solution through a membrane) of fluid into the interstitium (found within an organ or tissue) and pericapillary (occurring within the tissues) astrocytes (star-shaped cells). Such

changes result in the development of hyperperfusion (decreased blood flow through an organ) syndromes, which are characterized by debilitating neurologic sequelae, including seizures, headaches, encephalopathy, and stroke.[27]

Therefore, it is essential to have strict regulation of CBF to maintain normal brain function. Cerebral autoregulation is a protective mechanism that prevents brain ischemia (insufficient blood supply to a body part) during hypotension; capillary (the smallest blood vessel) damage and brain edema (swelling because of excess fluid) during hypertension. If autoregulation were not present, an otherwise insignificant decrease in the pressure, for example, during sleep, might cause tissue ischemia and, possibly, cell damage. Likewise, a sudden rise in arterial pressure, for example, during any kind of exercise, in the absence of autoregulation, would lead to passive vasodilatation (vasodilatation when the joint is moved by an external force) of arterioles (any of the small terminal twigs of an artery that ends in capillaries) and capillaries and a potential for brain edema to develop.[28]

BLOOD PRESSURE RANGE AND LIMITS OF AUTOREGULATION

In healthy adults, under normal conditions, these limits are MAPs of 60 and 160 mmHg and CPP of 50 and 150 mmHg, respectively.[25,26] It is important to note that cerebral autoregulation responds not only to blood pressure changes but also to changes in ICP.[29,30] In an upright position in a normal brain, ICP and central venous pressure (CVP) at head level are negative and, therefore, not considered. Changes in MAP will thus largely drive the perfusion pressure and CPP will be roughly equivalent to MAP. The limits of autoregulation are not fixed and can be modulated in different physiological situations.

Mechanisms

The mechanisms of cerebral autoregulation may involve a combination of myogenic (response by smooth muscles), metabolic, neurogenic (coming from the nerves) processes and endothelial cell-related factors.

THE MYOGENIC HYPOTHESIS

The myogenic theory states that the basal tone of the vascular smooth muscle is affected by change in perfusion (the passage of fluid through the circulatory system) or transmural (passing through the anatomic wall) pressure, and the small arteries and arterioles are constricting or dilating in response to increases or decreases in transmural pressure. The short latency (time to response) and rapidity of autoregulatory response, which is initiated within a few seconds after a change in the transmural pressure of the resistance vessels[31,32] and largely completed within 15 to 30 seconds, favors a myogenic response.

Experimentally, changes in transmural pressure correlate positively with changes in smooth muscle action potentials and membrane potentials that result in smooth muscle activation.[31,33] Studies have shown that this smooth muscle activation is blocked by removing calcium ions and adding ethylene glycol tetraacetic acid (EGTA).[34] Essentially, stretching vascular smooth muscles activates stretch-sensitive ion channels, which, in turn, depolarizes the membrane through nonselective cation channels, resulting in the entry of calcium through voltage-gated calcium channels, and, consequently, smooth muscle contraction.[35,36] Some investigators believe that the myogenic mechanism limits autoregulation, whereas the metabolic mediators are responsible for cerebral autoregulation itself.

THE METABOLIC HYPOTHESIS

The metabolic mechanism reduces local blood flow, which results in the release of chemical factors that result in dilatation of cerebral blood vessels. That is, CBF is maintained through the release of vasoactive mediators that tie the neuronal activity to blood flow. Regional CBF is then regulated by constriction and dilation of cerebral arterioles and the opening and closing of precapillary sphincters (a sphincter of smooth muscle tissue located at the arterial end of a capillary and serving to control the flow of blood to the tissues) in the metarterioles (delicate blood vessels that branch from the smallest arterioles and connect with the capillary bed—also called precapillary), which are responsible for distributing blood through the cerebrovascular bed. Accepted mediators include CO_2, H^+, O_2, adenosine and adenine nucleotides, K^+, and Ca^{2+}.[37] Among the mediators, adenosine is the only mediator with experimental support.

Adenosine is a known vasodilator[38] and its levels increase in the brain with minor reduction in blood pressure. In moderate to severe hypotension, its levels increase almost sixfold.[39] The failure of the adenosine antagonist caffeine to affect the pressure-flow relationship is accepted as evidence that contradicts the major role of adenosine in autoregulation.[31,40,41] Although the rapidity of the autoregulatory responses has been considered to favor the myogenic hypothesis, the changes in flow to metabolic demand also occur immediately.

Additionally, Nitric Oxide (NO) influences basal- and stimulus-mediated cerebrovascular tone. NO mediates its effect through cGMP and through a decrease in intracellular calcium. Other proposed substances include protein kinase C, melatonin, prostacyclin-activated potassium channels, and intracellular second messengers.[42]

THE NEUROGENIC MECHANISM

The cerebral blood vessels, extraparenchymal (unrelated to the specific tissues of an organ) and intraparenchymal (within the tissues of an organ), are innervated by nerves comparable to that of blood vessels in the periphery.[43] The nerves that are innervating cerebral vessels contain transmitters of several chemical classes along with a variety of cognate (related) receptors expressed on the vasculature. However, the exact role and mechanism of this innervation is still being investigated. The neurotransmitters involved include acetylcholine (most abundant), norepinephrine, neuropeptide Y, cholecystokinin, vasoactive intestinal peptide, and calcitonin gene-related peptide.[44] Stimulation or denervation (loss of nerve supply) of the sympathetic nerve supply slightly changes cerebral blood flow even though it has a marked effect on cerebral blood volume, cerebral capacitance,[45] intracranial pressure,[46] and cerebrospinal fluid formation.[47] Furthermore, sympathetic stimulation shifts the limits of autoregulation to higher pressures, resulting in a shift to the right of the autoregulatory curve. This shields the brain against severe elevation of MAP by affecting the increase in blood flow.[48–50]

ENDOTHELIAL CELL-RELATED FACTORS

Endothelial cell-related factors have also been implicated in autoregulation. Increments in flow without changes in transmural pressure in isolated vessels, both in situ (confined to its original location) and in vitro induce vasodilatation that is eliminated by the removal of endothelium.[51,52] These observations suggest the release of a vasodilatory mediator by the endothelium as a result of an increase in the flow. Harder et al.[33] studied the role of the endothelium in mediating or modulating the vascular responses to transmural pressure elevation. With an intact endothelium, high transmural pressure resulted in membrane depolarization, generating action potential, and vasoconstriction. Following disruption of the endothelium using collagenase or elastase, these responses were lost while contractile response to high potassium and serotonin was preserved. This suggests the endothelial dependence of responses of isolated cerebral blood vessels to changes in transmural pressure. Some are of the opinion that endothelial cells may serve as a transducer in the autoregulatory response to pressure.

Endothelium-derived relaxing factor (EDRF) has been identified as nitric oxide (NO) or a NO-containing substance that is produced in cerebral blood vessels. Its action is mediated by the activation of guanylate cyclase and formation of cyclic GMP. An impaired endothelium-dependent response with a decreased production of EDRF but increased release of endothelium-derived contracting factors, such as endothelin and arachidonic acid, has been reported in subarachnoid hemorrhage.

PATHOPHYSIOLOGY OF TRAUMATIC BRAIN INJURY

Traumatic brain injury (TBI) is a form of acquired brain damage due to external force. TBI pathophysiology is complex and encompasses two sequelae—one is the result of a direct mechanical impact and the other involves the cascade of reactive biochemical, molecular, and genomic responses as a consequence of the primary insult. Interplay of various molecular mechanisms, including excitotoxicity (a process in which nerve cells are damaged), ionic imbalance, oxidative damage, inflammation, and apoptosis (self-destruction of the cells) are involved in TBI. Holistic knowledge of the underlying pathophysiology of TBI would help to present new therapeutic options as well as credible use and refinement of the treatment that is already being used.

TBI represents one of the major epidemics that is responsible for huge morbidity and mortality (disease and death) in the world, especially in the younger age group (<45 years of age). Numerous studies—experimental and clinical—have contributed to our current understanding of the pathophysiology of TBI. This section focuses in detail on the different facets of the pathophysiology of TBI along with some newer, emerging ideas in this field.

The neurovascular unit

The concept of the neurovascular unit is an operative model that is conducive to understanding the intercellular signaling communication between the microvasculature and the cells in the brain parenchyma, including neurons, endothelial cells, astrocytes, pericytes, and oligodendrocytes (Figure 3.6). The functions of this physiologic unit include brain blood flow regulation, maintenance of integrity of the blood–brain barrier, and an important predictor of the outcomes following TBI,[53–55] as well. Recently, the interactions with the immune

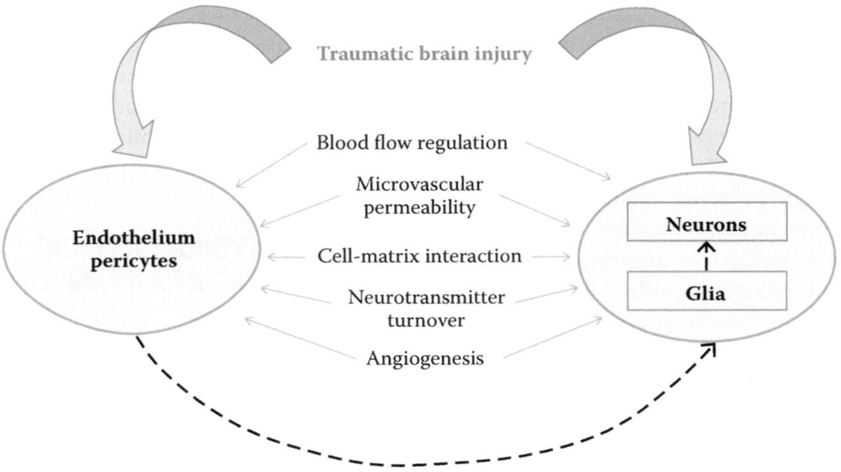

Figure 3.6 Depicts the different component cell types forming the neurovascular unit, their possible interactions, and physiological roles of this unit. Traumatic brain injury results in direct mechanical damage to all of the cells in the neurovascular unit (depicted by light brown, curved arrows) while the dotted arrows represent the indirect damage of the neurons.

cells have been included to have a holistic approach. This unit can become damaged in TBI and plays a critical role in protection and repair after TBI and thus is a target for many emerging, new therapies.

BIOMECHANICAL CHARACTERISTICS OF TRAUMATIC BRAIN INJURY (TBI)

There are different types of mechanical forces that act on the brain after a blow to the head and those forces determine the type and degree of damage after TBI. They include[56]

1. *Impact*, which sends a shockwave throughout the brain. It is common with almost all types of TBI and results in patchy, neuronal damage, which could range from mild to widespread.
2. *Deceleration*, which swings and stretches the cerebrum on the brain stem. This mechanical force is usually found in most TBIs and is known to strain the connections with reticular formation and with the corticospinal tract. Specifically and clinically, it manifests as loss of consciousness and spasticity.
3. *Rotation* principally twists the axons, which connect the two cerebral hemispheres.
4. *Vibration (resonance) of the skull* after impact bruises the underlying cortex.

Another way of classifying these mechanical forces in the literature is into the category of *contact* force, which signifies injury that has been caused by direct contact between the brain and the skull (which includes the impact in the above classification) and forces of inertia, which include the remaining three of the above classification: deceleration and rotational and vibrational forces.[57]

There are a few projections regarding the types of biomechanical forces and their impact.[58,59]

- Presence of loss of consciousness in TBI is a reflection of involvement of the cortex and subcortical system.
- Mesencephalon is the last structure to be affected in TBI; therefore, rostral brain stem injury is mainly seen with severe brain damage of the cortex and subcortical structures.
- Cognitive symptoms (confusion and memory disturbances) can be observed without loss of consciousness; nevertheless, the reverse is not experienced.
- The direction of impulse affects the severity of the injury; the rotational forces have especially been found to result in the most severe injuries.
- The direction of rotation also influences the severity of the injury and predicts recovery. Lateral injuries (side-to-side) are the most damaging, leading to coma or severe debility;

oblique (slanting) injuries fall in between while sagittal (front-to-back) have a good chance of recovery and thus are the least severe.

CLASSIFICATION OF TBI

Furthermore, to broaden the understanding of the underlying pathophysiology of TBI, it has been widely classified, either on the basis of the biomechanical findings or the neuropathologic mechanisms that are involved.

Biomechanical classification

1. Focal brain damage due to contact injury (eg, contusion, laceration, and intracranial hemorrhage).
2. Extensive brain damage due to acceleration/deceleration injury (eg, diffuse axonal injury a brain injury in which damage in the form of extensive lesions in white matter tracts occurs over a wide area).[60–62]

Neuropathological classification

1. Primary damage—The one that occurs directly during the point of impact due to mechanical forces.
2. Secondary damage—The delayed presentation of a cascade of the pathological processes that occur as a result of the initial impact.

EXPERIMENTAL MODELS OF TBI

Our current understanding of the biomechanical, cellular, and molecular aspects of TBI is based on the study of various animal models, in vitro models, and computational models of TBI. Among these approaches, the animal models are most critical to addressing the complex pathophysiologic mechanisms that are associated with TBI, developing and characterizing new therapeutic agents, and closing the therapeutic gap between preclinical studies and patient medical care. Many animal models have been built, among them—the most common include controlled cortical impact, weight loss, fluid percussion injury (experimentally induced TBI) and blast injury model (Table 3.2). Small animals have been used for most experimental protocols due to their modest cost, small size, and standardized outcome measurements. Although these models provide an excellent platform to precisely describe the key injury mechanisms, they have many limitations as well. Table 3.2 depicts the common animal models of TBI, type of injury that they simulate, their strengths, weaknesses, and the species used for these models, respectively.[63,64]

BASIC PATHOPHYSIOLOGY OF TBI

TBI-associated brain damage principally has two stages. First is the primary-injury phase, which occurs at the time of the impact. This is followed by a delayed, secondary stage, caused by a range of

Table 3.2 Experimental models of traumatic brain injury (TBI)

Model	Type of injury	Strengths	Weaknesses	Species
Controlled cortical impact	Mainly focal	Highly reproducible	Need for craniotomy	Mouse, rat, monkey
Weight drop (Feeney, Shohami, Marmarou, Maryland)	Feeney & Shohami – Focal; Marmarou & Maryland – Diffuse	Inexpensive, easy to perform and capable of producing graded DAI that closely mimics human TBI	High variability in injury severity	Cat, rabbit, rat
Fluid percussion injury (midline, parasagittal, lateral)	Mixed	Highly reproducible	Need for craniotomy, high mortality	Cat, rabbit, rat
Blast injury	Mainly diffuse	Close to military TBI	Need standardization	Mouse, rat, swine

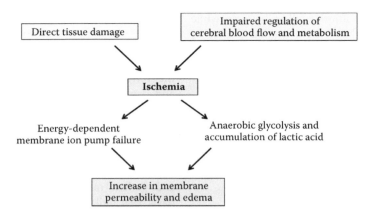

Figure 3.7 Shows the sequence of probable alterations that occur directly after mechanical trauma. Direct damage of neurons, glia, endothelium, and other neighboring cells is observed along with flow-metabolism uncoupling. This might result in ischemic changes resulting in an energy crisis and thus an increase in anaerobic metabolism to meet the requirements leading to lactate accumulation. All of these pathological changes finally culminate in an increase in membrane permeability and edema.

biochemical, cellular, and molecular responses. This is done in an effort to potentially repair the damaged tissue but often results in further damage to the primary injury. The primary phase involves direct mechanical damage to neurons, glia, and surrounding cells, along with flow-metabolism uncoupling, culminating mainly in tissue ischemia and brain swelling (Figure 3.7). The secondary phase may include glutamate excitotoxicity, oxidative stress, neuroinflammation, blood–brain barrier disruption and cell death (necrosis and/apoptosis) (Figure 3.8).

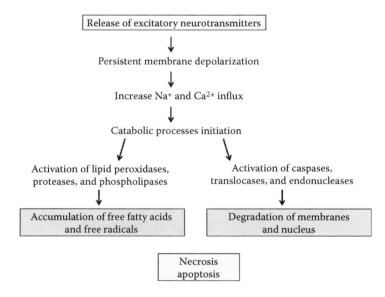

Figure 3.8 Depicts the pathophysiological changes observed in the secondary stage of traumatic brain injury. The excessive release of excitatory neurotransmitters results in persistent membrane depolarization and massive ionic fluxes across the membrane. Intracellular calcium overload results in downstream signaling and activation of enzymes and initiation of cell death (either apoptosis or necrosis).

SPECIFIC PATHOPHYSIOLOGY OF PRIMARY STAGE OF TBI

The preliminary pathologic changes in the primary stage of TBI are varied, depending on the type and severity of the external mechanical force. The cerebral circulation encounters marked alterations in blood flow, autoregulatory capacity, carbon dioxide reactivity, and changes in metabolism and brain swelling.

Cerebral blood flow changes

Cerebral blood flow measurement studies of TBI in animals and humans have found ischemia to be a common feature.[65–68] This leads to a common assumption that ischemic stroke and TBI might share the same pathophysiology. Although this might be partially true, there are some considerable differences between the two clinical conditions.

1. The critical threshold of cerebral blood flow for development of irreversible damage of brain tissue for ischemic stroke patients is lower (5–8.5 mL/100 g/min) than TBI patients (15 mL/100 g/min).[69]
2. The common pathologic features in these two conditions include metabolic stress and ionic perturbations, while over and above this—TBI also involves the mechanical shear force-induced structural damage of neurons, glia, endothelial cells, and microvasculature.[70–71]

Interestingly, early stages of TBI may even be associated with cerebral hyperperfusion (CBF >55 mL/100 g/min).[72–75] The probable etiology (the cause of the disease) of this phenomenon is mainly attributed to the vasodilatory metabolites (like lactic acid and adenosine) in TBI, which cause a decrease in distal cerebrovascular resistance,[65,73] thus resulting in an increase in the cerebral blood flow, which ultimately ends with an increase in ICP and further harmful effects.[76] Flow and metabolism are normally coupled in brain tissue, as discussed in an earlier section. Thus, it is necessary to measure CBF and oxygen consumption together to detect cerebral hypo- or hyperperfusion. Because only a mismatch between blood flow and metabolic demand in either direction will represent hypo- or hyperperfusion, flow changes in the same direction

as the cerebral metabolic rate is a normal physiologic phenomenon.

Cerebrovascular autoregulation and carbon dioxide (CO_2) reactivity

Autoregulation and reactivity of vasculature to CO_2 are crucial regulatory mechanisms for maintenance of cerebral blood flow (as discussed in an earlier section). If these mechanisms are disrupted, there is a definite risk of secondary brain damage. Numerous studies have reported reduced or absent cerebral autoregulatory responses in TBI patients.[68,77–83] Lower cerebral perfusion pressure is more damaging in TBI patients because the reserve for vasodilatation is more severely affected.[71] Impaired cerebral autoregulation would result in a passive relationship between MAP and CBF, implying that a decrease in MAP would result in a decrease in CBF, making a subject susceptible to cerebral ischemia (not enough blood to the brain). Patients with functioning autoregulation but reduced intracranial compliance may also be at risk of cerebral ischemia. In such a situation, a decrease in MAP causes cerebral vasodilatation, an increase in CBV, and, consequently, an increase in ICP. An increase in ICP further decreases the CPP, leading to further cerebral vasodilation, causing a vicious cycle, the vasodilator cascade. Thus theoretically, empirically augmenting MAP in such a situation would result in cerebral hemorrhage[84,85] and can be potentially harmful. However, the relationship between cerebral autoregulation and clinical outcome after TBI can be complicated. Impaired autoregulation might be indicative of a severe form of TBI and thus a poor clinical outcome or impaired cerebral autoregulation might have a direct impact on the clinical outcome independent of the degree of severity of the TBI.

CO_2 reactivity emerges as a more robust physiologic mechanism than autoregulation, usually only seen in severe brain injury[77]; it remains essentially unaltered or even heightened in many TBI patients. In fact, for this reason, it has actually been used for intracranial pressure management in hyperemic (an increase in blood flow to tissues) patients.[86,87]

Cerebral vasospasm

The presence of cerebral vasospasm (a condition in which an arterial spasm leads to vasoconstriction) is considered to be a sign of a poor prognosis and severe brain damage.[88,89] The proposed mechanisms for this significant secondary damage include:

1. Vasoconstriction due to persistent depolarization of vascular smooth muscle, caused by altered potassium channel activity[90]
2. Vasodilator (like NO) to vasoconstrictor (like endothelin) imbalance[91]
3. Depletion of cGMP of vascular smooth muscle[92]
4. Accentuation of prostaglandin-induced vasoconstriction[93]
5. Excessive generation of free radicals[71,87]

Alteration in cerebral metabolism

Conventionally, the brain relies principally on aerobic metabolism for its energy requirements (as discussed in an earlier section on Cerebral blood flow and metabolic rate). Nevertheless, there is an emergence of current literature that supports the role of astrocytes and glia-mediated anaerobic metabolism in meeting the energy needs of the brain. Neurons and glial cells are functionally coupled so that anaerobic glycolysis in glial cells in TBI provides the energy to neurons. There is a modification in the available energy supply in TBI (decreased concentrations of phosphocreatine and ATP along with increased lactate/pyruvate ratio) and with changes in the cerebral metabolism (reduction in cerebral oxygen and glucose consumption).[69,94–96] Metabolic failure is principally a consequence of the mitochondrial dysfunction that is mediated by primary brain damage. Mitochondrial damage is associated with calcium overload, reduced nicotinic coenzyme levels, and reduced ATP production in TBI.[97–98] Interestingly, cerebral blood flow changes do not reflect the changes in cerebral metabolism in TBI patients. That is, the decrease in cerebral metabolism may not be associated with reduction in CBF. Accumulation of adenosine (due to excessive ATP breakdown) and its action (via A2a receptor) in TBI results in an increase in CBF, even though there is a decrease in cerebral metabolism.[94,99] Along similar lines, early post-traumatic hypermetabolism of glucose in TBI may not be linked to an increase in CBF. Immediate changes in TBI include massive ionic fluxes; glucose hypermetabolism emerges as a protective response in order to restore this ionic imbalance.[100] This flow-metabolism uncoupling

seen in TBI has been linked to further progression of secondary ischemic injuries.[101]

Cerebral oxygenation

Tissue hypoxia due to a mismatch between cerebral oxygen delivery and consumption is characteristic of TBI. Brain-tissue oxygen (ptiO2) <10–15 mmHg is a critical threshold for brain infarction.[102,103] While managing TBI patients, an important consideration is that even with normal CPP or ICP, secondary brain damage with oxygen deprivation may be observed.[104] Therefore, in addition to CPP and ICP, tissue oxygen levels should also be monitored in TBI.[80,82,105,106] The probable mechanisms responsible for tissue hypoxia in TBI are listed below (any one or all of them could be present in patients).

1. Reduction in CBF
2. Decreased oxygen uptake by lungs (due to either adult respiratory distress syndrome or severe lung injury)
3. Impaired oxygen delivery by hemoglobin (due to a decrease in hemoglobin content, eg, anemia or altered functionality of hemoglobin, eg, carbon monoxide poisoning)
4. Defective unloading of oxygen to the tissues (eg, hypothermia)

Edema

There are two types of edema observed in TBI—vasogenic and cytotoxic. Albeit, these two differ in their underlying pathophysiology and site of tissue fluid accumulation. Vasogenic edema occurs due to disruption of the blood–brain barrier, resulting in extravasation and accumulation of fluid and albumin in the interstitial space.[71,107] Disruption of the blood–brain barrier could either be due to a hypertensive response to TBI[59] or due to an increase in the endothelial cell permeability by release of inflammatory mediators, such as arachidonic acid.[108] While in cytotoxic edema, there is an increase in neuron and glial cell membrane permeability, ionic pump failure, and intracellular accumulation of fluid.[107,109] Hypoxia during TBI results in the failure of the Na^+/K^+ pump, which would ultimately lead to intracellular Na and water accumulation.[110,111] Another cause of cellular swelling is an increase in excitatory glutamate and glycine levels, which lead to the persistent opening of ion channels, which lead to Na^+ entry, depolarization, and secondary influx of Cl^- and water.[59] Although both of these edemas are related to ICP and secondary ischemic events, there is far more prevalence of cytotoxic than vasogenic edema in TBI.[112,113]

SPECIFIC PATHOPHYSIOLOGY OF SECONDARY STAGE OF TBI

Secondary injuries of TBI occur because of an intricate interaction between multiple interdependent intracellular and molecular mechanisms. The hallmark of this stage includes glutamate toxicity, excessive accumulation of intracellular calcium, high levels of lactate, and neuroinflammation.[114,115] These pathophysiologic mechanisms ultimately change the gene expression and end with a variety of cell responses, including inflammation, apoptosis, and cell death.

Excitotoxicity and oxidative stress

An essential pathophysiology of TBI includes the substantial accumulation of extracellular excitatory neurotransmitters, principally glutamate.[99,116] Over-activation of their receptors (especially N-Methyl-D-Aspartate (NMDA) receptors) cause massive Ca^{2+}, Na^+, and K^+ fluxes.[117,118] These events result in persistent membrane depolarization, calcium overload, and cellular toxicity. Additionally, this increase in intracellular calcium load enhances the activity of catabolic enzymes, which can cause the cell to self-destruct by either apoptosis or necrosis.

TBI is also characterized by an imbalance between generating reactive oxygen species and depleting an endogenous anti-oxidant system, which leads to

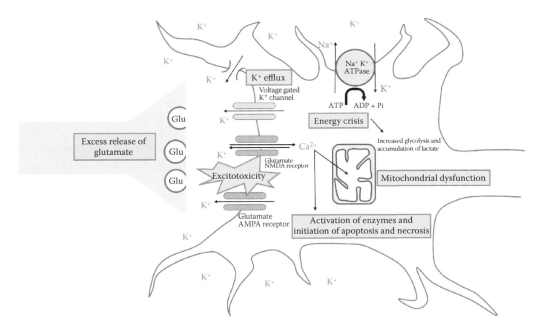

Figure 3.9 Depicts the neurometabolic cascade of pathological changes after traumatic brain injury. There is an excessive release of excitatory neurotransmitters especially glutamate, which acts through its receptors to result in membrane depolarization leading to opening of voltage gated K^+ channel, resulting in an increase in K^+ efflux, Ca^{2+}, and Na^+ influx and thus, an overall increase in K^+ extracellularly and Ca^{2+} intracellularly. There is increased activity of membrane ionic pumps to restore ionic homeostasis. This is followed by hyperglycolysis to meet the energy requirements of this enhanced pump function. Due to ischemic changes, the increase in ATP requirement is met principally by anaerobic metabolism, resulting in accumulation of lactate. Calcium overload in mitochondria results in mitochondrial dysfunction and a further energy crisis. Excess intracellular calcium also activates various enzymes responsible for apoptosis and necrosis. In addition to these pathological changes, inflammatory milieu observed in TBI also plays a very important role in its pathophysiology (this has not been shown in the above figure).

oxidative stress. The reactive oxygen species lead to a series of cellular-damaging events (irreversible modification of proteins, lipids, and/or DNA) originating from either cell death or apoptosis.[119] Free radicals frequently generated include superoxide, peroxynitrate, and the hydroperoxyl radical. Cerebral ischemia in TBI ends with acidosis due to a shift to anaerobic metabolism, which ultimately activates pH-dependent calcium channels.[120] This leads to increased intracellular calcium levels and induces an activation of phospholipases and the downstream arachidonic acid cascade, xanthine oxidase activity, mitochondrial leak, enzymatic or autoxidation of biogenic amine neurotransmitters, oxidation of hemoglobin, and NADPH oxidase activation. All of these events finally end with a tremendous increase in free radical production.[121,122]

Inflammation

Inflammation plays a major role in the complex array of pathology in TBI. A pro-inflammatory milieu with cytokines, prostaglandins, free radicals, and complement factors act as mediators to induce various chemokines and adhesion molecules and, subsequently, mobilize the immune and glial cells in a parallel and synergistic manner.[123,124] Neuroinflammation is a double-edged sword—at one end, it promotes repair of injured tissue while on the other hand, it promotes further destruction. There are stages of the inflammatory response following TBI. Initially, neutrophils and monocytes enter the brain parenchyma through the damaged blood–brain barrier. This is followed by the reactive phase, in which macrophages become activated and begin to phagocytose the cellular debris. During this phase, effector T-cells are increased while neuroprotective regulatory T-cell populations are low. Microglial cells and astrocytes undergo proliferation and secrete inflammatory mediators, such as cytokines and prostaglandins. This inflammatory milieu in the background of toxic concentrations of excitatory neurotransmitters results in massive neuronal damage. The last stage is the resolution phase, which is characterized by an increase in the production of anti-inflammatory mediators, such as TGF-β, IL-10, and IL-4. This results in an expansion of the regulatory T-cell population and a change in microglia phenotype to a neuroprotective (M2) state.[125]

Necrosis and apoptosis

There are two spectra of cell death after TBI, which include necrosis and apoptosis. Severe tissue damage with enormous accumulation of excitatory neurotransmitters, calcium overload, and ischemia leads to activation of enzymes like phospholipases, proteases, and lipid peroxidases, which culminates in necrosis.[126] However, apoptosis occurrence is delayed and cells undergoing apoptosis are initially morphologically intact. This process stops working due to an altered balance of pro- to anti-apoptotic proteins (as a result of altered gene expression) and requires energy.[126] Triggers of apoptosis include oxygen free radicals, death receptor ligation, DNA damage, protease activation, and ionic imbalance.[127,128]

SUMMARY AND CONCLUSION

TBI pathophysiology involves a neurometabolic cascade of biochemical and molecular changes with a unique temporal profile (Figure 3.9), which includes a mismatch between flow and metabolism, excitotoxicity, lactate accumulation, calcium overload, edema, inflammation, oxidative stress, and ultimately, apoptosis and necrosis. Extensive research into the investigation of this multidimensional vicious cycle continues, in an attempt to identify and manipulate pathophysiologic processes to help manage TBI effectively.

REFERENCES

1. Hawthorne C, Piper I. Monitoring of intracranial pressure in patients with traumatic brain injury. *Front Neurol.* 2014;5:121.
2. Wilson MH. Monro-Kellie 2.0: The dynamic vascular and venous pathophysiological components of intracranial pressure. *J Cereb Blood Flow Metab.* 2016;36(8):1338-1350.
3. Blomquist HK, Sundin S, Ekstedt J. Cerebrospinal fluid hydrodynamic studies in children. *J Neurol Neurosurg Psychiatry.* 1986;49(5):536-548.
4. Kandel ER, Schwartz JH, Jessell TM, Siegelbaum SA, Hudspeth AJ. *Principles of Neural Science.* 5th ed. New York: McGraw-Hill Education; 2012:1760.

5. Shapiro HM. Intracranial hypertension: Rherapeutic and anesthetic considerations. *Anesthesiology*. 1975;43(4):445-471.

6. Dunn LT. Raised intracranial pressure. *J Neurol Neurosurg Psychiatry*. 2002;73 (suppl 1):i23-i27.

7. Czosnyka M, Pickard JD. Monitoring and interpretation of intracranial pressure. *J Neurol Neurosurg Psychiatry*. 2004;75 (6):813-821.

8. Wiegand C, Richards P. Measurement of intracranial pressure in children: A critical review of current methods. *Dev Med Child Neurol*. 2007;49(12):935-941.

9. Lundberg N, Troupp H, Lorin H. Continuous recording of the ventricular-fluid pressure in patients with severe acute traumatic brain injury. A preliminary report. *J Neurosurg*. 1965;22(6):581-590.

10. Shapiro K, Marmarou A, Shulman K. Characterization of clinical CSF dynamics and neural axis compliance using the pressure-volume index: I. The normal pressure-volume index. *Ann Neurol*. 1980;7(6):508-514.

11. Avezaat CJ, van Eijndhoven JH, Wyper DJ. Cerebrospinal fluid pulse pressure and intracranial volume-pressure relationships. *J Neurol Neurosurg Psychiatry*. 1979; 42(8):687-700.

12. Vavilala MS, Lee LA, Lam AM. Cerebral blood flow and vascular physiology. *Anesthesiol Clin North America*. 2002;20(2):247-264, v.

13. Kennedy C, Sokoloff L. An adaptation of the nitrous oxide method to the study of the cerebral circulation in children; normal values for cerebral blood flow and cerebral metabolic rate in childhood. *J Clin Invest*. 1957;36(7):1130-1137.

14. Biagi L, Abbruzzese A, Bianchi MC, Alsop DC, Del Guerra A, Tosetti M. Age dependence of cerebral perfusion assessed by magnetic resonance continuous arterial spin labeling. *J Magn Reson Imaging*. 2007; 25(4):696-702.

15. Madsen PL, Schmidt JF, Wildschiødtz G et al. Cerebral O2 metabolism and cerebral blood flow in humans during deep and rapid-eye-movement sleep. *J Appl Physiol*. 1991;70(6):2597-2601.

16. Lam AM, Matta BF, Mayberg TS, Strebel S. Change in cerebral blood flow velocity with onset of EEG silence during inhalation anesthesia in humans: Evidence of flow-metabolism coupling? *J Cereb Blood Flow Metab*. 1995;15(4):714-717.

17. Karsli C, Luginbuehl I, Farrar M, Bissonnette B. Cerebrovascular carbon dioxide reactivity in children anaesthetized with propofol. *Paediatr Anaesth*. 2003;13(1):26-31.

18. Kontos HA, Raper AJ, Patterson JL. Analysis of vasoactivity of local pH, PCO2 and bicarbonate on pial vessels. *Stroke*. 1977;8 (3):358-360.

19. Schmetterer L, Findl O, Strenn K et al. Role of NO in the O2 and CO2 responsiveness of cerebral and ocular circulation in humans. *Am J Physiol*. 1997;273(6 pt 2):R2005-R2012.

20. Wagerle LC, Degiulio PA. Indomethacin-sensitive CO2 reactivity of cerebral arterioles is restored by vasodilator prostaglandin. *Am J Physiol*. 1994;266(4 pt 2):H1332-H1338.

21. Morii S, Ngai AC, Ko KR, Winn HR. Role of adenosine in regulation of cerebral blood flow: Effects of theophylline during normoxia and hypoxia. *Am J Physiol*. 1987;253 (1 pt 2):H165-75.

22. Hudetz AG, Shen H, Kampine JP. Nitric oxide from neuronal NOS plays critical role in cerebral capillary flow response to hypoxia. *Am J Physiol*. 1998;274(3 pt 2): H982-H989.

23. Berger C, von Kummer R. Does NO regulate the cerebral blood flow response in hypoxia? *Acta Neurol Scand*. 1998;97(2): 118-125.

24. Paulson OB, Waldemar OB, Schmidt JF, Strandgaard S. Cerebral circulation under normal and pathologic conditions. *Am J Cardiol*. 1989;63(6):2C-5C.

25. Lassen NA. Cerebral blood flow and oxygen consumption in man. *Physiol Rev*. 1959;39 (2):183-238.

26. Paulson OB, Strandgaard S, Edvinsson L. Cerebral autoregulation. *Cerebrovasc Brain Metab Rev*. 1990;2(2):161-192.

27. Van Mook WNKA, Rennenberg RJMW, Schurink GW et al. Cerebral hyperperfusion syndrome. *Lancet Neurol.* 2005;4(12):877-888.

28. Strandgaard S, Paulson OB. Cerebral autoregulation. *Stroke.* 1984;15(3):413-416.

29. Häggendal E, Johansson B. Effects of arterial carbon dioxide tension and oxygen saturation on cerebral blood flow autoregulation in dogs. *Acta Physiol Scand Suppl.* 1965;258:27-53.

30. Sadoshima S, Thames M, Heistad D. Cerebral blood flow during elevation of intracranial pressure: Role of sympathetic nerves. *Am J Physiol.* 1981;241(1):H78-H84.

31. Kontos HA, Wei EP, Navari RM, Levasseur JE, Rosenblum WI, Patterson JL. Responses of cerebral arteries and arterioles to acute hypotension and hypertension. *Am J Physiol.* 1978;234(4):H371-H383.

32. Symon L, Held K, Dorsch NWC. A study of regional autoregulation in the cerebral circulation to increased perfusion pressure in normocapnia and hypercapnia. *Stroke.* 1973; 4(2):139-147.

33. Harder DR, Kauser K, Roman RJ, Lombard JH. Mechanisms of pressure-induced myogenic activation of cerebral and renal arteries: Role of the endothelium. *J Hypertens Suppl.* 1989;7(4):S11-S15; discussion S16.

34. Osol G, Halpern W. Myogenic properties of cerebral blood vessels from normotensive and hypertensive rats. *Am J Physiol.* 1985;249(5 pt 2):H914-H921.

35. Hill MA, Davis MJ, Meininger GA, Potocnik SJ, Murphy TV. Arteriolar myogenic signalling mechanisms: Implications for local vascular function. *Clin Hemorheol Microcirc.* 2006;34(1-2):67-79.

36. Jackson WF. Ion channels and vascular tone. *Hypertension.* 2000;35(1 pt 2):173-178.

37. Kuschinsky W, Wahl M. Local chemical and neurogenic regulation of cerebral vascular resistance. *Physiol Rev.* 1978;58(3):656-689.

38. Wahl M, Kuschinsky W. The dilatory action of adenosine on pial arteries of cats and its inhibition by theophylline. *Pflugers Arch.* 1976;362(1):55-59.

39. Winn HR, Welsh JE, Rubio R, Berne RM. Brain adenosine production in rat during sustained alteration in systemic blood pressure. *Am J Physiol.* 1980;239(5):H636-H641.

40. Phillis JW. Adenosine in the control of the cerebral circulation. *Cerebrovasc Brain Metab Rev.* 1989;1(1):26-54.

41. Phillis JW, DeLong RE. The role of adenosine in cerebral vascular regulation during reductions in perfusion pressure. *J Pharm Pharmacol.* 1986;38(6):460-462.

42. Faraci FM, Sobey CG. Role of potassium channels in regulation of cerebral vascular tone. *J Cereb Blood Flow Metab.* 1998;18 (10):1047-1063.

43. Edvinsson L. Neurogenic mechanisms in the cerebrovascular bed. Autonomic nerves, amine receptors and their effects on cerebral blood flow. *Acta Physiol Scand Suppl.* 1975;427:1-35.

44. Zervas NT, Lavyne MH, Negoro M. Neurotransmitters and the normal and ischemic cerebral circulation. *N Engl J Med.* 1975;293(16):812-816.

45. Edvinsson L, Nielsen KC, Owman C, West KA. Evidence of vasoconstrictor sympathetic nerves in brain vessels of mice. *Neurology.* 1973;23(1):73-77.

46. Edvinsson L, Owman C, West KA. Changes in continuously recorded intracranial pressure of conscious rabbits at different time-periods after superior cervical sympathectomy. *Acta Physiol Scand.* 1971;83(1):42-50.

47. Lindvall M, Edvinsson L, Owman C. Sympathetic nervous control of cerebrospinal fluid production from the choroid plexus. *Science.* 1978;201(4351):176-178.

48. Mueller SM, Heistad DD, Marcus ML. Effect of sympathetic nerves on cerebral vessels during seizures. *Am J Physiol.* 1979;237(2): H178-H184.

49. D'Alecy LG, Rose CJ, Sellers SA. Sympathetic modulation of hypercapnic cerebral vasodilation in dogs. *Circ Res.* 1979;45 (6):771-785.

50. Edvinsson L, Owman C, Siesjö B. Physiological role of cerebrovascular sympathetic nerves in the autoregulation of cerebral blood flow. *Brain Res.* 1976;117(3):519-523.

51. Busse R, Trogisch G, Bassenge E. The role of endothelium in the control of vascular tone. *Basic Res Cardiol.* 1985;80(5):475-490.

52. Holtz J, Förstermann U, Pohl U, Giesler M, Bassenge E. Flow-dependent, endothelium-mediated dilation of epicardial coronary arteries in conscious dogs: Effects of cyclooxygenase inhibition. *J Cardiovasc Pharmacol.* 1984;6(6):1161-1169.

53. del Zoppo GJ, Mabuchi T. Cerebral microvessel responses to focal ischemia. *J Cereb Blood Flow Metab.* 2003;23(8):879-894.

54. Simard M, Arcuino G, Takano T, Liu QS, Nedergaard M. Signaling at the gliovascular interface. *J Neurosci.* 2003;23(27):9254-9262.

55. Nedergaard M, Ransom B, Goldman SA. New roles for astrocytes: Redefining the functional architecture of the brain. *Trends Neurosci.* 2003;26(10):523-530.

56. Martin GT. Acute brain trauma. *Ann R Coll Surg Engl.* 2016;98(1):6-10.

57. McAllister TW. Neurobiological consequences of traumatic brain injury. *Dialogues Clin Neurosci.* 2011;13(3):287-300.

58. Ommaya AK, Gennarelli TA. Cerebral concussion and traumatic unconsciousness. Correlation of experimental and clinical observations of blunt head injuries. *Brain.* 1974;97(4):633-654.

59. Gaetz M. The neurophysiology of brain injury. *Clin Neurophysiol.* 2004;115(1):4-18.

60. Marshall LF. Head injury: Recent past, present, and future. *Neurosurgery.* 2000;47(3):546-561.

61. McIntosh TK, Smith DH, Meaney DF, Kotapka MJ, Gennarelli TA, Graham DI. Neuropathological sequelae of traumatic brain injury: Relationship to neurochemical and biomechanical mechanisms. *Lab Invest.* 1996;74(2):315-342.

62. Nortje J, Menon DK. Traumatic brain injury: Physiology, mechanisms, and outcome. *Curr Opin Neurol.* 2004;17(6):711-718.

63. Xiong Y, Mahmood A, Chopp M. Animal models of traumatic brain injury. *Nat Rev Neurosci.* 2013;14(2):128-142.

64. Bondi CO, Semple BD, Noble-Haeusslein LJ et al. Found in translation: Understanding the biology and behavior of experimental traumatic brain injury. *Neurosci Biobehav Rev.* 2015;58:123-146.

65. Bouma GJ, Muizelaar JP, Stringer WA, Choi SC, Fatouros P, Young HF. Ultra-early evaluation of regional cerebral blood flow in severely head-injured patients using xenon-enhanced computerized tomography. *J Neurosurg.* 1992;77(3):360-368.

66. Coles JP, Fryer TD, Smielewski P et al. Defining ischemic burden after traumatic brain injury using 15O PET imaging of cerebral physiology. *J Cereb Blood Flow Metab.* 2004;24(2):191-201.

67. Inoue Y, Shiozaki T, Tasaki O et al. Changes in cerebral blood flow from the acute to the chronic phase of severe head injury. *J Neurotrauma.* 2005;22(12):1411-1418.

68. Lam JM, Hsiang JN, Poon WS. Monitoring of autoregulation using laser Doppler flowmetry in patients with head injury. *J Neurosurg.* 1997;86(3):438-445.

69. Cunningham AS, Salvador R, Coles JP et al. Physiological thresholds for irreversible tissue damage in contusional regions following traumatic brain injury. *Brain.* 2005;128(pt 8):1931-1942.

70. Rodríguez-Baeza A, Reina-de la Torre F, Poca A, Martí M, Garnacho A. Morphological features in human cortical brain microvessels after head injury: A three-dimensional and immunocytochemical study. *Anat Rec A Discov Mol Cell Evol Biol.* 2003;273(1):583-593.

71. DeWitt DS, Prough DS. Traumatic cerebral vascular injury: The effects of concussive brain injury on the cerebral vasculature. *J Neurotrauma.* 2003;20(9):795-825.

72. Kelly DF, Kordestani RK, Martin NA et al. Hyperemia following traumatic brain injury: Relationship to intracranial hypertension and outcome. *J Neurosurg.* 1996;85(5):762-771.

73. Langfitt TW, Weinstein JD, Kassell NF. Cerebral vasomotor paralysis produced by intracranial hypertension. *Neurology.* 1965;15:622-641.

74. Martin NA, Patwardhan RV, Alexander MJ et al. Characterization of cerebral hemodynamic phases following severe head trauma:

Hypoperfusion, hyperemia, and vasospasm. *J Neurosurg.* 1997;87(1):9-19.

75. Sakas DE, Bullock MR, Patterson J, Hadley D, Wyper DJ, Teasdale GM. Focal cerebral hyperemia after focal head injury in humans: A benign phenomenon? *J Neurosurg.* 1995;83(2):277-284.

76. Kelly DF, Martin NA, Kordestani R et al. Cerebral blood flow as a predictor of outcome following traumatic brain injury. *J Neurosurg.* 1997;86(4):633-641.

77. Enevoldsen EM, Jensen FT. Autoregulation and CO2 responses of cerebral blood flow in patients with acute severe head injury. *J Neurosurg.* 1978;48(5):689-703.

78. Hauerberg J, Xiaodong M, Willumsen L, Pedersen DB, Juhler M. The upper limit of cerebral blood flow autoregulation in acute intracranial hypertension. *J Neurosurg Anesthesiol.* 1998;10(2):106-112.

79. Hlatky R, Furuya Y, Valadka AB et al. Dynamic autoregulatory response after severe head injury. *J Neurosurg.* 2002;97 (5):1054-1061.

80. Jaeger M, Schuhmann MU, Soehle M, Meixensberger J. Continuous assessment of cerebrovascular autoregulation after traumatic brain injury using brain tissue oxygen pressure reactivity. *Crit Care Med.* 2006;34(6):1783-1788.

81. Jünger EC, Newell DW, Grant GA et al. Cerebral autoregulation following minor head injury. *J Neurosurg.* 1997;86(3):425-432.

82. Lang EW, Czosnyka M, Mehdorn HM. Tissue oxygen reactivity and cerebral autoregulation after severe traumatic brain injury. *Crit Care Med.* 2003;31(1):267-271.

83. Schmidt EA, Czosnyka M, Steiner LA et al. Asymmetry of pressure autoregulation after traumatic brain injury. *J Neurosurg.* 2003;99 (6):991-998.

84. Mandera M, Larysz D, Wojtacha M. Changes in cerebral hemodynamics assessed by transcranial Doppler ultrasonography in children after head injury. *Childs Nerv Syst.* 2002;18(3-4):124-128.

85. Bruce DA, Alavi A, Bilaniuk L, Dolinskas C, Obrist W, Uzzell B. Diffuse cerebral swelling following head injuries in children: The syndrome of "malignant brain edema." *J Neurosurg.* 1981;54(2):170-178.

86. Lee JH, Kelly DF, Oertel M et al. Carbon dioxide reactivity, pressure autoregulation, and metabolic suppression reactivity after head injury: A transcranial Doppler study. *J Neurosurg.* 2001;95(2):222-232.

87. McLaughlin MR, Marion DW. Cerebral blood flow and vasoresponsivity within and around cerebral contusions. *J Neurosurg.* 1996;85(5):871-876.

88. Lee JH, Martin NA, Alsina G et al. Hemo-dynamically significant cerebral vasospasm and outcome after head injury: A prospective study. *J Neurosurg.* 1997;87(2):221-233.

89. Oertel M, Boscardin WJ, Obrist WD et al. Posttraumatic vasospasm: The epidemiol-ogy, severity, and time course of an under-estimated phenomenon: A prospective study performed in 299 patients. *J Neurosurg.* 2005;103(5):812-824.

90. Sobey CG. Cerebrovascular dysfunction after subarachnoid haemorrhage: Novel mecha-nisms and directions for therapy. *Clin Exp Pharmacol Physiol.* 2001;28(11):926-929.

91. Zuccarello M, Boccaletti R, Romano A, Rapoport RM. Endothelin B receptor antag-onists attenuate subarachnoid hemorrhage-induced cerebral vasospasm. *Stroke.* 1998; 29(9):1924-1929.

92. Todo H, Ohta S, Wang J et al. Impairment in biochemical level of arterial dilative capa-bility of a cyclic nucleotides-dependent pathway by induced vasospasm in the canine basilar artery. *J Cereb Blood Flow Metab.* 1998;18(7):808-817.

93. Armstead WM. Differential activation of ERK, p38, and JNK MAPK by nociceptin/ orphanin FQ in the potentiation of prosta-glandin cerebrovasoconstriction after brain injury. *Eur J Pharmacol.* 2006;529(1-3):129-135.

94. Clark RS, Carcillo JA, Kochanek PM et al. Cerebrospinal fluid adenosine concentra-tion and uncoupling of cerebral blood flow and oxidative metabolism after severe head injury in humans. *Neurosurgery.* 1997;41 (6):1284-1292.

95. Diringer MN, Yundt K, Videen TO et al. No reduction in cerebral metabolism as a

result of early moderate hyperventilation following severe traumatic brain injury. *J Neurosurg.* 2000;92(1):7-13.

96. Glenn TC, Kelly DF, Boscardin WJ et al. Energy dysfunction as a predictor of outcome after moderate or severe head injury: Indices of oxygen, glucose, and lactate metabolism. *J Cereb Blood Flow Metab.* 2003;23(10):1239-1250.

97. Tavazzi B, Signoretti S, Lazzarino G et al. Cerebral oxidative stress and depression of energy metabolism correlate with severity of diffuse brain injury in rats. *Neurosurgery.* 2005;56(3):582-589.

98. Verweij BH, Muizelaar JP, Vinas FC, Peterson PL, Xiong Y, Lee CP. Impaired cerebral mitochondrial function after traumatic brain injury in humans. *J Neurosurg.* 2000;93(5):815-820.

99. Robertson CL, Bell MJ, Kochanek PM et al. Increased adenosine in cerebrospinal fluid after severe traumatic brain injury in infants and children: Association with severity of injury and excitotoxicity. *Crit Care Med.* 2001;29(12):2287-93.

100. Bergsneider M, Hovda DA, Shalmon E et al. Cerebral hyperglycolysis following severe traumatic brain injury in humans: A positron emission tomography study. *J Neurosurg.* 1997;86(2):241-251.

101. Chen SF, Richards HK, Smielewski P et al. Relationship between flow-metabolism uncoupling and evolving axonal injury after experimental traumatic brain injury. *J Cereb Blood Flow Metab.* 2004;24 (9):1025-1036.

102. Johnston AJ, Steiner LA, Coles JP et al. Effect of cerebral perfusion pressure augmentation on regional oxygenation and metabolism after head injury. *Crit Care Med.* 2005;33(1):189-195; discussion 255-257.

103. Rose JC, Neill TA, Hemphill JC. Continuous monitoring of the microcirculation in neurocritical care: An update on brain tissue oxygenation. *Curr Opin Crit Care.* 2006;12 (2):97-102.

104. Stiefel MF, Udoetuk JD, Spiotta AM et al. Conventional neurocritical care and cerebral oxygenation after traumatic brain injury. *J Neurosurg.* 2006;105(4):568-575.

105. Menzel M, Doppenberg EM, Zauner A et al. Cerebral oxygenation in patients after severe head injury: Monitoring and effects of arterial hyperoxia on cerebral blood flow, metabolism and intracranial pressure. *J Neurosurg Anesthesiol.* 1999;11(4):240-251.

106. Stiefel MF, Spiotta A, Gracias VH et al. Reduced mortality rate in patients with severe traumatic brain injury treated with brain tissue oxygen monitoring. *J Neurosurg.* 2005;103(5):805-811.

107. Unterberg AW, Stover J, Kress B, Kiening KL. Edema and brain trauma. *Neuroscience.* 2004;129(4):1021-1029.

108. Wahl M, Schilling L. Regulation of cerebral blood flow—A brief review. *Acta Neurochir Suppl.* (Wien). 1993;59:3-10.

109. Stiefel MF, Tomita Y, Marmarou A. Secondary ischemia impairing the restoration of ion homeostasis following traumatic brain injury. *J Neurosurg.* 2005;103(4):707-714.

110. Fishman RA. Brain edema. *N Engl J Med.* 1975;293(14):706-711.

111. Bullock R, Maxwell WL, Graham DI, Teasdale GM, Adams JH. Glial swelling following human cerebral contusion: An ultrastructural study. *J Neurol Neurosurg Psychiatry.* 1991;54(5):427-434.

112. Marmarou A, Fatouros PP, Barzó P et al. Contribution of edema and cerebral blood volume to traumatic brain swelling in head-injured patients. *J Neurosurg.* 2000;93 (2):183-193.

113. Marmarou A, Signoretti S, Fatouros PP, Portella G, Aygok GA, Bullock MR. Predominance of cellular edema in traumatic brain swelling in patients with severe head injuries. *J Neurosurg.* 2006;104(5):720-730.

114. Von Gertten C, Flores Morales A, Holmin S, Mathiesen T, Nordqvist AC. Genomic responses in rat cerebral cortex after traumatic brain injury. *BMC Neurosci.* 2005;6:69.

115. Lenzlinger PM, Morganti-Kossmann MC, Laurer HL, McIntosh TK. The duality of the inflammatory response to traumatic brain injury. *Mol Neurobiol.* 2001;24(1-3):169-181.

116. Bullock R, Zauner A, Woodward JJ et al. Factors affecting excitatory amino acid release following severe human head injury. *J Neurosurg.* 1998;89(4):507-518.

117. Floyd CL, Gorin FA, Lyeth BG. Mechanical strain injury increases intracellular sodium and reverses Na+/Ca2+ exchange in cortical astrocytes. *Glia.* 2005;51(1):35-46.

118. Yi J-H, Hazell AS. Excitotoxic mechanisms and the role of astrocytic glutamate transporters in traumatic brain injury. *Neurochem Int.* 2006;48(5):394-403.

119. Chong ZZ, Li F, Maiese K. Oxidative stress in the brain: Novel cellular targets that govern survival during neurodegenerative disease. *Prog Neurobiol.* 2005;75(3):207-246.

120. Xiong ZG, Zhu XM, Chu XP et al. Neuroprotection in ischemia: Blocking calcium-permeable acid-sensing ion channels. *Cell.* 2004;118(6):687-698.

121. Kontos HA, Wei EP. Superoxide production in experimental brain injury. *J Neurosurg.* 1986;64(5):803-807.

122. Sastre J, Pallardó FV, Viña J. The role of mitochondrial oxidative stress in aging. *Free Radic Biol Med.* 2003;35(1):1-8.

123. Lucas SM, Rothwell NJ, Gibson RM. The role of inflammation in CNS injury and disease. *Br J Pharmacol.* 2006;147(suppl 1): S232-S240.

124. Potts MB, Koh SE, Whetstone WD et al. Traumatic injury to the immature brain: Inflammation, oxidative injury, and iron-mediated damage as potential therapeutic targets. *NeuroRx.* J 2006;3(2):143-153.

125. Kelso ML, Gendelman HE. Bridge between neuroimmunity and traumatic brain injury. *Curr Pharm Des.* 2014;20 (26):4284-4298.

126. Werner C, Engelhard K. Pathophysiology of traumatic brain injury. *Br J Anaesth.* 2007;99(1):4-9.

127. Quillinan N, Herson PS, Traystman RJ. Neuropathophysiology of brain injury. *Anesthesiol Clin.* 2016;34(3):453-464.

128. Giza CC, Hovda DA. The new neurometabolic cascade of concussion. *Neurosurgery.* 2014;75(suppl 4):S24-S33.

PART IV

Preanesthetic evaluation

Prehospital care

MARIA J. COLOMINA, MAYLIN KOO, AND JOSÉ MARÍA SOTO-EJARQUE

INTRODUCTION

Traumatic brain injury (TBI), which particularly affects the young population, is an important cause of morbidity and mortality (injury and death) worldwide and is a public health issue with increased socioeconomic consequences. Unfortunately, the additional knowledge of the medical community in the field of pathophysiology of TBI has not led to substantial developments in therapeutic options for TBI patients, and currently, the medical community lacks effective neuroprotectors to treat the often-severe lesions that occur.[1,2]

Initial resuscitation of TBI, focused on prompt, specific management, has resulted in a significant decrease in mortality from 50% to less than 25% over the last few decades. The treatment that is provided in the acute phase has an impact on preventing secondary brain injury, morbidity, and mortality in these patients. This initial treatment includes prehospital care, which begins with processes of evaluation, stabilization, and other therapeutic interventions that continue up to the time that the actual in-hospital treatment is administered, based on protocols whose main objective is maintaining adequate cerebral perfusion pressure at all times.[3]

The general priorities in prehospital care, which were proposed by the Brain Trauma Foundation,[4] focus on preventing the common insults (events or occurrences that cause damage to a tissue or organ) that occur after TBI: hypoxemia and hypotension. Several studies have reported a link between hypoxemia (low oxygen in the blood) and a poor clinical outcome; the number and duration of hypotension episodes has shown a correlation with mortality. Even a single episode of hypotension is related to greater morbidity and a twofold increase in mortality.[2,4]

In this chapter, we will examine the most relevant pathophysiologic factors (the functional changes that accompany a specific syndrome or disease) to consider in the prehospital management of patients who have experienced severe TBI and the various treatment options available in the initial resuscitation phase.

ON-SITE TREATMENT: UNDERSTANDING THE ETIOPATHOGENESIS OF TBI

Gathered evidence has shown that a vital and functional outcome following TBI depends on the severity of the initial biomechanical impact (primary injury) as well as the presence and severity of the systemic and intracranial insults that appear minutes, hours, or days following the traumatic event. These subsequent insults can magnify or produce new brain lesions, which are commonly known as secondary brain injury.

Experimental and clinical data have supported the susceptibility of the post-trauma brain in several situations, with the common denominator being a decrease in cerebral oxygen transport (movement of oxygen through the brain) and an increase in metabolic needs. Hypoxemia, arterial hypotension, and intracranial hypertension (increased pressure within the skull due to trauma, tumor, or disease) are the most extensively investigated secondary events that can negatively affect a prognosis by producing ischemic injury, which can cause a blood deficiency to a body part (as in the heart or brain) due to obstruction of the inflow of arterial blood, in regions that have reduced blood flow.[5] An increase in intracranial pressure (ICP) or a decrease in the cerebral perfusion pressure (CPP) can lead to overall or localized brain ischemia, whereas severe systemic hypertension (excess pressure that affects the body) can cause edema in the injured brain tissue. Hypercapnia results in an ICP increase due to increased cranial blood flow (CBF) and blood volume in the brain. On the other hand, severe hypocapnia can decrease the cerebral blood and oxygen supply.[3,4]

INITIAL MANAGEMENT: MAIN POINTS TO CONSIDER

Initial treatment of severe TBI begins at the site of the injury and includes maintenance of blood pressure (BP), oxygenation, and ventilation,[6–8] all avoidable risk factors independently related to an unfavorable prognosis. The CPP should be maintained at 50 to 70 mmHg and all prehospital treatments should be administered as quickly as possible.[9]

The main physiologic (normal function) parameters to determine in the initial evaluation are the Glasgow Coma Scale (GCS) score, systolic BP, and respiratory rate, which are outcome predictors used in the prehospital triage (the process of sorting people based on their need for immediate medical treatment compared with their chance of benefiting from such care). The GCS is a fast, universally accepted, reproducible scoring system used to define

TBI severity (GCS ≤8 indicates severe TBI), which includes evaluation of eye opening, verbal response, and motor response. Prompt GCS assessment in a nonsedated patient is a proven predictor of outcome. The lowest total score (GSC=3) indicates a potentially severe lesion, particularly when ocular and vestibulo-ocular (a normal reflex in which eye position compensates for movement of the head) responses are lacking. Initially higher scores (GSC ≥13) tend to predict a better prognosis.[10] Information from the National Trauma Data Bank (NTDB) shows that after adjusting for age, sex, race, Injury Severity Score (ISS), and time in the hospital, TBI patients who have higher GCS scores have a higher probability of survival.[11] Another, less widely used assessment system is the prehospital simplified motor score (SMS).[12] In a retrospective review of 52,412 patients, the sensitivity, specificity, and area under the curve (AUC) of the SMS were similar to that of the GCS. The sensitivity for mortality was 72.2% for the SMS and 74.6% for the GCS, and the sensitivity for TBI was 40.8% and 45.4%, respectively.[11,13]

Airway management: Ventilation and hypoxemia

One important consideration in TBI is maintaining a patent airway without obstructions, as hypoxemia is a major predictive factor of an unfavorable prognosis and requires urgent attention. The protocols established for this purpose should be clear and defined according to the training, skills, and qualifications of the professionals on medical teams that are providing trauma care.[4,14–18] The priority in all such protocols is securing a patent airway (an airway that is open and clear) to provide adequate oxygenation and avoid secondary brain injury.[3,15,18–23]

The necessity for prehospital endotracheal intubation (a medical procedure in which a tube is placed into the windpipe [trachea] through the mouth or nose) in TBI is a subject of debate, and reported findings in the related studies vary considerably (Table 4.1). The effect of this measure on the patient's outcome is multifactorial and influenced by the type and severity of the patient's condition, the experience of the attending medical professional, and the use of sedatives and muscle relaxants. In general, these studies indicate that badly not indicated or poorly executed prehospital endotracheal intubation may be worse than basic

Table 4.1 Review of prehospital intubation studies in severe TBI patients

Authors	Definition criteria	Patient number	Overall mortality	Outcome
Winchell and Hoyt 1997[24]	Head AIS ≥4 and GCS ≤8	671 TBIs, with 351 isolated TBIs	57%	Field intubation reduced mortality from 57% to 36% in patients with severe TBI and from 50% to 23% in isolated TBI
Murray et al. 2000[21]	Severe TBI (field GCS <8 and head AIS >3)	894 TBIs, with 570 isolated TBIs	47.2%	PHI failed to demonstrate survival benefits in patients with severe TBI
Bochicchio et al. 2003[25]	Severe TBI (GCS score ≤8 and head AIS score ≥3) Patients who died within 48 hours of admission were excluded	191 TBIs, with 68 isolated TBIs	16.8%	PHI associated with significantly higher mortality (23% vs. 12.4%, P=0.05). Also, mortality risk was 1.85 times higher in the PHI group compared with ED-intubated patients
Wang et al. 2004[26]	Severe TBI (head/neck AIS ≥3)	4098	37%	PHI associated with increased risk of mortality (OR 3.99; 95%CI 3.21–4.93) and poor neurologic outcome (OR 1.61; 95% CI 1.15–2.26)
Davis et al. 2005[27]	Moderate to severe TBI (head/neck AIS score of ≥3)	13,625	22.9%	PHI associated with higher mortality (55% vs. 15%) compared with non-intubated patients with moderate to severe TBI
Warner et al. 2007[28]	Severe TBI (head AIS score >3), isolated TBI (head AIS score >3 but no other AIS score >2)	187 TBIs, with 95 isolated TBIs	24.4%	Targeted PHI associated with lower mortality after severe TBI
Vandromme et al. 2011[29]	Severe TBI (prehospital GCS ≤8)	149	46.9%	PHI associated with severe TBI, but no increased risk of mortality over ED intubation
Tuma et al. 2014[30]	Field GCS ≤8 and head AIS ≥3 Patients who died within first 24 hours were excluded	160 severe isolated TBIs	46%	No added benefit in PHI group. Field GCS motor score (OR 0.55; 95%CI 0.41–0.73) significantly associated with mortality
Denninghoff et al. 2017[31]	ProTECT III study Moderate to severe TBI (GSC 4–12)	882	17%	Mortality also lower in PHI group (13.8% vs. 19.5%, P=0.03)

Abbreviations: AIS: Abbreviated Injury Scale; ED: emergency department; GCS: Glasgow Coma Scale score; PHI: prehospital intubation; TBI: traumatic brain injury.

Table 4.2 Airway management in traumatic brain injury patients

Proposal		Device	Objective	Considerations
STEP 1	Oxygenation and ventilation with cervical spine stabilization	• Face mask • Self-inflating bag with O_2 reservoir • Oro-nasopharyngeal cannula and aspirator	Avoid hypoxia SpO_2 <90%[34]	Important to detect tension pneumothorax, which requires immediate drainage before starting an invasive airway procedure
STEP 2	Ventilation with either supraglottic or infraglottic devices	Supraglottic devices (laryngeal tube, King, combitube, laryngeal mask) in patients without reflexes	Avoid hypoxia SpO_2 <90%	
STEP 3	Tracheal intubation with intravenous drug support	Orotracheal tube, laryngeal mask fast rack, video-laryngoscopy [23,32,33]	Difficult intubation assessment (LEMON and 3-3-2 rule)[18] -Rapid sequence induction (RSI) and checklist [17,35] -Ventilation control (pulse oximetry SpO_2, capnography $EtCO_2$)	Protocol 3:2:1 (stable patient) Fentanyl: 3 µg/kg Ketamine: 2 mg/kg Rocuronium: 1 mg/kg Protocol 1:1:1 (unstable patient) Fentanyl: 1 µg/kg Ketamine: 1 mg/kg Rocuronium: 1 mg/kg
STEP 4	Surgical access (cricothyroidectomy)	Intubation not possible and no ventilation (maximum severity)	Avoid hypoxia SpO_2 <90% Avert death	

airway care and the patient's own oxygenation and ventilation capability.[19,22,32,34]

Patients with severe TBI should be intubated by specialized personnel using rapid sequence induction (RSI) (Table 4.2) and systems for cervical spine protection. Using the RSI technique with appropriate anesthetic agents is necessary to prevent bronchoaspiration and side effects related to sympathetic stimulation (this causes the trachea muscle to relax) following airway manipulation. Hypotension should also be avoided. The steps that should be followed for airway and oxygenation management and the appropriate pharmacologic agents to use are described in Table 4.2.

The role of lidocaine in RSI is controversial. Nonetheless, one recent retrospective study performed in a cohort of 101 patients has shown that lidocaine can be used without producing adverse hemodynamic changes.[36]

Ventilation management: Hypercapnia and hypocapnia

Patients that have been intubated should be properly ventilated to maintain normocapnia (a normal level of carbon dioxide pressure) [$PaCO_2$ 35–40 mmHg]. Hyperventilation commonly occurs in patients with severe TBI because an increase in alveolar ventilation decreases the $PaCO_2$ and induces a cerebrospinal fluid pH increase, which, in turn, produces cerebral vasoconstriction and a reduction in the brain blood content and CBF.

However, the decreased CBF due to vasoconstriction (constriction of the vessels) and its ischemic effects have led some medical professionals to question this therapy because of the side effects that can occur.[34]

As a guide to therapy, the gathered scientific evidence recommends avoiding prophylactic hyperventilation ($PaCO_2$=35 mmHg) in the first 24 hours following trauma because it can compromise cerebral perfusion pressure, which can drop to less than half of the value seen in healthy individuals. When hyperventilation is induced, brain oxygenation must be monitored in a hospital environment to detect whether brain ischemia develops. However, in cases of possible cerebral herniation (a potentially deadly side effect of very high pressure within the skull that occurs when a part of the brain is squeezed across structures within the skull), temporary hyperventilation could be a useful option in the prehospital setting.[14,16,34,37]

Hypotension and hypertension

Hypotension contributes substantially to the development of secondary brain injury[4,7,9,31,38–41] and should be treated with resuscitation fluids, and, if needed, vasopressor agents to maintain optimal systolic BP. Nonetheless, it is difficult to define the value indicating hypotension in this population. In one study, which was conducted in 15,733 patients with moderate or severe TBI, a systolic BP value of ≤110 mmHg was determined to be the most fitting model for defining hypotension when mortality was taken as the outcome measure.[38] Another study found that maintaining a systolic BP of approximately 120 mmHg is effective for minimizing secondary brain injury. Although additional, large clinical trials are needed to support the findings from these studies, it is recommended that BP control should be achieved as soon as possible in patients with severe TBI.[13]

Hypertension can be a physiologic response to sympathetic activation (an increase in cardiac output) and may indicate that the CPP is compromised. Hypertension should not be treated unless the cause has been identified and the patient's systolic BP is >180–200 mmHg or the medium BP is >110–120 mmHg. If BP is lowered as a compensatory mechanism to maintain adequate CPP, cerebral ischemia may be exacerbated (may become worse). Continuous infusion of short-acting beta-blockers can be effective for hypertension and they can achieve the correct CPP. As opposed to nitrates and calcium channel blockers, these agents do not cause cerebral vasodilatation and, therefore, do not lead to an increase in cerebral blood volume or ICP.[42]

Prehospital fluid resuscitation in patients with TBI

1. Physiology of the blood–brain barrier in brain injury. In physiologic conditions, the endothelium (the layer of cells that lines the cavities of the heart and blood and lymph vessels, and the cavities of the body that assist digestion, excretion, and respiration) of the brain capillaries shows sporadic intercellular pores 5 to 7Å in size; that is, 10-fold smaller than those found in other tissues. This characteristic is the basis for the blood–brain barrier (BBB), which, under normal conditions, prevents the passage of many types of hydrophilic molecules and electrically charged molecules across the capillary endothelium.[43]

The BBB has the ability to restrict the passage of substances in both directions in order to maintain cerebral homeostasis (a constant condition). In addition to endothelial cells, the BBB is composed of other cells that are located in the internal vessel walls, such as neurons, glial cells, and muscle tissue cells. These components form a complex functional group known as the neurovascular unit.[44]

When there is acute brain injury, edema (swelling) develops, and because of the anatomic characteristics of the neuronal tissue that is within the cranium, the fluid accumulation leads to an increase in the ICP, cerebral herniation, and in the final phase of the lesion, death. Two types of cerebral edema have been defined: cytotoxic and vasogenic. Cytotoxic edema occurs when there is an injury to the cell membrane, with sodium-potassium-ATPase changes that disrupt the transmembrane gradient (the concentration of a solution is higher on one side of a membrane than the other side). The cells, mainly astrocytes, begin to swell and the interstitial space shrinks. In this type of edema, the BBB remains intact.[45]

Vasogenic edema occurs when there is BBB disruption and fluid passes from the vascular space to the interstitial compartment, following the hydrostatic pressure gradient. Usually, both types of cerebral edema are common in an intracranial injury.[45]

2. The aim of prehospital fluid therapy. The main objective of fluid therapy in the prehospital phase is to maintain adequate BP that will ensure tissue perfusion pressure of 50 to 70 mmHg.[40] However, administering fluid should be limited to comply with the second objective of preventing cerebral edema from developing, increased ICP, and hemodilution, which favors bleeding. Therefore, it is important to achieve a close balance between the first and second objectives.

   In the initial prehospital management of severe hemorrhagic shock, medical professionals should understand the necessity of avoiding excessive fluid resuscitation and maintaining systolic BP between 80 and 90 mmHg (permissive hypotension [the use of fluid therapy that increases systemic blood pressure without reaching normal blood pressure]). Administering excessive fluid can lead to problems with coagulation and exacerbate bleeding, in addition to other complications that worsen the patient's prognosis. In patients with hemorrhagic shock and severe TBI (GSC ≤8), managing fluid therapy should aim for a mean BP of 90 mmHg to avoid the detrimental effect of hypotension.[46]

3. Types of fluids. The pharmacokinetic properties and ability of the available fluids to be absorbed should be taken into account when choosing the one that will provide the greatest benefits in unstable TBI patients who require prehospital volume resuscitation. The optimal type of fluids for these patients is currently a subject of debate.

Based on the pathophysiology of brain injury colloids may be the optimal fluid therapy because of their osmotic effect and capacity to maintain the transvascular oncotic gradient. In a *post hoc* study, the multicenter SAFE[47] group carried out a randomized, double-blind comparison between 4% albumin and 0.9% saline solution as fluid resuscitation therapy in patients with severe TBI. Mortality at 24 months was higher in the group treated with albumin (relative risk, 1.88; 95% CI, and 1.31–2.70). A posterior analysis showed that patients receiving albumin had higher ICP values during the first week after the injury, suggesting that this factor may have contributed to their higher mortality.[48]

The mechanism that explained this phenomenon may be extravasation (leakage) of albumin in areas with BBB changes, thus facilitating interstitial edema and a consequent ICP increase. Another determinant is the fact that 4% albumin solution has an osmolarity (the measure of the solution) of 274 mOsm/L and osmolality (the concentration of a solution that can be absorbed by osmosis) of 266 mOsm/Kg, which makes the solution hypo-osmolar relative to plasma.[49]

Therefore, the presence of BBB changes should prompt us to avoid hypo-osmolar solutions in order to prevent the occurrence of edema and increased ICP. Because of its hypotonicity (low muscle tone), Ringer's lactate (a fluid and electrolyte replenisher) should also be avoided in severe TBI. It is recommended to administer balanced solutions, and not hypo-osmolar solutions, in these patients.[46,49]

Using a hypertonic 7.5% saline solution has proven to be effective osmotherapy for treating intracranial hypertension. Nonetheless, prehospital use of this option as fluid resuscitation therapy in TBI patients has not demonstrated improved survival rates in those with concomitant hypotension[50] or in those with normal blood pressure.[51]

Additionally, we have to consider the effect of hypertonic fluids on coagulation, particularly solutions mixed with dextrans (a water-soluble polysaccharide of glucose). Prehospital administration of these fluids in situations of severe shock (systolic BP ≤70 mmHg) has been associated with laboratory parameters that are consistent with hypocoagulability (decreased or deficient ability of blood to clot) and hyperfibrinolysis (marked increase of subdural hematomas).[52]

Temperature management

Incidental hypothermia tends to develop spontaneously in the prehospital phase and has been associated with increased mortality in TBI and trauma patients. A recent prospective, multicenter study has provided further evidence of this association (OR 1.8).[9]

Currently, hypothermia induction is under consideration as a basic therapeutic option, mainly in the experimental setting, with the most work carried out in two areas: neuronal injury and hemorrhagic shock, both currently in the clinical trial phase. Recent findings in TBI have indicated that hypothermia can be beneficial, but only in certain patients. Several studies conducted in adults and children have failed to show improvements in the outcome. However, in one subgroup analysis in adults, patients (younger than 46 years of age) with hypothermia upon admittance who were not rewarded, but instead maintained hypothermia, showed a better prognosis.[53] In general, studies where hypothermia is used as a therapeutic measure in TBI patients have shown favorable effects on the ICP. Nonetheless, the neuroprotective value of hyperthermia resulting from inhibition of the biochemical/inflammatory cascade triggered by TBI has not been confirmed at this point.

CONCLUSION

Evidence continues to accumulate from research that is focused on the prevention of secondary brain injury in the prehospital phase in patients with TBI, and it is likely that this effort will continue in the future. It is essential that medical professionals involved in the care of these patients continue to offer their experience and results in this ongoing process of improvement.

REFERENCES

1. Lee JC, Rittenhouse K, Bupp K et al. An analysis of Brain Trauma Foundation traumatic brain injury guideline compliance and patient outcome. *Injury.* 2015;46(5):854-858.
2. Cancelliere C, Coronado VG, Taylor CA, Xu L. Epidemiology of isolated versus nonisolated mild traumatic brain injury treated in emergency departments in the United States, 2006-2012. *J Head Trauma Rehabil.* 2016;1. doi:10.1097/HTR.0000000000000260
3. Hoogmartens O, Heselmans A, Van de Velde S et al. Evidence-based prehospital management of severe traumatic brain injury: A comparative analysis of current clinical practice guidelines. *Prehosp Emerg Care.* 2014;18(2):265-273.
4. Carney N, Totten AM, O'Reilly C et al. Guidelines for the management of severe traumatic brain injury, fourth edition. *Neurosurgery.* 2016;80(1):6-10.
5. Merlano-almanza MJ, Rubiano AM, Alcalá-cerra G, Alvis-miranda HR, Moscote-salazar LR. [Trauma craneoencefálico severo: Atención prehospitalaria, manejo quirúrgico y monitoreo multomodal.] 2015:149-161.
6. Rincon F, Kang J, Vibbert M, Urtecho J, Athar MK, Jallo J. Significance of arterial hyperoxia and relationship with case fatality in traumatic brain injury: A multicentre cohort study. *J Neurol Neurosurg Psychiatry.* 2014;85(7): 799-805.
7. Moppett IK. Traumatic brain injury: Assessment, resuscitation and early management. *Br J Anaesth.* 2007;99(1):18-31.
8. Talley Watts L, Long JA, Manga VH, Huang S, Shen Q, Duong TQ. Normobaric oxygen worsens outcome after a moderate traumatic brain injury. *J Cereb Blood Flow Metab.* 2015;35(7):1137-1144.
9. Wijayatilake DS, Jigajinni S V, Sherren PB: Traumatic brain injury: Physiological targets for clinical practice in the prehospital setting and on the Neuro-ICU. *Curr Opin Anaesthesiol.* 2015;28(5):517-524.
10. Stein SC, Georgoff P, Meghan S, Mizra K, Sonnad SS. 150 years of treating severe traumatic brain injury: A systematic review of progress in mortality. *J Neurotrauma.* 2010;27 (7):1343-1353.
11. Pearson WS, Ovalle F, Faul M, Sasser SM. A review of traumatic brain injury trauma center visits meeting physiologic criteria from the American College of Surgeons Committee on Trauma/Centers for Disease Control and Prevention Field Triage Guidelines. *Prehospital Emerg Care.* 2012;16(3):323-328.
12. Caterino JM, Raubenolt A. The prehospital simplified motor score is as accurate as the prehospital Glasgow Coma Scale: Analysis of a statewide trauma registry. *Emerg Med J.* 2012;29(6):492-496.
13. Chowdhury T, Kowalski S, Arabi Y, Dash HH. Pre-hospital and initial management of head injury patients: An update. *Saudi J Anaesth.* 2014;8(1):114-120.
14. Hammell CL, Henning JD. Prehospital management of severe traumatic brain injury. *BMJ.* 2009;338:b1683.
15. Aubuchon MM, Hemmes B, Poeze M, Jansen J, Brink PR. Prehospital care in patients with severe traumatic brain injury: Does the level

of prehospital care influence mortality? *Eur J Trauma Emerg Surg.* 2013;39(1):35-41.

16. Dinsmore J. Traumatic brain injury: An evidence-based review of management. *Contin Educ Anaesthesia, Crit Care Pain.* 2013;13:1-7.

17. Rehn M, Hyldmo PK, Magnusson V et al. Scandinavian SSAI clinical practice guideline on pre-hospital airway management. *Acta Anaesthesiol Scand.* 2016;60(7):852-864.

18. Sherren PB, Tricklebank S, Glover G. Development of a standard operating procedure and checklist for rapid sequence induction in the critically ill. *Scand J Trauma Resusc Emerg Med.* 2014;22:41.

19. Bernard SA, Nguyen V, Cameron P et al. Prehospital rapid sequence intubation improves functional outcome for patients with severe traumatic brain injury: A randomized controlled trial. *Ann Surg.* 2010;252 (6):959-965.

20. Bukur M, Kurtovic S, Berry C et al. Pre-hospital intubation is associated with increased mortality after traumatic brain injury. *J Surg Res.* 2011;170(1):e117-e121.

21. Murray JA, Demetriades D, Berne TV et al. Prehospital intubation in patients with severe head injury. *J Trauma.* 2000;49(6):1065-1070.

22. Crewdson K, Lockey DJ, Røislien J, Lossius HM, Rehn M. The success of pre-hospital tracheal intubation by different pre-hospital providers: A systematic literature review and meta-analysis. *Crit Care.* 2017;21(1):31.

23. Jensen AG, Callesen T, Hagemo JS et al. Scandinavian clinical practice guidelines on general anaesthesia for emergency situations. *Acta Anaesthesiol Scand.* 2010;54 (8):922-950.

24. Winchell RJ, Hoyt DB. Endotracheal intubation in the field improves survival in patients with severe head injury. Trauma Research and Education Foundation of San Diego. *Arch Surg.* 1997;132(6):592-597.

25. Bochicchio GV, Ilahi O, Joshi M, Bochicchio K, Scalea TM. Endotracheal intubation in the field does not improve outcome in trauma patients who present without an acutely lethal traumatic brain injury. *J Trauma.* 2003;54(2):307-311.

26. Wang HE, Peitzman AB, Cassidy LD, Adelson PD, Yealy DM. Out-of-hospital endotracheal intubation and outcome after traumatic brain injury. *Ann Emerg Med.* 2004;44(5):439-450.

27. Davis DP, Peay J, Sise MJ et al. Prehospital airway and ventilation management: A trauma score and Injury Severity Score-based analysis. *J Trauma.* 2010;69(2):294-301.

28. Warner KJ, Cuschieri J, Copass MK, Jurkovich GJ, Bulger EM. The impact of prehospital ventilation on outcome after severe traumatic brain injury. *J Trauma.* 2007;62(6):1330-1338.

29. Vandromme MJ, Melton SM, Griffin R et al. Intubation patterns and outcomes in patients with computed tomography-verified traumatic brain injury. *J Trauma.* 2011;71 (6):1615-1619.

30. Tuma M, El-Menyar A, Abdelrahman H et al. Prehospital intubation in patients with isolated severe traumatic brain injury: A 4-year observational study. *Crit Care Res Pract.* 2014;2014:135986.

31. Denninghoff KR, Nuño T, Pauls Q et al. Prehospital intubation is associated with favorable outcomes and lower mortality in ProTECT III. *Prehosp Emerg Care.* 2017;21(5) 539-544.

32. Seder DB, Riker RR, Jagoda A, Smith WS, Weingart SD. Emergency neurological life support: Airway, ventilation, and sedation. *Neurocrit Care.* 2012;17(suppl 1):S4-S20.

33. Harris T, Davenport R, Hurst T, Jones J. Improving outcome in severe trauma: Trauma systems and initial management: Intubation, ventilation and resuscitation. *Postgrad Med J.* 2012;88(1044):588-594.

34. Beckers SK, Brokmann JC, Rossaint R. Airway and ventilator management in trauma patients. *Curr Opin Crit Care.* 2014;20 (6):626-631.

35. Lyon RM, Perkins ZB, Chatterjee D, Lockey DJ, Russell MQ, Kent, Surrey & Sussex Air Ambulance Trust. Significant modification of traditional rapid sequence induction improves safety and effectiveness of pre-hospital trauma anaesthesia. *Crit Care.* 2015;19:134.

36. Lin CC, Yu JH, Lin CC, Li WC, Weng YM, Chen SY. Postintubation hemodynamic effects of intravenous lidocaine in severe traumatic brain injury. *Am J Emerg Med.* 2012;30(9):1782-1787.

37. Vijay B, Bajwa S. Causes of tracheal re-intubation after craniotomy: A prospective study. *Saudi J Anaesth.* 2013;6:152-154.

38. Berry C, Ley EJ, Bukur M et al. Redefining hypotension in traumatic brain injury. *Injury.* 2012;43(11):1833-1837.

39. Brenner M, Stein DM, Hu PF, Aarabi B, Sheth K, Scalea TM. Traditional systolic blood pressure targets underestimate hypotension-induced secondary brain injury. *J Trauma Acute Care Surg.* 2012;72(5):1135-1139.

40. Boer C, Franschman G, Loer SA. Prehospital management of severe traumatic brain injury. *Curr Opin Anaesthesiol.* 2012;25(5):556-562.

41. Franschman G, Peerdeman SM, Andriessen TM et al. Analysis of Results and Methods—Traumatic Brain Injury (ALARM-TBI) Investigators: Effect of secondary prehospital risk factors on outcome in severe traumatic brain injury in the context of fast access to trauma care. *J Trauma Inj Infect Crit Care.* 2011;71:826-832.

42. Ghaffarpasand F, Dehghankhalili M. Current concepts and advancements in management of traumatic brain injury; a glimpse at the recently published evidence. *Bull Emerg Trauma.* 2017;5(2):67-69.

43. Drummond JC. Colloid osmotic pressure and the formation of posttraumatic cerebral edema. *Anesthesiology.* 2010;112(5):1079-1081.

44. Muoio V, Persson PB, Sendeski MM: The neurovascular unit—Concept review. *Acta Physiol (Oxf).* 2014;210(4):790-798.

45. Lukaszewicz AC, Soyer B, Payen D. Water, water, everywhere: Sodium and water balance and the injured brain. *Curr Opin Anaesthesiol.* 2011;24(2):138-143.

46. Rossaint R, Bouillon B, Cerny V et al. The European guideline on management of major bleeding and coagulopathy following trauma: Fourth edition. *Crit Care.* 2016;20:100.

47. SAFE Study Investigators, Australian and New Zealand Intensive Care Society Clinical Trials Group, Australian Red Cross Blood Service et al. Saline or albumin for fluid resuscitation in patients with traumatic brain injury. *N Engl J Med.* 2007;357(9):874-884.

48. Cooper DJ, Myburgh J, Heritier S et al. Albumin resuscitation for traumatic brain injury: Is intracranial hypertension the cause of increased mortality? *J Neurotrauma.* 2013;30(7):512-518.

49. Van Aken HK, Kampmeier TG, Ertmer C, Westphal M. Fluid resuscitation in patients with traumatic brain injury: What is a SAFE approach? *Curr Opin Anaesthesiol.* 2012;25(5):563-565.

50. Cooper DJ, Myles PS, McDermott FT et al. Prehospital hypertonic saline resuscitation of patients with hypotension and severe traumatic brain injury: A randomized controlled trial. *JAMA.* 2004;291(11):1350-1357.

51. Bulger EM, May S, Brasel KJ et al. A randomized controlled trial. *JAMA.* 2010;304:1455-1464.

52. Delano MJ, Rizoli SB, Rhind SG et al. Prehospital resuscitation of traumatic hemorrhagic shock with hypertonic solutions worsens hypocoagulation and hyperfibrinolysis. *Shock.* 2015;44(1):25-31.

53. Bukur M, Kurtovic S, Berry C, Tanios M, Ley EJ, Salim A. Pre-hospital hypothermia is not associated with increased survival after traumatic brain injury. *J Surg Res.* 2012;175(1):24-29.

5

Preanesthetic evaluation

JULIA MARTINEZ OCÓN, ANA RUIZ PARDOS, AND RICARD VALERO

INTRODUCTION

Traumatic brain injury (TBI) is a major health problem and a leading cause of death and disability.[1] Current TBI management is based on prevention of the primary injury and avoidance of secondary injuries. The perioperative period (the entire period of medical treatment from contemplating the surgery all the way through recovery after the surgery) provides an opportunity to continue and refine ongoing resuscitation during the treatment of the primary injury and to correct preexisting secondary insults.

Perioperative management implies rapid evaluation, continued resuscitation (cerebral and systemic), early surgical intervention, intensive monitoring, and an anesthetic plan.[2] In this setting, the goal of preanesthetic evaluation is the detection and correction of all of those factors that can contribute to worsening brain injury and, therefore, the prognosis of TBI.[2]

Preventing secondary injury is one of the main goals of anesthetic management. Surgery and anesthesia may make patients susceptible to these new injuries, which may contribute adversely to the outcome. While the severity of the primary injury is the major factor that determines outcome, secondary injury that is caused by physiologic insults, such as hypotension, hypoxemia, hypercarbia, hypocarbia, hyperglycemia, and hypoglycemia, which develop over time; causes further damage to brain tissue. All of these can appear both early and late in the course of a TBI. Moreover, the consequences of TBI may apply to other organ systems in addition to the brain and may require prompt attention.[2] The prevention of secondary injury is based on physiologic optimization of the insults.

PREANESTHETIC EVALUATION

The perioperative management of a patient after TBI necessitates a rapid evaluation, the continuation of systemic and cerebral resuscitation, early surgical intervention, intensive monitoring, and an appropriate anesthetic plan (Table 5.1).[2]

In the perioperative period, we must continue the resuscitation that began in the emergency department. The anesthesia team should perform a quick assessment of the patient and establish an anesthetic plan when the patient enters the operating room. Assessment will follow the ABC (airway, breathing, circulation) resuscitation plan

Table 5.1 Preanesthetic evaluation

Airway	Blood pressure	Blood transfusion	Coagulation	Neurologic assessment
• Rapid sequence intubation • Avoid nasal intubation • VL in difficult airway • Consider cervical spine injury	• SBP ≥100 mmHg in patients 50–69 y.o. or ≥110 mmHg in patients between 15–49 or >70 y.o. • Use of isotonic crystalloids • Use of colloids is controversial • Consider vasopressors	• Target Hb of 7–9 g/dL • No relationship between RBC transfusion and outcome • Anemia causes secondary ischemic damage	• Reversal of coagulopathy is a priority • PCC for rapid reversal of vit. K antagonists • Platelets in patients treated with APA	• GCS assessment • Pupillary assessment • Signs of herniation

Abbreviations: APA: antiplatelet agents; GCS: Glasgow Coma Scale; PCC: prothrombin complex concentrates; RBC: red blood cells; SBP: systolic blood pressure; VL: videolaryngoscope; y.o.: years old.

of any critical patient (ABC and then neurologic status assessment). We must bear in mind that the patient may have other injuries, such as thoracic, abdominal, spinal, and bone injuries that may cause hemodynamic instability and hypoxemia, requiring prompt evaluation and treatment.

Airway management

Airway management in TBI is complicated by several factors, including the urgency of the situation. Patients with TBI who require surgery will inevitably require endotracheal intubation. Patients with a GCS (Glasgow Coma Scale) labeled as severe will reach the operating room still intubated, while patients with a better GCS may reach the operating room breathing normally.[1]

If the patient is already intubated, the correct position of the endotracheal tube should be checked, because transfers from the emergency room or from the CT-scan machine can move the tube and cause endobronchial intubation (greatly diminished lung ventilation).

If the patient is not intubated and requires urgent surgery, it is important to remember that the TBI patient is thought to have a full stomach. In addition to this, it is essential to be ready for the possible presence of blood or vomit in the oral cavity. Finally, TBI often goes along with cervical spine injury, and this possibility must always be considered when performing endotracheal intubation in TBI patients. Rapid sequence intubation is recommended with

adequate sedative or analgesics, as well as a neuromuscular blocking agent to prevent increasing intracranial pressure during intubation.

The appropriate drug choice is important for airway management that is free from complications. Hypnotics decrease cerebral metabolic oxygen rate of and weaken increments in intracranial pressure caused by intubation. Ketamine has been associated with increased cerebral blood flow (CBF) and increased intracranial pressure (ICP) and may be contraindicated in patients with intracranial hypertension.

With respect to neuromuscular blocking agents, the choice for rapid sequence induction lies between succinylcholine and rocuronium. Succinylcholine increases ICP without significant side effects, so it is recommended in TBI cases where the patient has airway difficulties.

Normocapnia and mild hyperoxemia should be maintained to prevent secondary brain injury.[3]

The choice of technique for tracheal intubation is determined by urgency, individual expertise, and available resources. The choice generally incorporates rapid sequence intubation with cricoid pressure and manual in-line stabilization.[4] The front part of the cervical collar can be removed when intubating, as manual in-line stability allows greater mouth opening and thus facilitates intubation. Nasal intubation should be avoided in patients with skull-base or facial fractures, as well as in those with bleeding diathesis. In difficult airway cases, new devices, especially video-laryngoscopes, can be very useful.[3] In general, difficult intubation cases require an alternative plan due to the high risk of intracranial hypertension that can be caused by increased CBF as a result of hypoxemia and hypercapnia.

Hemodynamic assessment: Blood pressure management

Blood pressure management, including the choice of fluids or vasopressors, is an important parameter. Perioperative hypotension should be treated promptly.[2]

With regard to blood pressure goals, the latest Brain Trauma Foundation (BTF) guidelines recommend maintaining systemic blood pressure (SBP) ≥100 mmHg in patients with TBI between 50–69 years of age or ≥110 mmHg in patients between 15–49 or >70 years old.[5] Current literature supports a higher blood pressure level, which may vary by age. The association between SBP, mean arterial pressure (MAP), and cerebral perfusion pressure (CPP) should be kept in mind when considering threshold recommendations from these guidelines.[5]

Arterial catheterization is recommended for continuous blood pressure monitoring, blood gas analysis, and glucose sampling in patients who require surgical intervention.[2] Central venous catheterization is advisable; however, its placement must not delay surgical intervention.

INTRAVENOUS FLUIDS AND VASSOPRESSORS

In order to maintain tissue oxygenation, the traditional treatment of TBI patients used aggressive fluid administration to restore blood volume. This approach may, however, increase the hydrostatic pressure on the wound, cause blood clots to become dislodged, cause coagulation factors to become diluted, and cause the undesirable cooling of the patient.[6] The concept of "damage control resuscitation" aims to achieve a lower than normal blood pressure, or "permissive hypotension," and thereby avoid the adverse effects of early aggressive resuscitation; using high doses of fluids during short time periods when there is a potential risk of tissue hypoperfusion.[7] Restrictive volume replacement is contraindicated in patients with TBI and spinal injuries because adequate perfusion pressure is crucial to ensure that the central nervous system tissue receives enough oxygen.[8]

Although fluid resuscitation is the first step in restoring tissue perfusion in TBI patients, it is still unclear whether crystalloids (such as saline) or colloids should be used, and, more specifically, *which* crystalloid or colloid. When considering crystalloids, hypotonic solutions such as Ringer's lactate should be avoided in patients with TBI to minimize the fluid shift into the damaged cerebral tissue. Whether an advantage for certain isotonic, balanced crystalloids with respect to a reduced morbidity or mortality exists is not clear and should still be evaluated.[9,10]

Colloid administration is controversial. A post hoc analysis of the Saline vs. Albumin Fluid Evaluation (SAFE) trial determined that resuscitation with albumin was associated with a higher mortality and unfavorable neurologic outcomes at 24 months.[11]

The BTF guidelines recommend treating hypotensive patients with isotonic fluids, with the option of administering hypertonic fluids in patients with GCS <8. Non-glucose-containing isotonic crystalloid solutions are indicated in patients with TBI.

Vasopressors may also be required to maintain tissue perfusion in the presence of hypotension, even when fluid expansion is in progress and hypovolemia has not yet been corrected. Norepinephrine (NE) is often used to restore arterial pressure in septic and hemorrhagic shock. Although NE has β-adrenergic effects, it acts predominantly as a vasoconstrictor. NE exerts both arterial and venous α-adrenergic stimulation. Arterial α-adrenergic stimulation increases arterial resistance and may increase cardiac afterload.[12] At the splanchnic level, NE induces venoconstriction, which increases the pressure in capacitance vessels and actively shifts splanchnic blood volume to the systemic circulation.[13] This venous adrenergic stimulation may recruit blood from the venous unstressed volume, which fills the blood vessels without generating intravascular pressure. Moreover, stimulation of β-adrenergic receptors decreases venous resistance and increases venous return.[14] Current evidence does not show superiority of any specific vasopressor over another in increasing cerebral perfusion, and the choice should be individualized to patients.[2]

BLOOD TRANSFUSION

Because anemia is a cause of secondary ischemic damage, doubts have been raised about the safety of restrictive transfusion strategies in TBI patients. Most clinical information comes from retrospective observational studies with methodologic limitations. These have produced inconsistent results on the effects of red blood cell (RBC) transfusion on markers of cerebral perfusion and metabolism in patients with isolated, severe TBI.[6] The lack of high-level scientific evidence for hemoglobin (Hb) transfusion trigger in TBI patients has been addressed in several reviews.[14,15]

Recent studies have focused on the effect of anemia and RBC transfusion on neurologic outcome after TBI.[16] No relationship between RBC transfusion and outcome was found in patients with an initial Hb <10 g/dL. Generally, patients with severe TBI should not be managed with Hb transfusion thresholds different from those of other critical patients. A target Hb of 7 to 9 g/dL is recommended.[6]

COAGULOPATHY MANAGEMENT

When coagulopathy is present, rapid reversal should be a high priority in the perioperative period in order to avoid an increase in bleeding, which can lead to secondary injury. A study from Carney et al. found progression of traumatic intracranial hemorrhage in 80% of coagulopathic TBI patients (INR <1.3, PPT >35, platelets <100,000) compared with 36% of noncoagulopathic TBI patients, with the intracranial hemorrhage (ICH) progression group having a fivefold increase in mortality.[5]

The administration of blood products and duration of mechanical ventilation are factors that are associated with in-hospital mortality in TBI patients.[17] European guidelines recommend early algorithm-based and goal directed coagulation management in order to reduce transfusion and improve outcomes.[18] Coagulation monitoring is performed with whatever means are available; ranging from traditional laboratory tests, such as prothrombin time, activated partial thromboplastin time, and platelet count; to fibrinogen determination and viscoelastic test.

Off-label use of recombinant VIIa factor is only considered if major bleeding and traumatic coagulopathy persist despite all other attempts for control.[6]

Vitamin K antagonist

The association between drugs that alter a patient's coagulation function and adverse trauma outcomes

continues to be an important area of interest and study.[19] As life expectancy increases, there is also an increase in the number of people who are treated with anticoagulant and antiplatelet agents.[19] These drugs are prescribed to prevent the thromboembolic complications of atrial fibrillation; prosthetic cardiac valves; cerebral, coronary, and peripheral vascular disease; as well as several other serious medical conditions.

The most frequently prescribed medications are the vitamin K antagonists, acenocoumarol and warfarin. These inhibit the II, VII, IX, X clotting factors and C and S proteins. In the perioperative period, it is recommended that anticoagulated patients with TBI undergo a rapid reversal of anticoagulant treatment with a prothrombin complex concentrate (PCC).

PCC has been proven to be superior to plasma for the rapid reversal of vitamin K antagonists, which causes fewer hematoma formations in those patients with head injury.[20–23] Therefore, it is the agent of choice to reverse the effects of vitamin K antagonists.[24]

New oral anticoagulants

The appearance of "new oral anticoagulants" has made anticoagulation reversal more complicated.

Dabigatran, a direct thrombin inhibitor, now has an available antidote, idarucizumab. It is a monoclonal antibody fragment, which binds to free and bound dabigatran, acting in less than 5 minutes. European guidelines recommend measuring plasma levels of Anti-Xa agents, such as dabigatran, when managing TBI patients. If measurement is not possible or available, a determination of thrombin time and APTT (activated partial thromboplastin time) should be performed to determine the quality of the presence of dabigatran (recommendation grade 2c). If bleeding is life-threatening, treatment with idarucizumab (5 g intravenously) is recommended.

However, the other direct factor Xa inhibitors still present a challenge. In a retrospective study of 18 TBI patients with intracranial or subarachnoid hemorrhage who were taking rivaroxaban or apixaban, PCC was a good option to potentially reduce hematoma expansion.[5] Andexanet alfa, Xa inhibitor, and ciraparantag, Xa factor, and II factor inhibitors are in phase III clinical trials.

Early monitoring of coagulation is essential to detect trauma-induced coagulopathy and to define its causes, including hyperfibrinolysis.[25]

ANTIPLATELET AGENTS

Platelet transfusion is recommended in TBI patients who are treated with antiplatelet agents, especially clopidogrel (Plavix®), because it poses a great risk for uncontrolled bleeding. European guidelines also suggest that desmopressin (0.3 µg/kg) be administered in patients treated with platelet-inhibiting drugs or with Von Willebrand disease. Desmopressin has been shown to improve platelet function in volunteers who received aspirin and clopidogrel, and perioperatively, in patients with mild inherited platelet defects. However, the use of desmopressin for acquired bleeding disorders is not supported by clinical evidence.[5,6]

NEUROLOGICAL ASSESSMENT

TBI presentation can be highly varied and may coexist with a diverse range of extracranial pathology. Neurologic assessment will be performed using the Glasgow Coma Scale (GCS) score and pupillary responses, with severe TBI being defined as GCS ≤8. Neuroimaging is used for diagnosis, decision-making (especially surgical interventions), and prognosis.[26]

Hyperosmolar therapy

Hyperosmolar therapy is reserved for those cases in which intracranial hypertension is suspected, either by CT scan findings or due to clinical signs of transtentorial herniation or progressive neurologic deterioration.

Hyperosmolar medications can decrease ICP by creating an osmolar gradient that draws water across the blood–brain barrier into the intravascular space and thus decreases interstitial volume. Commonly used agents are mannitol (0.25–1 g/kg) and hypertonic saline solution at 7.5% (bolus administration seems superior to continuous infusion).[27]

Hypertonic saline is effective and may be preferred over mannitol, because it expands intravascular volume, and (unlike mannitol) is not associated with a subsequent diuresis that could cause hypovolemia and hypotension.[28] It is important to control osmolarity and to determine sodium plasma level in these patients.

Prophylactic antiepileptic treatment

Seizures can make secondary brain injury worse, causing an increase in cerebral metabolism and ICP and a decrease in cerebral blood flow. Prophylactic treatment with antiepileptic drugs has been shown to reduce the incidence of the early seizures.[29]

Guidelines recommend a 7-day antiepileptic drug therapy to reduce early seizures after TBI in patients with risk factors (GCS score <10; cortical contusion; depressed skull fracture; subdural, extradural or intracranial hematoma; and penetrating head wound).[30] During preanesthetic evaluation, these indications must be checked and antiepileptic medication should be administered, if required.

Levetiracetam has a better safety profile compared with phenytoin.[31]

Glycemic control

Admission hyperglycemia (blood glucose >180 mg/dL) contributes to metabolic acidosis through anaerobic metabolism and increased blood–brain barrier permeability; it has been associated with worse outcomes after TBI.[32] However, tight glycemic control is associated with an increased risk of hypoglycemia.[33] The ideal blood glucose level should range between 80 and 180 mg/dL. Glycaemic levels must be checked, to avoid both hyper- and hypoglycemia.

Temperature management

Hypothermia, or core body temperature <35°C, is associated with acidosis, hypotension, and coagulopathy in polytraumatic patients. The effects of hypothermia include altered platelet function, impaired coagulation, enzyme inhibition, and fibrinolysis.[6] European guidelines recommend perioperative early application of measures to reduce heat loss and active warming of hypothermic patients in order to maintain normothermia.[6] However, whereas hypothermia should clearly be avoided in patients without TBI, opposing results have been reported in patients with TBI. A recent meta-analysis by Crossley et al., which included several single-center studies, demonstrated a reduction in mortality and poor outcomes in those patients submitted to hypothermia.[34] These observations support the use of mild hypothermic therapy for TBI under specific circumstances.[5]

THROMBOPROPHYLAXIS

Patients with TBI are theoretically at an increased risk of venous thromboembolic events (VTE).[35] However, in complex trauma patients admitted to the intensive care unit (ICU) who were screened for high VTE risk, TBI did not add to this risk. The most likely explanation is that no single risk factor is necessary or sufficient for VTE development, especially in those patients who routinely receive chemical and mechanical thromboprophylaxis.[36] In TBI and solid organ injury, initiation of pharmacologic thromboprophylaxis 48 hours after injury is not associated with an increase of bleeding complications. There is no agreement or clear data showing which dosing regimen of low-molecular-weight heparin (LMWH) is most effective or whether routine laboratory measurements are beneficial for determining effective thromboprophylaxis.[37]

REFERENCES

1. Coronado VG, Xu L, Basavaraju SV et al. Surveillance for traumatic brain injury-related deaths—United States, 1997-2007. *MMWR Surveill Summ.* 2011;60(5):1-32.
2. Sharma D, Vavilala MS. Perioperative management of adult traumatic brain injury. *Anesthesiol Clin.* 2012;30(2):333-346.
3. Jung JY. Airway management of patients with traumatic brain injury/C-spine injury. *Korean J Anesthesiol.* 2015;68(3):213-219.
4. Crosby ET. Airway management in adults after cervical spine trauma. *Anesthesiology.* 2006;104(6):1293-1318.
5. Carney N, Totten AM, O'Reilly C et al. Guidelines for the management of severe traumatic brain injury, Fourth Edition. *Neurosurgery.* 2017;80(1):6-15.
6. Rossaint R, Bouillon B, Cerny V et al. The European guideline on management of major bleeding and coagulopathy following trauma: Fourth edition. *Crit Care.* 2016;20:100.
7. Waydhas C, German Society of Trauma Surgery (DGU). [Preclinical management of multiples injuries: S3 guideline.] *Unfallchirurg.* 2012;115(1):8-13.
8. Berry C, Ley EJ, Bukur M et al. Redefining hypotension in traumatic brain injury. *Injury.* 2012;43(11):1833-1837.
9. Smith CA, Duby JJ, Utter GH, Galante JM, Sherer CR, Shermer CR. Cost-minimization analysis of two fluid products for resuscitation of critically injured trauma patients. *Am J Health Syst Pharm.* 2014;71(6):470-475.
10. Orbegozo Cortés D, Rayo Bonor A, Vincent JL. Isotonic crystalloid solutions: A structured review of the literature. *Br J Anaesth.* 2014;112(6);968-981.
11. SAFE study investigators, Australian and New Zealand Intensive Care Society Clinical Trials Group; Australian Red Cross Blood Service et al.; Saline or albumin for fluid resuscitation in patients with traumatic brain injury. *N Engl J Med.* 2007;357(9):874-884.
12. Thiele RH, Nemergut EC, Lynch C 3rd. The physiologic implications of isolated alpha(1) adrenergic stimulation. *Anesth Analg.* 2011;113(2):284-296.
13. Gelman S, Mushlin PS. Catecholamine-induced changes in the splanchnic circulation affecting systemic hemodynamics. *Anesthesiology.* 2004;100(2)434-439.
14. Desjardins P, Turgeon AF, Tremblay MH et al. Hemoglobin levels and transfusions in neurocritically ill patients: A systematic review of comparative studies. *Crit Care.* 2012;16(2)R54.
15. Bellapart J, Boots R, Fraser J. Physiopathology of anemia and transfusion thresholds in isolated head injury. *J Trauma Acute Care Surg.* 2012;73(4):997-1005.
16. Robertson CS, Hannay HJ, Yamai M et al. Effect of erythropoietin and transfusion threshold on neurological recovery after traumatic brain injury: A randomized clinical trial. *JAMA.* 2014;312(1):34-37.
17. Almeida KJ, Rodrigues ÂB, Lemos LE et al. Hemotransfusion and mechanical ventilation time are associated with intra-hospital mortality in patients with traumatic brain injury admitted to intensive care unit. *Arg Neuropsiquiatr.* 2016;74(8):644-649.
18. White NJ, Contaifer D Jr, Martin EJ et al. Early hemostatic responses to trauma identified with hierarchical clustering analysis. *J Thromb Haemost.* 2015;13(6):978-988.
19. Smith K, Weeks S. The impact of pre-injury anticoagulation therapy in the older adult

patient experiencing a traumatic brain injury: A systematic review. *JBI Libr Syst Rev.* 2012;10(58):4610-4621.

20. Quinlan DJ, Eikelboom JW, Weitz JL. Four-factor prothrombin complex concentrate for urgent reversal of vitamin K antagonists in patients with major bleeding. *Circulation.* 2013;128(11):1179-1181.

21. Goldstein JN, Refaai MA, Milling TJ Jr et al. Four-factor prothrombin complex concentrate versus plasma for rapid vitamin K antagonist reversal in patients needing urgent surgical or invasive interventions: A phase 3b, open-label, non-inferiority, randomised trial. *Lancet.* 2015;385(9982):2077-2087.

22. Huttner HB, Schellinger PD, Hartmann M et al. Hematoma growth and outcome in treated neurocritical care patients with intracerebral hemorrhage related to oral anticoagulant therapy: Comparison of acute treatment strategies using vitamin K, fresh frozen plasma, and prothrombin complex concentrates. *Stroke.* 2006;37(6):1465-1470.

23. Edavettal M, Rogers A, Rogers F, Horst M, Leng W. Prothrombin complex concentrate accelerates international normalized ratio reversal and diminishes the extension of intracranial hemorrhage in geriatric trauma patients. *Ann Surg.* 2014;80(4):372-376.

24. Baglin TP, Keeling DM, Watson HG, British Committee for Standards in Haematology. Guidelines on oral anticoagulation (warfarin): Third edition—2005 update. *Br J Haematol.* 2006;132(3):277-285.

25. Cardenas JC, Rahbar E, Pommerening MJ et al. Measuring thrombin generation as a tool for predicting hemostatic potential and transfusion requirements following trauma. *J Trauma Acute Care Surg.* 2014;77(6):839-845.

26. Menon DK, Ercole A. Critical care management of traumatic brain injury. *Handb Clin Neurol.* 2017;140:239-274.

27. Hinson HE, Stein D, Sheth KN. Hypertonic saline and mannitol therapy in critical care neurology. *J Intensive Care Med.* 2013;28 (1):3-11.

28. Lazadiris C, Neyens R, Bodle J, DeSantis SM. High-osmolarity saline in neurocritical care: Systematic review and meta-analysis. *Crit Care Med.* 2013;41(5):1353-1360.

29. Volovici V, Haitsma IK, Dirven CMF, Steyerberg EW, Lingsma HF, Maas AIR. Letter: Guidelines for the management of severe traumatic brain injury, fourth edition. *Neurosurgery.* 2017;81(2):E21.

30. Chang BS, Lowenstein DH, Quality Standards Subcommittee of the American Academy of Neurology. Practice parameter: Anti-epileptic drug prophylaxis in severe traumatic brain injury: Report of the Quality Standards Subcommittee of the American Academy of Neurology. *Neurology.* 2003;60 (1):10-16.

31. Xu JC, Shen J, Shao WZ et al. The safety and efficacy of levetiracetam versus phenytoin for seizure prophylaxis after traumatic brain injury: A systematic review and meta-analysis. *Brain Inj.* 2016;30(9):1054-1061.

32. Liu-DeRyke X, Collingridge DS, Orme J, Roller D, Zurasky J, Rhoney DH. Clinical impact of early hyperglycemia during acute phase of traumatic brain injury. *Neurocrit Care.* 2009;11(2):151-157.

33. NICE-SUGAR Study Investigators for the Australian and New Zealand Intensive Care Society Clinical Trials Group and the Canadian Critical Care Trials Group, Finfer S, Chittock D et al. Intensive versus conventional glucose control in critically ill patients with traumatic brain injury: Long-term follow-up of a subgroup of patients from the NICE-SUGAR study. *Intensive Care Med.* 2015;41 (6):1037-1047.

34. Crossley S, Reid J, Maclatchie R et al. A systemic review of therapeutic hypothermia for adult patients following traumatic brain injury. *Crit Care.* 2014;18(2):R75.

35. Jamjoom AA, Chari A, Salijevska J, Meacher R, Brennan P, Statham P. A national survey of thromboprophylaxis in traumatic brain injury in the United Kingdom. *Br J Neurosurg.* 2016;30(2):240-245.

36. Valle EJ, Van Haren RM, Allen CJ et al. Does traumatic brain injury increase the risk for venous thromboembolism in polytrauma patients. *J Trauma Acute Care Surg.* 2014;77 (2):243-250.

37. Van PY, Schreiber MA. Contemporary thromboprophylaxis of trauma patients. *Curr Opin Crit Care.* 2016;22(6):607-612.

6

Emergency room resuscitation

MARTA MAGALDI, LUIS REYES, MARINA VENDRELL, AND RICARD VALERO

INTRODUCTION

Severe trauma is an increasing global problem among young adults (<45 years of age) and in children (1–15 years of age).

Patient evaluation and care administered prior to the arrival at the hospital, as well as the development of a regional system of specialized attention, has improved prognoses considerably. However, the role of an established trauma team that is specifically dedicated to the care of this type of patient is even more crucial, as it may reduce mortality by up to 40%.[1] When treating patients with severe traumatic brain injury (TBI), those admitted to non-neurosurgical centers have 26% greater mortality than those admitted at adequately prepared centers.[2]

INITIAL ASSESSMENT

Assessment of all trauma patients should begin, just like in the prehospital care setting, by evaluating the airway, breathing, and circulation (ABC) followed by a rapid assessment of the patient's neurologic status (D, disability) and associated extracranial injuries (E, exposure); further attention to specific secondary injury mechanisms and ongoing treatment of them should also be evaluated.[3] Despite this being similar to the approach in prehospital care, the condition of trauma patients is constantly changing and requires reevaluation upon arrival in order to establish the absence of lesions that compromise life and require immediate attention before specific tests and treatments can be administered.

Airway

Inadequate airway management is an avoidable cause of morbidity and mortality (injury and death). Ensuring proper oxygenation is important for all severe trauma patients; however, in the specific case of TBI, it is essential in order to prevent further brain damage. Moreover, in these patients, upper-airway obstruction is rather common, as well as bronchial aspiration, hypoxia, and respiratory compromise. Hence, early management is even more important.[4]

Breathing

It is necessary to eliminate the possibility of lesions that compromise adequate ventilation. Special attention should be paid to tension pneumothorax, which decreases airway entry and causes hemodynamic instability due to cava vein compression. In this case, both hypoxia and hypotension will increase the brain damage that may be present. Unless there are clear signs that emergent decompression is required, such as hypoxia (Sat O_2<92%) or hypotension (TAS<90 mmHg), a chest x-ray should be obtained in the emergency room (ER) before performing any other intervention.[1]

Circulation

Hemorrhage is still the main cause of mortality after trauma. The main goal after the resuscitation of a TBI patient is to avoid additional blood loss. However, recognizing active bleeding may be challenging. It is important to remember that TBI patients are usually young and changes in vital parameters may not show up until blood loss is greater than 30%.[5]

Long bone fractures should be splinted, and if there is a suspicion of significant pelvic injury, fixation should be applied here too. Any points of external hemorrhage should be controlled by direct compression.

Disability/Neurologic assessment

A cursory evaluation of the neurologic state must be performed, including a pupillary evaluation and Glasgow Coma Scale (GCS) score. Despite there being confounding factors (hypotension, hypoxia, intoxication) for proper neurologic evaluation, information obtained is nonetheless valuable. The goal of the assessment is to recognize significant brain injury early, which will modify resuscitation targets; and ascertain the existence of mass lesions, the treatment of which is surgical evacuation.[6]

It is important to remember that in-line cervical immobilization should always be performed until a cervical lesion has been rejected.

Exposure

The patient should be completely undressed (often, the patient's garments will have to be cut off). Normothermia should always be the goal with hemodynamically unstable trauma patients. Therapeutic hypothermia for better outcomes in TBI is controversial, with many trials not showing a clear benefit.[7]

PROGNOSTIC FACTORS

Historically, the mechanism of TBI has been divided into two types: primary (as a result of direct mechanical forces) and secondary (a consequence of further physiologic insults). Morbidity, mortality, and long-term disability were thought to depend largely on the management of this secondary type. Nowadays, this distinction can be vague, because experimental evidence suggests that managing the secondary injury may alter the length of the primary injury and that the secondary injury may also begin when the trauma occurred.[8]

Whatever the underlying physiopathology, the severity of the primary injury is the major factor that determines the outcome for TBI patients; the secondary injury is amplified even more by various cofactors, including hypoxemia, hypotension, hypercapnia, hypo/hyperglycemia, hypo/hyperthermia, seizures, and so on.

Thus, the management of the TBI in the ER has the potential to initiate interventions that may improve patient outcome.[9]

Physiologic parameters, including GCS, systolic blood pressure, and respiratory rate are useful outcome predictors and can be used in the ER triage in patients with TBI.

However, severity and prognosis are predicted more effectively if additional factors are also considered, including an altered pupillary reflex, hypotension, and computed tomography (CT) scan findings. Other tests, such as an x-ray and ultrasound, are also helpful to rule out other major injuries. A CT scan facility located in the trauma unit or emergency room reduces the time to acquire CT images and improves overall mortality.[10]

Glasgow Coma Scale: An update

The Glasgow Coma Scale (GCS) first appeared in print by Teasdale and Jennett in *Lancet* in 1974. The article was an attempt to unify the evaluation of patients with altered consciousness, thus facilitating a transfer of information among the professionals who were treating them.[11] Two years later, it was modified into the GCS that is used today, with three items that are assigned specific values, the total sum of which adds up to 15. This is the scale that is used to classify the severity of TBI.[12]

More than 40 years later, the GCS, in combination with other elements of diagnosis, is still an instrument of great importance and credibility, both for the on-site decision-making process as well as for evaluating the need for additional exams or surgery once the patient is in the hospital.[13] Furthermore, the GCS is a strong predictor of in-hospital mortality, duration of coma, and post-traumatic amnesia, as well as of mid- and long-term disability post-TBI.[14] Despite the practically linear correlation between a low GCS score and poor outcomes, this scale should never be used by itself as an outcome guide. Many studies have questioned the applicability of the GCS nowadays, stressing its limitations:

- Studies demonstrate an inaccurate GCS scoring in more than one-third of the assessments. Inter-rater reliability depends on experience and on consistency of assessment technique. More training translates into more accuracy, especially for GCS <13.[15]
- Confounding factors can determine that one or more components of the GCS cannot be tested (Table 6.1). Some of these have even increased since 1974, as patients with severe trauma are now often sedated and intubated at the site of the incident.[13,16]
- Providing only the GCS score implies a significant loss of information and may reduce predictive validity. Healey et al. demonstrated different prognoses in patients with the same global GCS on arrival to the ER. For example, the combination of *Eye 1—Verbal 2—Motor 1* had a mortality of 28%, whereas *Eye 1—Verbal 1—Motor 2* had a mortality of 56%.[17] Also, several studies have shown that the best motor response has relevant prognostic significance for mortality.[13]

Table 6.1 Confounders that influence GCS

Trauma	- Hypovolemic shock
	- Spinal cord injury
	- Thoracic trauma with hypoxia
	- Facial/eye trauma
Previous disease	- Cerebral disorders
	- Neuromuscular disorders
	- Psychiatric disorders
	- Hearing impairment
Drugs	- Sedatives and hypnotics
	- Opioids
	- Neuromuscular blockers
Intoxicants	- Alcohol
	- Drugs
Mechanical devices	- Endotracheal tubes
	- Immobilization devices
Others	- Language and culture

Sources: Adapted from Zuercher M et al., *Brain Inj.* 2009;23(5):371-384; Teasdale G et al., *Lancet Neurol.* 2014;13(8): 844-854.

The development of tools and prognostic models is necessary to guide the decision-making process, including discontinuing certain therapies. Despite several attempts to create these, like the one suggested by Murray et al. or the new FOUR coma scale, the IMPACT (*International Mission for Prognosis and Analysis of Clinical Trials in TBI*) study still considers the motor response of the GCS, along with pupillary reflex, the TBI characteristics, and age as the most reliable independent prognostic factors.[18,19]

A consensus statement should encourage quality improvement programs to reduce the limitations of the GCS.

CT scan: Indications and Marshall classification

After an initial evaluation and resuscitation of the trauma patient, additional tests must be performed to determine the severity of the injury. Which patients require a CT scan following head injury is always a source of controversy, especially in remote areas that are some distance from hospital centers. In the case of severe trauma, there is no doubt, but in moderate or mild brain injury, it may not be as clear and is still a source of debate.

Some indications for a CT scan, in addition to severe TBI, include[20]:

- Patients who remain confused for 2 hours after the initial insult
- Severe headache with nausea or vomiting
- Known coagulopathy or anticoagulant/antiagregant therapy
- Any focal neurologic deficit, including agitation
- "High-energy" accidents (high-speeding vehicles, drops from over 3 feet)

In patients with TBI, CT findings help to classify the severity of brain trauma and guide therapeutic decisions. They also help to estimate a neurologic prognosis and outcomes.

Various grading systems have been developed in an attempt to standardize the reporting of TBI in CT findings. The most widely used is the Marshall system[21] (Table 6.2).

However, like the GCS, this scale has its drawbacks:

- Significant interobserver variability. Measurement of mass volumes is not an exact science.
- Normal CT images, which may be present in mild head injuries, are not considered.
- If it is a retrospective CT reading, as clinical course must be known.

Despite these limitations, the Marshall classification is almost always reported in the literature and remains the standard for CT classification in TBI.

INITIAL MANAGEMENT AND ONGOING RESUSCITATION

The guidelines of Advanced Trauma Life Support (ATLS) provide a standardized protocol for management of the severely injured patient, with special attention on airway, breathing, and circulation, disability, and exposure, following the ABCDE scheme. Therefore, functional outcome may be improved by intensive medical care and prompt surgical interventions.

After the initial assessment upon hospital admission, resuscitation must be continued during the administration of additional tests and transfer to the operating room or the ICU.

The initial management goals of TBI patients are:

1. Stabilization of the patient, if still unstable
2. Prevention of intracranial hypertension
3. Maintenance of an adequate and stable cerebral perfusion pressure (CPP)
4. Avoidance of systemic, secondary brain insults
5. Optimization of cerebral hemodynamics and oxygenation

Table 6.2 Marshall CT classification

Category	Diffuse injury I	Diffuse injury II	Diffuse injury III	Diffuse injury IV	Evacuated mass lesion	Nonevacuated mass lesion
Incidence	2.1%	37.2%	20.2%	2.1%	24.5%	13.8%
CT findings	No visible lesions	Centered midline, visible ventricles	Bilateral swelling (absence of basal cisterns)	Unilateral swelling (>5 mm midline deviation)	Any surgically evacuated lesion	Lesion >25 mL, not surgically evacuated
Images						
Intracranial hypertension	–	28.6%	63.2%	100%	65.2%	64.6%
Bad outcome	0%	33.3%	55.6%	100%	52.6%	76.9%

Source: Marshall LF et al., *J Neurotrauma*. 1992;9(suppl 1):S287-S292.

Table 6.3 Comparison of induction agent effects on ICP and hemodynamics

	Propofol	Etomidate	Ketamine	Thiopental
Hypotension	X	–	–	X
ICP	–	–	Increase[a]	Decrease
Others	Vasodilator	Suppression of cortisol synthesis	Tachycardia	Brain protective effect Venodilator Negative inotrope

[a] Recent evidence suggests that it may be safe in patients with elevated ICP.[25]

Airway management

Airway management is central to the resuscitation of the neurologically ill. In these patients, it is important to maintain adequate oxygenation and ventilation and to prevent aspiration, but the process of induction and intubation is not risk free (it can cause brain herniation, enlargement of a massive infarction, etc.) and should not be performed without a risk-benefit assessment.

The best predictor of aspiration/hypoventilation is a low GCS score. Experts suggest that a GCS <9 has an elevated risk of aspiration; however, there is little evidence for this. In patients with GCS >9, intubation may be necessary because of agitation, inadequate ventilation (especially in chest trauma), or to permit the executing of certain procedures.[1]

When it comes to intubation, some considerations must be taken into account. During airway manipulation, organism responses may result in an increase of intracranial pressure (ICP). This should be controlled by minimizing the amount of time of airway manipulation and the use of specific drugs. Although induction agents decrease the systemic response to intubation and the cerebral metabolic extraction rate for oxygen, they may cause cardiovascular depression.[22]

The **technique** for tracheal intubation depends on the severity of the situation, individual skills, and available resources; however, it usually incorporates rapid sequence intubation with cricoid pressure and manual cervical in-line stabilization.

The choice of **induction drugs and neuromuscular blockers** is important to ensure the safety of the patient, providing good intubation conditions in a short period of time. As for neuromuscular blockers, the choice is between succinylcholine and rocuronium for rapid sequence intubation. It is said that succinylcholine may cause an increase of ICP, but its clinical significance is questionable.[9]

Other drugs, such as lignocaine [1.5 mg/kg] or fentanyl 3 µg/kg administered 1 minute before the induction, is used in order to avoid an increase in ICP.

Table 6.3 shows the characteristics of each induction agent.

Ventilation

After intubation, ventilation should be adjusted to ensure adequate oxygenation and gas exchange, trying to avoid hypoxemia as well as hyper- and hypocapnia, which act as secondary insults to the brain.

Most, but not all, observational studies in TBI have determined an association between early **hypoxia** and poor outcome.[8,23] This association is not as strong as it is for hypotension and may be less significant in children.

Regarding **hyper- and hypocapnia,** both are associated with a substantial increase in in-hospital mortality.[24] Recent evidence has shown that monitoring end-tidal CO_2 (ETCO$_2$) with capnography affects the outcome, thus, current guidelines strongly recommend continuous capnography monitoring, beginning in the prehospital period, in all ventilated patients.[10] As ETCO$_2$ values may be altered by low blood perfusion, ventilation in traumatic patients should be guided by frequent blood gas analysis.

HYPERVENTILATION TO TREAT BRAIN HERNIATION AND INCREASED ICP?

In any case, when patients present signs of incipient brain herniation, hyperventilation may be used as an immediate intervention to decrease ICP and to prevent subsequent neuronal death. Maximal cerebral vasoconstriction is achieved at a pCO$_2$ of 20 mmHg, so it makes no sense to hyperventilate the patient below this level. It is important that, as soon as other treatments to control ICP are performed (osmotherapy, surgery, hypothermia), normocapnia should be rapidly restored.[8,9,26]

The goals of mechanical ventilation should be:

- Normalization of oxygenation, at the lowest FiO_2 that will maintain oxygen saturation >94%.
- Normalization of ventilation, trying to maintain the systemic pH between 7.35–7.45, pCO_2 between 35–45 mmHg or end-tidal CO_2 between 30–40 mmHg.
- Normalization of breathing.
- Prevention of ventilator-induced lung injury.

Achieving these goals may be challenging in trauma patients if there are other major injuries, particularly chest injuries, aspiration of gastric contents, or acute pulmonary edema. A lung-protective ventilation strategy is required in that case. Most clinicians use tidal volumes of approximately 5 to 8 mL/kg of ideal body weight, a respiratory rate of 12 to 14 per minute, a plateau airway pressure below 30 cm H_2O, and, hemodynamic situation permitting, a minimum positive end expiratory pressure of 5 cmH_2O to ensure adequate oxygenation.[1,8,26]

Hemodynamic stability

Maintaining hemodynamic stability in the trauma patient is challenging, especially when various injuries have occurred. It is recommended that patients with severe TBI have arterial and central venous lines started as soon as possible.

Hypotension is a major secondary brain insult, and even an isolated episode of hypotension dramatically worsens the outcome. Hypotension should be treated primarily with fluid resuscitation to restore volemia and, if necessary, vasopressors. The Brain Trauma Foundation (BTF) guidelines recommend a median arterial pressure (MAP) ≥80 mmHg, especially before the insertion of an ICP monitoring device, in an attempt to maintain cerebral perfusion pressure (CPP) ≥60 mmHg for a treatment threshold of ICP >20 mmHg. After ICP monitoring has been achieved, the management of blood pressure will be driven by the ICP/CPP values. Individual decisions should be made to balance the requirements of cerebral oxygenation against the risk of worsening hemorrhage.[27]

Hypertension occurs less frequently but may be a physiologic sympathetic response, translating to compromised cerebral perfusion. An increase in arterial blood pressure could be a compensatory mechanism to maintain an adequate CPP and reducing it could cause cerebral ischemia to become worse. Thus, it should not be treated unless there is a justifiable cause for it or if systolic blood pressure is >180–200 mmHg or MAP is >110–120 mmHg.[28] The drugs of choice are short-acting beta-blockers, as these do not cause cerebral vasodilation, and thus, an increase of cerebral blood volume and ICP is avoided.

Fluid therapy and vasopressors

The initial resuscitation fluid of choice is still a matter of controversy. Many studies have attempted to demonstrate the superiority of one fluid over another. Some studies suggest that Hartmann's solution avoids the acidosis of 0.9% saline; but is slightly hypotonic, which may contribute to cerebral edema and fluid overload. Other studies recommend the use of hypertonic fluids because they might suppress the biomarkers of TBI and are associated with a better outcome. Hypertonic saline is often used for rapid restoration of CPP and reduction of intracranial pressure without affecting coagulation[29]; however, no studies have reported better survival and functional outcomes than the use of isotonic crystalloids. The multicentric Saline versus Albumin Fluid Evaluation (SAFE) trial demonstrated that the use of albumin was associated with the higher mortality data in patients with severe head injury.[30] After these findings, experts recommend a practical approach that includes, on one hand, the avoidance of colloids, as these are associated with coagulopathy; and on the other hand, to use Hartmann's for most trauma cases and 0.9% saline for patients with severe head injury.[30]

Vasopressors are commonly used to avoid or to treat hypotension or potentially inadequate CPP along with volume replacement. There are few studies comparing the use of different vasopressors in TBI, and results are inconclusive. It seems that norepinephrine has a more predictable and consistent effect; however, current evidence does not support recommending one vasopressor over another.[9,31]

Osmotherapy

The use of osmotic agents, like mannitol (0.25–1 g/kg body weight) and 7.5% hypertonic saline, is an effective option for lowering ICP by reducing blood viscosity. However, it is important to remember that it also causes (especially mannitol) osmotic diuresis, which can result in hypovolemia and subsequent hypotension. Hence, osmotherapy is usually recommended only when there are signs of transtentorial herniation or progressive neurologic deterioration that is not attributable to extracranial causes.[8,9,32]

Blood transfusion and coagulopathy

Anemia and the presence of coagulation disorders are common problems in trauma patients and are associated with increased in-hospital mortality and poor outcome in TBI.

However, regarding anemia, there is little evidence to support packed red blood cell (PRBC) transfusion to treat anemia, as current literature suggests that both anemia and PRBC transfusions are associated with poor neurologic outcome.[33] The optimal hemoglobin (Hb) level is still unclear, but a liberal transfusion strategy, defined as transfusion whenever Hb <10 g/dL, has no proven benefits.

As for coagulopathy, there are no guidelines for its management in TBI, and each case must be individualized, depending on hemodynamic state, degree of coagulopathy, associated injuries, and the need for surgery.[9]

Commonly recommended goals for some physiologic parameters are summarized in Table 6.4.[32]

Antifibrinolytic therapy

Tranexamic acid (ATX) is typically administered in surgical patients to diminish the risk of bleeding and the need for blood transfusions. It decreases the number of patients who require a blood transfusion by approximately one-third, the amount of PRBC required in one unit, and the need for repeated surgery (for blood control, in those patients undergoing elective surgery) in half.[34]

More recently, ATX has proven its effect in reducing mortality in trauma patients with extracranial bleeding. The CRASH-2 (*Clinical Randomization of an Antifibrinolytic in Significant Hemorrhage*) study demonstrated that the administration of ATX within the first 8 hours after insult significantly decreased deaths due to bleeding or due to any cause compared with placebo, with no apparent increase in occlusive vascular events.[35] Among those patients who were treated immediately after the injury, the decrease in mortality was even greater.[36]

After these results, ATX has been incorporated in the protocols of trauma management at the global level and it has been included in the list of essential medications of the World Health Organization (WHO). Resuscitation guidelines for the trauma patient with active bleeding recommendations can be seen in Table 6.5.

When referring specifically to the TBI patient, two studies have evaluated the effects of ATX. Despite results not being statistically significant, a CT scan 24 to 48 hours afterward found less intracranial hemorrhage and fewer ischemic lesions in those patients who had received ATX.[37] A second study in patients with isolated TBI also detected a decrease in hemorrhage and mortality with ATX, but this study didn't record data on ischemic lesions. The meta-analysis of both assays shows a significant reduction in hemorrhage and

Table 6.4 Physiologic target in TBI patients

Physiologic parameter	Goal
CPP (*cerebral perfusion pressure*)	≥60 mmHg
Hemoglobin	≥7g/dL
INR (*international normalized ratio*)	≤1.4
PaCO$_2$ (*arterial partial pressure of carbon dioxide*)	35–45 mmHg
PaO$_2$ (*arterial partial pressure of oxygen*)	≥100 mmHg
pH	7.35–7.45
Platelets	≥75,000
Pulse oximetry	≥95%
MAP (*median arterial pressure*)	≥80 mmHg

Source: Whitaker-Lea WA, Valadka AB, *Phys Med Rehabil Clin N Am.* 2017;28(2):227-243.

Table 6.5 Dose of tranexamic acid recommended for the trauma patient with active bleeding

Treatment	Ampules	Dose	Infusion and duration
Loading dose	2	1 gr	Add to a 100 mL bag of 0.9% saline and infuse over 10 minutes
Maintenance dose	2	1 gr	Add to a 500 mL bag of isotonic fluid and infuse over 8 hours

It is recommended not to mix with blood or solutions that contain penicillin or mannitol.

mortality when using ATX. Conclusions were promising; however, results were imprecise and there were not enough data on the effect that antifibrinolytic treatment has on disability after TBI. Moreover, the patients in the CRASH-2 study with TBI also had significant extracranial blood loss, thus, the extrapolation of results to isolated TBI patients is still open for discussion.

Currently, the CRASH-3 (*Clinical Randomization of an Antifibrinolytic in Significant Head Injury*) study is under way. It began in 2011; the plan was to recruit 10,000 patients. This study aims to quantify the effects that the early (within the first 8 hours) administration of ATX has on mortality and disability in patients with TBI.[38] It also aims to evaluate the effect of ATX on occlusive cardiovascular events and convulsions.

Corticosteroids

Corticosteroids have been used to treat head injuries for more than 30 years. In 1997, findings of a systematic review suggested that these drugs reduced risk of death in 1% to 2%.[39] Patients with medullary lesion treated with steroids instead of placebo have been found to improve their motor function, as well as pain and tactile stimuli,[40] and this led to a renewed interest in their role in the treatment of head injury. A multicenter international trial

(CRASH—*Corticosteroid Randomization After Significant Head injury*) was conducted to confirm or refute such an effect. Aiming to recruit 20,000 patients with head injuries and a GCS ≤14, patients received either a 48-hour infusion of corticosteroid (methylprednisolone) or placebo. However, the study was halted in May of 2004, as data demonstrated that, compared to placebo, the risk of death from all causes within 2 weeks and at 6 months was higher in the corticosteroid group,[41] as was the risk of severe disability.[42] In conclusion, after these results, guidelines suggest that corticosteroids should not be used routinely to treat head injury, no matter the severity of the injury.

Indications for emergent surgery

The CT scan findings can help the neurosurgeon decide on whether surgical treatment is necessary. Surgically, significant lesions are relatively uncommon; with incidences of 0.1%–3.2% for GCS 15 and 0.5%–6.5% for GCS 14. Acute neurosurgical intervention is required in less than 1%.[43–46] Surgical indication varies according to the type of hemorrhage:

- In subdural hematoma, clot thickness greater than 10 mm, or a mid line shift greater than 5 mm are suggested as critical parameters for surgery.
- In extradural hematoma, volume of hematoma greater than 30 cm should undergo surgical evacuation.[44]
- In brain contusion, patients with GCS 6–8, with frontal or temporal lesions greater than 20 cc, a midline shift ≥5 mm, and/or compression of the basal cisterns; and all patients with lesions greater than 50 cc, should undergo surgery.[28,47]

If there is uncontrolled intracranial hypertension despite medical treatment, procedures of choice are:

Cerebrospinal fluid (CSF) drainage: Use of a CSF drain to lower ICP in patients with an initial GCS <6 during the first 12 hours after injury may be considered.

Decompressive craniectomy (DC): Bifrontal DC does not improve outcome. However, it does reduce

ICP and minimizes ICU stay; frontotemporoparietal DC reduces mortality and improves neurologic outcomes in patients with severe TBI.[27]

PROCEDURES ACCORDING TO INJURY SEVERITY

Initial treatment of the patient with brain injury often depends on the severity of the head trauma, findings on the CT scan, and associated noncranial injuries. Initial evaluation by a multidisciplinary team is fundamental for correct medical management and will define additional treatment.

Depending on TBI severity and associated lesions, the lines of action are:

Mild brain injury

In a patient with **mild brain injury**, without other body injuries, several clinical indicators help us to know when it is necessary to perform a CT scan upon arrival. These are: Persistent abnormal mental status manifested by either abnormal GCS or

Table 6.6 Surgical recommendations by the Brain Trauma Foundation

Topic	Recommendation
Intracranial pressure monitoring	Management of severe TBI using ICP monitoring is recommended to reduce in-hospital and 2-week postinjury mortality.
	ICP should be monitored in all salvageable patients with a TBI (GCS 3–8 after resuscitation) and an abnormal CT scan.
Cerebral perfusion pressure monitoring	Guideline-based recommendations for CPP monitoring are recommended to decrease 2-week mortality.
Cerebrospinal fluid drainage	An external drain catheter system zeroed at the midbrain with continuous drainage of CSF may be considered to lower ICP burden more effectively than intermittent use.
	Use of CSF drainage to lower ICP in patients with an initial GCS 6 during the first 12 hours after injury may be considered.
Decompressive craniectomy (DC)	Bifrontal DC is not recommended for outcome improvement (as measured by the GOS-E score at 6 months postinjury) in severe TBI patients with diffuse injury, and with ICP elevation to 20 mmHg for more than 15 minutes within a 1-hour period that are refractory to first-tier therapies. However, ICP reduction and less ICU stay has been demonstrated.
	A large frontotemporoparietal DC (no less than 12 x 15 cm or 15 cm diameter) is recommended over a small frontotemporoparietal DC to reduce mortality and improve neurologic outcomes in patients with severe TBI.

Source: Carney N et al., *Neurosurgery.* 2017;80(1):6-15.

abnormal alertness, behavior, or cognition; known coagulopathy (particularly supratherapeutic anticoagulation); and initial symptoms like seizure, prolonged loss of consciousness (more than 5 minutes), worsening of GCS, persistent vomiting, and focal neurologic deficit.[20,48]

If the image studies are normal, the patient can be discharged after a few hours of neurologic observation. The correct discharge requires adequate home support and appropriate advice on when to return to the hospital.[49]

Moderate brain injury

Patients with **moderate brain injury** should undergo an urgent CT scan upon admission. In 10% to 20% of patients with moderate brain injuries, the tendency is to deteriorate (10%–20%); and then injury should be managed as a severe head injury. These patients have higher rates of intracranial lesions.[48] Sherman C et al., describe a 40.3% of abnormal CT scans with 30.6% intracranial lesions.[50]

CT scan findings can help the medical professional to decide about surgical indications.

Severe brain injury

In **severe head injury,** the most important aspect of initial care is the systematic resuscitation (ABCDE), with appropriate measures taken to prevent secondary brain injury. An ICU is essential for the appropriate management of these patients. Recommendations are published and are continually being updated: The Brain Trauma Foundation published a fourth edition of the guidelines for the management of severe traumatic brain injury in 2016. Some of the surgical recommendations are summarized in Table 6.6.[27]

REFERENCES

1. Harris T, Davenport R, Hurst T, Jones J. Improving outcome in severe trauma: Trauma systems and initial management: Intubation, ventilation, and resuscitation. *Postgrad Med J.* 2012;88(1044):588-594.
2. Patel HC, Bouamra O, Woodford M et al. Trends in head injury outcome from 1989 to 2003 and the effect of neurosurgical care: An observational study. *Lancet.* 2005;366(9496):1538-1544.
3. ATLS Subcommittee, American College of Surgeons' Committee on Trauma, International ATLS working group. Advanced trauma life support: The ninth edition. *J Trauma Acute Care Surg.* 2013;74(5):1363-1366.
4. Davis DP. Early ventilation in traumatic brain injury. *Resuscitation.* 2008;76(3):333-340.
5. Victorino GP, Battistella FD, Wisner DH. Does tachycardia correlate with hypotension after trauma? *J Am Coll Surg.* 2003;196(5):679-684.
6. McCullough AL, Haycock JC, Forward DP, Moran CG. Early management of the severely injured major trauma patient. *Br J Anaesth.* 2014;113(2):234-241.
7. Sydenham E, Roberts I, Alderson P. Hypothermia for traumatic head injury. *Cochrane Database Syst Rev.* 2009;(2):CD001048.
8. Moppett IK. Traumatic brain injury: Assessment, resuscitation and early management. *Br J Anaesth.* 2007; 99(1):18-31.
9. Curry P, Viernes D, Sharma D. Perioperative management of traumatic brain injury. *Int J Crit Illn Inj Sci.* 2011;1(1):27-35.
10. Chowdhury T, Kowalski S, Arabi Y, Dash HH. Pre-hospital and initial management of head injury patients: An update. *Saudi J Anaesth.* 2014;8(1):114-120.
11. Teasdale G, Jennett B. Assessment of coma and impaired consciousness. A practical scale. *Lancet.* 1974; 2(7872):81-84.
12. Teasdale G, Jennett B. Assessment and prognosis of coma after head injury. *Acta Neurochirurgica.* 1976;34(1-4):45-55.
13. Zuercher M, Ummenhofer W, Baltussen A, Walder B. The use of Glasgow Coma Scale in injury assessment: A critical review. *Brain Inj.* 2009;23(5):371-384.
14. Sherer M, Struchen MA, Yablon SA, Wang Y, Nick TG. Comparison of indices of traumatic brain injury severity: Glasgow Coma Scale, length of coma and post-traumatic amnesia. *J Neurol Neurosurg Psychiatry.* 2008;79 (6):678-685.
15. Reith FC, Van den Brande R, Synnot A, Gruen R, Maas A. The reliability of the Glasgow Coma Scale: A systematic review. *Intensive Care Med.* 2016;42(1):3-15.
16. Teasdale G, Maas A, Lecky F, Manley G, Stocchetti N, Murray G. The Glasgow Coma Scale at 40 years: Standing the test of time. *Lancet Neurol.* 2014;13(8): 844-854.

17. Healey C, Osler TM, Rogers FB et al. Improving the Glasgow Coma Scale score: Motor score alone is a better predictor. *J Trauma.* 2003;54(4):671-678.

18. Stead LG, Wijdicks EF, Bhagra A et al. Validation of a new coma scale, the FOUR score, in the emergency department. *Neurocrit Care.* 2009;10(1):50-54.

19. Murray GD, Butcher I, McHugh GS et al. Multivariable prognostic analysis in traumatic brain injury: Results from the IMPACT study. *J Neurotrauma.* 2007;24(2):329-337.

20. Honeybul S, Woods P. Initial management of traumatic brain injury in the rural setting. *J Neurosci Rural Pract.* 2013;4(1):33-38.

21. Marshall LF, Marshall SB, Klauber MR et al. The diagnosis of head injury requires a classification based on computed axial tomography. *J Neurotrauma.* 1992;9(suppl 1): S287-S292.

22. Turner BK, Wakim JH, Secrest J, Zachary R. Neuroprotective effects of thiopental, propofol, and etomidate. *AANA J.* 2005;73(4): 297-302.

23. Manley G, Knudson MM, Morabito D, Damron S, Erickson V, Pitts L. Hypotension, hypoxia, and head injury: Frequency, duration, and consequences. *Arch Surg.* 2001; 136(10):1118-1123.

24. Dumont TM, Visioni AJ, Rughani AI, Tranmer BI, Crookes B. Inappropriate prehospital ventilation in severe traumatic brain injury increases in-hospital mortality. *J Neurotrauma.* 2010;27(7):1233-1241.

25. Bar-Joseph G, Guilburd Y, Tamir A, Guilburd JN. Effectiveness of ketamine in decreasing intracranial pressure in children with intracranial hypertension. *J Neurosurg Pediatr.* 2009;4(1):40-46.

26. Seder DB, Riker RR, Jagoda A, Smith WS, Weingart SD. Emergency neurological life support: Airway, ventilation, and sedation. *Neurocrit Care.* 2012;17(suppl 1):S4-S20.

27. Carney N, Totten AM, O'Reilly C et al. Guidelines for the management of severe traumatic brain injury, fourth edition. *Neurosurgery.* 2017;80(1):6-15.

28. Haddad SH, Arabi YM. Critical care management of severe traumatic brain injury in adults. *Scand J Trauma Resusc Emerg Med.* 2012;20:12.

29. Baker AJ, Rhind SG, Morrison LJ et al. Resuscitation with hypertonic saline-dextran reduces serum biomarker levels and correlates with outcome in severe traumatic brain injury patients. *J Neurotrauma.* 2009;26 (8):1227-1240.

30. SAFE Study Investigators, Australian and New Zealand Intensive Care Society Clinical Trials Group, Australian Red Cross Blood Service et al. Saline or albumin for fluid resuscitation in patients with traumatic brain injury. *N Engl J Med.* 2007;357(9):874-884.

31. Steiner LA, Johnston AJ, Czosnyka M et al. Direct comparison of cerebrovascular effects of norepinephrine and dopamine in head-injured patients. *Crit Care Med.* 2004;32 (4):1049-1054.

32. Whitaker-Lea WA, Valadka AB. Acute management of moderate-severe traumatic brain injury. *Phys Med Rehabil Clin N Am.* 2017;28 (2):227-243.

33. Salim A, Hadjizacharia P, DuBose J et al. Role of anemia in traumatic brain injury. *J Am Coll Surg.* 2008;207(3):398-406.

34. Henry DA, Carless PA, Moxey AJ et al. Anti-fibrinolytic use for minimising perioperative allogeneic blood transfusion. *Cochrane Database Syst Rev.* 2011;(1): CD001886.

35. CRASH-2 Trial collaborators, Shakur H, Roberts I et al. Effects of tranexamic acid on death, vascular occlusive events, and blood transfusion in trauma patients with significant haemorrhage (CRASH-2): A randomised, placebo-controlled trial. *Lancet.* 2010; 376(9734): 23-32.

36. CRASH-2 collaborators, Roberts I, Shakur H et al. The importance of early treatment with tranexamic acid in bleeding trauma patients: An exploratory analysis of the CRASH-2 randomised controlled trial. *Lancet.* 2011;377 (9771):1096-1101.

37. CRASH-2 Collaborators, Intracranial Bleeding Study. Effect of tranexamic acid in traumatic brain injury: A nested randomised, placebo controlled trial (CRASH-2 Intracranial Bleeding Study). *BMJ.* 2011;343: d3795.

38. Dewan Y, Komolafe EO, Mejía-Mantilla JH et al. CRASH-3—Tranexamic acid for the treatment of significant traumatic brain

injury: Study protocol for an international randomized, double-blind, placebo-controlled trial. *Trials.* 2012;13:87.

39. Alderson P, Roberts I. Corticosteroids in acute traumatic brain injury: A systematic review of randomised trials. *BMJ.* 1997;314 (7098):1855-1859.

40. Bracken MB, Shepard MJ, Collins WF et al. A randomized, controlled trial of methylprednisolone or naloxone in the treatment of acute spinal cord injury. Results of the Second National Acute Spinal Cord Injury Study. *N Engl J Med.* 1990;322(20):1405-1411.

41. Roberts I, Yates D, Sandercock P et al. Effect of intravenous corticosteroids on death within 14 days in 10008 adults with clinically significant head injury (MRC CRASH trial): Randomised placebo-controlled trial. *Lancet.* 2004;364(9442):1321-1328.

42. Edwards P, Arango M, Balica L et al. Final results of MRC CRASH, a randomised placebo-controlled trial of intravenous corticosteroid in adults with head injury-outcomes at 6 months. *Lancet.* 2005;365(9475):1957-1959.

43. Haydel MJ, Preston CA, Mills TJ, Luber S, Blaudeau E, DeBlieux PM. Indications for computed tomography in patients with minor head injury. *N Engl J Med.* 2000;343 (2):100-105.

44. Ibañez J, Arikan F, Pedraza S, Sánchez E et al. Reliability of clinical guidelines in the detection of patients at risk following mild head injury: Results of a prospective study. *J Neurosurg.* 2004;100(5):825-834.

45. Dunham C, Coates S, Cooper C. Compelling evidence for discretionary brain computed tomographic imaging in those patients with mild cognitive impairment after blunt trauma. *J Trauma.* 1996;41(4):679-686.

46. Teasdale GM, Murray G, Anderson E et al. Risks of acute traumatic intracranial haematoma in children and adults: Implications for managing head injuries. *BMJ.* 1990;300 (6721):363-367.

47. Soon WC, Marcus H, Wilson M. Traumatic acute extradural haematoma—Indications for surgery revisited. *Br J Neurosurg.* 2016;30(2):233-234.

48. *Initial Management of Closed Head Injury in Adults*, 2nd Edition, NSW Institute of Trauma and Injury Management, 2011 Sydney, Australia.

49. Hugenholtz H, Stuss DT, Stethem LL, Richard MT. How long does it take to recover from a mild concussion? *Neurosurgery.* 1988;22 (5):853-858.

50. Stein SC, Ross SE. Moderate head injury: A guide to initial management. *J Neurosurg.* 1992;77(4):562-564.

PART V

Neurosurgery

7

Extradural hematoma

EMMA TEMPLE AND ASHA NANDAKUMAR

INTRODUCTION

Extradural (or epidural) hematoma (EDH) is the term given to a collection of blood that accumulates in the potential space between the periosteal dura and the skull. It is well accepted that any delay in the decompression of a rapidly expanding, or large volume, intracranial hematoma can result in significant morbidity and mortality (disability and death) and; therefore, neurosurgery and clot evacuation are time critical.

Traumatic brain injury (TBI) is the leading cause of disability and death in young adults across developed countries[1,2] with an estimated 1.2 million people living with some degree of disability from TBI in the United Kingdom (UK). This results in significant socioeconomic costs for the individual, the family, and the community. EDH is relatively common, occurring in around 2.7% to 4%[3] of all patients who present with TBI. In fact, EDH is higher among those presenting with severe or fatal head injury. The literature offers a wide range of mortality estimates with some reporting a mortality of up to 40%, although this is likely to be heavily influenced by easy access to diagnostic imaging and proximity to neurosurgical expertise.[4]

Anesthesiologists and intensive care physicians are often involved with TBI patients at an early stage and, therefore, play a key role in diagnosing EDH quickly and, subsequently, saving lives. For this reason it is imperative to develop a sound knowledge base and skills in order to nurture the optimal management of traumatic EDH.

ANATOMY AND PATHOPHYSIOLOGY

In addition to the definition of the term for the potential space between the periosteum (dense membrane composed of fibrous connective tissue that closely wraps all bone except that of the articulating surfaces in joints) dura and the skull, the epidural space also extends from the foramen magnum (the opening in the skull through which the spinal cord passes) to the sacral hiatus. Traumatic EDH can occur at any point along its path, however, spinal EDH will be discussed at some other time.

EDH occurs most commonly as a result of disruption or injury to the middle meningeal artery (or its branches) due to its path beneath the temporal bone of the skull in adults. Around 75% of EDHs are associated with skull fractures. Temporo or temporo-parietal hamatomas (hematomas that appear in the area of the brain where the temporal and parietal lobes meet) are the most common and represent 66% of all EDHs. Frontal EDHs represent approximately 26% of EDHs and are associated with injuries to branches of the ethmoidal artery (branches of the ophthalmic artery that supply blood to the paranasal sinuses and the walls of the nasal cavity).[4] The occipital location (the back of the head or skull) is the least common, occurring in only 1.5% of cases.

The posterior fossa (a depression or hollow, usually in bone) bleeds are much less common than their supratentorial (the region of the brain that contains the cerebellum) counterparts. They represent approximately 2% to 10% of all EDH and 25% to 35% of all SOLs (space-occupying lesion) of the posterior cranial fossa and are usually associated with fractures of the occipital bone of the skull. Unlike temporoparietal or frontal bleeds, 85% of posterior fossa EDHs originate from venous bleeding and are often secondary to damage to the transverse (crosswise) or sigmoid (curved) venous sinuses. This results in a slower, expanding hematoma and thus a more subtle and atypical clinical picture. Posterior fossa EDHs are subsequently often diagnosed late, with harmful consequences.[5]

Isolated EDHs are associated with good prognoses provided that they are managed appropriately. This is because there is minimal injury to the underlying brain parenchyma (all of the functioning tissue of the brain) until the EDH causes a significant SOL and increased intracranial pressure (ICP), which will result in a midline shift, and tentorial and cerebellar herniation.

ETIOLOGY AND EPIDEMIOLOGY

Although traumatic EDH can present at any age, it is most common in patients in their 20s and 30s. Similar to most other categories of adult major trauma, it is more common in males than females (approximately 6:1). This is most likely because of the differences of leisure activities, occupational hazards, and risky behaviors.

The etiology of EDH is dependent on age. Over 10 years of age, road traffic collisions (RTCs) are the most common mode of injury (45%–53%) followed closely by assaults and falls from heights.[3,4]

CLINICAL FEATURES

Presentation

Adult patients will typically present with a history of a "blow to the head" or polytrauma with a mechanism consistent with significant head trauma, such as an RTC. Typically, with an isolated EDH, there is a history of a transient loss of consciousness that, in approximately 20% to 50% of adult patients is followed by a falsely reassuring "lucid interval." The lucid interval can last from a few to many hours following the injury before neurologic deterioration occurs due to compression of the brain and increased ICP, which, if not managed well, can lead to cerebral/tonsillar herniation (coning) and death. Other common symptoms include: headache and nausea and vomiting (63%), which are thought to be caused by the dura stripping from the skull periosteum. There is focal neurological deficit (a problem with nerve, spinal cord, or brain function) in around 30% of patients at the time of presentation (hemiparesis, decerebration [loss of cerebral function], seizures), 60% have a Global Coma Score (GCS) <15[3]; pupillary abnormalities occur in approximately 18% to 44% of patients presenting with EDH.

As previously mentioned, posterior fossa bleeds are less common due to the slower accumulation of blood from venous sinus bleeding. They are more subtle in their presentation and are associated with bradycardia and abnormalities of respiration due to direct brainstem injury and compression.[6]

It is important to remember that in up to 50% of cases, EDH will occur along with other associated lesions. They can be linked to other types of traumatic brain injury, including; subdural hematomas, parenchymal hemorrhage, subarachnoid hemorrhage, diffuse axonal injury (DAI) (a brain injury in which damage in the form of extensive lesions in white matter tracts occurs over a widespread area) and contusions.[4] This will complicate the clinical picture as well as the surgical management of the patient. Cases of patients who seek medical treatment for polytrauma and significant extracranial injuries will generally present atypically and are likely to have additional and often-conflicting management priorities.

Radiologic appearances of extradural hematoma (EDH)

The preferred test is a noncontrast computed tomography (CT) scan because it can quickly identify life-threatening complications of suspected TBI.[7] Magnetic resonance imaging (MRI) tests are more sensitive when it comes to detecting small EDHs and associated intraparenchymal conditions, such as DAI; however, MRI is rarely used for acute TBI or polytrauma because it is logistically more complex and takes longer to conduct, which may delay the treatment of the injury. CT scanners are now common in most emergency departments (ERs) and as such, the National Institute of Clinical Excellence (NICE) has issued guidelines for CT head scans for adults following a head injury.[8] Additionally, CT head imaging is also a part of the majority of local trauma protocol scans for high risk polytrauma patients.

The nonenhanced CT image of an EDH is typically a biconvex (convex on both sides [or lentiform—lens-shaped]) SOL, which adheres to the inside of the skull, often causing a local mass effect on the underlying brain parenchyma. Typically, supratentorial EDHs do not cross suture lines, although, in one study of traumatic EDHs in children, 11% did cross suture lines. In the majority of cases, EDHs form secondary to acute bleeding and, as such, the SOL is extremely dense. With heavy bleeding, the swirl sign can be seen as fresh blood mixes with older blood within the hematoma, creating less dense areas within the clot that is forming.[6,9] As the hematoma spreads, it can cause a midline shift, ventricular effacement and cerebral/tonsillar herniation, all of which may be evident on an initial CT head scan. This result should alert the attending physician to the need for neurosurgery.

Although originally designed to calculate intracerebral hemorrhage volume, EDH volume can be approximated at the bedside by using the Peterson and Espersen equation $(A \times B \times C/2)$.[10–12] This is a calculation based on CT images and is a simplified ellipsoid volume equation, which can be calculated as follows;

A = Maximum length of hemorrhage (in cm)

B = Width of hemorrhage (measured perpendicular to A on the same CT head slice, in cm)

C = CT slice thickness x number of slices (where slice with >74% area of hemorrhage = 1 slice, 25%–74% area of hemorrhage = 0.5 slice, <25% area of hemorrhage = 0 slice)

Although useful, it is important for the clinician to remember that this is an estimation of volume and, therefore, may be inaccurate. When comparing to planimetry (the measurement of surface areas and perimeters by tracing the boundaries), studies have shown that the ABC/2 calculation tends to overestimate EDH volume.[11]

Determinants of outcome

There have been multiple important factors identified in the search for determining long-term outcome of EDH in adults.

- **Age:** The influence of age on outcome in a subgroup of patients with EDH is not as pronounced as it is in TBI patients overall, however, it has been determined that older patients with EDH have a mortality rate three times that of younger adults. Due to increased space within the skull secondary to age-related cerebral atrophy (wasting or decrease of brain tissue), it has been suggested that elderly patients may tolerate conservative management better than younger patients despite EDH >30 cm^3 in volume.[13]
- **GCS:** Presenting or preoperative GCS is a good predictor of outcome in EDH. Gennarelli et al., discovered that patients who have undergone surgery for an isolated EDH with a GCS of 3–5 had a mortality rate of 36% whereas patients with a GCS of 6–8 had a mortality rate of only 9%.[14] This has been corroborated by a number of other studies that identified GCS as the single most important predictor of outcome in patients with EDH who have undergone surgery.[15]
- **Pupillary abnormalities:** This occurs in approximately 20% to 30% of patients with EDH who have undergone surgery and in 62% of patients who are comatose (GCS <9) on admission.[15] Ipsilateral mydriasis (dilation of the pupil on the same side) is not associated with adverse outcome if hematoma evacuation is performed within 70 minutes of pupillary dilatation. Contralateral and bilateral (opposite side and both sides) mydrias are both associated with a less-unfavorable

outcome due to increasing herniation and brainstem injury. However, this has recently been subject to debate. Scotter et al.[16] published a systematic review and a meta-analysis of studies examining the mortality and neurologic outcomes in patients with acute SDH (subdural hemorrhage) or EDH and bilateral fixed and dilated pupils (BFDP). The authors determined that despite popular opinion, BFDP is a poor prognostic tool and that good neurologic recovery is possible in some patients. In the authors' analysis, 54% of patients with EDH and BFDP made a good recovery following surgery. This suggests that a prediction of the patient's physical condition based on pupillary abnormalities alone is challenging and prone to inaccuracies.

- **Associated Lesions:** Associated lesions are found in approximately 30% to 50% of patients who require surgery for EDH. Subdural hemorrhage (SDH) and/or parenchymal lesions in association with EDH lower the chance of a favorable outcome and, in a number of studies, have been found to be an independent predictor of an unfavorable outcome.[17] This is likely due to additional underlying parenchymal damage that does not occur in isolated EDH. The impact of skull fractures on the outcome in EDH is uncertain because several studies that have been published have conflicting results.
- **CT Findings and Hematoma Volume:** There is currently no evidence to suggest that the location of the hematoma is related to neurologic outcome. However, hematoma volume, midline shift (MLS), and mixed-density blood clot are thought to be significant factors in determining outcome. Larger EDH volumes are linked to worse neurologic outcomes, although at what volume this occurs, is up for debate. Currently, the Brain Trauma Foundation (BTF) recommends surgical evacuation for volumes >30 cm^3, irrespective of GCS. Two studies found that a MLS >10–12 mm was associated with significantly increased mortality.[15]

MANAGEMENT OF EDH

The management of a rapidly expanding EDH is time critical. A delay in surgical decompression can result in significantly increased morbidity and mortality (disability and death) and can occur anywhere along the patient pathway.[18] Since the

time from injury to evacuation of an intracranial hematoma is critical for a favorable outcome, all components of the healthcare system must aim to avoid a delay. Anesthesiologists and intensive care physicians often help to reduce avoidable delays while ensuring good, ongoing clinical management and basic resuscitation of the patient with TBI.

Initial management

The initial management of traumatic brain injury will largely depend on the history and mechanism of injury. In the majority of cases, patients should undergo an immediate, full assessment and examination of the trauma to identify and treat the life-threatening condition according to the Advanced Trauma Life Support (ATLS) guidelines.[1] The treatment of the polytrauma patient is complex and senior decision makers should be involved early on to guide treatment priorities.

The initial management of an acute TBI focuses on interventions to prevent secondary brain injury while managing or observing the primary injury, if indicated. Targeted resuscitation and early injury management have resulted in a decline in morbidity and mortality over the last few decades. Although optimal management of the TBI patient is controversial, it is well accepted that episodes of hypotension (systolic BP <90 mmHg) and hypoxia <10 KpA (exact value is debated) have a negative effect on patient outcome. The number and duration of episodes of hypotension and hypoxia are known to correspond with mortality. Seizures should be treated early and aggressively although there is no indication of an urgent need for prophylactic anticonvulsant medication.

Patients with TBI should have oxygen titrated to maintain PaO$_2$ >10 KpA.[19] If there are concerns regarding airway patency, inadequate ventilation, or concerns about increased ICP, intubation and ventilatory support is often required. Tracheal intubation remains the gold standard for airway management for patients with TBI.[1] The risks associated with this are not insignificant (hypertensive response to laryngoscopy, aspiration, cardiovascular instability) and in the context of polytrauma, may be challenging. It should be considered that these patients have a full stomach and; therefore, they should receive rapid-sequence induction. There is much debate surrounding the most appropriate anesthetic agents and technique to use in this scenario; however, anesthesiologists should use their knowledge and skills to intubate the trachea for maximal cardiovascular stability and avoid hypoxia and hypercapnia. This may require a different combination of medications and equipment in different clinical scenarios. The risks and benefits of this decision should be assessed by a senior anesthesiologist or intensive care specialist in conjunction with the trauma team.

Consideration should be given to cervical immobilization due to associated risks between cervical cord injury and TBI. This can be challenging considering the inclination of the TBI patient to move; additionally, cervical collars often cause a reduction in venous flow and hence contribute to increased ICP.

Anticoagulant medication should be stopped immediately and attempts should be made to normalize coagulation in an effort to prevent further increases in hematoma volume. This should be initiated with the local hematology and neurosurgical protocols or advice in mind. It is essential to determine the reason for anticoagulation because, in many cases (such as patients with metallic cardiac valves), there is significant risk to normalizing coagulation and this needs to be weighed against the morbidity and risk to the outcome of an expanding EDH.

In cases in which there are concerns about significantly increased ICP and all first-line management targets are being met, osmotherapy may be considered as a temporary measure whilst the patient is being transferred for surgery. Mannitol $0.25–1 \text{ g Kg}^{-1}$ repeated as necessary, as needed, or hypertonic saline (5%) $1–2 \text{ mL/Kg}^{-1}$ (q 4–6 hourly max 8 mL/kg^{-1} in 24 h) can be used if the patient has a normal blood volume and serum osmolality <320.

Operative vs. nonoperative management of EDH

EDH can be managed surgically by hematoma evacuation, or conservatively (nonoperative management). The indications for surgery are dependent on hematoma characteristics in addition to the patient's clinical presentation and imaging studies. The patient's neurologic path over time is also an important factor, which influences the decision to operate and thus should be carefully observed and documented. When indicated, rapid surgical evacuation of EDH is associated with an excellent prognosis and is thus the most cost-effective neurosurgical operation.[12] However, there is insufficient

data at present to support one surgical treatment method over another; however, craniotomy is thought to provide a more complete hematoma evacuation than a burr hole method.

In the 2007 National Confidential Enquiry into Patient Outcome and Death (NCEPOD) report, *Trauma: Who Cares?*[19] 23% of the TBI patients included in the study underwent a surgical procedure as a consequence of their head trauma, the majority of which involved an insertion of an ICP monitoring device (54%). Fifty-four additional surgeries were performed related to decompression of a SOL or decompressive craniectomies for raised ICP. Of these surgeries, 19.3% were for evacuation of EDH.

The BTF has produced informative guidelines on the management of EDH. Conservative management under close observation in a neurosurgical center can be considered if all of the following conditions are met:

- Noncomatose (GCS >8)
- No focal neurologic deficit
- No pupillary abnormalities
- EDH volume <30 cm^3
- EDH thickness <15 mm
- Midline shift <5 mm
- Ability to undergo serial CT scanning (repeated scan should occur 6–8 hours postinitial scan or in the event of any deterioration)

Surgical management is indicated if either the criteria for conservative management is not met or for any patient presenting with EDH volume >30 cm^3, irrespective of his or her GCS.

This guidance was based on early case studies and cohort studies published over 20 years ago and, consequently, has recently become a subject of debate in the literature. Soon et al.[12] reported that more recent studies suggest that EDH volume does not contribute to prognostic value and, therefore, an isolated EDH with volume >30 cm^3 should not automatically result in surgery. They comment that this may be of particular importance when considering the management of EDH in the elderly. Due to the increased space inside the skull secondary to age-related cerebral atrophy, older patients may potentially tolerate a greater EDH volume without neurologic deterioration, thus avoiding the increased risks of surgery and anesthesia in older age.

Timing of surgery and transfer

It is strongly recommended that a patient with an acute EDH and neurologic deterioration, as defined by onset of coma and/or pupillary abnormalities, should undergo hematoma evacuation as soon as possible; ideally, within 70 minutes of pupillary dilatation. Every hour delay is associated with progressively worse outcome.[15] For patients without neurologic deterioration,[17] there is less justification for expedited surgery.

In situations in which patients requiring time-critical surgery are more than 70 minutes from a neurosurgical center, there is an ongoing debate about whether clot evacuation should be performed locally by non-neurosurgeons prior to transfer. There are a number of recommendations published on emergency burr holes for non-neurosurgeons; however, studies examining this are limited and uncontrolled with respect to patient selection because those patients who require immediate surgery are likely to have more severe injuries and are, therefore, subject to bias.[20] Current studies suggest that patients undergoing surgery at a non-neurosurgical center have a significantly worse outcome than those admitted directly to a neurosurgical center. However, this has to be weighed against the risks of unnecessary neurologic deterioration caused by surgery delay due to transfer. Following a study of 107 patients operated on for EDH, Poon and Li discovered that patients who were transferred from an outside institution had a significantly greater delay from neurologic deterioration to surgery than patients admitted directly (3.2 ± 0.5 hours vs. 0.7 ± 1 hour). At 6 months, neurologic outcome was significantly better in patients who experienced a minimal delay between deterioration and surgery.[21]

Although this is likely to be less of a concern for most areas of the UK where neurosurgical expertise can be accessed relatively quickly, transfer of critically ill or unstable patients carries risk and, therefore, ideally, patients with suspected severe TBI should be triaged directly to a neurosurgical center. If transfer occurs, the patient should receive the same level of expert critical care required throughout his or her experience.

The need to transfer can also be complicated by a lack of capacity at the neurosurgical center, often due to a lack of critical care capacity, as highlighted in the recent NCEPOD report. It is vitally important that clear protocols are put in place locally in order to make the process of accessing neurosurgical care smooth in order to reduce delay.

PERIOPERATIVE CONSIDERATIONS

Anesthetic considerations are similar to that of any time-critical emergency neurosurgery requiring craniotomy for decompression of increased ICP. The process should be a seamless continuation of ongoing resuscitation. Care must be taken to maintain adequate cerebral perfusion pressure (CPP) throughout by avoiding hypotension through considered anesthetic agent choices in addition to careful titration of fluid or blood product resuscitation and vasopressors. Adequate analgesia and anesthesia therapy can also help to improve the outcome by reducing cerebral oxygen consumption ($CMRO_2$). There is much debate about the *best* anesthetic for such patients; however, it is understood that while rapidly evaporating agents may reduce $CMRO_2$, they may also cause cerebral vasodilatation and loss of autoregulation with respect to CO_2. However, this effect is thought to be minimal at concentrations below 1 MAC and Sevoflurane (used for maintenance of general anesthesia) is thought to have the most favorable profile. Total intravenous anesthesia (TIVA) with Propofol and Remifentanil offer an excellent alternative as it reduces $CMRO_2$, CBF, and ICP. However, the anesthesiologist must be aware of the significant risk of hypotension with the technique. Neuromuscular blocking agents can be used to reduce movement and offer a good surgical field.

Secondary cerebral insults (the result of the injury) can be prevented by adequate oxygenation, normocapnia, and strict avoidance of hyper- or hypoglycemia and hyperthermia. Monitoring should be used in line with the Association of Anaesthetists of Great Britain Ireland (AAGBI) guidelines with the addition of invasive blood pressure monitoring, which allows beat-to-beat monitoring of blood pressure and regular arterial blood gas and glucose sampling.

The positioning in surgery will depend on the location of the hematoma and the surgical preference; however, in most cases, the surgery can be performed supine (lying on the back) with a degree of lateral (side) head tilt. Posterior fossa bleeds (bleeds at the back of the skull) may be more challenging to access and may require prone (lying face down) positioning.

Anesthesiologists should be alert from the moment that the skull is opened and the increased ICP is alleviated. In some cases, this can result in significant cardiovascular instability due to the fall in sympathetic stimulation from intracranial hypertension.

EXTRADURAL HEMORRHAGE IN CHILDREN

Overall, the incidence of EDH in children is less than that found in adults. This has been attributed to the tighter adherence of the dura to the inner table of the skull.[12] There is a wide range of reported mortality estimates but they are approximately 0% to 17%. It has been reported that younger children who present with EDH have a higher mortality rate than older children.[3]

Children typically present EDH less often and thus the injury is often examined late and with fewer typical, nonspecific symptoms. This may be due to the higher incidence of venous bleeding, which causes EDH in addition to the unfused sutures, open fontenelles, large extracerebral spaces, and basal cisterns, which allow children to cope better with increased ICP. There is a higher incidence of EDH without skull fracture in children, likely due to their increased bone plasticity and flexibility. They predominantly present with vomiting and/or a reduced level of consciousness. Seizures occur early in approximately 8% of children. In younger children (younger than 10 years of age), falls are the most common type of traumatic EDH. Even a fall from a height of less than 1 meter [3.3 feet]) can cause an EDH with a fatal outcome.

Above 10 years of age, RTC becomes the most common type of injury after falls. With increasing age, injuries become increasingly more common, comprising up to 30% of EDHs in the 16+ years age group.[3] The medical team must always consider the possibility of nonaccidental injury (NAI) in the younger child.

NICE has issued guidelines for indications for the immediate/emergency department management of children with a head injury.[22] Any positive findings on imaging or clinical concerns should be discussed with the neurosurgical center without delay.

There is no current consensus on when to perform surgery on the child with an asymptomatic EDH.[12,23] There are a number of studies that have reported excellent outcomes following conservative management[24]; however, others have argued that, in this age group, in particular, the risks of surgery and anesthesia are low and early surgery may prevent EDH complications from occurring.

SUMMARY

EDHs are common among patients presenting with moderate-to-severe TBIs. If managed correctly and quickly, especially when presenting with GCS <9 and anisocoria (pupils of different sizes in the same person), an excellent neurologic outcome can often be achieved. Predicting neurologic outcome in the context of EDH is challenging and may be inaccurate; even patients presenting with BDFP should be considered for emergency surgery.

The attending anesthesiologist or intensive care physician should focus on minimizing delays of diagnosis and obtaining expert neurosurgical advise and/or treatment while minimizing potential secondary brain injury by optimizing the patient's physiology according to current BTF/NICE guidelines. If the patient needs to be transferred to a neurosurgical center, this should be done without delay and the patient should be provided with the same level of care as he or she would receive in a critical care unit.

Surgical management is guided by numerous factors, including neurologic status, progress of neurologic status, and characteristics of the hematoma and underlying brain on a CT scan.

REFERENCES

1. Dinsmore J. Traumatic brain injury: An evidence-based review of management. *Continuing Education in Anaesthesia, Critical Care & Pain.* 2013;13(6):189-195.
2. Yates PJ, Williams WH, Harris A, Round A, Jenkins A. An epidemiological study of head injuries in a UK population attending an emergency department. *J Neurol Neurosurg Psychiatry.* 2006;77(5): 699–701.
3. Irie F, Le Brocque R, Kenardy J, Bellamy N, Tetsworth K, Pollard C. Epidemiology of

traumatic epidural hematoma in young age. *J Trauma.* 2011;71(4):847-853.

4. Chowdhury NK, Raihan MZ, Chowdhury FH, Ashadullah ATM, Sarkar MH, Hussain SS. Surgical management of traumatic extradural haematoma: Experiences with 610 patients and prospective analysis. *Indian Journal of Neurotrauma.* 2008;5(2):75-79.

5. Khwaja HA, Hormbrey PJ. Posterior cranial fossa venous extradural haematoma: An uncommon form of intracranial injury. *Emerg Med J.* 2001;18(6):496-497.

6. Dirim BV, Orük C, Erdoŭan N, Gelal F, Uluc E. Traumatic posterior fossa hematomas. *Diagn Interv Radiol.* 2005;11(1):14-18.

7. Kolias A, Guilfoyle M, Helmy A, Allanson J, Hutchinson P. Traumatic Brain Injury in Adults. *Pract Neurol.* 2013;13:228-235.

8. Yates D, Aktar R, Hill J, Guideline Development Group. Assessment, investigation, and early management of head injury: Summary of NICE guidance. *BMJ.* 2007;335(7622):719-720.

9. Hopkins R, Peden C, Ghandhi S. Radiology for Anaesthesia and Intensive Care. *Cambridge University Press.* 2010.

10. Kothari RU, Brott T, Broderick JP et al. The ABCs of measuring intracerebral hemorrhage volumes. *Stroke.* 1996;27(8):1304-1305.

11. Hu TT, Yan L, Yan PP, Wang X, Yue GF. Assessment of the ABC/2 method of epidural hematoma volume measurement as compared to computer-assisted planimetric analysis. *Biol Res Nurs.* 2016;18(1):5-11.

12. Khan MB, Riaz M, Javed G, Hashmi FA, Sanaullah M, Ahmed SL. Surgical management of traumatic extra dural hematoma in children: Experiences and analysis from 24 consecutively treated patients in a developing country. *Surg Neurol Int.* 2013;4:103.

13. Soon W, Marcus H, Wilson M. Traumatic acute extradural haematoma - indications for surgery revisited. *Br J Neurosurg.* 2016;30(2):233-234.

14. Gennarelli TA, Spielman GM, Langfitt TW et al. Influence of the type of intracranial lesion on outcome from severe head injury. *J Neurosurg.* 1982;56(1):26-32.

15. Bullock MR, Chesnut R, Ghajar J et al. Surgical management of acute epidural hematomas. *Neurosurgery.* 2006;58(suppl 3):S7-S15.

16. Scotter J, Hendrickson S, Marcus HJ, Wilson MH. Prognosis of patients with bilateral fixed dilated pupils secondary to traumatic extradural or subdural haematoma who undergo surgery: A systematic review and meta-analysis. *Emerg Med J.* 2015;32(8):654-659.

17. Lee EJ, Hung YC, Wang LC, Chung KC, Chen HH. Factors influencing the functional outcome of patients with acute epidural hematomas: Analysis of 200 patients undergoing surgery. *J Trauma.* 1998;45(5):946-952.

18. Mendelow AD, Karmi MZ, Paul KS, Fuller GA, Gillingham FJ. Extradural haematoma: Effect of delayed treatment. *Br Med J.* 1979;1(6173):1240-1242.

19. NCEPOD. Trauma: Who cares? *National Confidential Enquiry into Patient Outcome and Death* (2007).

20. Wilson MH, Wise D, Davies G, Lockey D. Emergency burr holes: "How to do it." *Scand J Trauma Resusc Emerg Med.* 2012;20:20-24.

21. Poon W, Li AK. Comparison of management outcome of primary and secondary referred patients with traumatic extradural haematoma in a neurosurgical unit. *Injury.* 1991;22(4):323-325.

22. National Institute for Health and Clinical Excellence. Head injury: Triage, assessment, investigation and early management of head injury in infants, children and adults. *NICE Clinical Guideline 56.* London: National Institute for Health and Clinical Excellence, 2007.

23. Bejjani GK, Donahue DJ, Rusin J, Broemeling LD. Radiological and clinical criteria for the management of epidural hematomas in children. *Pediatr Neurosurg.* 1996;25(6):302-308.

24. Chen TY, Wong CW, Change CN et al. The expectant treatment of "asymptomatic" supratentorial epidural hematomas. *Neurosurgery.* 1993;32(2):176-179.

8

Subdural hematoma

SHANALI THIRUNAVUKKARASU AND MORFAIZAN AHMAD

INTRODUCTION

Subdural hematomas (SDHs) are one of the most common neurosurgical disorders that require surgical intervention. They represent an extracerebral blood collection, which can be formed as a solid clot or in liquid form, located between the dura mater and middle layer of the meninges (arachnoid) and which does not expand in the subarachnoid area or in the basal cistern. This is usually caused by trauma but can be spontaneous or result from an intervention or procedure such as lumbar puncture as well.[1,2] The compressive effect on the brain produces localizing neurologic signs, signs of increased intracranial pressure (ICP) and a change in the level of consciousness.

The pathophysiology of subdural hemorrhages has a time-dependent, heterogeneous nature. Approximately 1% to 6% of untreated, acute subdural hematomas (ASDHs) experience transformation into chronic subdural hematomas (CSDHs) by 3 weeks after the initial injury.[3,4] ASDHs and CSDHs display significantly different behaviors and dynamics. Approximately 10% to 20% of patients are admitted to the hospital with traumatic brain injury (TBI).[4,5]

Infants, the elderly, and patients with alcoholism are groups at risk for developing SDHs. In the infant brain, SDHs are caused by the tearing of the bridging veins in the subdural space.[3,6–8] Cerebral atrophy can occur in people over the age of 60,

causing tension on the veins, which may then also be weaker and more susceptible to injury as a consequence of age.[9] Arachnoid cysts are more commonly associated with CSDH in patients younger than 40 years.[3] Alcohol misuse leads to a risk of thrombocytopenia (an abnormally low level of platelets), prolonged bleeding times, and blunt head trauma and is a risk factor for SDHs.

Depending on the amount of time that passes from the initial trauma to the onset of symptoms and signs, subdural hematomas can be classified into the following groups:[10]

- Acute subdural hematoma: The manifestations appear during the first 3 days
- Subacute subdural hematoma: Clinically manifests between 4 and 21 days
- Chronic subdural hematoma: The clinical manifestations appear after 21 days

As the population ages, we are confronted with a growing number of elderly patients with TBI who often suffer from delayed onset of symptoms of intracranial hematomas associated with prehospital, anticoagulant medication and antiplatelet therapy.

Epidemiology

SDHs can occur in about one-third of people with TBI. It is more common with increasing age. Meagher and Young found a prevalence of 7.35 cases per 100,000 population in those aged 70 to 79 years.[11] A United Kingdom (UK)-based epidemiologic study determined that the annual incidence of SDH/effusion in infants is approximately 12.5 cases per 100,000 population in 0 to 2 year olds and approximately 24 cases per 100,000 in 0 to 1 year olds.[12] The majority of cases were determined to be due to nonaccidental injury (57%). Spontaneous intracranial hypotension has also been reported as a rare cause.[13]

CHRONIC SUBDURAL HEMATOMA

With an approximate incidence of 2% to 3% in neurosurgical centers, SDHs usually have a traumatic etiology and are most often the result of a fall from standing or from a greater height.[10,14] The trauma is usually minor, with an anteroposterior direction and causes the rupture of the emissary veins to the superior saggital sinus.

In TBI, between the acceleration and deceleration of the skull and the encephala, there is a short interval, and then the brain quickly follows the movement and then stops the skull. The moment the skull stops moving, the brain, which has inertia, continues its movement while determining the

stretching and subsequent rupture of the bridging veins in the subdural space. If the traumas have a lateral direction, the subdural hematoma can rarely form, in which case, in addition to the subdural hematoma, there are also brain contusions or brain dilacerations.[13,14]

The incidence of CSDH is estimated at 18 in 100,000 people and increases to 58 in 100,000 in those over 65 years of age. The median age of patients with chronic subdural hematomas is 63 years.[14–17]

Chronic subdural hematomas are more common in the male gender—64% vs. 33%, according to some studies, 72% vs. 28% according to other studies. As far as the localization of CSDHs is concerned, studies have shown a higher frequency of CSDHs in the left brain hemisphere (52%) compared with the ones of the right brain hemisphere (30%) and in 18% of the cases, the CSDH is bilateral (on both sides).[10,14,18,19]

ACUTE SUBDURAL HEMATOMA

Karibe et al. have reported on the analysis by the Traumatic Coma Data Bank (TCDB), in the United States; and the Japan Neurotrauma Data

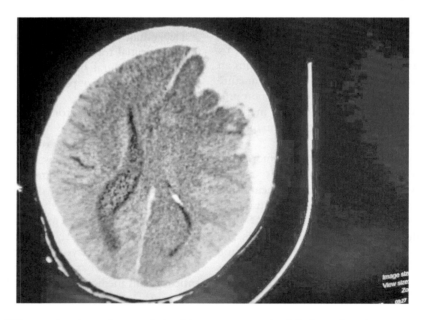

Figure 8.1 A CT scan showing a large subdural hematoma on the left frontal region.

Bank (JNTDB), that most ASDHs are caused by motor vehicle–related accidents (MVAs) and falls; frequency of assaults or other mechanisms is significantly less. MVAs are most frequent in the younger (15–30-year-old) age group.[20–22] Falls are most frequent in the older (45–80-year-old) age group. Studies involving comatose patients have demonstrated MVAs as the mechanism of injury in most ASDHs, suggesting that MVAs not only cause more severe injuries but also accompany diffuse axonal injury (Figure 8.1).

Approximately 40% to 80% of patients with ASDHs present with a Glasgow Coma Scale (GCS) score of 8 or less. Mortality in those patients with a GCS score of 3–15 is in the range of approximately 30% to 60% and those with a GCS of 8 or less have a mortality of 55% to 70%.[20,23–26]

PROGNOSIS

Timing and the nature of neurosurgical intervention in a patient with an SDH depends on multiple factors, including the size of the clot(s), age, and the location of the hematoma, in addition to the medical and neurologic condition of the patient. Surgery may be urgently required, yet even emergency surgery does not guarantee a satisfactory outcome.[27–29]

Studies have shown an increase in favorable outcome in younger patients. A patient younger than 40 years was associated with a mortality rate of 20%, whereas ages 40 to 80 years was associated with a mortality rate of 65%. A patient older than 80 years carried a mortality rate of 88%.[27,30–32]

The final prognosis depends on the amount of associated direct brain damage and the damage resulting from the mass effect of the hematoma. A simple ASDH (without parenchymal injury) accounts for about half of all cases and is associated with a mortality rate of approximately 20%. A complex subdural hematoma (accompanying a contusion or laceration of the cerebral hemisphere) is associated with a mortality rate of approximately 60%.[32,33]

Surgical evacuation via craniotomy is often considered in patients with an ASDH thicker than 5 mm (as measured with axial computed tomography [CT]) and those who have any neurologic

signs, such as lethargy, change in mental status, or a focal neurologic deficit. Bullock et al. reported that for ASDH with a thickness greater than 10 mm, or a midline shift greater than 5 mm on a CT scan, the patient's hematoma should be surgically evacuated, regardless of the patient's GCS score.[28,29,33–35]

Surgery for a chronic SDH may also be indicated if the hematoma is symptomatic or is producing a significant mass effect, as evaluated by diagnostic imaging. Diagnostic imaging that shows an expanding hematoma may also indicate the need for surgery, even in some patients whose neurologic status is almost normal.

Acute subdural hematoma

The mortality of a patient with an acute subdural hematoma (SDH) has been reported to be in the range of 36% to 79%. Many survivors do not regain previous levels of function, especially after an acute SDH that is severe enough to need surgical drainage. Favorable outcome rates after an acute SDH range from 14% to 40%.[30–32]

Hanit et al. demonstrated that mortality was significantly higher in older patients (50% above 70 years, 25% between 40 to 70 years, and 26% below 40 years). Overall outcome was poorer (Glasgow outcome score 3–5) for elderly patients, even after intervention.[36]

Other poor prognostic indicators for acute SDH have been reported to include the initial and postresuscitation GCS, the GCS motor score on admission, pupillary abnormalities, alcohol use, injury by motorcycle, ischemic damage, hypoxia (too little oxygen in the body) or hypotension, and overall ability to control ICP.[30,37–39]

Chronic subdural hematoma

Outcome after drainage of a chronic SDH has also been found to correlate with preoperative neurologic status. Early diagnosis before a significant neurologic deterioration may correlate with a more favorable prognosis. However, no correlation has been found between CT findings before surgery and postoperative outcome.[14,18,19]

The mortality within 30 days of surgery is 3.2% to 6.5%. Approximately 80% of patients resume their prehematoma level of function and favorable outcomes occur in 61% of patients aged 60 years or younger and in 76% of patients older than 60 years.[31,32,40,41]

Management

The crucial element that is needed to manage SDHs is prompt evaluation of these patients as emergency cases. This depends on early recognition of potential intracranial injuries of those patients; the immediate correction of factors leading to secondary injuries; the rapid diagnosis of intracranial pathology; and immediately administering the most appropriate treatment for the patients, which is often surgery.

A surgical guideline for decompression of SDHs is well established. Subdural hemorrhages with a thickness greater than 10 mm and/or a midline shift greater than 5 mm on a CT scan should be surgically evacuated regardless of the patient's GCS. There is also a consensus on draining CSDHs if they are symptomatic and if they present with a thickness greater than 1 cm.[28,29,35–39]

Cautious management is generally considered appropriate for SDHs that are small, do not cause a significant midline shift or cisternal encroachment and do not cause significant neurologic impairment. Typically, this includes a patient with:

- GCS 9 to 15 with a subdural hematoma <10 mm and midline shift <5 mm
- GCS <9 with a hematoma <10 mm and midline shift of <5 mm who has been stable between the time when the injury occurred and when the patient came to the emergency department; with reactive, symmetric pupils and ICP <20 mmHg

ACUTE SUBDURAL HEMATOMA

Craniotomy

Surgery to manage an ASDH usually consists of a craniotomy to decompress the brain; to stop any active subdural bleeding; and, if indicated, to evacuate any intraparenchymal hematoma in the immediate vicinity. ASDHs usually have a firm consistency, which does not permit removal through burr holes alone. Including the Sylvian fissure in the craniotomy, exposure should be considered, because this is likely the location of a ruptured cortical vessel. If brain injury and edema

are associated with the SDH, an ICP monitor can be activated at this time. Bullock et al. stated that "All patients with acute SDH in a GCS score of less than 9 should undergo intracranial [ICP] pressure monitoring."[27–29]

Craniectomy

Craniectomy is also sometimes required, especially when an increase in ICP is present or anticipated. A meta-analysis by Zhang et al. showed that early decompressive craniectomy (DC) [time to surgery after injury <24 h] may be more helpful in improving the long-term outcome of patients with refractory, raised ICP after moderate or severe TBI than late DC. Bilateral pupillary abnormality generally indicates an unfavorable outcome and increased mortality in those patients with a DC after moderate or severe TBI.[28,42]

Theoretically, from the time of the injury to the time of the surgery may be an important factor in rescuing brain tissue from secondary ischemia due to compression and/or intracranial hypertension (ICH) by an ASDH. In general, prompt evacuation of an ASDH is recommended in patients with any indications for surgery.

A study in 1981 demonstrated 30% mortality in patients with an ASDH who were operated on within 4 hours after the injury occurred and 90% mortality in those patients who waited more than 4 hours after injury.[43] It has also been determined that the time from when the injury occurred to the time when the surgery was performed was significantly shorter in patients with a functional recovery than with a fatal outcome, suggesting the importance of prompt evacuation of an acute subdural hematoma.[28,32,44] It has also been reported that there are trends indicating that earlier surgery improves outcome, although the time from injury to operative evacuation of an ASDH with regard to outcome morbidity and mortality were not statistically significant, even when examined at hourly intervals.[28,44]

There is still uncertainty regarding DC for the primary evacuation of ASDHs. In 2011, a collaborative group was formed in the UK with the goal of answering the following question: "What is the clinical- and cost-effectiveness of decompressive craniectomy, in comparison with craniotomy for adult patients undergoing primary evacuation of an ASDH?" The proposed RESCUE-ASDH trial (Randomized Evaluation of Surgery with

Craniectomy for patients Undergoing Evacuation of Acute Subdural Hematoma) is a multicenter, pragmatic, parallel-group, randomized trial of DC vs. craniotomy for adult TBI patients with an ASDH. The trial results demonstrate that there is significant uncertainty as to the optimal surgical technique for primary evacuation of ASDH.[45]

With data now available from DC and RESCUE ICP, there is concern that lifesaving surgery may not leave the patient with normal function. Further investigations, which explore patient selection, longer-term recovery, and quality of life may be indicated.[46,47]

CHRONIC SUBDURAL HEMATOMA

The three main surgical techniques used for the treatment of SDHs consist of the following:

1. Craniotomy: Most often used in the past, it has the advantage of exposing an important part of the brain for clot evacuation. It is usually performed under general anesthesia and it is the most invasive of the treatment options as it is a longer procedure and it anticipates a lot of blood loss during surgery. However, it remains the chosen option in cases of old, organized, multiseptated subdural hematomas (hematomas that require surgery). In Markwalder's study[16] on chronic subdural hematomas, craniotomy, which was considered a radical approach, was reserved for cases in which: (a) the subdural hematoma had relapsed; (b) the hematoma seemed to be very well organized on CT examination and was of a solid consistency; (c) the brain did not re-expand and obliterated the subdural area.[10,48]
2. Minimal craniotomy (trephination): One of the most-often-used surgical techniques in cases of current CSDHs. According to a national Canadian study in 2005, 85% of the respondents indicated that this technique is the most commonly used initial surgical treatment. However, in cases of relapse, 1% preferred the craniotomy and only trephination.[10,49] It is usually done under general anesthesia, some surgeons preferring only one trephination, others two. Nevertheless, neither of the two options demonstrated a clear advantage, although, in one study, it was shown that patients who received only one trephination had a high relapse rate, a longer hospitalization period, and high rates of postoperative wound infection.[10,50]

3. Single-twist drill trephination: The greatest advantage of this procedure is that it can be performed in the hospital bed while using local anesthesia or in an operating room under local or general anesthesia. It is considered useful in those patients with multiple diseases or conditions, often the elderly, in whom the risks of a complex surgery are very high. Single-twist drill trephination is efficient only in cases in which the subdural hematoma is completely liquefied and, therefore, drainable.[10]

A closed drainage system may remain in the subdural space for 24 to 72 hours postoperatively. Santarius et al. found that the placement of drains after drainage of CSDHs reduces recurrence and improves clinical outcome. The randomized, controlled trial of 269 adult patients with a chronic SDH for burr-hole drainage was stopped prematurely due to the recurrence being reduced with drain placement. The hematoma recurred in 10 of 108 (9.3%) patients with a drain compared with 26 of 107 (24%) patients without a drain. At 6 months, mortality was 8.6% in treated patients and 18.1% in controls.[51]

Bilateral CSDHs may require drainage from both sides, usually during the same operation by means of burr holes placed on each side of the head. However, the recurrence rate of a chronic hematoma after surgical evacuation remains at least at 30%, and the use of glucocorticoids to lower the incidence of this complication remains controversial despite their long, effective history.[52] A multicenter, phase III trial, the DRESH study aimed to evaluate the efficacy of dexamethasone (an anti-inflammatory, anti-allergic agent) in reducing the reoperation rate of CSDH, which was started in Austria and China in February 2014.[53] The Steroids in Chronic Subdural Hematomas (SUCRE) study—a double-blind, randomized, controlled trial comparing methylprednisolone with placebo in the treatment of CSDH without clinical and/or radiologic signs of severity—was also started in June 2016 to clarify the role of corticosteroids in the management of CSDH.[54]

HEMOSTATIC THERAPY

Recent evidence suggests that rapid correction of coagulopathy and the enhancement of coagulation variables in the absence of coagulopathy can play a significant role in acute treatment of subdural hematoma and is associated with improvement outcomes.

In the PLATelet inhibition and patient Outcomes (PLATO) trial, the incidence of ICH was 0.34% and 0.19% for ticagrelol- and clopidogrel-treated patients, respectively. Although the absolute incidence of ICH in patients on dual antiplatelet therapy (DAPT) is low, the mortality is very high (55%). Accordingly, the management of a patient on DAPT in the setting of an ICH is driven by the patient's risk of neurologic deterioration and permanent injury vs. the risk of coronary stent thrombosis.[55]

The oral administration of tranexamic acid in a daily dose of 750 mg has provided the basis for studies that indicate that fibrinolysis and the kinin-kallikrein inflammatory system play an important role in the growth of chronic subdural hematomas. The study involving tranexamic acid was conducted over 4 years; the clinical follow-up and the image analysis of the patients in the study were, on average, 58 days and the medium volume of the chronic subdural hematoma was reduced to 55.6 mL. After treatment with tranexamic acid, the volume of the hematoma was reduced to a medium size of 3.7 mL, with no reccurrence or growth in size.[52]

ANTICONVULSIVE TREATMENT

The use of prophylactic anticonvulsive treatment has numerous opinions for and against this approach; studies indicate that between 2% and 19% of the patients who present with CSHs will have an epileptic crisis before or after surgery. The majority's opinion is that the prophylactic administration of anticonvulsants is reasonable, mostly because the patients with CSDHs frequently present other traumatic brain injuries, which is a well-known risk factor for seizures. However, the idea that anticonvulsant medication represents an additional risk factor for falls in the population of over 65-years-old, which also represents the main presenting age group for chronic subdural hematomas, should not be ignored.[56,57]

STATIN AND TRANEXAMIC ACID

Atorvastatin is reported to promote angiogenesis and suppress inflammation. The ATOCH study protocol by Jian et al. are currently undergoing an evaluation of the therapeutic effects of atorvastatin on CSDH. Jian et al. have recently shown that atorvastatin is effective for nonsurgical reduction and elimination of CSDHs with minimal side effects but its effectiveness and safety as an alternative plan to surgical treatment of a CSDH has still not been proven.[58]

The Tranexamic Acid (TXA) in Chronic Subdural Hematomas (TRACS) trial will be the first prospective study of TXA for CSDH. The trial aims to determine if TXA can increase the rate of CSDH resolution following conservative management, lower the number of required surgical procedures, and decrease the rate of CSDH recurrence following surgical evacuation.[59]

TARGETED TEMPERATURE MANAGEMENT

Hyperthermia, by as little as 1°C, has been shown to worsen outcome in a variety of cerebral ischemia settings. It is generally accepted that hyperthermia must be avoided when cerebral injuries have occurred. However, Eurotherm has demonstrated in patients with elevated intracranial pressure after TBI, therapeutic hypothermia, in addition to standard treatment, results in a greater risk of death and worse neurologic outcomes in survivors compared with standard measures.[60] Currently, there is a phase II, multicenter trial (REACTOR) to be conducted in Australian and New Zealand Intensive care units, which aims to determine if active temperature control reduces body temperature compared with standard care. It is primarily being conducted to establish whether a phase III trial with a patient-centered endpoint of day 90 mortality is justified and feasible.[61]

BLOOD GLUCOSE

Hyperglycemia is an independent predictor of mortality within the first 28 days of ICH, however, "tight" glucose control has been found to be associated with depleted cerebral glucose levels and also increased mortality compared with conventional glucose control.[62,63]

REFERENCES

1. Louhab N, Adali N, Laghmari M, Hymer WE, Ben Ali SA, Kissani N. Misdiagnosed spontaneous intracranial hypotension complicated by subdural hematoma following lumbar puncture. *Int J Gen Med*. 2014;7:71-73.
2. Mashour GA, Schwamm LH, Leffert L. Intracranial subdural hematomas and cerebral

herniation after labor epidural with no evidence of dural puncture. *Anesthesiology*. 2006;104(3):610-612.

3. Vezina G. Assessment of the nature and age of subdural collections in nonaccidental head injury with CT and MRI. *Pediatr Radiol*. 2009; 39(6):586-590.

4. Servadei F, Nasi MT, Giuliani G et al. CT prognostic factors in acute subdural haematomas: The value of the 'worst' CT scan. *Br J Neurosurg*. 2000;14(2):110-116.

5. Kameyama M, Karibe H, Onuma T, Tominaga T. Epidemiological study of head injury in miyagineurotrauma data bank: Age, cause of injury, pathophysiology and outcome [in Japanese]. *Neurotraumatology*. 2008;31:46-56.

6. Jayawant S, Parr J. Outcome following subdural haemorrhages in infancy. *Arch Dis Child*. 2007;92(4):343-347.

7. Squier W. Shaken baby syndrome: The quest for evidence. *Dev Med Child Neurol*. 2008; 50(1):10-14.

8. Salehi-Had H, Brandt JD, Rosas AJ, Rogers KK. Findings in older children with abusive head injury: Does shaken-child syndrome exist? *Pediatrics*. 2006;117(5):e1039-e1044.

9. Adhiyaman V, Asghar M, Ganeshram KN, Bhowmick BK. Chronic subdural haematoma in the elderly. *Postgrad Med J*. 2002;78(916):71-75.

10. Iliescu IA. Current diagnosis and treatment of chronic subdural haematomas. *J Med Life*. 2015;8(3):278-284.

11. Meagher RJ, Young, WF. Subdural hematoma, *Medscape*. https://emedicine.medscape.com /article/1137207-overview. Accessed July 12, 2017.

12. Hobbs C, Childs AM, Wynne J et al. Subdural haematoma and effusion in infancy: An epidemiological study. *Arch Dis Child*. 2005;90(9):952-955.

13. Ali O, Srikantha M, Bhat W, Uzoigwe CE; Postural headache. *BMJ*. 2009;338:b911.

14. Iliescu IA, Constantinescu AI. Clinical evolutional aspects of chronic subdural haematomas - literature review. *J Med Life*. 2015;8 (spec issue):26-33.

15. McArthur DL. Traumatic brain injury: Some history and some epidemiology. In: Levin H, Shum D, Chan R, eds. *Understanding Traumatic Brain Injury: Current Research and Future Directions*. Oxford University Press; 2014: 8-25.

16. Markwalder TM. Chronic subdural hematomas: A review. *J Neurosurg*. 1981;54(5):637-645.

17. Fogelholm R, Waltimo O. Epidemiology of chronic subdural haematoma. *Acta Neurochir (Wien)*. 1975;32(3-4):247-250.

18. Chen JC, Levy ML. Causes, epidemiology, and risk factors of chronic subdural hematoma. *Neurosurg Clin N Am*. 2000;11(3):399-406.

19. Thotakura AK, Marabathina NR. Nonsurgical treatment of chronic subdural hematoma with steroids. *World Neurosurg*. 2015;84(6): 1968-1972.

20. Karibe H, Hayashi T, Hirano T, Kameyama M, Nakagawa A, Tominaga T. Surgical management of traumatic acute subdural hematoma in adults: A review. *Neurol Med Chir (Tokyo)*. 2014;54(11):887-894.

21. Howard MA, Gross AS, Dacey RG, Winn HR. Acute subdural hematomas: An age-dependent clinical entity. *J Neurosurg*. 1989;71(6):858-863.

22. Sawauchi S, Murakami S, Ogawa T, Abe T. [Acute subdural hematoma associated with diffuse brain injury: Analysis of 526 cases in Japan neurotrauma data bank]. *No Shinkei Geka*. 2007;35(1):43-51.

23. Servadei F, Nasi MT, Giuliani G et al. CT prognostic factors in acute subdural haematomas: The value of the 'worst' CT scan. *Br J Neurosurg*. 2000;14(2):110-116.

24. Umezawa K, Kimura S, Ogita S, Takegami T, Ikeda E: [Analysis of 469 cases of acute subdural hematoma: The characteristics of "talk and deteriorate" patients]. *Neurotraumatology*. 2011;34:132-138.

25. Dent DL, Croce MA, Menke PG et al. Prognostic factors after acute subdural hematoma. *J Trauma*. 1995;39:36-42; discussion 42-43.

26. van den Brink WA, Zwienenberg M, Zandee SM, van der Meer L, Maas AI, Avezaat CJ. The prognostic importance of the volume of traumatic epidural and subdural haematomas revisited. *Acta Neurochir (Wien)*. 1999; 141(5):509-514.

27. Shima K, Aruga T, Onuma T et al. JSNT-guidelines for the management of severe head injury (abridged edition). *Asian J Neurosurg*. 2010;5(1):15-23.

28. Bullock MR, Chesnut R, Ghajar J et al. Surgical management of acute subdural hematomas. *Neurosurgery.* 2006;58(3 suppl):S16-S24; discussion Si–Siv.

29. Mathew P, Oluoch-Olunya DL, Condon BR, Bullock R. Acute subdural haematoma in the conscious patient: Outcome with initial non-operative management. *Acta Neurochir (Wien).* 1993;121(3-4):100-108.

30. Servadei F. Prognostic factors in severely head injured adult patients with acute subdural haematoma's. *Acta Neurochir (Wien).* 1997;139(4):279-285.

31. Servadei F, Nasi MT, Giuliani G et al. CT prognostic factors in acute subdural haematomas: The value of the 'worst' CT scan. *Br J Neurosurg.* 2000;14(2):110-116.

32. Wilberger JE Jr, Harris M, Diamond DL. Acute subdural hematoma: Morbidity and mortality related to timing of operative intervention. *J Trauma.* 1990;30(6):733-736.

33. Hanif S, Abodunde O, Ali Z, Pidgeon C. Age related outcome in acute subdural haematoma following traumatic head injury. *Ir Med J.* 2009;102(8): 255-257.

34. Wong CW. Criteria for conservative treatment of supratentorial acute subdural haematomas. *Acta Neurochir (Wien).* 1995;135(1-2):38-43.

35. Ducruet AF, Grobelny BT, Zacharia BE et al. The surgical management of chronic subdural hematoma. *Neurosurg Rev.* 2012;35(2):155-169; discussion 169.

36. Lega BC, Danish SF, Malhotra NR, Sonnad SS, Stein SC. Choosing the best operation for chronic subdural hematoma: A decision analysis. *J Neurosurg.* 2010;113(3):615-621.

37. Abe M, Udono H, Tabuchi K, Uchino A, Yoshikai T, Taki K. Analysis of ischemic brain damage in cases of acute subdural hematomas. *Surg Neurol.* 2003;59(6):464-472; discussion 472.

38. Massaro F, Lanotte M, Faccani G, Triolo C. One hundred and twenty-seven cases of acute subdural haematoma operated on. Correlation between CT scan findings and outcome. *Acta Neurochir (Wien).* 1996;138(2):185-191.

39. Brain Trauma Foundation, AANS, Joint Section on Neurotrauma and Critical Care. Guidelines for the management of severe head injury. *J Neurotrauma.* 1996;13(11):641-734.

40. Mori K, Maeda M. Surgical treatment of chronic subdural hematoma in 500 consecutive cases: Clinical characteristics, surgical outcome, complications, and recurrence rate. *Neurol Med Chir (Tokyo).* 2001;41(8):371-381.

41. Stanisic M, Lund-Johansen M, Mahesparan R. Treatment of chronic subdural hematoma by burr-hole craniostomy in adults: Influence of some factors on postoperative recurrence. *Acta Neurochir (Wien).* 2005;147(12):1249-1256; discussion 1256-1257.

42. Zhang K, Jiang W, Ma T, Wu H. Comparison of early and late decompressive craniectomy on the long-term outcome in patients with moderate and severe traumatic brain injury: A meta-analysis. *Br J Neurosurg.* 2016;30(2):251-257.

43. Seelig JM, Becker DP, Miller JD, Greenberg RP, Ward JD, Choi SC. Traumatic acute subdural hematoma: Major mortality reduction in comatose patients treated within four hours. *N Engl J Med.* 1981;304(25):1511-1518.

44. Nirula R, Millar D, Greene T et al. Decompressive craniectomy or medical management for refractory intracranial hypertension: An AAST-MIT propensity score analysis. *J Trauma Acute Care Surg.* 2014;76(4):944-952.

45. Kolias AG, Scotton WJ, Belli A et al. Surgical management of acute subdural haematomas: Current practice patterns in the United Kingdom and the Republic of Ireland. *Br J Neurosurg.* 2013;27(3):330-333.

46. Cooper DJ, Rosenfeld JV, Murray L et al. Decompressive craniectomy in diffuse traumatic brain injury. *N Engl J Med.* 2011;364(16):1493-1502.

47. Hutchinson PJ, Kolias AG, Timofeev IS et al. Trial of decompressive craniectomy for traumatic intracranial hypertension. *N Engl J Med.* 2016;375(12):1119-1130.

48. Cenic A, Bhandari M, Reddy K. Management of chronic subdural hematoma: A national survey and literature review. *Can J Neurol Sci.* 2005;32(4):501-506.

49. Taussky P, Fandino J, Landolt H. Number of burr holes as independent predictor of postoperative recurrence in chronic subdural

haematoma. *Br J Neurosurg.* 2008;22(2): 279-282.

50. Fukuhara T, Gotoh M, Asari S, Ohmoto T, Akioka T. The relationship between brain surface elastance and brain reexpansion after evacuation of chronic subdural hematoma. *Surg Neurol.* 1996;45(6):570-574.

51. Santarius T, Kirkpatrick PJ, Ganesan D et al. Use of drains versus no drains after burr-hole evacuation of chronic subdural haematoma: A randomised controlled trial. *Lancet.* 2009; 374(9695):1067-1073.

52. Kageyama H, Toyooka T, Tsuzuki N, Oka K. Nonsurgical treatment of chronic subdural hematoma with tranexamic acid. *J Neurosurg.* 2013;119(2): 332-337.

53. Emich S, Richling B, McCoy MR et al. The efficacy of dexamethasone on reduction in the reoperation rate of chronic subdural hematoma–the DRESH study: Straightforward study protocol for a randomized controlled trial. *Trials.* 2014;15(1):6.

54. Henaux PL, Le Reste PJ, Laviolle B, Morandi X. Steroids in chronic subdural hematomas (SUCRE trial): Study protocol for a randomized controlled trial. *Trials.* 2017;18(1):252.

55. Becker RC, Bassand JP, Budaj A et al. Bleeding complications with the P2Y12 receptor antagonists clopidogrel and ticagrelor in the PLATelet inhibition and patient Outcomes (PLATO) trial. *Eur Heart J.* 2011; 32(23):29332944.

56. Rubin G, Rappaport ZH. Epilepsy in chronic subdural haematoma. *Acta Neurochir.* 1993; 123(1-2):39-42.

57. Ratilal BO, Pappamikail L, Costa J, Sampaio C. Anticonvulsants for preventing seizures in patients with chronic subdural haematoma. *Cochrane Database Syst Rev.* 2013;6(6): CD004893.

58. Jiang R, Wang D, Poon WS et al. Effect of ATorvastatin On Chronic subdural Hematoma (ATOCH): A study protocol for a randomized controlled trial. *Trials.* 2015;16:528.

59. Iorio-Morin C, Blanchard J, Richer M, Mathieu D. Tranexamic acid in chronic subdural hematomas (TRACS): Study protocol for a randomized controlled trial. *Trials.* 2016;17(1):235.

60. Andrews PJ, Sinclair HL, Rodriguez A et al. Hypothermia for intracranial hypertension after traumatic brain injury. *N Engl J Med.* 2015;373(25):2403-2412.

61. Young PJ, Bailey MJ, Beasley RW et al. Protocol and statistical analysis plan for the Randomised Evaluation of Active Control of Temperature versus Ordinary Temperature Management (REACTOR) trial. *Crit Care Resusc.* 2017;19(1):81-87.

62. Messé SR, Sansing LH, Cucchiara BL et al. Prophylactic antiepileptic drug use is associated with poor outcome following ICH. *Neurocrit Care.* 2009;11(1):38-44.

63. Fogelholm R, Murros K, Rissanen A, Avikainen S. Admission blood glucose and short term survival in primary intracerebral hemorrhage: A population based study. *J Neurol Neurosurg Psychiatry.* 2005;76(3):349-353.

9

Subarachnoid hemorrhage

EMILY G.Y. KOO, MANDY H.M. CHU, PATRICIA K.Y. KAN, EUNICE Y.L. DAI, AND MATTHEW T.V. CHAN

INTRODUCTION

Traumatic brain injury (TBI) is a global health problem, affecting 50 to 350 per 100,000 people.[1-4] It is a major cause of disability and death. In the United States alone, traumatic brain injury was the primary diagnosis for over 3 million admissions to emergency departments in 2013, with a mortality rate approaching 17 per 10,000 patients.[1]

Subarachnoid hemorrhage (SAH), defined as the presence of blood in the subarachnoid space, is a common diagnosis among patients with head injuries. With the advances in brain imaging in the emergency department and in the intensive care unit (ICU), it is estimated that over 40% of patients with TBI had evidence of SAH in the initial computed tomography (CT) scan.[5,6] This chapter focuses on the pathophysiology (conditions typically described during a disease state), diagnosis, management, and outcome of traumatic SAH.

PATHOPHYSIOLOGY

Research on the pathogenesis, management, and outcome of isolated traumatic SAH has been very limited because of the heterogeneous nature of TBI.

In particular, trauma occurs in patients across all age groups with different comorbidities (additional diseases or conditions). Additionally, traumatic SAH is most likely not the only pathology in the brain and the patient often sustains traumatic injuries to other vital organs as well. Therefore, animal models specifically designed to study traumatic SAH do not currently exist. Nevertheless, there are several proposed mechanisms where traumatic SAH may have originated from[7-9]:

1. Stretching of the vertebrobasilar (poor blood flow to the posterior [back] of the brain) artery during hyperextension of the neck with the initial trauma.
2. Tearing of cortical veins, bridging sinusoids or pial vessels (the delicate innermost layer of the meninges, the membranes surrounding the brain and spinal cord) with rotational acceleration and oscillatory movements during the impact.
3. Rupture of preexisting vascular anomalies in the cervical carotid artery[8]
4. Dispersion of blood from intracranial hemorrhage or cerebral contusion into the subarachnoid space

The presence of dexoyhemoglobin (the oxygen-carrying pigment of red blood cells that gives them their red color and supplies oxygen to the tissues) in the extracellular (the space outside of the cells) space from subarachnoid blood promotes the release of excitatory amino acids (eg, glutamate), oxygen free radicals, and cytotoxic chemicals, such as cytokines. In addition to the direct stretching and mechanical irritation of arteries during the initial impact, these molecules trigger cerebral vasospasm (sharp, often persistent contraction of a blood vessel, reducing its caliber and blood flow) and subsequent ischemia (deficient blood supply).[5,10] In postmortem studies, angiographic and transcranial Doppler reports, anatomic or radiologic vasospasm appears to be common (19%–68%) after traumatic SAH

(Table 9.1).[11] Specifically, vasospasm from traumatic SAH occurred sooner after head injury (within 12 hours), and the duration was generally shorter and lasted <2 weeks.[11,12] However, the significance of vasospasm after traumatic SAH remains unclear because only 3.9% to 16.6% of patients suffering traumatic SAH actually develop significant neurologic deficits, compared with 17% to 40% of patients having vasospasm from SAH due to cerebral aneurysms rupture.[11,13–16]

PRESENTATION

Traumatic SAH tends to occur in patients with more severe brain contusions and subdural hemorrhage. It may indicate early cortical microbleeding, and is

Table 9.1 Vasospasm in traumatic and aneurysmal subarachnoid hemorrhage

	Traumatic subarachnoid hemorrhage	Aneurysmal subarachnoid hemorrhage
Timing (days)		
Onset time	<2	3–7
Peak vasospasm	5–7	7–14
Incidence of vasospasm (%)		
Diagnosed by transcranial Doppler	19%–68%	38%–45%
Diagnosed by cerebral angiography	19%–41%	40%–45%
Percent with neurologic deficits	3.9%–16.6%	17%–40%
Location	Over the cerebral convexity, tentorium, superficial sulci, and fissures	Basal cisterns
Mechanism of vasospasm	Bleeding cortical arteries or veins or diffusion from surface brain contusions	Bleeding from ruptured cerebral aneurysm in the circle of Willis
	Vasoconstriction due to stretch or mechanical injury to vessels, blood and its degradation products	Vasoconstriction mainly due to blood and its degradation products
Cerebral ischemic pattern	Diffuse and relate to sites of contusions	Relate to discrete vascular territories
Treatment	Efficacy of nimodipine is inconclusive Induced hypertension can be hazardous because of cerebral edema, intracranial bleed, and bleeding from other parts of the body involved in trauma	Commonly used therapies include nimodipine and induced hypertension after occlusion of aneurysm

a marker of severe traumatic head injury.[6,16,17] Nevertheless, isolated traumatic SAH is also seen in mild head injury.[2]

The bleeding pattern of traumatic SAH differs from rupture of aneurysms of the large cerebral artery (ie, aneurysmal SAH, Table 9.1). Traumatic SAH is commonly seen over the cerebral convexity, tentorium (a fold that separates the cerebellum from the cerebrum), superficial sulci (a depression or groove in the cerebral cortex), and fissures (a deep fold). It is generally found adjacent to a skull fracture and cerebral contusions. In contrast, aneurysmal SAH is typically located in basal cisterns (one of the three major openings of the brain's subarachnoid space) that originates in the circle of Willis. Given that the subarachnoid space and the ventricles communicate, delayed scans may show an extension to intraventricular hemorrhage. It should be noted that hypodensities, representing ischemic damage, on CT scans are also common and coincide with concurrent contusions but are not related to a particular vascular territory.[9]

Other features that distinguish traumatic from aneurysmal SAH include the fact that ischemia is generally diffuse (spread out) and not restricted to one particular vascular territory. Additionally, hydrocephalus (an abnormal buildup of cerebrospinal fluid) as a result of traumatic SAH occurred in 30% of patients, and is related to the conscious state on admission to the ED and presence of intraventricular hemorrhage.[18]

DIAGNOSIS

Considering the widespread availability and speed of acquisition, patients who have TBI can easily have a noncontrast CT scan performed.[19] CT scans are currently the imaging method of choice to diagnose traumatic SAH. The CT scan is also sensitive enough to detect fractures of the skull, radiopaque foreign body (an object that blocks radiation) and other injuries that require urgent neurosurgical attention, such as hemorrhage, herniation, and hydrocephalus.[6,20]

Specifically, traumatic SAH appears as curvilinear (consisted of or bounded by curved lines) hyperdensities within cortical sulci, Sylvian fissures, and basal cisterns on a CT scan (Figure 9.1). The density of the hematoma decreases with time. Subacute hemorrhages may appear isodense (evenly or uniformly dense) to the surrounding brain

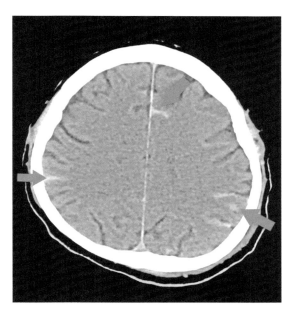

Figure 9.1 Computed tomography scan showing traumatic subarachnoid hemorrhage in superficial sulci in left frontal and bilateral parietal regions (arrows).

parenchyma. It should be noted that acute hemorrhage may also appear isodense when hemoglobin is less than 8 g/dL.

In contrast, magnetic resonance imaging (MRI) is less sensitive than CT when detecting traumatic SAH. It is also more cumbersome and time-consuming to obtain a MRI in the acute brain-injured patient. Nevertheless, with the development of new imaging sequences, modern MRIs can be useful in diagnosing traumatic SAH. Since T1 and T2 relaxation times of a blood clot changes over time in a standardized fashion, the time of hemorrhage from the initial impact can be estimated.[21] There are three MRI sequences that may help to highlight traumatic SAH:

1. Fluid-attenuated inversion recovery (FLAIR) sequence is designed to null signals from cerebrospinal fluid. A subtle amount of blood located at the periphery of the hemispheres and in the periventricular (white matter near the lateral ventricles) region can be easily outlined as hyperintense signal (Figure 9.2). FLAIR sequences are influenced by artefacts, such as supplemental oxygen and vascular pulsations. Other pathology that increases the protein content in the

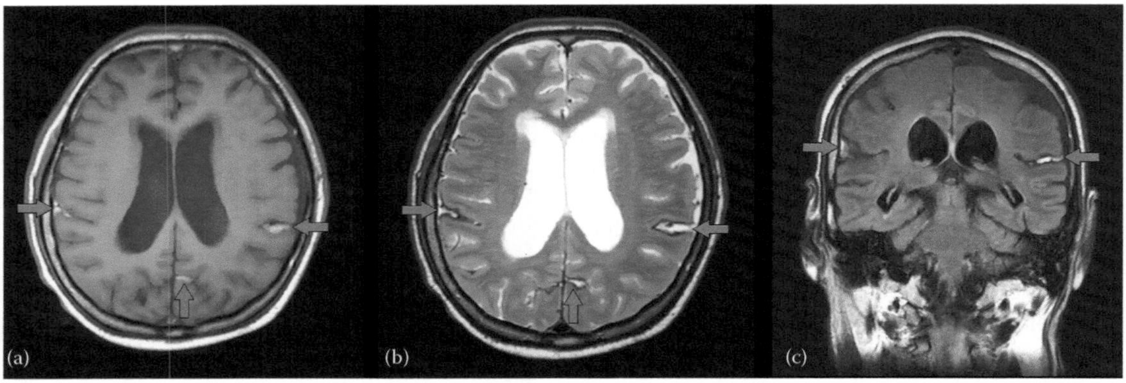

Figure 9.2 Subacute subarachnoid hemorrhage at bilateral parietal and left occipital sulcal spaces (arrows) on MRI: (a) T1-weighted, (b) T2-weighted, (c) Fluid attenuated inversion recovery (FLAIR) sequence.

cerebrospinal fluid, such as meningitis and leptomeningeal carcinomatosis (cancer of the membranes surrounding the brain), may also appear as a hyperintensity lesion.

2. Gradient echo (GRE) sequences is used to expedite signal acquisition. The presence of blood and its degradation products (ferritin or hemosiderin) will appear as a signal void (ie, dark) on the scan (Figure 9.3). However, bone at the base of the skull may interfere with the ability to interpret the signal.

3. Susceptibility weighted imaging (SWI) uses flow compensated, long echo, and GRE sequences to acquire images.[22] SWI is extremely sensitive to blood (Figure 9.4). Images from the filtered phase that were acquired from SWI show differentiation of blood from calcification, which will appear as opposite signal intensities.

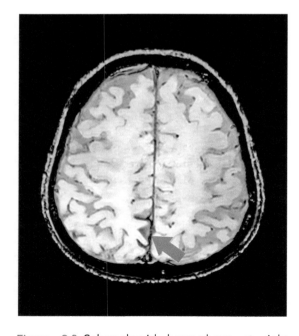

Figure 9.3 Subarachnoid hemorrhage at right occipital sulcal spaces (arrow) on gradient echo (GRE) sequence.

PROGNOSIS

In the International Mission for Prognosis and Analysis of Clinical Trials in traumatic brain injury (IMPACT) study,[23–25] the presence of traumatic SAH is an independent risk factor for mortality and an unfavorable neurologic outcome among patients with moderate-to-severe TBI, odds ratio (95% confidence intervals): 2.1 (1.9–2.4).[24] Similar findings are reported from other large databases, such as the Corticosteroid Randomization After Significant Head injury (CRASH) trial[26,27] and the Tirilazad trials.[28] Table 9.2 shows the other risk factors that predict unfavorable neurologic deficits and mortality after severe traumatic brain injury.

However, the association between the extent of traumatic SAH and unfavorable deficit or mortality is controversial. Nevertheless, a number of classifications have been proposed to define the severity of traumatic SAH (Table 9.3). Essentially, higher severity traumatic SAH is associated with poorer outcome. It should also be noted that, in contrast to aneurysmal SAH, the relationship between

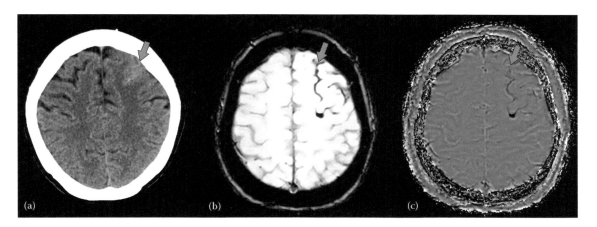

Figure 9.4 Computed tomography scan (a) shows subtle curvilinear hyperdensity at the left frontal sulcal spaces (arrow). Susceptibility weighted imaging (b) confirms the presence of subarachnoid hemorrhage (arrow). Filtered phase image (c) shows hypointense signal consistent with presence of blood (arrow).

Table 9.2 Risk factors for severe traumatic brain injury

Risk factors	Adjusted odds ratios (95% confidence intervals)
Age (per year)	1.7 (1.5–1.9)
Motor score of the GCS	
Flexion	1.7 (1.1–2.4)
Abnormal flexion	3.3 (2.1–5.2)
Extension	5.7 (3.7–9.0)
No response	6.6 (4.7–9.2)
Pupillary response	
None reactive	4.4 (3.8–5.2)
One reactive	1.9 (1.6–2.2)
Hypoxia with arterial tension <60 mmHg or hemoglobin oxygen saturation <90%	1.3 (1.1–1.6)
Hypotension with systolic arterial pressure <90 mmHg	2.1 (1.8–2.5)
Compressed or absent basal cisterns	1.9 (1.6 – 2.2)
Midline shift	1.3 (1.1–1.5)
Traumatic subarachnoid hemorrhage	2.1 (1.9–2.4)

Table 9.3 Classification of traumatic subarachnoid hemorrhage (SAH)

Greene et al. Classification

Grade	CT scan findings
1	Thin traumatic SAH (≤5 mm)
2	Thick traumatic SAH (>5 mm)
3	Thin traumatic SAH with mass lesion
4	Thick traumatic SAH with mass lesion

Morris and Marshall Classification

Grade	CT scan findings
0	No CT evidence of traumatic SAH
1	Traumatic SAH present at only one location
2	Traumatic SAH present at only one location but quantity of blood fills that structure or traumatic SAH at two sites, filling neither of them
3	Traumatic SAH at two sites, one of which is the tentorium, filled with blood
4	Traumatic SAH present at three or more sites, any quantity

traumatic SAH and vasospasm is less precise. Interestingly, in patients with mild TBI, only 3% demonstrated radiographic deterioration of traumatic SAH. Nevertheless, progression to other intracerebral lesions may occur,[16,17] and quality of life could be impaired for weeks or months. Patients with isolated traumatic SAH should be monitored after hospital discharge for potential postconcussive symptoms and should also be counseled to avoid repeated head injury.[17]

MANAGEMENT

Management of traumatic SAH goes along with the overall treatment for TBI. In this respect, patients with severe TBI, defined as Glasgow Coma Scale (GCS) score ≤8 on admission, should be monitored and treated aggressively. These patients, often with multiple intracranial lesions in addition to isolated traumatic SAH, should be managed in specialized ICUs with dedicated neurosurgical services.[29] Monitoring of the conscious state closely, arterial and cerebral hemodynamics (the mechanism involved with circulation) should be performed to detect and prevent secondary injury.[30] Intracranial pressure (ICP) monitoring should be considered.[31,32] Repeated brain imaging (CT or, less commonly, MRI) should also be performed to monitor the progression of intracranial lesions.

Isolated traumatic SAH in mild head injury (GCS score >12) is generally benign.[16] Many of these patients may be nursed in a general neurosurgical ward. Neurologic deterioration may occur but is usually self-limiting. It has not been determined how long these patients should be monitored. However, deterioration had been reported 57 hours after injury.[16] A moderate head injury (GCS score of 9–12) indicates a more complex primary insult and should be managed in a specialized neurosurgical center.

Specific management of traumatic SAH has been evaluated to target three complications:

1. Electrolyte disturbance with hyponatremia (dangerously low levels of sodium) or hypernatremia (dangerously high levels of sodium) may occur with salt-losing nephropathy or diabetes insipidus (excessive urination and extreme thirst), respectively. Damage to the hypothalamic-pituitary axis appears to be a major contributing factor. Management should aim to maintain euvolemia (appropriate hydration) or modest hypervolemia, with a plasma sodium concentration up to 150–155 mmol/L. Enteral (through the intestine) feeding is preferred, unless contraindicated. In general, monitoring of central venous pressure and renal function are required for patients with severe TBI.

2. Prophylactic treatment for vasospasm after traumatic SAH with calcium channel blockers has been studied in eight randomized trials,[33–40] including 2101 patients with severe head injury.[38,41] Intravenous nimodipine (a calcium channel blocker) (seven trials, 2079 patients) did not reduce the risk of unfavorable outcome after severe head injury (nimodipine 42.5% vs. controls 40.7%); relative risk (95% confidence intervals): 0.92 (0.78–1.10), $p = 0.37$; random effect model (34–40). Similarly, nicardipine (one trial, 22 patients) had no effect on outcome in severe head injury, relative risk (95% confidence intervals): 0.43 (0.15–1.24), $p = 0.12$.[40] These data suggested that calcium channel blockers should not be prescribed routinely in patients with traumatic SAH. Currently, there are no studies that evaluate other agents, such as an endothelial antagonist (eg, clazosentan), to counteract vasospasm after traumatic SAH. It should be clear that therapeutic techniques that are commonly used in aneurysmal SAH, including induced hypertension, hypervolemia, and hemodilution,[42] may be detrimental in the treatment of severe TBI.

3. Finally, as much as 30% of patients with traumatic SAH developed obstructive hydrocephalus (cerebrospinal fluid in the brain) as the cerebrospinal fluid pathways are blocked with subarachnoid blood. When hydrocephalus is detected, it should be promptly treated with external drainage or by ventriculo-peritoneal shunting.

CONCLUSIONS

In summary, traumatic SAH is common after severe head injury. Although neurologic outcome is likely to be associated with the extent of the underlying brain contusion and intracranial and intraventricular hemorrhage, traumatic SAH remains a significant contributing risk factor to unfavorable outcome. Rigorous monitoring should be conducted to detect common complications such as electrolyte disturbance, vasospasm, and hydrocephalus, so that appropriate management of these complications can be performed quickly.

REFERENCES

1. Roozenbeek B, Maas AI, Menon DK. Changing patterns in the epidemiology of traumatic brain injury. *Nat Rev Neurol.* 2013;9(4):231-236.

2. Brazinova A, Rehorcikova V, Taylor MS et al. Epidemiology of traumatic brain injury in Europe: A living systematic review. *J Neurotrauma.* 2016;33:1-30.

3. El-Fiki M, El-Ghandour N. Traumatic subarachnoid hemorrhage in developed and developing communities. *World Neurosurg.* 2015;83(2):170-173.

4. Menon DK, Schwab K, Wright DW, Maas AI, Demographics, Clinical Assessment Working Group of the International and Interagency Initiative toward Common Data Elements for Research on Traumatic Brain Injury and Psychological Health. Position statement: Definition of traumatic brain injury. *Arch Phys Med Rehabil.* 2010;91(11):1637-1640.

5. Servadei F, Murray GD, Teasdale GM et al. Traumatic subarachnoid hemorrhage: Demographic and clinical study of 750 patients from the European brain injury consortium survey of head injuries. *Neurosurgery.* 2002;50(2):261-267; discussion 267-269.

6. Eisenberg HM, Gary HE Jr, Aldrich EF et al. Initial CT findings in 753 patients with severe head injury. A report from the NIH Traumatic Coma Data Bank. *J Neurosurg.* 1990;73(5):688-698.

7. Greve MW, Zink BJ. Pathophysiology of traumatic brain injury. *Mt Sinai J Med.* 2009;76(2):97-104.

8. Kim BJ, Kim SH, Lim DJ, Ha SK. Traumatic subarachnoid hemorrhage originating from mid-cervical arterial injury. *World Neurosurg.* 2015;84(4):1177 e13-6.

9. Armin SS, Colohan AR, Zhang JH. Traumatic subarachnoid hemorrhage: Our current understanding and its evolution over the past half century. *Neurol Res.* 2006;28(4):445-452.

10. Chan MTV, Chu MHM, Lam CKM, Jia B, Tsang S, Wu WKK. Deep anesthesia: Too much of a good thing? *Can J Anaesth.* 2017;64(6):574-580.

11. Kramer DR, Winer JL, Pease BA, Amar AP, Mack WJ. Cerebral vasospasm in traumatic brain injury. *Neurol Res Int.* 2013;2013:415813.

12. Fehnel CR, Wendell LC, Potter NS, Klinge P, Thompson BB. Severe cerebral vasospasm after traumatic brain injury. *R I Med J (2013).* 2014;97(7):45-46.

13. Wong GK, Chan DY, Siu DY et al. High-dose simvastatin for aneurysmal subarachnoid hemorrhage: Multicenter randomized controlled double-blinded clinical trial. *Stroke.* 2015;46(2):382-388.

14. Wong GK, Chan MT, Poon WS, Boet R, Gin T. Magnesium therapy within 48 hours of an aneurysmal subarachnoid hemorrhage: Neuro-panacea. *Neurol Res.* 2006;28(4):431-435.

15. Wong GK, Poon WS, Chan MT et al. Intravenous magnesium sulphate for aneurysmal subarachnoid hemorrhage (IMASH): A randomized, double-blinded, placebo-controlled, multicenter phase III trial. *Stroke.* 2010;41(5):921-926.

16. Phelan HA, Richter AA, Scott WW et al. Does isolated traumatic subarachnoid hemorrhage merit a lower intensity level of observation than other traumatic brain injury? *J Neurotrauma.* 2014;31(20):1733-1736.

17. Lee JJ, Segar DJ, Asaad WF. Comprehensive assessment of isolated traumatic subarachnoid hemorrhage. *J Neurotrauma.* 2014;31(7):595-609.

18. Tian HL, Xu T, Hu J, Cui YH, Chen H, Zhou LF. Risk factors related to hydrocephalus after traumatic subarachnoid hemorrhage. *Surg Neurol.* 2008;69(3):241-246.

19. Mattioli C, Beretta L, Gerevini S et al. Traumatic subarachnoid hemorrhage on the computerized tomography scan obtained at admission: A multicenter assessment of the accuracy of diagnosis and the potential impact on patient outcome. *J Neurosurg.* 2003;98(1):37-42.

20. Mutch CA, Talbott JF, Gean A. Imaging evaluation of acute traumatic brain injury. *Neurosurg Clin N Am.* 2016;27(4):409-439.

21. Bradley WG, Jr. MR appearance of hemorrhage in the brain. *Radiology*. 1993;189(1): 15-26.

22. Wu Z, Li S, Lei J, An D, Haacke EM. Evaluation of traumatic subarachnoid hemorrhage using susceptibility-weighted imaging. *Am J Neuroradiol*. 2010;31(7):1302-1310.

23. Steyerberg EW, Mushkudiani N, Perel P et al. Predicting outcome after traumatic brain injury: Development and international validation of prognostic scores based on admission characteristics. *PLoS Med*. 2008;5 (8):e165; discussion e165.

24. Maas AI, Steyerberg EW, Butcher I et al. Prognostic value of computerized tomography scan characteristics in traumatic brain injury: Results from the IMPACT study. *J Neurotrauma*. 2007;24(2):303-314.

25. Hukkelhoven CW, Steyerberg EW, Habbema JD et al. Predicting outcome after traumatic brain injury: Development and validation of a prognostic score based on admission characteristics. *J Neurotrauma*. 2005;22(10):1025-1039.

26. Roberts I, Yates D, Sandercock P et al. Effect of intravenous corticosteroids on death within 14 days in 10008 adults with clinically significant head injury (MRC CRASH trial): Randomised placebo-controlled trial. *Lancet*. 2004;364(9442):1321-1328.

27. Edwards P, Arango M, Balica L et al. Final results of MRC CRASH, a randomised placebo-controlled trial of intravenous corticosteroid in adults with head injury-outcomes at 6 months. *Lancet*. 2005;365 (9475):1957-1959.

28. Maas AI, Hukkelhoven CW, Marshall LF, Steyerberg EW. Prediction of outcome in traumatic brain injury with computed tomographic characteristics: A comparison between the computed tomographic classification and combinations of computed tomographic predictors. *Neurosurgery*. 2005;57(6):1173-1181.

29. Lombardo S, Scalea T, Sperry J et al. Neuro, trauma, or med/surg intensive care unit: Does it matter where multiple injuries patients with traumatic brain injury are admitted? Secondary analysis of the American Association for the Surgery of Trauma Multi-Institutional Trials Committee decompressive craniectomy study. *J Trauma Acute Care Surg*. 2017;82(3):489-496.

30. Prins M, Greco T, Alexander D, Giza CC. The pathophysiology of traumatic brain injury at a glance. *Dis Model Mech*. 2013;6(6):1307-1315.

31. Chesnut RM, Temkin N, Carney N et al. A trial of intracranial-pressure monitoring in traumatic brain injury. *N Engl J Med*. 2012; 367(26):2471-2481.

32. Brain Trauma Foundation, American Association of Neurological Surgeons, Congress of Neurological Surgeons et al. Guidelines for the management of severe traumatic brain injury. VI. Indications for intracranial pressure monitoring. *J Neurotrauma*. 2007;24(suppl 1):S37-S44.

33. Bailey I, Bell A, Gray J et al. A trial of the effect of nimodipine on outcome after head injury. *Acta Neurochir (Wien)*. 1991;110(3-4): 97-105.

34. The European Study Group on Nimodipine in Severe Head Injury. A multicenter trial of the efficacy of nimodipine on outcome after severe head injury. *J Neurosurg*. 1994;80 (5):797-804.

35. Harders A, Kakarieka A, Braakman R. Traumatic subarachnoid hemorrhage and its treatment with nimodipine. German tSAH Study Group. *J Neurosurg*. 1996;85(1): 82-89.

36. Feng D, Ma Y, Zhang Y, Plets C, Goffin J, Chen J. Controlled study of nimodipine in treatment of patients with diffuse axonal injury. *Chin J Traumatol*. 2000;3(2):85-88.

37. Pillai SV, Kolluri VR, Mohanty A, Chandramouli BA. Evaluation of nimodipine in the treatment of severe diffuse head injury: A double-blind placebo-controlled trial. *Neurol India*. 2003;51 (3):361-363.

38. Vergouwen MD, Vermeulen M, Roos YB. Effect of nimodipine on outcome in patients with traumatic subarachnoid haemorrhage: A systematic review. *Lancet Neurol*. 2006;5 (12):1029-1032.

39. Farhoudi M, Asghari A, Aghajanloo M, Zeinali A. Effects of nimodipine on cerebral hemodynamics, and prognosis of diffuse axonal injury patients. *Neurosciences (Riyadh)*. 2007;12(4):285-288.

40. Sahuquillo J, Robles A, Poca A, Ballabriga A, Mercadal J, Secades JJ. [A controlled, double-blind, randomized pilot clinical trial

of nicardipine as compared with a placebo in patients with moderate or severe head injury]. *Rev Neurol.* 2000;30(5):401-408.

41. Xu GZ, Wang MD, Liu KG, Bai YA, Wu, W Li W. A meta-analysis of treating acute traumatic brain injury with calcium channel blockers. *Brain Res Bull.* 2013;99:41-47.

42. Lee KH, Lukovits T, Friedman JA. "Triple-H" therapy for cerebral vasospasm following subarachnoid hemorrhage. *Neurocrit Care.* 2006;4(1):68-76.

10

Diffuse axonal injury

MARCO ECHEVERRIA

INTRODUCTION

Traumatic brain injury (TBI) is the leading cause of morbidity and mortality in the modern world, with major socioeconomic implications. In the United States alone, it has been reported that over 1.7 million people sustain a TBI each year, which represents healthcare expenses of more than $60 billion.[1,2] Additionally, sufficient evidence exist that a single TBI may be associated with late-onset occurrence of neurodegenerative disorders, such as Alzheimer's disease.[3]

Damage to central nervous system (CNS) tissue as a result of a closed, repetitive, or penetrating injury to the cranial cavity can produce mild to severe neurologic disability or death. Diffuse axonal injury (DAI) typically results from a rotational acceleration/deceleration force of the head, as well as the force spreading through the brain. It is often characterized as a structural lesion, with irreparable breakdown of the axonal architecture. Among the various forms of cerebral lesions, DAI is a major component of primary TBI and is associated with a complex chain of mechanical effects of the impact of the trauma, which leads to disruption of the axonal cytoskeleton, axonal transport interruption, swelling and proteolysis (the breakdown of proteins), secondary disconnection, and, finally, Wallerian degeneration (the degeneration of nerve fibers that occurs following an injury). Axons can reach 10,000 times the volume of the parent neuronal cell body and their elongated structure places them at particular risk of mechanical injury.

However, other pathophysiologic factors such as metabolic, electrochemical, and inflammatory events triggered by the initial or secondary trauma also play a definitive role in the resulting microstructural damage. In a wide range of extensions and severity of the effects of trauma, the patient may experience an acute loss of consciousness or confusion, which can progress to a coma or cognitive dysfunction. Nevertheless, recent studies suggest that TBI may induce long-term neurodegenerative disorders as a result of progressive axonal damage.[3]

DAI is typically characterized as coma without small, identifiable lesions; it is defined pathologically by axonal disruption in multiple areas of the brain parenchyma, which interrupts interneuronal (neurons that communicate with each other) connectivity, which impairs cognitive autonomic motor and sensory functions.[4,5] Some areas of the brain are more commonly affected than others, such as the brainstem, the parasagital white matter near the cerebral cortex, and the corpus callosum (the nerve tract that connects the two cerebral hemispheres of the brain).[6] The histopathologic pattern (tissue changes characteristic of disease or trauma) of DAI shows worsening swelling and distortion of the normal axonal architecture with the occurrence of retraction bulbs and helical structures.[7] Based on these histopathologic findings, Adams et al. proposed a classification for grading DAI.[7]

DAI typically results from head rotational acceleration/deceleration forces, as well as the propagation of the force through the brain following the impact. Axonal lesions of the brainstem and corpus callosum are indicators of an unfavorable prognosis, and the location of the axonal lesions are related to the severity of the condition and the plane on which the force occurred.[8] Many studies have demonstrated that the plane of the head, by the time a rotational acceleration force is applied in reference to the brainstem, is a critical element; which determines the induction and duration of the loss of consciousness (LOC) or coma following an injury. It has been determined that a rotational transverse force to the brainstem is associated with coma, whereas an equivalent rotation circumferential force is not.[9,10] Browne et al. has found that the duration of LOC or coma following the application of a rotational transverse force to the brainstem after TBI was directly proportional to the extent of DAI to the brainstem, also determining the clinical severity following brain injury because, when the brainstem had no lesions, there was no LOC, although extensive axonal damage through the white matter occurred. Therefore, it appears that location, rather than the extent of axonal damage, is the most important factor in determining LOC or coma after TBI.[11]

PATHOLOGIC FEATURES OF DAI

Adams et al. propose the classification of DAI for histopathologic findings.[7] Grade I (mild DAI) includes pathologic features restricted to "retraction balls" or axonal swelling at characteristic brain sites like the cortical white matter, corpus callosum, brainstem, and cerebellum. Grade II (moderate DAI) is composed of the features of Grade I along with hemorrhagic or necrotic lesions of the corpus callosum, involvement of the interventricular wall, and, possibly, intraventricular hemorrhage. Grade III (severe DAI) involves lesions of the dorsolateral areas of the rostral region (located toward the oral or nasal region) of the brainstem.[7] A subsequent study found a variable frequency of lesions in separate regions of the brain.[12]

The deformation that is formed in the white matter tracts by the trauma forces applied to the brain is the interruption of axonal transport and the consequent accumulation of transported material at axonal swellings after the first few hours after the head trauma occurred. The swelling appears at the injury site, referred to as axonal varicosities, 2 to 3 hours after the impact occurred with a disconnection 6 to 12 hours later. Also, a large, single swelling is generally found soon after the injury occurred, described as an "axonal bulb" or "retraction ball," as previously named because of the shape of the swelling at the end of the axonal axis, which represents a complete axonal disconnection, interrupting the protein transport.[10,11,13,14] Currently, the diagnostic confirmation of DAI is only possible with postmortem histopathologic examination; however, increasing evidence suggests that advanced neuroimaging techniques such as diffusion tensor imaging (DTI) seems to be a promising technique that assesses white matter integrity in vivo by measuring the anisotropic diffusion of water molecules.[15]

The trauma forces and movements of different regions of the brain during TBI not only produce axonal tearing but also small cerebral vessel damage at the site where movements occur. These vascular lesions produce petechial hemorrhages preferentially in the white matter of the frontal lobe and are referred to as diffuse vascular injury.[13] Hypothalamic injury can occur as a result of shearing damage of the pituitary stalk caused by high kinetic energy, particularly during basilar skull fractures, presenting as panhypopituitarism.[16,17] Notably, with axonal pathology in long-term survivors, the damaged axons displayed the phenotype of axonal bulbs, potentially representing a complete disconnection, rather than that of varicose, connected axons, indicating a distinct mechanism.

MECHANISMS OF INJURY

Primary mechanical damage (primary axotomy)

There is cumulative evidence that biomechanical mechanisms of TBI are closely related to clinical symptoms of mechanical axonal damage. The human brain is viscoelastic in nature and is mechanically compliant to normal and gradual acceleration loads that occur in daily life. Nevertheless, due to inertia, when the CNS experiences a sudden acceleration over an interval of less than 50 ms, this force overcomes the viscoelastic properties of the brain, causing shearing of the membrane and cytoskeleton structure that may be followed, in most cases, by a delayed elastic return to the normal morphology (form and structure). The white matter axons are particularly vulnerable when a mechanical loading force is applied to them, most probably due to its anisotropy (not having properties or characteristics that are the same in every direction) and structural design. Within axons, microtubules and neurofilaments are linear, with perpendicular protein projections and cross-links. A large surface-to-volume ratio of the axon membrane (axolemma) to the axoplasm is also unique. The selective injury to axons in TBI appears to be related to their viscoelastic nature, reflecting a unique ultrastructure and collective anisotropic arrangement in the tracts. The complex network of fiber families, fiber orientations, and fiber-tract distribution in the brain are responsible for many states of deformation as a result of a traumatic insult, including local tension, focal compression, and shearing. The axons, according to their cerebral anisotropic property, have several physically different orientations. Cellular-level heterogeneities have an important influence on the axonal strain, leading to an orientation and location-dependent sensitivity of the tissue to mechanical loads. With a sudden application of a mechanical shearing force or compression at the moment of the head trauma, axons lose their natural compliance and ductility, becoming essentially fragile, which is also referred to as "primary axotomy," which does not always occur. Instead, the swelling that follows cytoskeleton disruption or, "secondary axotomy," is highly frequent.[18] Animal studies have shown that after TBI, axonal breakage might not occur; therefore, the myelin of axons remains intact.[19] Another form of axonal injury is characterized by increased axolemmal permeability, mitochondrial swelling, and cytoskeletal compaction, leading to microtubule and microfilament damage.[20] Although axonal varicosities resolve with time, the retraction balls may persist for years, reflecting axonal separation following TBI. Currently, primary axotomy seems to be a minor contributor to axonal damage compared with secondary post-traumatic mechanisms that are triggered after brain trauma,[21] as opposed to a stretch injury without complete axotomy. Although a large number of axons immediately become disrupted (primary axotomy) when they are exposed to the mechanical force, this leads to a temporal response, resulting in a progressive loss of neural connectivity that is responsible for physical and cognitive disability following TBI. The axonal cytoskeleton of axon is a complex network of proteins with a variety of configurations whose main role is to provide functional and structural stability to the axons. Anatomically, an axon contains microtubules that are disposed in longitudinal tracks, arranged in overlapping strands, offering structural support, and functioning as polarized tracks for motor proteins. The other major somatic components, the neurofilaments, provide tensile strength and determine axon diameter. Their actin filaments maintain membrane stability through ring-like structures that run circumferentially along the axon and hold together with spectrin links and adduction caps. The neurofilaments are responsible for the mechanical strength and stability and axon diameter. Microtubules determine intracellular transport and structural rigidity. Secondary axotomy is associated to the disruption microtubule and microfilament network.[22,23] There is sufficient evidence supporting microtubule breakdown as a primary mechanism for axonal bulb formation and eventual axon degeneration; however, in a recent study, Fournier et al. has shown that changes in neurofilaments precede structural damage in microtubules.[24] Microtubules are the strongest component of the axonal cytoskeleton and are more resistant to degeneration in response to a mechanical load, as opposed to less-rigid components such as neurofilaments.[25] Although it is well known that the axonal cytoskeleton is subject to shearing and torsional and compression forces during and after TBI, it is not clear how this primary process triggers the following secondary insult, which is produced by chemical and molecular changes.

Some studies have demonstrated that when a large-scale traumatic force is applied uniformly across a brain region, the initial histologic examination shows scattered axonopathy in the traumatized area, which can be explained because myelination varies between neighboring axons, and myelinated small axons are probably more susceptible to damage.[26] Another important observation from animal models and patients is the fact that the proportion of histologic abnormal axons is incongruent (not compatible) with the magnitude of the clinical picture seen after TBI, suggesting that some axons appear morphologically normal but are functionally incapacitated after trauma.[27]

Secondary axonal injury (secondary axotomy)

Primary brain damage occurs at the time of the head impact, has an almost immediate clinical effect, and is refractory to most treatment. By contrast, secondary brain damage occurs at varying times after the impact and may be preventable and responsive to treatment, although it can occur very rapidly after the impact to the head. For patients who survive the initial traumatic injury, morbidity and mortality are largely determined by the severity of the secondary injury process. Secondary, or delayed, DAI develops over hours, days, weeks, or even years after the initial injury as a complication of the different types of primary brain damage and exacerbates the already-altered homeostasis of the injured brain. Below is a summary of the most important mechanism or process determining the secondary axonal damage after TBI and TAI.

ALTERED CALCIUM HOMEOSTASIS

After trauma, axons that were not destroyed by primary axotomy may remain injured as a result of mechanical stretch, resulting in axolemmal disruption and increased permeability, which, in turn, precipitates depolarization and the entry of large amounts of calcium, increasing intra-axonal calcium levels. Along with axolemmal breaching (tearing or rupturing), activation of the transmembrane calcium channels also contributes to the migration of extracellular calcium to the interior of the axons. The activation of mechanosensitive sodium channels by axonal deformation reverses

the natural flux of sodium/calcium transporters and activates voltage-gated calcium channels (L-type and T-type), increasing the influx of extracellular calcium.[28] Nevertheless, there is also evidence for intracellular calcium release by the axoplasmic reticulum in stretch axonal injury.[3,29,30] A study by Staal et al. showed a biphasic calcium elevation in primary neuron cultures subjected to axonal stretch injury, indicating that intracellular as well as extracellular calcium contribute to the overall increase in axoplasmic calcium.[29] High levels of cytosolic calcium damage axons through destruction of cytoskeletal components[29] and mitochondrial dysfunction.

EXCITOTOXIC CASCADE ACTIVATION

When a CNS axon is stretched, there is an acute increase in intracellular calcium, primarily derived from intracellular stores. This is followed by a more gradual and long-lasting dysregulation of intracellular calcium metabolism. Depolarization that occurs with axolemmal disruption causes a change in the electrochemical equilibrium of the damaged axonal membrane, which triggers the release of excitatory amino acids, such as glutamate, up to concentrations of 50 times normal after TBI, and worsened by a dysfunctional glutamate reuptake mechanism by astrocytes in brain injury. Glutamate molecules bond to N-methyl-d-aspartate (NMDA) and AMPA receptors increase the influx of calcium into the cytosol that activate calcium-dependent second messenger systems, disrupt transmembrane ion gradient and the osmotic load of the neuronal cytosol, among other mechanisms that worsen axonal injury.[31,32] The excitotoxic response also triggers axonal degeneration, caspase-3 activation, and distal axon swelling.[33–35] Cytosolic calcium overload induces the opening of the mitochondrial permeability transition pore, which leads to the neutralization of the electrochemical gradients necessary for mitochondrial function and allows water influx and mitochondrial death. Intramitochondrial sequestration of calcium leading to mitochondrial dysfunction and destruction is one of the final stages in the injury process.

HYDROLYSIS OF STRUCTURAL PROTEIN

Calpain baseline activity is low and in normal physiologic conditions, calpains are predominantly involved in cell signaling and plasticity. Elevated concentrations of glutamate and intracellular calcium, as a result of post-traumatic excitotoxic cascade activation, stimulate the activity of calpains and caspases; both have been calcium-dependent enzymes promoting cytoskeletal destruction (calpain) and the apoptotic process. Calpain activity begins shortly after TBI and a second peak has been observed with axonal necrosis and the acceleration of the cellular apoptotic process, suggesting that calpains are an early mediator of neural damage and also considered a potential therapeutic target in TBI.[36] Spectrin is a structural protein found on the inner side of the membrane, functioning as a support of the lipid bilayer; it also maintains the concave shape of the blood red cells. In the earlier stage after head trauma, calpain mediates the hydrolysis of axonal spectrin 1 to 2 hours after injury. The most important consequence of spectrin hydrolysis is loss of microtubules, mitochondrial swelling, and neurofilament knots.[35,37–39] Calpain is also partially responsible for excitotoxic cell injury. When axonal injury and excessive calcium shifts occur, calpains respond by moving from cytosol to producing plasma membranes, by sustained activation and widespread proteolysis, particularly of spectrin. Calpain-induced spectrin breakdown may contribute to the axolemmal permeability found in DAI. Calpain activation can cause long-term dysfunction of axonal transport and plasticity and can be involved in the degranulation of distal (distant) segments of the injured axon by proteolysis of neurofilaments. It has been shown that calpains are strongly implicated in Wallerian degeneration (WD) in both peripheral and CNS.[40] The failure of glutamate antagonists to prevent or ameliorate TBI-induced axonal damage has shifted the therapeutic interest toward downstream targets like calpains,[41] driven by the evidence that calpain activation is an early mediator of secondary axonal injury in DAI, and because calpains cause spectrin breakdown, they provide a specific molecular biomarker of the process.[37] Inhibition of intra-axonal calpains is likely a necessary component of any effective therapeutic strategy for a wide spectrum of human diseases. Regarding the potential role of calpain in axonal degeneration, an interest in using a calpain inhibitor to protect the cytoskeleton has emerged. Calpain-inhibiting agents have been tested in animal models with some success; however, its use has many limitations such as severe adverse reactions and logistic difficulties around the need for early drug intervention.[36]

ACTIVATION OF CASPASE-MEDIATED APOPTOSIS

Mitochondrial damage after diffuse axonal damage is the result of the excessive calcium influx and intracellular overload, which leads to changes in permeability in the mitochondrial membrane, swelling, and breakage of the mitochondrial crest and membrane.[42] The mitochondrial death is followed by an energy failure, ionic imbalance, and disconnection; however, this mitochondrial damage may also lead to the release of cytochrome c (cyto-c), which then activates caspases with significant adverse intra-axonal consequences.[43] Caspase-activation by cyto-c mediates degradation of spectrin and increases permeability in plasma membranes.[44] After cytochrome c is released from damaged mitochondria, in conjunction with Apaf-1, which contains a caspase recruitment domain, it activates caspase-3, the primary-effect enzyme in neuronal and axonal apoptosis.[45] Once the apoptotic process is initiated, other propapoptotic factors can be released or activated, such as caspase -2,-3 and -9, as well a a57kDa flavoprotein, capable of directly activating caspase-3.[43,45]

MITOCHONDRIAL ENERGY FAILURE IN DAI

Axonal distortion by mechanical stress is associated with mitochondrial derangements like reduction of cristae, swelling, coalescence, or fragmentation followed by an acute energy failure and ATP depletion. Diffuse stretching of axons increases membrane permeability and allows an ionic flux, which increases intracellular calcium and sodium as well as extracellular potassium. The result is a membrane depolarization, activation of voltage, or ligand-gated ion channels and an excessive release of excitatory amino acids, such as glutamate. The binding of these neurotransmitters to synaptic receptors leads to further depolarization and a feedback loop, resulting in a spreading depression-like state. Once neurons are depolarized, use ATP-dependent ionic pumps to restore membrane potential, with the restocking of neuronal and axonal ATP stores requiring oxidative respiration and glycolisis. The vascular disruption produced by TBI reduces local blood flow and impairs autoregulation, resulting in mitochondrial energy failure. This decline in ATP levels severely affects the axon's ability to sustain membrane action potentials, ionic gradients, regulation of calcium influx, and normal axonal transport, resulting in irreversible axonal damage.[46,47]

Under energy failure conditions, axons increase reactive oxygen species (ROS) and the generation of mitochondrial permeability pores (mPTP), which are inner membrane proteins that have been induced in response to high calcium concentration and allow movement of small molecules in or out of the mitochondria; this is a process that results in swelling and death.[48,49] Mitochondrial permeability pores has been studied as a potential therapeutic target to avoid axon degeneration. Cyclosporine A, an immunotherapeutic agent that binds and inhibits cyclophilin D, is a protein complex involved in the opening of the mPTP.[50] Results of the use of cyclosporin A in animal models remain inconclusive. While pretreatment with cyclosporin A may not prevent axonal swelling in neuronal cultures exposed to ROS, this drug attenuate cytoskeleton breakdown and axon degeneration after stretch axonal injury.[51] Human Phase II trials are currently ongoing. An analogue to cyclosporin A, NIM811, which also binds to cyclophilin D and prevents the formation of mPTP, is under investigation. NIM811 decreases spectrin degradation induced by calpain and cognitive deficit when administered 15 minutes to 12 hours after TBI.[52,53] Readnower et al. has shown that neuroprotection with NIM811 is dose dependent, with the 10 mg/kg being the most effective dose to improve cognition, mitochondrial functioning, and reduce oxidative damage following TBI in a rat model.[54] Other pharmacologic and nonpharmacologic strategies targeting mitochondrial energetics include the use of N-acetyl cysteine (NAC), methylene blue, creatine, and low-level laser light. N-acetyl cysteine has shown antioxidant and neurovascular protective effects after TBI. Chen et al. has reported that NAC administration after TBI may attenuate the inflammatory response by decreasing the levels of proinflammatory cytokines, NF-kB, IL-1β, TNF-α, and ICAM-1, by this mechanism, ameliorating secondary axonal and neuronal damage.[55,56] A recent study by Eakin et al., comparing the use of NAN with placebo in TBI resulting from blast injury in a combat setting demonstrated that NAC had a beneficial effect on the severity and resolution of neurologic sequelae.[57] Another study that was conducted by the same group in a rodent model with TBIs found that administering NAC 30 to 60 minutes after the injury showed significant behavioral recovery after injury.[57] The experimental drug FK506 (tracolimus) may have a role as a cellular energetics modulator, inhibiting calcineurin

and hence reducing translocation of BAD to BCL-X in mitochondria and the mPTP opening.[58] The exposure to low-level laser light (670-nm light) represents a nonpharmacologic approach to improving mitochondrial energetics by inducing changes in the redox state, transcription factor expression, and increasing nitrous oxide (NO). This technique can be applied to humans and has had beneficial effects on animals.[59] Methylene blue (MB) has a biochemical redox property acting as an electron cycler on the mitochondrial transport system, enhancing mitochondrial respiration as an electron donor to the electron transport chain by means of an autoxidizing redox property. This property of MB to maintain redox equilibrium by serving as an electron donor and acceptor permits the cycling of electrons from inside the mitochondrial matrix to electron transport proteins in the mitochondria. Oxygen, the final acceptor of electrons in the respiratory chain, is obtained from oxyhemoglobin that is transported in the blood.[60] Near-infrared light from a low-power laser and LEDs stimulates mitochondrial respiration by a bioenergetic process called photoneuromodulation, which occurs in the CNS tissue and consists of donated protons that are absorbed by cytochrome oxidase.[60] The absorption of luminous energy results in increased brain cytochrome oxidase enzymatic activity and oxygen consumption, which is coupled with oxidative phosphorylation and ATP production.[60] It has been proposed by Gonzalez-Lima et al. that the combined therapy of low-dose MB and near-red light, by sharing a common mechanism of enhancing mitochondrial respiration, may provide better neuroprotection against neuronal and axonal degeneration in TBI and other human neurobehavioral disorders.[60] Zhao et al., in a recent study using a mouse model of controlled cortical impact injury of TBI, reported that animals treated with MB after trauma showed a significant increase of Beclin-1, LC3-II to LC3-I ratio, indicating a high rate of autophagy, lower brain water content (BWC), and blockage of microglial activation.[61] Thus, some recent studies have shown promising evidence that immediate MB intravenous administration (15–30 minutes after TBI) attenuated microglial activation of neuroinflammatory gene expression (IL-1β, TNF-α), cerebral edema, and depressive, post-traumatic behavior up to 7 days after the injury.[62] Creatine (methylguanidoacetic acid) is a naturally produced nitrogenous organic acid, stored predominately in skeletal muscles but also present in the brain. Creatine administration after TBI can enhance supplies of phosphocreatine, a high energy intracellular compound, which can also have a direct effect on CNS axons blocking calcium-induced activation of mPTP, sustain ATP levels, maintain normal mitochondrial membrane potentials, and reduce calcium concentration inside the mitochondria.[63] The creatine system enables cells to regenerate ATP quickly, efficiently, and without the need for oxygen. All of these properties would help reduce the generalized energy crisis that occurs after TBI, where ATP is in high demand for restoration of membrane potentials and ion gradients, neurotransmitter release and reuptake, and intracellular transport.[63]

POST-TRAUMATIC NEUROINFLAMMATORY AND IMMUNE RESPONSE

There exists sufficient scientific evidence that DAI sparks a complex neuroinflammatory response with the release of inflammation mediators such as cytokines, chemokines, and growth factors by microglia, astrocytes, and neurons. Neuroinflammation starts shortly after TBI, expands rapidly, and remains in the damaged brain areas long term. Indeed, clinical and preclinical research shows that neuroinflammation activity after TBI may have detrimental and beneficial effects, depending on whether the examination was done in the acute or delayed phase post injury.[64] The cornerstone of developing neuroprotective treatments to counteract neuroinflammation after TBI is to minimize the deleterious neurotoxic effects and promote the beneficial and neurotrophic effects in order to promote conditions for repair and regeneration after trauma damage. It is well established that neuroinflammation represents a key pathologic response to brain injury and non-neuronal cells, such as endothelial cells, microglial, astrocytes, and oligodendrocytes; they all play an important role in secondary injury-mediated response. Post-traumatic neuroinflammatory reaction is characterized by glial cell activation, leukocyte recruitment, and upregulation of inflammatory mediators. Brain trauma results in rupture of the blood–brain barrier (BBB), allowing recruitment of bloodborne immune cells, such as neutrophils, macrophages, and lymphocytes to the injury site. Additionally, microglial cells activate and migrate to the damaged tissue in response to extracellular ATP, which is released by the damaged cells.[65] Activation of microglia after TBI appears to currently be the most important event that is initiating the neuroinflammatory chain reaction. Nevertheless, it shows a multiphasic pattern with early and late peaks of microglial macrophage concentration in the injured brain tissue.[66] The activated microglia releases microglial-derived microparticles (MP) loaded with proinflammatory mediators (IL-1β, miR-155), which can activate additional microglial cells and promote the spreading of the neuroinflammatory reaction in the injured brain, as well as stimulate systemic immune response.[67] If the inflammatory process cannot be controlled in the short term or become dysregulated, it may be an important contributing factor to chronic activation of neurotoxic microglia and chronic neurodegeneration.[67] The accumulation of myelin debris may be a major contributor to the inflammatory response after diffuse axonal injury, resulting from delayed accumulation and incomplete clearance of myelin; it is another important mediator of inflammation and it inhibits axon regeneration. It may lead to persistent secondary immune damage to the brain if it exists long term.[68] Post-trauma hypoxic episodes, very common after TBI, may exacerbate neurologic deficit after traumatic axonal injury (TAI) and it may prolong secondary injury mechanisms such as microglial activation, neuroinflammation, and axonal damage.[69] Neuroinflammation post-TAI and microglial activation may persist for years and may be a mechanism underlying chronic neurodegenerative disease, such as Alzheimer's disease, even after mild traumatic brain injury. Griffin et al. has suggested that chronic microglial activation and maintained production of glia-derived cytokines and other proteins originates a cytokine circle of cellular and molecular events, resulting in neurodegenerative changes and disease. Interleukin-1β production promotes neuronal synthesis and processing of the beta-amyloid protein, also maintaining the process of its deposition in neurons and axons.[70]

TAI AND NEURODEGENERATIVE DISEASE

Multiple factors contribute to amyloid beta (Aβ)-plaque formation after TBI. The presence of the Aβ precursor, APP, in damaged axons is the main potential source of Aβ. The Aβ precursor protein (APP) is a transmembrane glycoprotein synthesized by neurons and directly involved in cell growth, adhesion, and response to injury. APP also has neurotrophic functions that promote axonal sprouting, neurite outgrowth, and synaptogenesis, which is an essential mechanism of post-traumatic injury repair. APP is transported in the axons by fast transport mechanisms and accumulates in areas of axonal disruption.[71] Most important factors determining APP concentrations are its production rate and the effectiveness of axonal transport.[71] A high amount of APP accumulates in the axon bulbs with the necessary enzymes (presenelin-1 and beta-site APP-cleaving enzyme) for Aβ cleavage. Aβ, a peptide that exists extracellularly as a monomer, polymerizes into neurotoxic plaques to surrounding tissue when axonal damage occurs, from the first day after injury through day 14. The amyloid plaqes can last for years, however, its regression is possible as a result of enzymatic catabolic mechanisms. Kamal et al. suggested that post-traumatic interruption of axonal transport has been implicated in the APP processing and formation of Aβ, through interaction of APP, β-Secretase, and PS-1 with kinesin-1.[72] A recent study done that was conducted in an Alzheimer disease mouse model demonstrated that disruption of axonal transport by decreased kinesin-1 results in severe axonal pathology associated with excessive intraneuronal and extracellular accumulation and deposition.[73] The posterior lysis and breakage of injured axons allows the outflow of Aβ into the parenchyma, where it aggregates to form plaques.[74] Additionally, disorders such as dementia pugilistica and chronic traumatic encephalopathy following single TBI or repetitive mild TBI are linked to Aβ plaque formation and the accumulation of microtubule-associated protein tau (MAP-tau).[74,75] MAP-tau is a microtubule-bound protein that has an important function in cytoskeletal organization and axonal transport. After axonal injury and cytoskeleton breakdown occur, tau protein is degraded by activated calpain and caspase-3 into cleaved tau (c-tau) fragments that act as mediators for AB-induced tau phosphorylation and produce phosphorylated tau complexes that accumulate as neurofibrillary tangles and promote cellular apoptosis. One hour after injury, tau fragments can be found in the CSF and peak at 24 hours, declining over the next 96 hours. CSF concentrations of c-tau can be useful as an outcome predictor, because higher amounts are associated with poor functional outcome.[76] Smith et al. have described tau pathology after TBI as predominantly localized in superficial cortical layers, accumulating preferentially in the depth of sulci, and in perivascular distribution. However, activated microglia showed a diffuse distribution and did not exhibit any particular accumulation in the areas previously mentioned. These findings suggest that there is no direct spatial relationship between activated microglia and neurons and axons showing abnormal tau protein accumulation.[77]

NEUROIMAGING DIAGNOSIS IN DIFFUSE AXONAL INJURY (DAI)

Neuroradiology data in the clinical setting is mostly evaluated in qualitative grounds (CT, MRI), which may miss, even to an expert neuroradiologist, significant and critical pathologic elements that are necessary to forecast outcome. With improvements in imaging technologies, radiographic analysis of the brain following TBI is improving outcome prediction.[78] DAI typically consists of focal white matter lesions of 1 to 15 mm with a characteristic pattern of distribution.[79] When the clinical picture of a patient with DAI is compared with typical findings seen in radiologic imaging (CT, MRI), a greater degree of microscopic damage is suggested to explain such disproportion.

Computed tomography

A CT scan, as a neuroimaging resource, has evident advantages over NMRI in terms of speed and accessibility in most acute trauma environments. Usually, a brain CT scan does not show specific pathologic features associated to DAI, therefore, false negatives are possible, though normal or almost normal CT-scan findings can be commonly seen in patients with DAI on initial presentation. In the acute setting, in approximately 10% of patients, hemorrhagic punctate lesions of the corpus callosum and gray-white matter junctions of the cerebrum and pontine-mesencephalic junction close to cerebellar peduncles can be observed. Delayed CT scanning may be helpful in demonstrating edema or atrophy as delayed findings.[80] Images of atrophy are more prominent in areas of high white-matter concentration and periventricular parenchyma; also ventriculomegaly may be found.[80,81]

Conventional nuclear magnetic resonance imaging (NMRI)

NMRI is more sensitive than a brain CT scan for the diffuse and small pathology in DAI. The shearing forces associated with TAI produce transection of small vessels running parallel to axons, forming microscopic hemorrhages in these areas. Signal-loss that is provoked by the iron-containing heme group in slow-flow areas can be detected by gradient echo and T2-weighted NMRI imaging. Distribution of microhemorrhages in areas most frequently associated with shearing axonal injury, such as corpus callosum, brainstem, and other white matter tracts, are highly suggestive of imaging diagnosis of DAI, as they appear as punctate, signal-free lesions in white matter and can be visualized for years after the initial injury occurred.[82] Gradient echo imaging has become the mainstay of NMRI for patients with suspected shearing-type axonal injury because it can show signal abnormalities in areas that appear normal in T1- and T2-weighted spin-echo sequences; also, these abnormal signals can persist for many years after trauma.[83] An additional factor is the strength of the magnet field, being 3TNMRI twice more sensitive than 1.5 Tesla devices for microhemorrhages.[83]

Susceptibility weight imaging (SWI)

Susceptibility weight imaging (SWI) is a high-resolution 3D imaging technique whose images are based on local magnetic field aberrations. However, it is six times more powerful than a conventional MRI that detects traumatic microhemorrhages and renders hemorrhage volume approximately twice the size of the conventional NMRI gradient echo.[84] In severe cerebral edema and associated venous stasis, slow venous blood flow produces SWI signal dropout in medullary cerebral vein distribution, as they appear irregular and radially distributed throughout the white matter.[84]

Diffusion-weighted imaging

Diffusion-weighted imaging (DWI) and the corresponding apparent diffusion coefficient (ADC) can identify lesions with high and low diffusion, based on the net movement of water molecules. It has demonstrated improved detection of nonhemorrhagic lesions over conventional MRI in areas of cytotoxic or vasogenic edema. DWI is very useful for diagnosing acute ischemic events, due to its high sensitivity for low-flow states. Nonetheless, this technique is also sensitive to other cerebral disease processes, including DAI.[85] In adult patients, DWI/ADC imaging has shown a close correlation between the high intensity of ADC signals in the corpum callosus, brainstem, and in pediatic patients, and deep frontal and temporal white matter, with duration of coma and poor outcome after traumatic brain damage and TAI.[86,87]

Nuclear imaging

Nuclear imaging has no practical role as part of the routine diagnostic workup of patients with TBI and diffuse axonal damage. Nevertheless, some studies have suggested that iodine-123 (^{123}I) single proton emission CT (SPECT) can show areas of hypoperfusion in known areas of lesion and visualize additional areas of injury that cannot be observed with NMRI.

CONCLUSION

Diffuse axonal damage is an extremely complex process that is initiated with the stretching and shearing of axons and may evolve into a long-term syndrome of cerbral dysconnection and functional impairment. A very high number of preclinical and clinical studies have been conducted to improve our knowledge of the neurophysiologic mechanisms involved in primary axotomy, but most of all, in secondary axotomy. The identification of biomarkers and its implications in potential therapeutic strategies to improve clinical and functional outcome of patients with DAI is underway. Technologic advances and innovations in neuroimaging, especially NMRI, are increasing our understanding of DAI outcome following TBI. However, in spite of all of these advances, a marked lack of translation into efficacious therapies still exists. Hopefully, an increased undertanding of the mechanistic process of axonal injury will lead to effective therapies and better clinical and functional outcomes.

REFERENCES

1. Meythaler JM, Peduzzi JD, Eleftheriou E, Novack TA. Current concepts: Diffuse axonal injury-associated traumatic brain injury. *Arch Phys Med Rehabil.* 2001;82(10):1461-1471.

2. Smith DH, Meaney DF. Axonal damage in traumatic brain injury. *Neuroscientist.* 2000;6 (6):483-495.

3. Povlishock JT, Katz DI. Update of neuropathology and neurological recovery after traumatic brain injury. *J Head Trauma Rehabil.* 2005;20(1):76-94.

4. Christman CW, Grady MS, Walker SA, Holloway KL, Povlishock JT. Ultrastructural studies of diffuse axonal injury in humans. *J Neurotrauma.* 1994;11(2):173-186.

5. Povlishock J, Becker DP, Cheng CL, Vaughan GW. Axonal change in minor head injury. *J Neuropathol Exp Neurol.* 1983;42(3): 225-242.

6. Johnson VE, Stewart W, Smith DH. Axonal pathology in traumatic brain injury. *Exp Neurol.* 2013;246:35-43.

7. Adams JH, Doyle D, Ford I, Gennarelli TA, Graham DI, McLellan DR. Diffuse axonal injury in head injury: Definition, diagnosis and grading. *Histopathology.* 1989;15(1):49-59.

8. Gupta RK, Przekwas A. Mathematical models of blast-induced TBI: Current status, challenges, and prospects. *Front Neurol.* 2013; 4:59.

9. Smith DH, Wolf JA, Lusardi TA, Lee VM, Meaney DF. High tolerance and delayed elastic response of cultured axons to dynamic stretch injury. *J Neurosci.* 1999;19(11): 4263-4269.

10. Smith DH, Nonaka M, Miller R et al. Immediate coma following inertial brain injury dependent on axonal damage in the brainstem. *J Neurosurg.* 2000;93(2):315-322.

11. Browne KD, Chen XH, Meany DF, Smith DH. Mild traumatic injury and diffuse axonal injury in swine. *J Neurotrauma.* 2011;28(9): 1747-1755.

12. Blumbergs PC, Jones NR, North JB. Diffuse axonal injury in head trauma. *J Neurol Neurosurg Psychiatry.* 1989;52(7): 838-841.

13. Polivshock JT. Traumatically induced axonal injury: Pathogenesis and pathobiological implications. *Brain Pathol.* 1992;2(1):1-12.

14. Smith DH, Meaney DT, Shull WH. Diffuse axonal injury in head trauma. *J Head Trauma Rehabil.* 2003;18(4):307-316.

15. Hunter JJ, Wilde EA, Shull WH. Emerging tools for use with traumatic brain research. *J Neurotrauma.* 2012;29(4):654-671.

16. Sundaram NK, Acer EB, Greenwood BD. The impact of traumatic brain injury in pituitary function. *EndocrinolMetab Clin North Am.* 2013;42(3):565-583.

17. Reifschneider K, Auble BA, Rose SR. Update of endocrine dysfunction following pediatric traumatic brain injury. *J Clin Med.* 2015;4(8): 1536-1560.

18. Christman SA, Grady MS, Walker SA, Holloway KL, Polivshock JT. Ultrastructural studies of diffuse axonal injuries in man. *J Neurotrauma.* 1994;11(2):173-186.

19. Reeves TM, Phillips LC, Polivshock JT. Myelinated and unmyelinated axons of the corpus callosum differ in vulnerability and functional recovery following traumatic brain injury. *Exp Neurol.* 2005;196(1):126-137.

20. Stone JR, Okonkwo DO, Dialo AO et al. Impaired axonal transport and altered axolemmal permeability occur in distinct populations of damaged axons following traumatic brain injury. *Exp Neurol.* 2004;190 (1)59-69.

21. Li J, Li XY, Feng DF, Pan DC. Biomarkers associated with diffuse traumatic axonal injury: Exploring pathogenesis, early diagnosis, and prognosis. *J Trauma.* 2010;69(6):1610-1618.

22. Mukhopadhyay R, Kumar S, Hoh JH. Molecular mechanisms for organizing the neuronal cytoskeleton. *Bioassays.* 2004;26(9): 1017-1025.

23. Maxwell WL, Domleo A, McColl G, Jaffari SS, Graham DJ. Post-acute alterations in the axonal cytoskeleton after traumatic axonal injury. *J Neurotrauma.* 2003;20(2):151-168.

24. Fournier AJ, Hogan JD, Rajbhandari L, Shrestha S, Venkatesan A, Ramesh KT. Changes in neurofilament and microtubule distribution following focal axon compression. *PLoS One.* 2015;10(6):e0131617.

25. Auyang H, Nauman E, Shi R. Contribution of cytoskeletal elements of mechanical property of axons. In Micro/Nano Symposium (UGIM) 2010; 18th Biennal University/Goverment/Industry:1-5.

26. Polivshok JT, Christman CW. The pathobiology of traumatically induced axonal injury in animals and humans: A review of current thoughts. *J Neurotrauma.* 1995;12(4):555-564.

27. Tomei G, Spagnoli D, Ducati A et al. Morphology and neurophysiology of focal axonal injury experimentally induced in the guinea pig optic nerve. *Acta Neuropathol.* 1990;80(5):506-513.

28. Knöferle J, Koch JC, Ostendorf T et al. Mechanisms of acute axonal degeneration in the optic nerve in vivo. *Proc Nat Acad Sci U S A.* 2010;107(13):6064-6069.

29. Staal JA, Dickson TC, Gasparini R, Lin Y, Foa L, Vickers JC. Initial calcium release from intracellular stores followed by calcium dysregulation is linked to secondary axotomy following transient axonal stretch injury. *J Neurochem.* 2010;112(5):1143-1155.

30. Stirling DP, Cummins K, Wayne Chen SR, Stys P. Axoplasmic reticulum Ca(2$^+$) release causes secondary degeneration in spinal axons. *Ann Neurol.* 2014;75(2):220-229.

31. Bullock R, Zauner A, Myseros JS, Marmarou A, Woodward JJ, Young HF. Evidence for prolonged release excitatory amino acids in severe human head trauma. Relationship to clinical events. *Ann NY Acad Sci.* 1995;765:290-297.

32. Bullock R, Zauner A, Woodward JJ et al. Factors affecting excitatory amino acid release following severe human head injury. *J Neurosurg.* 1998;89(4):507-518.

33. Hosie KA, King AE, Blizzard CA, Vickers JD, Dickson TC. Chronic excitotoxin-induced axon degeneration in a compartmented neuronal culture model. *ASN Neuro.* 2012;4(1):e00076.

34. King AE, Dickson TC, Blizzard CA et al. Excitotoxicity mediated by non-NMDA receptors causes distal axonopathy in long-term cultured spinal motor neurons. *Eur J Neurosci.* 2007;26(8):2151-2159.

35. King AE, Southon KA, Dittman I, Vickers JC. Excitotoxin-induced caspase-3 activation and microtubule disintegration in axons is inhibited by taxol. *Acta Neuropathol Commun.* 2013;1:59.

36. Saatman KE, Creed J, Raghupathi R. Calpain as a therapeutic target in traumatic brain injury. *Neurotherapeutics.* 2010;71(1):31-42.

37. Mondello S, Robiesek SA, Gabrielli A et al. all-Spectrin breakdown products (SBDis): Diagnosis and outcome in severe traumatic brain injury patients. *J Neurotrauma.* 2010;27(7):1203-1213.

38. Saatman KE, Abai B, Grosvenor A, Vorwerk CK. Traumatic axonal injury results in biphasic calpain activation and retrograde transport impairment in mice. *J Cereb Blood Flow Metab.* 2003;23(1):34-42.

39. Xu K, Cruishen Z, Xiaowei Z. Actin, spectrin and associated protein from a periodic cytoskeletal structure in axons. *Science.* 2013;339(6118):452-456.

40. Ma M, Ferguson TA, Schoch KM, Li QY et al. Calpains mediate axonal cytoskeleton disintegration during Wallerian degeneration. *Neurobiol Dis* 2013;56:34-46.

41. Maas AIR, Roozenbeek B, Manley GT. Clinical trials in traumatic brain injury: Past experience and current developments. *Neurotherapeutics.* 2010;7(1):115-126.

42. Thornberry NA, Lazebnik Y. Caspases: Enemies within. *Science.* 1998;281(5381):1312-1316.

43. Susin SA, Lorenzo HK, Zamzani M et al. Molecular characterization of mitochondrial apoptosis-inducing factor. *Nature.* 1996;397(6718):441-446.

44. Büki A, Okonkwo DO, Wang KK, Polivshock JT. Cytochrome c release and caspase activation in traumatic axonal injury. *J Neurosci.* 2000;20(8):2825-2834.

45. Wang KK, Postmantur R, Nath R et al. Simultaneous degradation of alphaII- and betaII-spectrin by caspase-3(CPP32) in apoptotic cells. *J Biol Chem.* 1998;273(35):22490-22497.

46. Shen H, Hyrc KL, Goldberg MP. Maintaining energy homeostasis is an essential component of Wld(S)-mediated axon protection. *Neurobiol Dis.* 2013;59:69-79.

47. Court FA, Coleman MP. Mitochondria as a central sensor for axonal degenerative stimuli. *Trends Neurosci.* 2012;35(6):364-372.

48. Halestrap AP. What is the mitochondrial transition pore? *J Mol Cell Cardiol.* 2009;46(6):821-831.

49. Mazzeo AT, Beat A, Singh A, Bullock MR. The role of mitochondrial transition pore, and its modulation, in traumatic brain injury

and delayed neurodegeneration after TBI. *Exp Neurol.* 2009;218(2):363-370.

50. Barrientos SA, Martinez NW, Yoo S et al. Axonal degeneration is mediated by the mitochondrial permeability pore. *J Neurosci.* 2011;31(3):966-978.

51. Staal JA, Dickson TC, Chung RS, Vickers JC. Cyclosporin-A treatment attenuates delayed cytoskeletal alterations and secondary axotomy following mild axonal stretch injury. *Dev Neurobiol.* 2007;67(14): 1831-1842.

52. Waldemeier PC, Feldtrauer JJ, Qian T, Lemasters JJ. Inhibition of the mitochondrial permeability transition by the nonimmuno-suppressive cyclosporine derivative NIM811. *Mol Pharmacol.* 2002;62(1):22-29.

53. Mbye LH, Singh IN, Sullivan PG, Springer JE, Hall ED. Attenuation of acute mitochondrial dysfunction after traumatic brain injury in mice by NIM811, a non-immunosuppressive cyclosporin A analog. *Exp Neurol.* 2008;209 (1):243-253.

54. Readnower RD, Pandya JD, McEwen ML, Pauly JR, Springer JE, Sullivan PG. Post-injury administration of the mitochondrial permeability transition pore inhibitor, NIM811, is neuroprotective and improves cognition after traumatic brain injury in rats. *J Neurotrauma.* 2011;28(9):1845-1853.

55. Chen G, Shi J, Hu Z, Hang C. Inhibitory effect on cerebral inflammatory response following traumatic brain injury in rats: A potential neuroprotective mechanism of N-acetylcysteine. *Mediators Inflamm.* 2008; 2008:716458.

56. Hoffer ME, Balaban C, Slade MD, Tsao JW, Hoffer B. Amelioration of acute sequelae of blast induced mild traumatic brain injury by N-acetyl cysteine: A double-blind, placebo controlled study. *PLoS One.* 2013;8(1): e54163.

57. Eakin K, Baratz-Goldstein R, Pick CG et al. Efficacy of N-acetyl cysteine in traumatic brain injury. *PLos One.* 2014:9(4):e90617.

58. Smith DH, Hicks R, Polivshock JT. Therapy development for diffuse axonal injury. *J Neurotrauma.* 2013;30(5):307–323.

59. Xuan W, Vatansever F, Huan L et al. Transcranial low-level laser therapy improves neurological performance in traumatic brain injury in mice: Effect of treatment repetition regimen. *PLos One.* 2013;8(1):e534454.

60. Gonzalez-Lima F, Auchter A. Protection against neurodegeneration with low-dose methylene blue and near-infrared light. *Front Cell Neurosci.* 2015;9:179.

61. Zhao M, Liang F, Xu H, Yan W, Zhang J. Methylene blue exerts a neuroprotective effect against traumatic brain injury by promoting autophagy and inhibiting microglial activation. *Mol Med Reo.* 2016;13(1):13-20.

62. Fenn AM, Skendelas JP, Moussa DW et al. Methylene blue attenuates traumatic brain injury-associated neuroinflammation and acute depressive-like behavior in mice. *J Neurotrauma.* 2015;32(2):127-138.

63. Dean PJ, Arikan G, Opitz B, Sterr A. Potential use of creatine supplementation following mild traumatic brain injury. *Concussion.* 2017; 2(2):CNC34.

64. Helmy A, De Simoni MG, Guilfoyle MR, Carpenter KL, Hutchinson PJ. Cytokines and innate inflammation in the pathogenesis of human traumatic brain injury. *Prog Neurobiol.* 2011;95(3):352-372.

65. Davalos D, Grutzendler J, Yang G et al. ATP mediates rapid microglial response to local brain injury in vivo. *Nat Neurosci.* 2005;8 (6):752-758.

66. Wang G, Zhang J, Xu X, Zhang et al. Microglial/macrophage polarization dynamics in white matter after traumatic brain injury. *J Cereb Blood Flow Metab.* 2013;33(12):1864-1874.

67. Kumar A, Stoica BA, Loane DJ, Yang M et al. Microglial-derived microparticles mediate neuroinflammation after traumatic brain injury. *J Neuroinflammation.* 2017;14(1): 47.

68. Wen L, Xu J, Zhan T et al. The occurrence of diffuse axonal injury in the brain: Associated with the accumulation and clearance of myelin debris. *Neural Regen Res.* 2014;9 (21):1902-1906.

69. Yan EB, Hellewell SC, Agyapomaa D, Morganti-Kossman MC. Post-trauma hypoxia excacerbates neuroinflammation and axonal damage in rat model of diffuse axonal damage. *Injury.* 2010;41(suppl 1):S61.

70. Griffin WS, Sheng JG, Royston MC et al. Glial-neuronal interactions in Alzheimer's disease: The potential role of a 'cytokine

cycle' in disease progression. *Brain Pathol.* 1998;8(1):65-72.

71. Su E, Bell M. Diffuse Axonal Injury. In: Laskowitz D, Grant G, eds. Translational Research in Traumatic Brain Injury. Boca Raton, FL: CRC Press/Taylor and Francis Group; 2016. Chapter 3. *Frontiers in Neuroscience.*

72. Kamal A, Almenar-Queralt A, LeBlanc JF, Roberts EA, Goldstein LS. Kinesin-mediated axonal transport of a membrane compartment containing beta-secretase and presenilin-1 requires APP. *Nature.* 2001;414(6864):643-648.

73. Stokin GB, Lillo C, Falzone TL et al. Axonopathy and transport deficits early in the pathogenesis of Alzheimer's disease. *Science.* 2005;307(5713):1282-1288.

74. Browne KD, Chen XH, Meaney DF, Smith DH. Mild traumatic brain injury and diffuse axonal injury in swine. *J Neurotrauma.* 2011; 28(9):1747-1755.

75. Hill CS, Coleman MP, Menon DK. Traumatic axonal injury: Mechanisms and translational opportunities. *Trends Neurosci.* 2016;39(5): 311-324.

76. Zemlam FP, Jauch EC, Mulchahey JJ et al. C-tau biomarker of neuronal damage in severe brain injured patients: Associations with elevated intracranial pressure and clinical outcome. *Brain Res.* 2002;947(1):131-139.

77. Smith G, Gentleman SM, Leclerq PD et al. The neuroinflammatory response in humans after traumatic axonal injury. *Neuropathol Appl Neurobiol.* 2013;39(6):654-666.

78. Murray GD, Butcher I, McHugh GS et al. Multivariable prognostic analysis in traumatic brain injury: Results from IMPACT study. *J Neurotrauma.* 2007;24(2):329-337.

79. Liu J, Kou Z, Tian Y. Diffuse axonal injury after traumatic cerebral microbleeds: An evaluation of imaging techniques. *Neural Regen Res.* 2014;9(12):1222-1230.

80. Mata-Mbemba, D, Mugikura S, Nakawa A et al. Intraventricular hemorrhage on initial computed tomography as marker of diffuse axonal injury after traumatic brain injury. *J Neurotrauma.* 2015;32(5):359-365.

81. Provenzale JM. Imaging of traumatic brain injury: A review of the recent medical literature. *AM J Roentgenol.* 2010;194(1): 16-19.

82. Imaizumi T, Chiba M, Honma T, Yoshikawa J. Niwa J. Dynamics of dotlike hemosiderin spots associated with intracerebral hemorrhage. *J Neuroimaging.* 2003;13(2):155-157.

83. Scheid R, Preul C, Gruber O, Wiggins SC, van Cramon DJ. Diffuse axonal injury associated with chronic traumatic brain injury: Evidence from T2*-weighted gradient-echo imaging at 3T. *Am J Neuroradiol.* 2003;24(6):1049-1056.

84. Iwamura A, Taoka T, Fukusumi A et al. Diffuse vascular injury: Convergent-type hemorrhage in the supratentorial white matter on susceptibility-weighted image in case of severe traumatic brain damage. *Neuroradiology.* 2012;54(4):335-343.

85. Schaefer RN, Grant PE, Gonzalez RG. Diffusion-weighted MR imaging of the brain. *Radiology.* 2000;217(2):331-345.

86. Zheng WB, Liu GR, Kong KM, Wu RH. Coma duration prediction in diffuse axonal injury: Analysis of apparent diffusion coefficient and clinical prognostic factors. *Conf Proc IEEE Eng Med Biol Soc.* 2006;1:1052-1055.

87. Galloway NR, Tong KA, Ashual S Ayayo U, Oberaus A. Diffusion-weighted imaging improves outcome prediction in pediatric traumatic brain injury. *J Neurotrauma.* 2008; 25(10):1153-1162.

11

Cervical spine injury

FERENC RABAI AND LAUREN BERKOW

INTRODUCTION

Cervical spine injury is a relatively common occurrence, with an estimated incidence of 3% to 6% in all trauma patients and nearly 8% in patients with significant head injury.[1,2] Most common etiologies are motor vehicle accidents and falls. Injury to the vital neuronal pathways passing through the cervical spinal cord can result in catastrophic morbidity, including quardriplegia, cardiorespiratory collapse, and death.

The two principal determining factors of the severity of injury are the extent to which the structural integrity of the spine has been compromised and the degree of spinal cord injury (SCI). When trauma causes the spine to be unstable, it is no longer able to reliably protect the spinal cord from further external trauma. SCI evolves in two phases: primary injury results from direct mechanical forces at the time of impact, and secondary injuries develop subsequently as a result of local and systemic physiologic derangements in response to the trauma, which further compromise the homeostasis of the spinal cord. The goals of care in cervical spine (C-spine) trauma revolve around mitigating (lessening the severity of) secondary injuries.

We provide an overview on functional anatomy, physiology, and biomechanics of the C-spine and spinal cord. We present the various types of C-spine and SCI, their clinical and radiologic assessment, and the principles of management with special emphasis on airway and anesthetic management.

FUNCTIONAL ANATOMY AND BIOMECHANICS OF THE CERVICAL SPINE

Understanding the complex anatomic and biomechanic features of the C-spine is critical for the successful assessment and management of a wide variety of C-spine injuries.

The first two vertebrae of the C-spine differ in appearance from the rest (Figure 11.1) The first vertebra (C1), called the "atlas," has a unique ring shape that comprises the anterior (front) and posterior (back) arches, which are connected by the lateral masses. It also has a wider diameter than the rest of the vertebrae because it accommodates the superiorly projecting peg-shaped process or

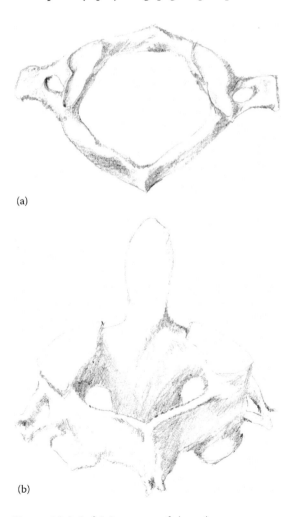

(a)

(b)

Figure 11.1 (a,b) Anatomy of the atlas.

"dens" of the body of the second vertebra (C2), which is known as the "axis." Aside from the presence of the dens, the appearance of the axis resembles the other vertebrae, which are signet ring-shaped and comprise the body anteriorly, the lateral masses on each side, and the laminae and the spinous process posteriorly (a bony projection off of the back of each vertebra). The vertebrae articulate with each other via tough fibrocartilaginous discs that are interpositioned between the bodies and via two small synovial joints arising from the lateral masses. The lateral masses of the cervical vertebrae contain the foramina transversaria, which protect and transmit the vertebral arteries on both sides.

Strong ligaments and cervical paraspinous muscles stabilize the C-spine, creating a physiologic lordosis (an arch in the spine). The anterior and posterior longitudinal ligaments originate at the occiput and run along the anterior and posterior aspects of the vertebral bodies. Posteriorly, the ligamentum flavum, interspinous, and supraspinous ligaments connect the laminae and stabilize the posterior elements of the vertebrae. A complex array of ligaments also join the C1 and C2 vertebrae to each other and to the occiput. The cruciate ligament attaches the dens to the occiput and the atlas. The transverse ligament of the atlas is the main stabilizer of the dens posteriorly inside the atlas. The right and left alar ligaments project from the dens superiorly to the occipital condyles (Figure 11.2).[3]

In addition to serving as a resilient structural support for the head and protecting the spinal cord, the C-spine also facilitates a wide range of movement for the head and neck. The atlanto-occipital junction is formed by a pair of synovial condyloid joints, which allow for significant freedom in head movement in all directions on the C-spine but mainly flexion, extension, and lateral tilt. Rotation is primarily achieved by the atlas rotating around the dens of the axis. The entire C-spine also contributes to flexion-extension, lateral tilt, and rotation of the head and neck.[4,5]

ANATOMY AND PHYSIOLOGY OF THE CERVICAL SPINAL CORD

The medulla continues as the cervical spinal cord caudal to the foramen magnum (the hole in the base of the skull through which the spinal cord passes). The cervical spinal cord has eight segments.

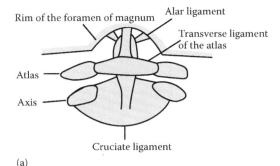

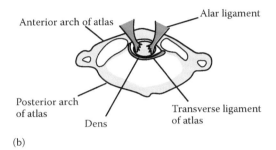

(a)

(b)

Figure 11.2 (a) Schematic illustration of the transverse and alar ligaments in the coronal plane. (b) Schematic illustration of the transverse and alar ligaments in the axial plane.

Nerve roots of each segment exit the spinal canal above their respective vertebra except for nerve roots of the 8th segment, which exits below C7. The neuronal elements that are responsible for motor functions occupy the anterior and lateral aspects of the spinal cord (eg, motor neurons in the ventral horn of the gray matter, corticospinal tracts, vestibulo-spinal and rubrospinal tracts, etc.). Sensory pathways are located posteriorly (dorsal columns) and laterally (spinothalamic tracts).[6]

Additionally, there are a number of other vital neural pathways contained within the cervical spinal cord, including motor pathways that innervate muscles of the diaphragm (which exit through C3–C5 segments) and the accessory muscles of respiration, sympathetic pathways that maintain systemic, sympathetic tone of the heart and the entire vasculature, inhibitory descending pathways, and pathways that regulate bowel and bladder function.[6]

The blood supply to the cervical spinal cord originates from the vertebral arteries and branches of the aortic arch, which feed into a single, anterior, spinal artery supplying the anterior two-thirds and a pair of posterior spinal arteries, supplying the posterior one-third of the spinal cord. The characteristics and determinants of spinal cord blood flow are similar to that in the brain. Autoregulation ensures constant blood flow (approximately 50 mL/min/100 g) over a wide range of mean arterial pressure (60–120 mmHg).[7] There is a vasodilatory response to hypercapnia and hypoxia to maintain the tightly regulated metabolic homeostasis necessary for normal neuronal function. This delicate balance may be subject to disturbances caused by primary and secondary injuries in the form of edema, diminished systemic oxygen delivery, inflammatory, and other toxic molecular insults. Spinal cord blood flow in SCI may be severely reduced.[8]

CERVICAL SPINE INJURY CLASSIFICATION

Anatomic classification of SCI is based on the location of the injury in relation to the cervical segment and specific anatomic structures. Combination injuries involving multiple bones and ligaments at adjacent or even different spinal levels are common. SCI severity ranges from minimal soft tissue strain (eg, whiplash) to catastrophic damage to the spine and spinal cord.

OCCIPUT TO C2 INJURIES

The complicated anatomic relationships between the skull, atlas, and axis renders this complex prone to a variety of injuries. The main determinants of stability of the atlanto-occipito-axial complex are the ligaments; thus most isolated bony injuries without injury to the supporting ligaments can be considered stable.

Atlanto-occipital injuries

Atlanto-occipital dislocation (AOD) is a rare injury resulting from disruption of the anterior and posterior atlanto-occipital membranes. Depending on the force of impact, the skull can be displaced anteriorly, posteriorly, laterally, and superiorly in relation to the atlas and the spine. In severe injuries, the junction between the medulla and the spinal cord can be severed, resulting in bulbospinal dissociation and sudden death. Depending on the degree of injury that is assessed by computed tomography (CT) and magnetic resonance imaging

(MRI), surgical stabilization may be indicated in the form of occipito-cervical fusion.[9]

Occipital condyle fractures are rare and may be associated with AOD. The evaluation is done through CT. Treatment usually consists of rigid collar immobilization, but rarely, halo immobilization or surgical intervention may be necessary.[10]

Atlas fractures

The ring of the atlas is wider than other vertebrae and only about one-third of the space enclosed by this ring is occupied by the spinal cord. Because of this, fractures are less likely to cause direct injury to the cord. Atlas fractures are also relatively rare and are one of three types. Type I includes single arch fractures. Type II are burst fractures involving two or more locations on the ring of the atlas. This type includes the classic "Jefferson fracture," which is a four-point fracture of the ring of C1 (Figure 11.3). These fractures usually occur as a result of axial loading and result in outward displacement of the bony fragments and are, therefore, rarely associated with neurologic deficits. Type III fractures include lateral mass fractures.[11]

Although neurologic injury is rare in C1 fractures, the stability of the spine may be compromised when the transverse ligament is injured and is no longer able to support the dens. In such cases, surgery may be indicated to restore stability.[12]

Atlanto-axial subluxation

Atlanto-axial subluxation usually occurs as a result of disruption or incompetence of the transverse ligament, which is no longer able to stabilize the peg of C2. This generally leads to anterior dislocation or rotatory dislocation (more commonly seen in children) of the atlas ring on the axis and narrowing of the spinal canal. Of note, the weakening of the transverse ligament or its attachments in patients with rheumatoid arthritis may lead to similar phenomena, even in the absence of trauma, which may put them at risk of SCI during intubation. The treatment of anterior atlanto-axial subluxation with associated transverse ligament disruption is usually surgical fusion. For rotatory subluxation, traction and halo immobilization may be attempted prior to surgical fixation.[13]

Axis injuries

Because C2 has extensive ligamentous attachments with nearby structures, any injury to it could potentially cause instability and carry significant risk for SCI. The axis is susceptible to fractures in two locations: (1) at the odontoid (a tooth-like projection from the second cervical vertebra on which the first vertebra pivots) process and (2) at the isthmus, between the pedicle and the articular process.

Odontoid fractures are relatively common and are classified into three major types (Figure 11.4).[14] Type I is rare and is a fracture at the tip of the peg above the transverse ligament. The alar ligaments attach the tip of the peg to the occiput. Therefore, a Type I fracture may represent an avulsion (pulling or tearing away) type AOD with other extensive ligamentous injuries of the atlanto-occipital dissociation complex with serious consequences. Type II is a fracture through the base of the odontoid process. Although the cruciate ligament of the dens may be preserved and provide some stability to the fragments, most Type II odontoid fractures are unstable. Type III fractures occur below the dens

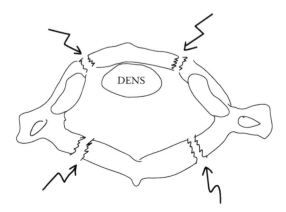

Figure 11.3 Jefferson fracture of the atlas.

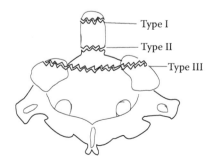

Figure 11.4 Odontoid fracture classification.

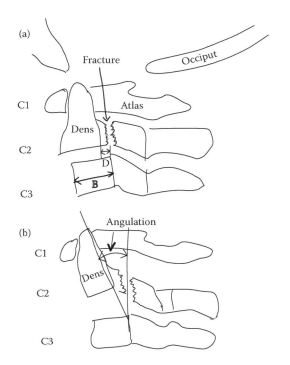

Figure 11.5 Two components of the Francis grading system of Hangman's fracture. **(a)** Degree of anterior displacement of the body of C2 vertebra on C3 and **(b)** degree of angulation of the dens of C2 vertebra relative to the body of C3. D: distance between posterior surface of dens of C2 and posterior surface of the body of C3; B: length of body of C3 measured in the sagittal plane.

and involve the superior part of the vertebral body and are usually stable.

Halo or rigid collar immobilization is usually attempted, but nonunion rates are high, especially for Type II fractures. Surgical fusion should, therefore, be strongly considered for all odontoid fractures, especially for displaced fractures and older patients with limited bone healing potential.[15]

A "Hangman's fracture" is sustained at the time of hanging as the result of a hyperextension-distraction type force. A much more common mechanism of this injury is related to motor vehicle accidents or diving head first with a hyperextension and axial loading-type of force, which impacts the C-spine. The resultant injury is typically a bilateral fracture of the pars interarticularis (a small segment of bone joining the facet joint and the dens) and various degrees of traumatic spondylolisthesis (one vertebra slides forward on the one below it) of C2 on C3. Grading is based on the degree of anterior

displacement of the body of C2 on C3 and the degree of angulation of the dens of C2 in relation to the body of C3 (Figure 11.5). The most severe form (grade V) represents disc disruption between C2 and C3 and complete loss of stability of the spine. Conservative treatment with external immobilization in a halo or rigid collar is usually successful with low nonunion rates. High-grade injuries require surgical stabilization.[15]

C3–C7 INJURIES

Unlike the first two cervical vertebrae, the vertebrae that comprise the subaxial C-spine (C3–C7) have a uniform anatomic appearance and biomechanical function; therefore, the patterns of injury, assessment, and treatment principles can be generalized within this spinal segment.

The classic assessment of instability of an acute traumatic spine injury is based on the three-column spine concept, which was first described in 1984 by Denis.[16] This model divides the spine into three columns in the sagittal plane. The anterior column is formed by the anterior longitudinal ligament, the anterior half of the vertebral bodies, and discs. The middle column is formed by the posterior vertebral bodies and discs, the posterior longitudinal ligament, and synovial joints. The posterior column is formed by the laminae, spinous processes, and posterior ligaments of the spine. An injury that disrupts any two or more of these conceptual columns makes the spine unstable.

A more recent classification system, known as the subaxial injury classification, assesses the morphology of bony injuries, the integrity of the disco-ligamentous complex of the spine, and the extent of the neurologic injury.[17] Level I evidence supports its use in determining if an injury should be treated surgically or nonsurgically, depending on the total score in all three categories (operative treatment for scores ≥5, nonoperative treatment for score 1–3) (Table 11.1).

Another classification describes typical patterns of injury based on the mechanism and impact on the C-spine.[18] Flexion forces may exert injury alone or may be compounded by axial loading or distraction. Flexion by itself or flexion with superimposed distraction can lead to unilateral and bilateral facet dislocations, and various degrees of neurologic deficit are commonly seen. Medical professionals may attempt to use traction or manipulation under

Table 11.1 Subaxial injury classification scoring

	Points
Morphology	
No abnormality	0
Compression	1
Burst	+1 = 2
Distraction (eg, facet perch, hyperextension	3
Rotation/translation (eg, facet dislocation, unstable teardrop or advanced staged flexion compression injury)	4
Disco-ligamentous complex (DLC)	
Intact	0
Indeterminate (eg, isolated interspinous widening, MRI signal change only)	1
Disrupted (eg, widening of disc space, facet perch, or dislocation)	2
Neurologic status	
Intact	0
Root injury	1
Complete cord injury	2
Incomplete cord injury	3
Continuous cord compression in setting of neuro deficit (neuro modifier)	+1

Source: Vaccaro AR et al. *Spine (Phila PA 1976)*. 2007;32:2365.)

anesthesia; however, open surgical reduction and stabilization is often required. Flexion with axial loading may result in anterior vertebral body fracture and disruption of posterior ligaments and locked facets. In severe cases (eg, "teardrop fracture"), surgery may be necessary. Similarly, extension forces on the C-spine may act alone or be compounded by axial compression or distraction and, in most cases, result in less severe injuries involving the spinous processes and laminae, as well as fractures through the lateral mass and facets. When the C-spine and head are in a neutral position, pure compression may result in burst fractures. Distraction forces, on the other hand, may cause complete ligamentous disruption with instability.[15]

WHIPLASH

Whiplash can be defined as an injury caused by any mechanical force affecting the soft tissues of the C-spine (cervical and paraspinous muscles, ligaments, discs, and synovial joints) in the absence of bone fractures, dislocations, or disc herniations.[19] Clinical grading of whiplash is based on the severity of symptoms, which may include neck pain, stiffness, tenderness, and reduced range of motion. When there are symptoms and signs that indicate higher grade injuries (grade II and III), patients should initially be treated for suspicion of an unstable spine and SCI, and C-spine x-ray, CT, or MRI should be considered according to assessment and imaging protocols. Treatment usually consists of range-of-motion exercises and stepwise analgesia. Prolonged cervical collar immobilization is not recommended.[15,20]

NEUROLOGIC INJURY AND ASSESSMENT

Neurologic injury evolves in two stages: The primary or immediate injury is followed by a cascade of pathophysiologic processes that lead to the secondary injury. The extent of the primary neurologic injury should be evaluated using standardized assessment tools. Management should be geared toward providing immediate resuscitative measures, stabilizing the spine, and mitigating the events that lead to secondary injury.

Pathophysiology of primary and secondary injury

Primary injury results from mechanical disruption of neuronal structures at the time of the accident and is determined by the mechanism and force of the trauma. The level and extent of the initial injury is a principal determinant of prognosis. The secondary injury is initiated by harmful biochemical and inflammatory processes in response to the primary injury and systemic derangements in response to the trauma. Tissue trauma results in disturbances to local blood supply and oxygen delivery, inflammatory response, and edema. At a cellular level, neurons may lose their ability to regulate and balance energy and transmembrane ion pumps may not function. This results in cellular swelling, calcium influx, and further cell damage, including necrosis and activation of protease-induced apoptosis (cell death). Inflammatory cytokines increase free-radical production and lipid peroxidation. Moreover, oxygen delivery to neurons may be compromised by anemia due to extreme blood loss, hypotension, and hypoxemia. Immobilizing the unstable spine and prompt resuscitation of the trauma patient is the principal approach to reducing the risk of secondary injury in the acute phase, followed by early surgical decompression when necessary.[21]

Cervical spinal cord injury classification and assessment

COMPLETE VS. INCOMPLETE SPINAL CORD INJURY AND AMERICAN SPINAL INJURY ASSOCIATION IMPAIRMENT SCALE

Complete SCI is the result of a disruption of the entire spinal cord and results in the immediate loss of all motor and sensory function below the injury. Depending on the level of injury, this may cause sudden death (eg, in cervico-bulbar disruption), quadriplegia, or paraplegia, with corresponding lack of feeling. In contrast, an incomplete lesion is defined as the presence of any residual motor or sensory function below the level of the injury, including sensation or voluntary movement distal to the segment of the injury and sacral sparing in the form of voluntary sphincter contraction and perianal sensation. The assessment of completeness of a SCI is based on the American Spinal Injury Association (ASIA) Impairment Scale, which describes five grades of injury (Table 11.2).[22]

AMERICAN SPINAL INJURY ASSOCIATION MOTOR AND SENSORY LEVEL ASSESSMENT

The ASIA motor and sensory scoring system is used to rapidly assess residual motor and sensory function. For motor scoring, 10 well-defined muscle groups (five in the upper extremity and five in the lower extremity) are assessed for strength on both sides and each are graded based on the Medical Research Council scale. A score of "0" on the Medical Research Council scale represents complete plegia (paralysis) and a score of "5" defines full strength of the tested muscle group. The maximum ASIA motor score is 100. Sensory-level assessment is performed by testing light touch and pinprick separately on either side at 28 key sensory landmarks or dermatomes (an area of skin that is mainly supplied by a single spinal nerve) using a 3-point grading scale ("0" absent, "1" impaired, and "2" intact) for each landmark.

Table 11.2 American Spinal Injury Association Impairment Scale

A	Complete	No motor or sensory function is preserved in the sacral segments S4–S5
B	Incomplete	Sensory but not motor function is preserved below the neurologic level and includes the sacral segments S4–S5
C	Incomplete	Motor function is preserved below the neurologic level, and the majority of key muscles below the neurologic level have a muscle grade less than 3
D	Incomplete	Motor function is preserved below the neurologic level, and at least half of the key muscles below the neurologic level have a muscle grade of 3 or more.
E	Normal	Motor and sensory function are normal

Source: Aarabi et al. *Neurosurgery.* 2013;72(suppl 2): 195–204.

The maximum ASIA sensory score is, therefore, 112 (Figure 11.6).[22]

The combination of these scoring systems together with the ASIA Impairment Scale provides a comprehensive description of the completeness and level of SCI. Establishing a baseline with these tools is essential for monitoring any progression or improvement of neurologic injury.[22]

PARTIAL SPINAL CORD INJURY AND SPINAL CORD SYNDROMES

In partial SCI, recognizing the characteristic patterns of neurologic signs can help define the site and extent of injury (Figure 11.7).

Central cord syndrome usually results from spinal cord contusion caused by hyperextension injuries that affect a spondylotic spine with preexisting cervical canal stenosis. Motor and sensory deficits mainly affect the upper extremities and generally spare the lower extremities. Management should focus on carefully maintaining spinal cord perfusion pressures and offering surgical decompression, as needed.[23]

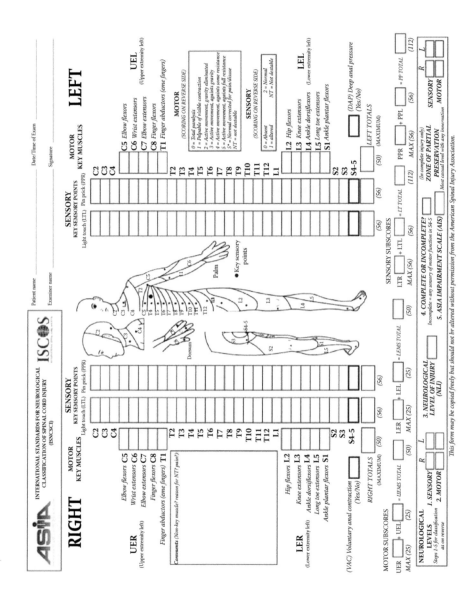

Figure 11.6 ASIA motor and sensory-level assessment.

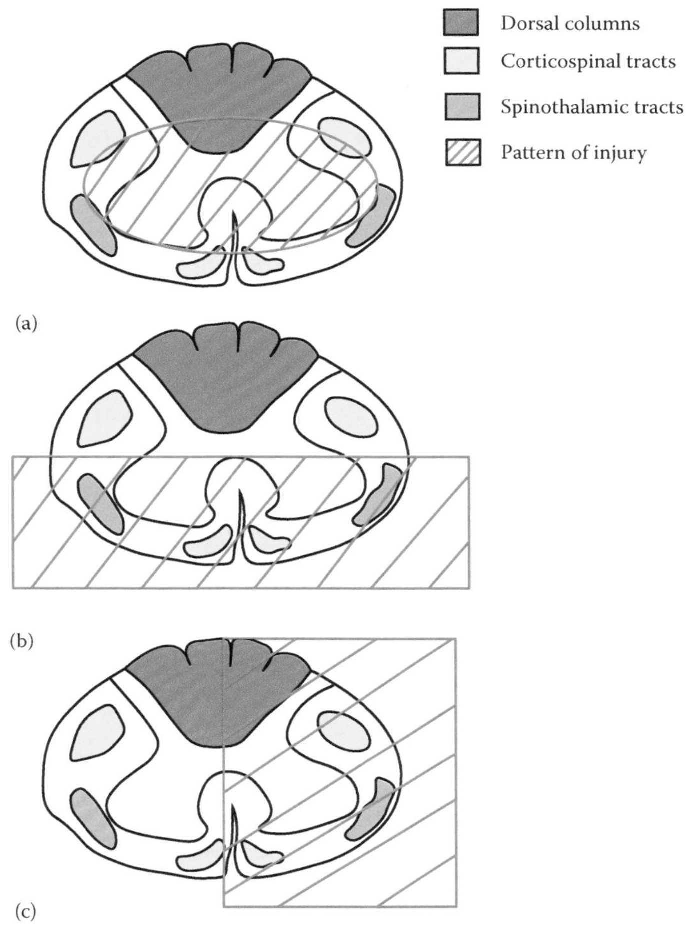

Legend:
- Dorsal columns
- Corticospinal tracts
- Spinothalamic tracts
- Pattern of injury

(a)

(b)

(c)

Figure 11.7 Spinal cord syndromes. **(a)** Central cord syndrome is associated with motor and sensory deficits of bilateral upper extremities. **(b)** Anterior cord syndrome is associated with variably decreased motor function and decreased pain and temperature sensation below the level of the injury. **(c)** Lateral cord syndrome (commonly known as "Brown-Sequard" syndrome) is associated with loss of motor function and proprioception on the same side of the lesion and loss of pain and temperature sensation on the opposite side below the level of injury.

Anterior cord syndrome may result from direct injury to the anterior spinal cord or indirectly as a result of traumatic occlusion of the anterior spinal artery. The symptoms include para- or quadriplegia, depending on the level of injury to the motor pathway and loss of pain and temperature sensation caused by injury to the spinothalamic tract but preservation of proprioception (the ability to sense stimuli arising within the body regarding position, motion, and equilibrium) by the dorsal columns in the posterior cord.

Brown-Sequard syndrome, also known as lateral cord syndrome, usually results from direct trauma. Symptoms include ipsilateral motor and proprioception deficits and contralateral impairment of pain and temperature sensation.

NEUROGENIC VS. SPINAL SHOCK

A near-complete SCI at the cervical level is commonly associated with neurogenic shock. This manifests as a loss of sympathetic outflow to the heart, peripheral resistance arteries, and capacitance veins that result in a loss of systemic vascular resistance, decreased preload, and an inability to increase heart rate. The parasympathetic tone conveyed by the vagus nerves prevails and results in profound hypotension and bradycardia.

Spinal shock refers to the transient loss of all neurologic function below the level of injury, which usually accompanies complete SCI. The initial phase of spinal shock results in flaccid paralysis (weakness or paralysis and reduced muscle tone without other obvious causes) and areflexia absent reflexes) and is caused by loss of function of descending motor and autonomic pathways. After the first 24 to 72 hours, partial recovery of spinal cord-level reflexes occurs. Subsequently, as a result of synaptic remodeling and a lack of descending inhibitory pathways, spasticity will occur. Partial SCI may also result in spinal shock in the initial phase of injury due to a "concussion" of the spinal cord, but with a potential for more complete recovery and a better prognosis.[24]

RADIOLOGIC ASSESSMENT

Determining the presence of a potentially unstable C-spine injury can be difficult, especially when the mechanism is unknown, in the presence of distracting injuries or in a patient with an altered mental status. Radiologic assessment is the cornerstone of evaluating SCI. The National Emergency X-ray Utilization Study Group criteria (NEXUS) and the Canadian C-spine rules (CCS) were developed to reduce unnecessary C-spine imaging in awake, asymptomatic trauma patients.[25,26] Both systems have Level I evidence of their clinical use, but the CSS rules are slightly more sensitive and specific than the NEXUS criteria.[27]

The CCS rules classify patients into two groups: low risk for C-spine injury or high risk for C-spine injury. Based on CCS rules, a patient is low risk for SCI and the C-spine can be cleared clinically if the patient does not meet any of the following three criteria (age ≥65 years, extremity paresthesias, or dangerous mechanism), and meets any of the low-risk factor criteria: sitting position in the emergency department, ambulatory at any time, delayed neck pain, no midline tenderness, simple rear-end motor vehicle collision (excludes: pushed into traffic, hit by bus/large truck, rollover, hit by high-speed vehicle), and is able to actively rotate the neck 45° left and right.

Likewise, to determine that imaging is not indicated based on the NEXUS criteria, a patient must meet all of the following criteria: no mental status changes and no intoxication, no neck pain or midline tenderness, no focal neurologic deficit, and no significant distracting injuries.

When imaging is indicated, C-spine immobilization should be maintained. Based on a Level I recommendation, high-quality CT scanning should be the first line of imaging when available.[28] CT scanning is very sensitive to bony injuries but is suboptimal for soft-tissue injuries, and significant disco-ligamentous injuries may go undetected. Therefore, in the absence of positive CT scan findings, clearing the C-spine remains controversial. When clinical suspicion is high, further evaluation could be considered by either MRI or flexion-extension X-rays, depending on a number of circumstances. MRI also more accurately assesses injury to neuronal elements. When CT scanning is unavailable, plain radiographs may be useful for ruling in C-spine injuries but can rarely be relied on to rule out C-spine injuries.[28,29]

NEUROSURGICAL MANAGEMENT PRINCIPLES

Immobilization, closed reduction and traction, and surgical fixation

In the presence of C-spine injury, immobilization of the head and neck and necessary resuscitative measures are of primary importance. The treatment plan is based on the initial evaluation of the severity of SCI and the radiographic findings. The goal is to prevent further neurologic injury, and to restore and maintain normal C-spine alignment by conservative or operative strategies.

Immobilization is generally performed with the application of an adjustable, rigid cervical collar; even correctly sized cervical collars may allow some movement of the head and neck. Immobilization can be enhanced by placing sandbags on both sides of the head and securely taping the head to the backboard. This effectively eliminates any movement during the workup and before treatment can be initiated.

In the presence of joint dislocation or significant displacement of the fracture site, early closed reduction with craniocervical traction may be attempted in selected patients. However, MRI may provide additional information and enhance the safety of this approach. When traction is indicated, tongs or halo rings are applied to the skull and weights are applied to the traction pulley. Small weights, not to exceed 5 to 10 lbs, can be used to stabilize the spine. The weights can be gradually increased in an attempt to achieve closed reduction.[29]

Emergency surgery may be indicated if closed reduction is unsuccessful or in the presence of neurologic deterioration, extrinsic spinal cord compression, or penetrating fragments. Emergency surgery is contraindicated in a medically unstable patient and when there is evidence of complete SCI.[29]

The choice of the surgical approach depends on the mechanism of injury, the extent of the damage to bony structures, and the presence of spinal-cord and nerve-root compression from extruded discs or bone fragments. The goal of surgical fixation is to decompress neuronal elements, restore anatomic alignment, and provide long-term stabilization of the C-spine. Posterior fixation may be indicated in most flexion-type injuries in which there is disruption of posterior elements and the anterior column of the spine is intact. Occasionally, pedicle screw fixation may be sufficient for simple fractures, however, more commonly, posterior fusion may be necessary. An anterior approach may be necessary when there is significant injury to the vertebral bodies or in the presence of disc extrusion or bony compression of the spinal cord. Options include decompression, corpectomy (a surgical procedure that involves removing all or part of the vertebral body, with the intention of decompressing the spinal cord and nerves), and fusion. In more extensive injuries with significant instability or to eliminate the need for external immobilization after surgery, a (combined) anterior/posterior approach may be the treatment of choice.[19]

Spinal cord protection strategies

Resuscitation, early spinal-cord decompression, and C-spine stabilization are the only effective options to prevent secondary injury.

In spite of earlier trials suggesting a clinical benefit from high-dose methylprednisone in the treatment of SCI, these trials had significant design flaws and their conclusions have been refuted. Due to the lack of evidence for a benefit from high-dose steroid use, their administration is no longer recommended in SCI.[30]

However, there is increased interest in searching for potential pharmacologic agents, yet no studies have produced any breakthroughs in this field.

Systemic or local hypothermia has been extensively studied in animal models, but there remains a lack of evidence for or against the use of hypothermia in acute SCI.

KEY CONSIDERATIONS FOR AIRWAY MANAGEMENT IN CERVICAL SPINE TRAUMA

The main focus of management of SCI is external immobilization of the C-spine to reduce the risk of secondary trauma to the spinal cord. However, the need to establish an airway under difficult circumstances may be just as urgent. The following section focuses on how best to approach these dueling management priorities in the emergency and elective settings.

Emergent airway management

Emergent airway management may be indicated for reduced Glasgow Coma Scale score, combativeness, severe craniofacial trauma, cardiorespiratory compromise, and/or evidence of elevated intracranial pressure. The approach to the airway in an emergency depends on a number of factors, including the patient, the experience of the anesthesiologist, the available equipment, and resources.

Patients with C-spine trauma usually present in a rigid collar. The rigid collar is unreliable in restricting C-spine movement and does not reliably prevent flexion and extension at the atlanto-occipital joint, where the majority of movement occurs during direct laryngoscopy. It also interferes with mouth opening, making oral instrumentation more difficult.[31] When done correctly, manual in-line immobilization (MILI) of the head and neck effectively reduces C-spine movement during any airway manipulation and allows for better mouth opening and visualization. Therefore, it is advisable to remove the front part of the rigid collar and perform MILI.[5]

A number of studies have shown that various airway maneuvers and intubating equipment cause various degrees of C-spine movement. Of all airway manipulations, mask ventilation was found to cause the most significant movement.[32] The degree of movement caused by direct laryngoscopy, either with a curved or a straight blade, has been shown to be no greater than basic airway maneuvers, such as mask ventilation, chin lift, and jaw thrust.[33] When performed carefully and diligently, these airway manipulations may be life-saving and can prevent serious complications and morbidity in a true airway emergency. The benefit of quickly securing the airway with rapid-sequence induction and direct laryngoscopy under such circumstances outweighs the small risk of SCI associated with the movement of an unstable C-spine.[5] Although there is an arsenal of various intubating technology and equipment, including indirect videolaryngoscopes, flexible bronchoscopes, and light wand stylets, no single technique or piece of equipment has been proven to have superior outcomes than another in emergency airway management for SCI. The experience and judgment of the provider generally remains the constant determinant of outcome.

Direct laryngoscopes are simple, readily available, and most providers are familiar and comfortable with their use.[34] However, when initial attempts at intubation are unsuccessful, alternative emergency airway plans should be initiated. These include attempting mask ventilation with airway adjuncts such as an oral or nasopharyngeal airway, insertion of a regular or intubating supraglottic airway, the use of a bougie, or lighted stylets; even blind nasal intubation techniques may be considered. When the index of suspicion for a basal skull fracture is high, no instrument should be used in nasal passages. Insertion of supraglottic airways may cause significant C-spine movement, and their successful placement may be limited by cricoid pressure.[35] Indirect videolaryngoscopes have been shown to cause less C-spine movement in some studies, but airway secretions or blood may limit their use in an emergency.[5]

When back-up airway plans fail, especially when ventilation remains inadequate, emergency surgical airway should be performed. Of note, a surgical airway may be the first-line option in rare cases of associated airway or craniofacial trauma, which precludes oral intubation. Options include cricothyroidotomy, transtracheal jet ventilation, or retrograde wire insertion.[21]

Nonemergent airway management

When there is no immediate need for emergency intubation, complete radiologic assessment of the C-spine injury may provide useful information and enhance the safety of airway management. Despite a lack of evidence, fiber-optic intubation is generally regarded as being the least associated with unwanted C-spine movement in unstable SCI. Indirect videolaryngoscopy techniques are acceptable alternatives. Although some studies suggest that they may cause less C-spine movement than direct laryngoscopy, the use of videolaryngoscopes usually result in longer intubation periods. Intubation may be performed following induction of anesthesia in patients without features that may predict a difficult intubation; MILI should be maintained. In patients with predictors of a difficult intubation or who present in a halo device, awake intubation may be the safer option. The main advantages of awake intubation are the preservation of spontaneous breathing and the ability to perform a neurologic examination following intubation and prior to when general anesthesia is administered.

ANESTHETIC CONSIDERATIONS FOR PATIENTS WITH CERVICAL SPINE INJURY

Management of patients with SCI poses a range of unique challenges to the anesthesiologist. SCI may be isolated or may present with other concomitant and potentially serious injuries. Neurogenic shock and loss of innervation to vital respiratory muscles may result in hemodynamic and respiratory disturbances. The traumatized spinal cord has impaired autoregulation, reduced physiologic reserves, and reduced tolerance for secondary conditions. Low systemic blood pressure, hypoxemia, and anemia may result in aggravation of secondary injury. Assessment for injury to other organ systems should also be performed. Furthermore, special anesthetic considerations apply to patients with a past history of SCI.

Preoperative considerations

An efficient and focused evaluation of the patient with C-spine trauma is essential to enhancing the safety of anesthetic management. Information pertaining to the circumstances of the accident and relevant past medical history may be valuable. The impact of SCI on neurologic status and concomitant traumatic injuries on vital organ systems should be evaluated carefully when formulating the anesthetic management plan.

In patients with a past history of SCI who undergo anesthesia for other indications, careful consideration should be given to specific anesthesia-related problems. First, due to chronic denervation of skeletal muscles, extrajunctional nicotinic acetylcholine receptors may be upregulated, which predisposes to an exaggerated, potentially life-threatening hyperkalemic response when succinylcholine is given, and it should be avoided. Second, patients with SCI are at risk for autonomic hyperreflexia (AH). Due to a lack of descending inhibitory pathways, pain signals carried by afferent fibers to the spinal cord below the level of the injury may elicit an exaggerated sympathetic response in the form of a diffuse vasoconstriction and severe hypertensive crisis. Common etiologies include distension of hollow viscera (bladder or bowel) and any painful stimulation below the level of injury. The higher the level of SCI, the more susceptible a patient will be to the development of AH. Preoperative assessment should focus on past episodes of AH, and anesthesia should be carefully planned.

Positioning

Positioning the patient with an unstable spine requires careful planning, coordination, and communication with the surgical team. Immobilization of the head and neck should be maintained during the transfer to the operating table, induction of anesthesia, and the preparatory and intraoperative phases of surgery. A baseline neurologic examination should be performed immediately before anesthesia induction. Final positioning depends on the surgical approach and may be supine (face up) or prone (face down). An anterior/posterior approach is conducted in two phases and requires repositioning the patient between phases. Fluoroscopic guidance is commonly used to ensure satisfactory alignment of the C-spine throughout. The shoulders may need to be pulled downward using tape to facilitate intraoperative fluoroscopic imaging, and when not done carefully, this maneuver may stretch the brachial plexus. Often, the arms are tucked and not accessible during the procedure, thus adequate intravenous access and,

possibly, arterial line placement should be established prior to final positioning.[21]

Induction, maintenance and monitoring, and emergence

Ensuring adequate homeostasis, restoring euvolemia (adequate volume status), and adequate preoxygenation prior to induction of anesthesia is vital. Induction medications should be administered carefully to reduce hemodynamic disturbances and should be customized to the airway management plan.

The combination of anesthetic agents should ensure adequate depth of anesthesia, avoidance of patient movement, and quick emergence when neurologic examination is necessary. The choice of anesthetic technique should also be conducive to electrophysiologic (EP) monitoring when it is used. Total intravenous anesthesia with propofol and an opioid with a short and predictable context-sensitive half-life usually achieve these goals. Titration may be facilitated by depth-of-anesthesia monitors. Balanced anesthesia with short-acting inhalants may also be used with the caveat that inhalational agents at higher concentrations may interfere with EP monitoring. Muscle relaxants may interfere with motor-evoked potentials (MEPs) and should be avoided in the maintenance phase when MEPs are monitored.

Hemodynamic stability should be maintained by optimizing preload, cardiac function, and afterload. This can be achieved by adequate goal-directed intravenous fluid and blood-product administration, and careful titration of vasopressors, inotropes, and vagolytic medications when necessary. Mean arterial pressure greater than 85 mmHg is recommended to avoid hypoperfusion of the injured spinal cord.[36] Frequent blood gas analyses, coagulation profile, invasive hemodynamic monitoring with an arterial line, pulse pressure variation, and cardiac output measurements may help achieve these goals. Controlled mechanical ventilation should be adjusted to maintain oxygenation and normocapnia.

The primary goal at the end of surgery is to achieve rapid emergence from anesthesia to facilitate a neurologic examination and safe extubation, when appropriate. In an anterior approach to C-spine surgeries, it is important to avoid coughing and straining to reduce bleeding into the soft tissues of the neck. Emergence on a low-dose remifentanil infusion may help reduce this risk by suppressing unwanted airway reflexes. Careful assessment of the extent and level of the spine and SCI, airway edema, respiratory, hemodynamic, and neurologic status should be made prior to proceeding with extubation.

Electrophysiologic monitoring for C-spine trauma

Electrophysiologic monitoring may be useful in detecting neuronal compromise in an anesthetized patient with SCI during positioning and the various phases of surgery. Somatosensory-evoked potentials (SSEPs) and MEPs can be recorded after induction of anesthesia but prior to positioning in unstable SCIs and satisfactory baseline recordings can be followed throughout surgery. The disappearance or reduction of evoked potentials may represent neuronal compromise, which can be caused by various intraoperative events but may also be due to signal artifacts. Positioning and surgical manipulation may result in direct or indirect injury to neuronal elements. Perturbation of neuronal homeostasis caused by hemodynamic instability, hypoxia, and/or anemia may lead to aggravation of secondary injury and neuronal compromise. Hypothermia, anesthetic agents, and technical problems may also interfere with EP recordings and complicate interpretation. It is, therefore, vitally important to maintain a stable anesthetic background and homeostasis not only to reduce secondary injury but also to optimize conditions for EP monitoring, especially during important phases of surgery (eg, surgical manipulation or spinal realignment) when the risk of neuronal injury is high.

REFERENCES

1. Ghafoor AU, Martin TW, Gopalakrishnan S, Viswamitra S. Caring for the patients with cervical spine injuries: What have we learned? *J Clin Anesth.* 2005;17(8):640-649.
2. Hills MW, Deane SA. Head injury and facial injury: Is there an increased risk of cervical spine injury? *J Trauma.* 1993;34(4):549-553.
3. Netter FH. Craniovertebral ligaments. In: Netter FH, ed. *Atlas of Human Anatomy,* 6th Ed. Philadelphia, PA: Saunders, 2013: plate 23.
4. Netter FH. Cervical spine posterior view. In: Netter FH, ed. *Atlas of Human Anatomy,* 6th Ed. Philadelphia, PA: Saunders, 2013: Plate 19.
5. Crosby ET. Airway management in adults after cervical spine trauma. *Anesthesiology.* 2006;104:1293-1318.
6. Haines DE. Internal morphology of the spinal cord and brain: Functional components, MRI, stained sections. In: Haines DE, ed. *Neuroanatomy in Clincial Context,* 9th Ed. Philadelphia, PA: Lippincott, Williams, & Wilkins, 2015:104-107.
7. Hickey R, Albin MS, Bunegin L, Gelineau J. Autoregulation of spinal cord blood flow: Is the cord a microcosm of the brain? *Stroke.* 1986;17(6):1183-1189.
8. Sandler AN, Tator CH. Review of the effect of spinal cord trauma on the vessels and blood flow in the spinal cord. *J Neurosurg.* 1976;45(6):638-646.
9. Horn EM, Feiz-Erfan I, Lekovic GP, Dickman CA, Sonntag VK, Theodore N. Survivors of occipitoatlantal dislocation injuries: Imaging and clinical correlates. *J Neurosurg Spine.* 2007;6(2):113-120.
10. Theodore N, Aarabi B, Dhall SS et al. Occipital condyle fractures. *Neurosurgery.* 2013;72(suppl 2):106-113.
11. Landells CD, Van Peteghem PK. Fractures of the atlas: Classification, treatment and morbidity. *Spine (Phila Pa 1976).* 1988;13(5):450-452.
12. Ryken TC, Hadley MN, Aarabi B et al. Management of isolated fractures of the axis in adults. *Neurosurgery.* 2013;72(suppl 2):132-150.
13. Dickman CA, Greene KA, Sonntag VK. Injuries involving the transverse atlantal ligament: Classification and treatment guidelines based upon experience with 39 injuries. *Neurosurgery.* 1996;38(1):44-50.
14. Anderson LD, D'Alonzo RT. Fractures of the odontoid process of the axis. *J Bone Joint Surg Am.* 1974;56(8):1663-1674.
15. Greenberg MS. Occipitoatlantoaxial injuries (occiput to C2). In: Greenberg MS, ed. *Handbook of Neurosurgery,* 8th Ed. Thieme: Stuttgart, Germany, 2016:972-981.

16. Denis F. Spinal instability as defined by the three-column spine concept in acute spinal trauma. *Clin Orthop Relat Res.* 1984;189: 65-76.

17. Vaccaro AR, Hulbert RJ, Patel AA et al. The subaxial cervical spine injury classification system: A novel approach to recognize the importance of morphology, neurology, and integrity of the disco-ligamentous complex. *Spine (Phila Pa 1976).* 2007;32(21):2365-2374.

18. Allen BL, Ferguson RL, Lehmann TR, O'Brien RP. A mechanistic classification of closed, indirect fractures and dislocations of the lower cervical spine. *Spine (Phila Pa 1976).* 1982;7(1):1-27.

19. Greenberg MS. Subaxial (C3-C7) injuries/fractures. In: Greenberg MS, ed. *Handbook of Neurosurgery*, 8th Ed. Thieme: Stuttgart, Germany, 2016:996-1000.

20. Spitzer WO, Skovron ML, Salmi L et al. Scientific monograph of the Quebec Task Force on Whiplash-Associated Disorders: Redefining "whiplash" and its management. *Spine (Phila Pa 1976).* 1995;20(8 suppl):1S-73S.

21. Cottrell JE, Patel P. Spinal cord injury in neurosurgical diseases and trauma of the spine and spinal cord: Anesthetic considerations. In: Cottrell JE, Patel P, eds. *Cottrell and Patel's Neuroanesthesia*, 6th Edition. Amsterdam, Netherlands: Elsevier, 2017:372-373.

22. Ditunno JF, Young W, Donovan WH, Creasey G. The international standards booklet for neurological and functional classification of spinal cord injury. American Spinal Injury Association. *Paraplegia.* 1994;32(2):70-80.

23. Aarabi B, Hadley MN, Dhall SS et al. Management of acute traumatic central cord syndrome (ATCCS). *Neurosurgery.* 2013;72 (suppl 2):195-204.

24. Atkinson PP, Atkinson J. Spinal shock. *Mayo Clin Proc.* 1996;71(4):384-389.

25. Hoffman J, Mower W, Wolfson A, Todd KH, Zucker MI. Validity of a set of clinical criteria to rule out injury to the cervical spine in patients with blunt trauma. National Emergency X-Radiography Utilization Study Group. *N Engl J Med.* 2000;343(2):94-99.

26. Stiell IG, Wells GA, Vandemheen KL et al. The Canadian C-spine rule for radiography in alert and stable trauma patients. *JAMA.* 2001;286(15):1841-1848.

27. Stiell IG, Clement CM, McKnight RD et al. The Canadian C-Spine Rule versus the NEXUS low-risk criteria in patients with trauma. *N Engl J Med.* 2003;349(26):2510-2518.

28. Como JJ, Diaz JJ, Dunham CM et al. Practice management guidelines for identification of cervical spine injuries following trauma: Update from the eastern association for the surgery of trauma practice management guidelines committee. *J Trauma.* 2009;67 (3):651-659.

29. Greenberg MS. Management of Spinal Cord Injury. In: Greenberg MS, ed. *Handbook of Neurosurgery*, 8th Ed. Thieme: Stuttgart, Germany, 2016:957-960.

30. Hurlbert RJ, Hadley MN, Walters BC et al. Pharmacological therapy for acute spinal cord injury. *Neurosurgery.* 2013;72(suppl 2):93-105.

31. Goutcher CM, Lochhead V. Reduction in mouth opening with semi-rigid cervical collars. *Br J Anaesth.* 2005;95(3):344-348.

32. Hauswald M, Sklar DP, Tandberg D, Garcia JF. Cervical spine movement during airway management: Cinefluoroscopic appraisal in human cadavers. *Am J Emerg Med.* 1991;9 (6):535-538.

33. Donaldson W 3rd, Heil B, Donaldson V. The effect of airway maneuvers on the unstable C1-C2 segment. A cadaver study. *Spine (Phila Pa 1976).* 1997;22(11):1215-1218.

34. Harris EA. Airway management for the patient with an unstable cervical spine. In: Ruskin KJ, Rosenbaum SH, Rampil IJ, eds. *Fundamentals of Neuroanesthesia: A Physiologic Approach to Clinical Practice.* New York, NY: Oxford University Press, 2014:288-298.

35. Keller C, Brimacombe J, Keller K. Pressures exerted against the cervical vertebrae by the standard and intubating laryngeal mask airways: A randomized, controlled, crossover study in fresh cadavers. *Anesth Analg.* 1999;89(5):1296-1300.

36. Levi L, Wolf A, Belzberg H. Hemodynamic parameters in patients with acute cervical cord trauma: Description, intervention, and prediction of outcome. *Neurosurgery.* 1993;33 (6):1007-1016; discussion 1016-1017.

12

Thoracolumbar spine injury

MONICA S. TANDON AND PRIYANKA KHURANA

INTRODUCTION

Thoracolumbar (T–L) spine trauma accounts for nearly half of the injuries of the spine.[1–3] Most of these injuries occur due to high energy mechanisms and often result in considerable morbidity, due to both vertebral column (VC) and spinal cord injury (SCI), and also because of concomitant injuries, especially of the cervical spine, head, thorax, and appendicular skeleton. SCI progresses through three stages: acute, intermediate, and chronic. Its severity is largely determined by the collective impact of the "primary injury," which occurs at the moment of impact, and the subsequent "secondary injury," which is typically characterized by ischemia and edema of the spinal cord (SC). While the primary injury is irreversible, secondary injury is potentially treatable. Anesthesiologists, with their innate, specialty-related skills, play an important role in limiting the extent of secondary SCI and in contributing to an improved outcome after T–L spine trauma. Optimal anesthetic management of patients with T–L spine trauma requires an integrated understanding of the epidemiology; functional anatomy and biomechanics of the spine; pathophysiologic and clinical consequences of SCI; and pertinent surgery-related concepts. The initial sections of this chapter provide an overview of these basic concepts; the latter sections describe the management of these patients when they present in the emergency department (ED), and the important anesthesia considerations when they require urgent decompression-stabilization surgery in the acute phase of SCI or a repeat/associated surgery in the chronic phase of SCI.

EPIDEMIOLOGY

T–L spine trauma accounts for approximately 30% to 50% of all spine injuries; approximately 50% to 60% of these occur at the T–L junction, 25% to 40% involve the thoracic spine, and 10% to 14% affect the lower lumbar spine and sacrum.[1–5]

These injuries usually occur due to a high-energy impact (acceleration/deceleration), mostly caused by blunt trauma to the T–L spine, for example, high-velocity motor vehicle accidents (36.7%), fall from a height (31.7%), mishaps during a recreational sport (diving, skiing, snowboarding, paragliding, horseback riding); and sometimes, because of penetrating gunshot injuries.[6,7] Motor vehicle accidents are the most common cause in younger patients. Falls account for most of the injuries in older adults (osteoporotic bones) and in patients with an underlying neoplastic or a metabolic spine disorder; in these patients, even a low-impact mechanism, for example, a ground-level fall from the standing position to the ground, can result in a T–L spine injury.[8]

Associated neurologic injury occurs in 20% to 40% of T–L spine fractures and can cause significant morbidity; up to 7% of patients who develop paraplegia because of thoracic spine fractures die within the first year of the injury.[6,9–11] Furthermore, multiple simultaneous injuries are not uncommon (47%) and include noncontiguous fractures, especially of the cervical spine (10.4%); head injuries (12.9%); thoracic (22.6%), abdominal (7.6%), pelvic (9.3%), and long bone (18.2%) injuries; and vascular injuries.[6,12]

Functional anatomy and physiology

The T–L spine consists of 12 thoracic and five lumbar vertebrae, which are interconnected by intervertebral (IV) discs and are stabilized by spinal ligaments. Biomechanically, the T–L spine is divided into three regions: a rigid, kyphotic thoracic spine (T1–T10); a relatively hypermobile, lordotic lumbar spine (L3-L5); and the T–L junction (T11–L2), the transition zone between these two regions.[13]

Thoracic spine

The thoracic spine has significant, inherent stability, because of its connections with the rib cage and sternum (by articulations between costal facets of T1–T10 vertebrae and costal heads of corresponding ribs); the thin intervertebral (IV) discs, coronally orientated facet articulations, and inferiorly directed spinous processes further increase its rigidity. Consequently, a higher amount of energy is required for injuries to occur in this region, and the incidence of thoracic spine fractures is much lower than the rest of the spine. However, dissipation of this high amount of kinetic energy results in a risk of injury to vital structures that are in proximity to the thoracic spine; conversely, sternal fractures can destabilize the thorax and have a strong association with thoracic spine fractures. Furthermore, because of the relatively narrow thoracic spinal canal, severity of cord damage is usually high, and T–L spine injuries almost always results in a complete SCI.[2]

Lumbar spine

In contrast to the thoracic spine, the thick IV discs, sagitally oriented articular lumbar facets, and absence of the rib cage increase the mobility, as well as the vulnerability of the lumbar spine to injury. However, because of the relatively wider neural canal and greater resilience of the cauda equina nerve roots, neurologic injuries are usually less severe, compared with the thoracic SC.

T–L junction

The T–L junction (T11–L2) marks an abrupt transition between the long, rigid, kyphotic thoracic spine and the shorter, more dynamic, lordotic lumbar spine. Most of the bending and axial loads of the spine are concentrated at the T–L junction, hence, this biomechanically vulnerable zone is one of the most common sites for spine fractures. The T–L junction also represents the termination of the SC as conus medullaris (T11–L2/L3 in adults) and a further continuation of the lumbosacral roots as "cauda equina" through the sacral canal.

Autonomic system

The sympathetic T–L outflow is formed by the preganglionic fibers arising from T1 to L2/L3 segments of the SC, and traverses along the length of the VC, on either side of the cord. The sacral preganglionic fibers of the parasympathetic system emerge from the cord, via the ventral rami of S2–S4 nerves. Damage to autonomic outflow during a T–L spine injury is associated with profound systemic consequences.

Blood supply of the SC

The SC receives its primary blood supply from the anterior spinal artery and two posterior spinal arteries; this supply is augmented by multiple anterior and posterior radicular arteries. The thoracic spine is highly vulnerable to ischemia because of its relatively tenuous blood supply (1–4 anterior radicular arteries for the entire thoracic spine, compared with 1–2 for the shorter lumbar spine). The midthoracic spine is particularly at risk because

of the creation of a "watershed zone" where the anterior radicular and anterior spinal artery merge; hence, it is also referred to as the "critical vascular zone" of the SC. The artery of Adamkiewicz, the largest anterior radicular artery, is the primary source of the blood supply to the lower thoracic and upper lumbar SC; a traumatic or iatrogenic injury (during a posterolateral approach to the anterior thoracic spine) to this vessel can result in profound neurologic damage.[10]

SC blood flow is autoregulated over a wide range of mean arterial pressures (MAP), 60 to 150 mmHg.[14] However, autoregulation is lost after SCI, which increases the vulnerability of the cord to hypotension-induced ischemia.[15]

BIOMECHANICS AND STABILITY OF THE SPINE

Stability of the spine fundamentally refers to "its ability to maintain normal intervertebral alignment and prevent any excessive movement between vertebrae during normal physiologic loading, so that there is no neurological injury (damage to SC or nerve roots), incapacitating deformity or pain, as a consequence of structural changes in the spine."[16]

Spinal motion unit

A "spinal motion unit," the fundamental biomechanical unit of the spine, is basically divided into an "anterior portion" and a "posterior portion." The anterior portion, formed by two aligned vertebral bodies (VB), IV discs, and anterior and posterior longitudinal ligaments, contributes to the stability of the spine in extension. The VBs support most of the axial loads and resist compressive loads on the spine; IV discs, in addition to supporting axial and lateral loads, also resist the tension and shearing forces on the spine. The posterior portion, which consists of vertebral arches, facet joints, and the posterior ligamentous complex (PLC), contributes more to the stability of the spine in flexion. The PLC is composed of the supraspinous ligament, interspinous ligaments, articular facet capsules, and ligamentum flavum. In the upright position, when gravity exerts a continual axial load on the VC and the axis of rotation is immediately anterior to, or just within the anterior half of the VB, the PLC serves as a "posterior tension band" to constantly counterbalance the compressive forces on the VBs, and hence, maintain the stability of the spine.[17] Conceptually, when the VB has been compressed to a critical point, the PLC can fail in tension. The PLC has a poor healing potential; therefore, a surgical intervention usually becomes necessary, if it is disrupted, in order to prevent the subsequent development of kyphosis and vertebral collapse.[10]

An abrupt increase in the load on the T–L spine, as can occur due to a high energy traumatic impact, can cause various components of the spinal motion unit to fail, and can consequently lead to a mechanical and neurologic instability (neurologic deficits due to compression and/or injury of the SC, nerve roots) of the spine. Generally, the anterior elements tend to get disrupted in hyperextension injuries; and posterior elements are more vulnerable to disruption in hyperflexion injuries; disruption of both elements can occur with extreme flexion/extension or if a compressive/rotational force is also added. An operative intervention is usually indicated in a patient who has an unstable T–L spine.

Classification of T–L spine instability

There are several classification systems for assessment of spinal instability, such as the two-column concept of the spine by Holdsworth, the three-column concept by Denis et al., and McAfee et al., Arbeitsgemeinschaft für Osteosynthesefragen (AO) classification by Magerl et al., and Thoracolumbar Injury Classification and Severity Score (TLICS) by the Spine Trauma Study Group.[18–23] However, since none of them has sufficient validity and reproducibility to reliably guide the clinical decision-making process, hence a conclusive and clinically relevant classification system still continues to evolve.

Denis three-column system

In this classification system, the VC is sagitally divided into three columns:

Anterior column: Anterior longitudinal ligament, anterior half of VB, anterior annulus fibrosus of IV disc
Middle column: Posterior longitudinal ligament, posterior half of VB, posterior annulus fibrosus of IV disc

Posterior column: Posterior arch, ligamentum flavum, and supraspinous and interspinous ligaments

The middle column, being in the neutral axis of the spine, tolerates the maximum axial loads during spine flexion or extension, and its integrity is considered to be essential for stability of the spine. A middle-column disruption, along with injury of the anterior and/or posterior column, is indicative of an unstable spine. Because of the subsequent realization that two-column unstable injuries are also amenable to conservative management (if PLC is intact), this classification is not very useful for guiding critical clinical decisions; nevertheless, it is still frequently used in clinical practice because it is relatively simple and includes most of the common T–L spine injury patterns. It classifies major T–L spine injuries on the basis of their morphology and injury mechanism, as wedge-compression fractures, burst fractures, flexion-distraction (seat-belt) injuries, and fracture dislocations (Table 12.1). Simple wedge compression fractures are usually stable and are managed conservatively; burst fractures may cause instability and may require surgical stabilization; flexion distraction and fracture dislocations are extremely unstable and almost always require surgical stabilization.

WEDGE COMPRESSION FRACTURES

These fractures occur because of compression and/or axial forces and usually involve only the anterior column. They produce a wedge-shaped deformity in the anterior VB; the amount of wedging is usually small (anterior portion of VB is rarely more than 25% shorter than the posterior half of VB) and is not associated with any ligamentous injury or neurologic deficits; the middle column and PLC are usually intact. Most of these fractures are stable; on the rare occasion, the injuries may be severe enough to cause significant disruption of the anterior and posterior columns.

BURST COMPRESSION FRACTURES

The majority of T–L spine injuries are usually caused by vertical-axial compression/flexion forces and involve both anterior and middle columns (Figure 12.1). They result in loss of height of the anterior column and disruption of the posterior wall of VB, often with retropulsion of the fractured fragments/disc material into the spinal

Table 12.1 Classification of fractures according to Denis' three-column system[23]

Type of injury	Mechanism of injury	Morphology	Management
Simple wedge fractures	Compression and/or axial forces	**Mostly stable** Usually involves only the anterior column (small wedge-shaped deformity in anterior portion of VB); usually no associated ligamentous injury or neurologic deficits	Conservative management
Burst compression fractures Account for a majority of T–L spine injuries	Vertical-axial compression/flexion forces	**Stable or unstable** Involve anterior and middle columns; affect posterior portion of VB, with retropulsion of fractured fragments into the spinal canal; deficits due to cord compression and/or neural injury	May require surgical intervention
Flexion-distraction injuries (seat-belt injuries) Most common site: T–L junction	Flexion about an axis anterior to or within the vertebral column, usually due to high-energy, motor-vehicle crashes in which the patient was restrained by only a lap belt, without the use of shoulder belt	**Unstable** Profound mechanical and neurologic instability because of disruption of two (posterior and middle)/all three spinal columns Chance fracture: Transverse injury through the VB, which involves all columns; associated neurologic injuries, concomitant retroperitoneal, and intra-abdominal visceral injuries often present	Surgical management
Fracture-dislocations	Various combinations of shear, torsion, distraction, flexion, and extension forces	**Highly unstable** Disruption of all three spinal columns; often result in serious neurologic compromise; concomitant chest, abdominal, and pelvic injuries often present	Surgical management

Abbreviations: T–L: thoracolumbar; VB: vertebral body.

canal, and consequently, damage to the neural elements.

FLEXION-DISTRACTION INJURIES (SEAT-BELT INJURIES)

These injuries are caused by flexion around an axis anterior to or within the VC and usually cause profound mechanical instability because of disruption of two or three spinal columns. They occur most commonly at the T–L junction and are often a consequence of high-speed automobile crashes in which the patient was restrained by only a lap belt, without the shoulder belt in place. Usually, the entire PLC is disrupted; the extent of anterior column involvement is determined by location of the axis of rotation of the flexed T–L spine. Distraction of the entire spine occurs if the axis of rotation is located anterior to the VB; if it is within

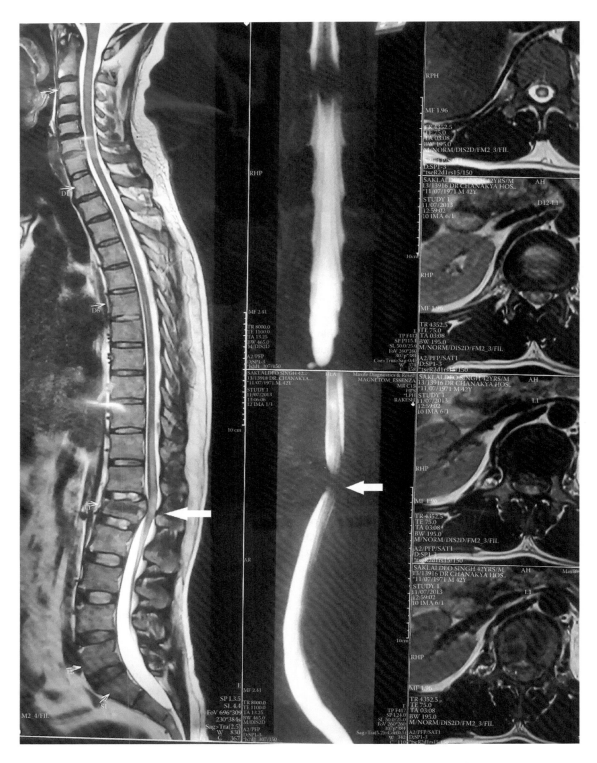

Figure 12.1 MRI of spine showing post-traumatic burst compression fracture of L1 vertebra, with a retropulsed bony fragment compressing the spinal cord.

the VB, it causes subluxation or dislocation of the VBs, along with a distractive disruption of the PLC. A Chance fracture is a transverse injury through the VB, which involves all of the columns and is frequently associated with neurologic deficits and retroperitoneal/intra-abdominal visceral injuries.[6,10]

FRACTURE-DISLOCATION INJURIES

These highly unstable injuries are usually a consequence of various combinations of shear, torsion, distraction, and flexion and extension forces and result in disruption of all three spinal columns. They are usually associated with a serious neurologic compromise as well as with significant concurrent chest, abdominal, and pelvic injuries.[1]

The AO classification system

This system broadly classifies spine injuries into three major categories: A-C, on the basis of the injury mechanism; osseous or ligamentous disruption; and direction of displacement.[21] The A-C categories represent a continuum of progressively worsening morphologic damage and instability, and consequently, an increasingly higher likelihood of a surgical intervention.

Type A: Compression injury; axial loading force results in vertebral compression and burst fractures.

Type B: Distraction injury; flexion distraction, or hyperextension force results in transverse disruption/distraction injury in the anterior and posterior columns

Type C: Translation or rotation injury; horizontal movement of one vertebra on another, results in a highly unstable injury with significant facet subluxation, fracture dislocation, and ligamentous disruption; neurologic injury occurs due to a cord compression or shear injury from repeated segmental translation

TLICS

One of the biggest advantages of this classification system is that it provides a quantitative evaluation of spinal instability and also facilitates the clinical decision-making process (Table 12.2).[22–24] This "clinical injury severity score" is based on three major categories: mechanism of injury, PLC integrity [detected by magnetic resonance imaging (MRI)], and neurologic status of the patient. Each category has four subcategories, which are graded on

Table 12.2 Thoracolumbar injury classification and severity score (TLICS)

Morphology	Compression	1	Diagnosis: Radiographs, CT
(immediate stability)	Burst	2	
	Translation/Rotation	3	
	Distraction	4	
Integrity of PLC	Intact	0	Diagnosis: MRI
(Long-term stability)	Suspected	2	
	Injured	3	
Neurologic status	Intact	0	Diagnosis: Physical examination
	Nerve root	2	
	Complete cord	2	
	Incomplete cord	3	
	Cauda equina	3	

Suggested Management	Suggested Surgical Approach
Total score	Incomplete neurologic injury,
0–3 -: Conservative management	neural compression from anterior structures:
4 -: Surgeon's decision	Anterior approach
>4 -: Surgery	PLC injury: Posterior approach
	Both anterior compression and PLC injury:
	Posterior and/or anterior approach

Abbreviations: PLC: Posterior ligamentous complex; CT: computerized tomography; MRI: magnetic resonance imaging.

a scale of 1 to 4 (from least to maximal severity of injury and potential instability); the sum of these values provides the comprehensive severity score. Conservative management is recommended if total score is 3 or less; a score of 5 or higher indicates the need for definitive surgical management; injuries with a score of 4 are managed surgically or conservatively, based on the surgeon's decision. The TLICS system is externally validated, has good interobserver reliability, and is presently the most widely used classification system.[24]

SCI: PATHOPHYSIOLOGY AND ITS CLINICAL IMPLICATIONS

Primary and secondary SCI injury

SCI develops in two stages: An initial primary injury (mechanical damage) and a subsequent secondary injury (nonmechanical mechanisms of damage).

Primary SCI injury

It occurs at the time of the trauma, due to biomechanical forces generated during the impact. These forces cause injury to the SC and nerve roots by direct damage, by causing compression, and/or due to interruption of the SC blood supply by the injured bony and disco-ligamentous structures. Four types of SC lesions are commonly seen: concussion; compression (associated with persistent spinal cord ischemia); contusion (associated with axonal destruction and hemorrhagic infiltration); and sectioning of the cord. Cord concussion resolves in a few hours; some neurologic recovery may occur in spinal cord compression, but cord contusion and sectioning have minimal and no possibility of a functional recovery, respectively.[15]

Secondary injury

Within minutes of when the primary injury occurs, a combination of events, including intramedullary vessel damage, small hemorrhages into and around the SC, and local vasospasm, lead to a critical decrease in SC perfusion. The ensuing cord ischemia triggers "secondary SCI," a cascade of systemic responses and biochemical processes that evolve over the next few days to weeks, to further aggravate the damage caused during the primary insult.

The hallmarks of this acute, inflammatory phase are tissue ischemia and cord edema. Tissue ischemia acts as a trigger for some of these processes and a final common pathway for others. It develops rapidly, particularly in the gray matter and the central white matter, and is further aggravated by SC edema, which typically peaks at 3 to 6 days and can persist for weeks after the injury.[14] Autoregulatory failure, abnormalities in venous drainage, systemic hypotension, and loss of the blood-SC barrier, which are often observed after SCI, further exacerbate the tissue ischemia. At the cellular level, some of the key destructive processes during this phase are: impaired microperfusion due to microvascular damage, vasospasm, thrombosis, and increased vascular permeability; ischemia/hypoxia, increased glucose use, decreased adenosine triphosphate production, metabolic acidosis; release of inflammatory and immune mediators; cellular dysfunction with membrane failure, ionic shifts, cellular swelling, mitochondrial insufficiency, free-radical production, lipid peroxidation, and apoptotic neuronal cell death. Consequently, neurologic transmission ceases below the level of the injury, and patients present with sensorimotor deficits, areflexic and autonomic imbalance. Since secondary SCI aggravates the original injury, it is not uncommon for the level of neurologic injury to ascend further in the first 48 hours after the injury. The chronic phase of SCI is characterized by cicatrization with glial scar formation, followed by neuronal regeneration.

These ischemic and biochemical phenomena have important clinical implications.

SC perfusion pressure is determined by the difference between the MAP and the intramedullary pressure; hence, an increase in intramedullary pressure due to edema and concomitant hypotension in the setting of an impaired autoregulation, can significantly decrease the perfusion of the SC and consequently aggravate neuronal ischemia.[15]

There is an ischemic "penumbra" of perinecrotic tissue that may evolve toward apoptosis or toward recovery.

There is also a "therapeutic window" during which it may be possible to limit the extent of the secondary SCI by aggressive prevention and/or correction of systemic factors that worsen SC ischemia and edema eg, hypotension, hypoxia, hypercapnia, anemia, hypothermia, acidosis, and hypo- and hyperglycemia; stabilization of unstable motion segments by spine immobilization and early decompression plays a vital role in preventing further SCI injury.

Several pharmacologic interventions have been evaluated extensively for attenuation of the severity of secondary SCI (corticosteroids, gangliosides, naloxone, riluzole, calcium channel blockers, free-radical scavengers, NMDA receptor antagonists, neurotropic agents, erythropoietin, minocycline, hypothermia, stem-cell therapy, etc.); however, the neuroprotective/neuroregenerative efficacy in humans has not been very encouraging.[25–29]

PHASES OF SCI: ACUTE, INTERMEDIATE, CHRONIC

Acute phase

PHASE 1: AREFLEXIA/HYPOREFLEXIA; 0–1 DAY

In the initial post-trauma phase, the cord caudal to the injury becomes isolated from the higher centers. The consequent loss of supraspinal descending facilitation results in "spinal shock," a temporary interruption of the physiologic functions of the cord, caudal to the injury. Clinically, patients develop flaccid paralysis with loss of autonomic and reflex activity (distal to the SCI level). The SCI injury can be complete (no demonstrable sensory, motor, bowel or bladder function) or incomplete (some preservation of function).[30] Neurogenic shock (NS) can occur during this phase.

Intermediate phase

PHASE 2: INITIAL REFLEX RETURN; 1–3 DAYS

This phase is characterized by denervation supersensitivity and receptor upregulation; clinically, spinal shock begins to resolve; cutaneous reflexes start returning [deep plantar reflex (DPR), bulbocavernous reflex, cremasteric reflex], but deep tendon reflexes (DTR), eg, ankle reflex, knee reflex, Babinski Sign are still absent.[30]

PHASE 3: INITIAL HYPER-REFLEXIA, 4 DAYS—1 MONTH

This phase is characterized by return of DTR, disappearance of DPR, and early hyper-reflexia. Autonomic function continues to improve, and there is a decrease in the incidence of vagally mediated bradyarrhythmias and hypotension. Autonomic

hyper-reflexia (AH) can begin to emerge at this time.[30]

Chronic phase

PHASE 4: SPASTICITY/HYPER-REFLEXIA (1–12 MONTHS)

The loss of descending inhibitory controls, along with the development of spasticity and hyper-reflexia, mark the transition to the fourth phase of SCI. Gradual functional recovery occurs during this phase. The extent of recovery is relatively poor in complete SCI; those with incomplete SCI have a better prognosis. The DPR should have disappeared by this time; its persistence is associated with a poor prognosis for neurologic recovery.[30] AH can complicate the chronic phase of patients with high thoracic SCI (T1–T6).

Neurogenic shock (NS)

Patients with high thoracic spine injuries (T1–T6) are at risk for developing NS during the initial phase of SCI. NS is characterized by hypotension [systolic blood pressure (SBP) <90 mmHg], with/without bradycardia. It occurs because of disruption of the descending sympathetic vasomotor pathways and the concomitant, unopposed parasympathetic system activity, which is caudal to the injury. The severity of clinical manifestations depends on the level and completeness of the SCI; cardiovascular compromise is more severe in patients with complete SCI above T6 than in those with an incomplete SCI; lesions below T6 usually do not result in NS. The risk of NS persists for up to 5 weeks after the injury.

In T4 to T6 level SCI, the hypotension occurs due to the loss of sympathetic vasoconstrictor tone in the arterioles and veins, and the consequent decrease in systemic vascular resistance (vasodilatation) and preload (venous pooling in the extremities). These effects are compounded in patients with higher cord injuries (T1–T4) because of the additional loss of sympathetic innervation to the heart (T1–T4) and to the splanchnic vasculature. Profound hemodynamic instability can occur because of the ensuing reduction in heart rate, myocardial contractility, preload and stroke volume; atrioventricular block, supraventricular tachycardia, ventricular tachycardia, and even cardiac arrest can occur due to the autonomic lability.

Autonomic hyper-reflexia (AH)

About 60% to 85% of patients with chronic, high thoracic (T1–T6) SCI[31] are at risk for developing AH, an exaggerated, reflex-sympathetic discharge that is triggered by a minor noxious stimulus, and which can result in potentially life-threatening hypertension. AH can occur any time within 3 to 12 weeks, up to 12 years or even later, after the initial injury.[31]

The chronic phase of SCI is characterized by alterations in the neuronal connections of the cord caudal to the injury (adrenergic receptor upregulation, neuronal alterations in the cord itself/ abnormal synaptic connections due to postinjury sprouting); these connections lack the usual descending inhibition from higher centers. Hence, when an afferent impulse generated by even a minor noxious stimulus is transmitted to the isolated SC, it triggers a massive, inappropriate sympathetic discharge from the adrenal medulla and sympathetic nervous system (no longer under central hypothalamic control); this results in profound vasoconstriction below the level of the injury, and consequently, severe systemic hypertension. Normally, carotid sinus activation (baroreceptor reflexes) sends inhibitory signals to the SC to stop the sympathetic firing, but because of the SCI, these signals do not reach the lower sympathetic outflow segments. Although activation of the baroreceptor reflexes produces rostral bradycardia and vasodilatation, this compensatory response is usually inadequate to overcome the severe precipitous rise in blood pressure (BP).

Common precipitating events are (noxious stimuli below the level of the injury) distension/ manipulation of hollow viscera (bladder, bowel, uterus, gallbladder) eg, urinary catheterization; cutaneous stimulation, eg, handling of a pressure sore; and surgical procedures, frequently involving pelvic organs or the lower extremities.

Clinically, AH is characterized by a cluster of symptoms, which include paroxysmal hypertension, bradycardia, dysrhythmia, headache, and, occasionally, loss of consciousness; profuse sweating, pallor, or flushing and nasal congestion occur above the level of the injury; cutaneous vasoconstriction, piloerection, and bladder spasm are observed below the level of the injury. AH is considered a medical emergency; untreated, it can lead to encephalopathy, stroke, seizures, intracerebral or retinal hemorrhage, heart block, myocardial infarction, congestive heart failure, arrhythmias, neurogenic pulmonary edema, and even death.

CLINICAL MANIFESTATIONS AND THEIR MANAGEMENT CONSIDERATIONS

The most common outcome of a T–L spine trauma is a T–L vertebral fracture; significant injuries can result in mechanical and/or neurologic instability of the spine. Concomitant systemic injuries and systemic manifestations of SCI further complicate the clinical course of patients with a T–L spine injury. In general, the morbidity is higher in patients with high thoracic spine injuries and/or complete SCI.

Mechanical instability of the spine

As previously described, T–L spine trauma can result in vertebral fractures (ranging from simple, undisplaced fractures to complex fracture dislocations); joint dislocation (eg, facet joints, IV joints); arthropathy (spondylosis, spondylolisthesis); ligamentous tears or herniation of IV discs; and, consequently, instability of the spine. Clinically, patients usually complain of axial, nonradiating, stabbing, back pain; the location of the pain usually correlates with the level of injury.

Neurologic injury

Patients with an injury to the thoracic SC, conus medullaris, or cauda equina can present with complete or incomplete paraplegia (quadriplegia indicates a SCI above T1 level). Complete paraplegia (no demonstrable sensory or motor function in the S4–S5 region) represents total disruption of the SC at one level and has an unfavorable prognosis with very minimal/no possibility of neurologic recovery; an incomplete SCI has a significantly better prognosis. A conclusive distinction regarding the completeness of an injury may not be possible in the immediate postinjury phase (first few days after injury) because of the presence of spinal shock; sometimes, sacral sparing (preservation of some sensory perception in the perianal region and/or voluntary contraction of the rectal sphincter may be the only sign of residual function.[1] An incomplete SCI produces a range of syndromes, such as central cord syndrome; anterior cord syndrome; conus medullaris syndrome; cauda equina syndrome; and rarely, posterior cord and Brown-Sequard syndrome; these can be identified by certain characteristic patterns of neurologic injury (Table 12.3).

Neurologic injuries above L1 typically produce an upper motor neuron injury (spasticity, clonus, hypertonia, hyper-reflexia, and positive

Table 12.3 Incomplete spinal cord syndromes

Name	Site	Clinical findings
Central cord syndrome	Central portion of spinal cord	Paraplegia, flaccid areflexic paralysis, variable sensory deficit below the lesion, anal sphincter atonia, urinary retention, and, in males, priapism
Posterior cord syndrome Least-common spinal cord injury syndrome	Posterior column injury	Ipsilateral loss of fine touch, vibration and proprioception (position sensation) below level of injury but preservation of pain, temperature sensation, and motor function, resulting in ataxia and faltering gait
Anterior cord syndrome	Malfunction of all tracts except posterior columns	Paraplegia, dissociated sensory loss below the lesion, bilateral loss of pain and temperature (spinothalamic tract) Preservation of posterior column function functions (proprioception, 2-point discrimination, joint position sense, vibration, and deep pressure)
Transverse lesion syndrome	Corticospinal, spinothalamic tracts, and posterior columns	Complete loss of sensation and paralysis below the level of the lesion; hyporeflexia at level of lesion; hyper-reflexia below the lesion; loss of sphincter function
Brown-Sequard syndrome (hemisection of the cord)	Lateral half of spinal cord, ie, corticospinal tract, spinothalamic tract, posterior column	Ipslateral paralysis (corticospinal tract lesion), ipsilateral loss of touch, position, and vibratory sensation proprioception (loss of posterior column function) Contralateral loss of pain and temperature sensation
Conus medullaris syndrome (CMS)	Injury of the sacral cord (conus) and lumbar nerve roots within the spinal canal	Combination of upper and lower motor neuron signs. Perianal and perineal loss of sensation (saddle anesthesia); erectile dysfunction; urinary retention, frequency, or incontinence; fecal incontinence; hypotonic anal sphincter Variable degrees of lower extremity paresis.
Cauda equina syndrome	Injury to the lumbosacral nerve roots within the neural canal	Can present similarly to CMS with saddle anesthesia, bladder, and bowel dysfunction, and variable lower extremity involvement; however, it is a pure lower motor neuron lesion with the absence of upper motor neuron signs, and it is characterized by asymmetric lower extremity weakness

Babinskis sign).[7] Injuries below L1 to L2 affect only the cauda equina roots and typically result in a lower motor neuron-type injury (flaccid paresis/paralysis, hypotonia, hyporeflexia), along with bladder and bowel dysfunction.[1,7] Because of the intrinsic resilience of the cauda equina, these injuries are usually incomplete and have a high potential for significant neurologic recovery.

Since the T–L junction marks the transition between central and peripheral nervous systems (junction of conus medullaris and cauda equina), injuries at this level produce a wide spectrum of neurologic injury patterns, with a varying combination of upper and lower motor-neuron signs (conus medullaris syndrome).

Concomitant nonspinal injuries

T–L spine injuries usually occur due to a high-energy impact; dissipation of this large amount of kinetic energy through the adjacent structures often results in concomitant, systemic injuries of the bone, soft tissues, and organs in proximity to the T–L spine.

Thoracic spine injuries may be associated with:

- Head injuries
- Cervical spine fractures
- Chest wall injuries: Rib fractures, sternal fractures, flail chest
- Pulmonary injuries: Pulmonary contusion/laceration, pneumothorax (simple/open/tension), hemothorax, hemo-pneumothorax
- Cardiac injuries: Blunt cardiac injury (cardiac contusion), hemopericardium, pericardial tamponade
- Great vessel injures: Aortic dissection or rupture
- Occult head injury is not uncommon in these patients[32]

Intra-abdominal visceral injuries and mesenteric avulsions usually occur in association with flexion distraction injuries of the lumbar spine; distraction-rotational injuries can be associated with abdominal aortic dissection.

Systemic manifestations of SCI (Table 12.4)

CARDIOVASCULAR SYSTEM

Hemodynamic instability can occur in these patients for several reasons:

1. Hemorrhagic shock: Associated injuries, eg, chest injuries; retroperitoneal or intra-abdominal trauma (visceral or vascular); pelvic and/or long bone fractures; external bleeding, eg, laceration of the scalp vessels, vascular injury
2. NS (in patients with T1–T6 level SCI)
3. Obstructive shock: Concomitant tension pneumothorax, cardiac tamponade
4. Cardiogenic shock: Associated blunt cardiac injury (myocardial contusion)

While hemorrhage is the most common etiology of traumatic shock, patients with high thoracic spine injuries (T1–T6) can also develop hypotension due to NS; in addition, the possibility of obstructive shock/cardiogenic shock also needs to be considered in patients who have incurred concurrent thoracic injuries as a result of high energy, blunt chest trauma.

The classic findings of NS are bradycardia with warm extremities; patients with hemorrhagic, cardiogenic, or obstructive shock typically have tachycardia and cool extremities. But these clinical signs often may not be pathognomonic because these conditions can coexist and, moreover, disruption of autonomic pathways in patients with high thoracic SCI can prevent the occurrence of tachycardia and peripheral vasoconstriction. Some important considerations that can aid in the differential diagnosis of these conditions are:

- Hypotension in a SCI below T6, or without an associated neurologic deficit or an apparent SCI is unlikely to be due to NS.
- Flattened neck veins are observed in hemorrhagic shock; patients with cardiogenic/obstructive shock usually have jugular venous distension and pulmonary edema.

Cardiac tamponade should be suspected if the patient has tachycardia, muffled heart sounds, dilated, engorged neck veins and hypotension that is resistant to fluids. Tension pneumothorax also has similar findings, but the additional features of acute respiratory distress, subcutaneous emphysema, absent breath sounds, tracheal deviation, and hyperresonance to percussion over the affected hemithorax can help to differentiate between the two conditions.

SCI is associated with a loss of autoregulation. In this situation, SC perfusion becomes dependent on systemic perfusion; and a fall in BP can further decrease the SC blood flow and exacer-

Table 12.4 Systemic manifestations of spinal cord injury

System	Manifestation	Mechanism
Cardiovascular More common in T1–T6 spinal cord injury	Neurogenic shock in acute SCI (hypotension, bradycardia, arrhythmias)	Due to loss of supraspinal control over thoracolumbar sympathetic outflow originating from T1–L2 segments; and unopposed parasymapathetic activity
	Autonomic hyper-reflexia in chronic SCI Episodes of severe hypertension	Massive, inappropriate sympathetic discharge due to loss of descending inhibitory control
Respiratory More severe in T1–T6 spinal cord injury	Paradoxical respiration, ↓ vital capacity, ↓ maximal inspiratory force, ventilatory insufficiency. Ineffective cough, atelectasis, pneumonia, respiratory failure	Loss of innervations to inspiratory intercostal muscles (T1–T11) and expiratory abdominal muscles (T6–L2),concomitant thoracic injuries; cervical extension of the neurologic deficits due to secondary SCI
	Pulmonary edema	Excessive fluid administration
	Increased airway hyper-reactivity (bronchoconstriction) and increased mucus production	Unopposed parasympathetic activity
Gastrointestinal	Paralytic ileus, delayed gastric emptying, aspiration risk, occult peritonitis, stress ulcer	Unopposed parasympathetic activity
Genitourinary Tract	Urinary retention, outflow incontinence, recurrent urinary tract infection, renal failure, nephrocalcinosis	Atonic bladder, reflex bladder, and detrusor contraction; prolonged catheterization
Skin	Decubitus ulcer	Insensate pressure areas; immobility and hypotonia due to sensorimotor deficits; alterations in cutaneous blood flow and autoregulation
Thermoregulation	Poikilothermia	Disruption of sympathetic pathways
	Tendency toward hypothermia	Rapid loss of heat from vasodilated skin; lack of thermogenesis from paralyzed muscles
Hemostatic system	Deep-vein thrombosis, pulmonary embolism	Venous stasis from paralyzed muscles; stimulation of thrombogenic factors following injury
Musculosketal system (in chronic SCI)	Osteoporosis, muscle calcification, joint immobility, contractures, pathologic fractures, hypercalcemia	Altered calcium metabolism and osteopenia
	Hyperkalemia with succinylcholine administration (between 3 days to 1 year of SCI)	Denervation supersensitivity
Hematologic system (in chronic SCI)	Normocytic hypochromic anemia	Chronic sepsis (recurrent pulmonary, urinary tract infections)

Abbreviation: SCI: spinal cord injury.

bate the secondary SCI. Several studies have reported worsening of neurologic function with hypotension; on the other hand, maintenance of normal hemodynamic parameters has been associated with improved axonal function and a better neurologic outcome after SCI.[33,34] Hence, hypotension mandates prompt treatment. The American Association of Neurological Surgeons (AANS) recommends a target MAP of 85 to 90 mmHg and avoidance of a SBP <90 mmHg (Class 3 evidence) for over 5 to 7 days after SCI. [33]

A stepwise approach is recommended for the management of hypotension:

Since hemorrhage is the most common etiology of shock in injured patients and most polytrauma patients have some degree of hypovolemia; and moreover, most nonhemorrhagic shock states also respond partially or briefly to volume resuscitation, the initial management of shock (irrespective of the etiology), begins with a trial of volume resuscitation (1–2 liters of warm, isotonic saline/Ringers Lactate).[1]

Subsequent management is based on the response to fluid administration; a partial response indicates either an active, undetected hemorrhage and/or a nonhemorrhagic etiology of shock.

Invasive central venous pressure (CVP) monitoring is recommended to guide the fluid administration and identify the potential cause of shock. A minimal rise in an initially low CVP or a declining CVP with fluid therapy suggests the need for additional fluid/blood replacement and a renewed search for the source of the bleeding. On the other hand, an abrupt, persistent elevation of CVP is indicative of overtransfusion/rapid transfusion; cardiac dysfunction because of neurogenic or cardiogenic shock; and/or increased intrathoracic pressures due to obstructive shock.[1]

Vasopressors/inotropes are added if there is a partial or insignificant response to fluid administration.[1] Patients with NS are at risk of fluid overload and pulmonary edema, hence, vasopressors are usually required for restoration of BP; phenylephrine hydrochloride, dopamine, norepinephrine, or epinephrine are preferred. Dopamine, norepinephrine, or epinephrine ($\alpha 1$- β_1-agonists) have inotropic, chronotropic, and vasopressor actions and are useful for upper thoracic spine injuries (T1–T6). Since phenylephrine predominantly has an α_1-agonist and minimal β_1 effects, it is useful for counteracting the

peripheral vasodilatation associated with lower thoracic and lumbar cord injuries; it can, however, cause reflex bradycardia. Dobutamine, with its prominent vasodilatory effects, has limited use in these patients. Atropine may be used to counteract hemodynamically significant bradycardia.

Vasopressors can be used as a temporizing measure, even in patients with "pure" hypovolemic shock, to serve as a "bridge" while fluids are being administered and the source of the hemorrhage is being identified.

Chronic SCI, patients with high thoracic lesions, are at risk of developing acute hypertensive episodes due to AH. Management includes removal of the precipitating stimulus, for example, checking for a blocked urinary catheter or impacted fecal matter; sitting the patient upright can help to reduce the BP. A wide range of antihypertensive drugs can be used to pharmacologically lower the BP, for example, labetalol, propranolol, esmolol, midazolam, magnesium sulfate, and nifedipine.

Respiratory system

Patients with upper thoracic, especially complete, SCI, are at increased risk of pulmonary complications in the acute phase of injury because of loss of innervation to the inspiratory (intercostals, T1–T11) and expiratory abdominal muscles (T6–L2).[35]

Paresis/paralysis of the intercostals results in paradoxic respiration, decreased vital capacity (30%–80%), and reduction in the maximal inspiratory force; this leads to increased work of breathing with risk of ventilatory insufficiency and prolonged postoperative ventilation.[36] Because of denervation of the expiratory muscles, patients cannot generate an effective cough to clear the secretions, and consequently, are prone to develop atelectasis, pneumonia, and respiratory failure. In addition, concomitant thoracic injuries; cervical extension of the neurologic deficits due to secondary SCI; development of pulmonary edema due to excessive fluid administration; increased airway hyper-reactivity (bronchoconstriction) and increased mucus production due to unopposed parasympathetic activity can further aggravate the respiratory morbidity.

Lung volumes tend to be the lowest at 3 to 4 days postinjury. A gradual improvement in respiratory function may occur with time because of the decrease in cord edema, strengthening of accessory muscles of respiration, and recovery from spinal shock.[37] Respiratory mechanics are minimally affected in patients with lower thoracic and lumbar SCI, hence, respiratory dysfunction is usually not observed in these patients.

Hypoxemia and hypercarbia can further worsen secondary SCI, hence, it is imperative to closely monitor the respiratory function in the early postinjury period. Clinical manifestations of respiratory impairment include tachypnea; paradoxic chest movements; use of accessory respiratory muscles; agitation, anxiety, decreased air entry; rhonchi; crepitations; pallor; cyanosis; decreasing oxygen saturation (SaO_2); increasing arterial carbon dioxide (CO_2) levels; and a reduction in the vital capacity to 30% to 50% of predicted values.[35] Mechanical ventilation may be required if PaO_2 (partial pressure of arterial oxygen) is <60 mmHg or is significantly decreasing despite supplemental oxygen; $PaCO_2$ (partial pressure of arterial CO_2) >60 mmHg; PaO_2/FiO_2 (fraction of inspired oxygen) is <250; vital capacity is <20% of predicted, <15 mL/kg or is approaching 1 L; maximal inspiratory force is < −20 cm H_2O, maximal expiratory force is > +20 cm H_2O, or there is evidence of atelectasis/infiltrates on chest radiography.[14,37]

Patients with a high thoracic SCI have a better respiratory function in the recumbent than in the sitting position. In the former, the diaphragm is pushed up into the chest by abdominal contents and, therefore, has a greater excursion in inspiration; whereas in the latter, it is pulled down by abdominal contents, which further impede excursion in inspiration.[36] Furthermore, the potential for hemodynamic instability is higher in the sitting position (because of NS). Therefore, the recumbent position is preferable for the first few days after the injury occurs. Subsequently, sitting up gradually can be allowed as the intercostal paralysis improves and the chest no longer collapses during inspiration, hence, preserving the smaller tidal volumes produced by diaphragmatic descent.[36]

Gastrointestinal system

The gastrointestinal effects of SCI are of particular concern to the anesthesiologist. The autonomic dysfunction predisposes to gastric atony and para-lytic ileus; the resulting abdominal distension can further compromise the ventilation and also increase the risk of aspiration. These patients are also susceptible to stress ulcers.

Genitourinary system

Patients with acute T–L spine injuries can have painless urinary retention and outflow incontinence due to an atonic bladder. Patients with chronic SCI have urinary incontinence due to a reflex (neurogenic or spastic) bladder. These problems increase the risk of recurrent, ascending urinary tract infections; subsequently, complications such as pyelonephritis can lead to renal insufficiency and renal failure.

Thermoregulation

Poikilothermia due to disruption of sympathetic pathways with rapid heat loss from vasodilated skin and lack of thermogenesis from paralyzed muscles increases the risk of hypothermia, especially in the cool environment of an operating room, and can worsen the secondary SCI injury in these patients.

Hemostatic system

Venous stasis due to paralysis of muscles and hypercoagulability because of stimulation of thrombogenic factors following injury significantly increases the risk of venous thromboembolism (VTE). Patients with SCI have one of the highest incidences of VTE among hospital admissions; the risk of deep-vein thrombosis and pulmonary embolism is particularly high in patients with complete SCI, upper thoracic spine injuries, and those undergoing prolonged surgeries, especially combined anterior-posterior surgeries.[14] Mechanical prophylaxis with sequential intermittent pneumatic compression devices for lower extremities, the cornerstone of VTE prevention, should be initiated in all SCI patients immediately after admission and should continue until ambulation, and even during the perioperative period.[38,39]

Combining pharmacologic prophylaxis (low molecular weight heparin) with mechanical prophylaxis further reduces the risk for VTE; it can be started on admission and can be withheld 1 day prior to and 1 day following surgical intervention.[38,39] However, this may be slightly controversial, taking into account any other trauma, coagulaopathy, or an impending surgery with increased risk of perioperative bleeding and hematoma formation; alternatively, pharmacologic prophylaxis can be started as early as deemed feasible by the surgeon. It should be continued for at least 6 to 12 weeks after the initial injury.[38]

Cutaneous manifestations

Insensate pressure areas, immobility and hypotonia due to sensorimotor deficits, along with alterations in cutaneous blood flow and autoregulation, increase the risk of ischemia and subsequent necrosis of the skin. Decubitus ulcers, especially on the heels, sacrum, scapulae, and ischium, can develop within minutes of the injury; hence, particular care is required in the early postinjury period, when there will be several patient interventions, movements, and manipulations. Pressure relief mattresses and turning beds help in the prevention of bed sores; in addition, pressure-relieving procedures must be carried out every 2 hours, unless contraindicated by physiological instability.

Metabolism

These patients have a markedly decreased basal metabolic rate and hence, a decreased metabolic CO_2 production; they require lower minute volumes to maintain eucapnia during perioperative controlled ventilation.[40]

Musculoskeletal system

Because of the upregulation of the acetylcholine receptors, administration of succinylcholine (depolarizing muscle relaxant) can cause massive efflux of potassium due to the simultaneous depolarization of the entire muscle surface. This hyperkalemia is mostly observed from the third day of injury, is maximal between 1 month and 5 months, and can persist up to 1 year in some patients; hence, use of succinylcholine is preferably restricted to the initial 48 hours after the occurrence of the injury.

Prolonged immobilization of chronic SCI patients leads to altered calcium metabolism and osteopenia. These patients are prone to develop osteoporosis, muscle calcification, joint immobility, contractures, pathologic fractures, hypercalcemia, and nephrocalcinosis with renal failure.

Hematologic system

Patients with chronic SCI are also likely to have normocytic hypochromic anemia (due to chronic infection, eg, pulmonary, urinary tract infection; decubitus ulcers) and lower-extremity edema (due to blood pooling).[37]

IMAGING

Imaging for T–L spine injuries includes plain radiographs (x-rays), computerized tomography (CT) scans, and MRI. Conventionally, spine radiographs have been the initial investigation for screening and diagnosing these injuries; however, a multidetector computed tomographic (MDCT) scan is superior to plain films for detection of T–L spine fractures, and presently, is the recommended initial imaging method of choice (if available) [level 1 evidence].[41] Nevertheless, plain radiographs continue to be useful for identifying the level of injury, characterizing bony injuries, assessing the relationship of one VB to another, and for evaluating the overall alignment of the spine.[10] MRI is complementary to CT scanning, while neural elements and discoligamentous soft tissues, especially related to PLC injury, are better visualized, however, it is less-sensitive than CT or plain films for distinguishing bony abnormalities, particularly of the posterior spinal elements. It may be indicated for screening of T–L spine injury if the patient has a neurologic deficit despite a normal appearance of the spinal CT scan (spinal cord edema, ligamentous injury, epidural hematoma, or disc protrusions causing spinal cord compression are visualized more clearly with MRI).

Radiograph T–L spine (anteroposterior [AP] and lateral spine films)

Anatomically, the spine resists significant rotation and an altered alignment of either spinous processes or pedicles is indicative of considerable anatomic destruction and instability; hence, measurements on x-rays should be made at the level of injury, and should be compared with the vertebrae at the more cranial and caudal levels.

A-P views are useful for identifying loss of lateral VB height, changes in horizontal and vertical interpedicular distance, widening of the interspinous spaces, asymmetry of the posterior structures, perpendicular or oblique fractures of the dorsal elements, facet joint separation, and lateral translation. Widening of interpedicular distance indicates a failure of posterior VB (middle column instability) eg, in burst fractures. Widening of the interspinous distances suggests a flexion-distraction injury.

Lateral views demonstrate superior endplate fracture, disruption of rostral endplate, anterior wedging deformity (loss of VB height), anterior wall-cortex irregularity, dorsal cortical wall fracture with retropulsed bone, fracture of spinous processes, widening of interspinous distance, and malalignment (subluxation or angulation) of VB. They are useful for detecting subluxations, compression fractures, and Chance fractures.

CT scan

Multiplanar reformations in MDCT provide excellent bone detail and permit visualization in any plane; three-dimensional constructions add a spatial appreciation of the fracture pattern. The vertebral arches, posterior elements (facet joints, pedicles, lamina, spinous processes, and neural canal), are very well visualized, hence, MDCT is particularly useful for detection of subluxation/fractures of facets and lamina, the integrity of the middle column, and assessment of the degree of canal compromise caused by burst fractures. CT also adds the benefit of visceral imaging, especially because associated chest, abdominal, and pelvic injuries are not uncommon in these patients; moreover, CT spine can be extracted from a chest and abdominal CT scan.

MRI

MRI evaluates PLC directly, and hence is the modality of choice for detecting PLC injury; as mentioned previously, discoligamentous, soft tissue, and neural injuries; epidural hematomas and their relationship to the SC are also well visualized. In addition, the artery of Ademkiwickz can be detected in the majority of patients with contrast-enhanced magnetic resonance angiography.[8,17]

Detection of PLC injury

Signs of PLC disruption on radiographs or CT images include a >50% decrease in the VB height,

more than 30 to 35 degrees of kyphotic deformity; increase in interspinous distance (splaying of spinous processes); avulsion fracture of superior or inferior aspects of contiguous spinous processes; widened, empty ("naked"), perched or dislocated facet joints; or subluxation, translation, or rotation of VB.

On an MRI, PLC injury is diagnosed by disruption of the low-signal-intensity black stripe on sagittal T1- or T2-weighted MR images (supraspinous ligament or ligamentum flavum tear); and fluid in the facet capsules (capsular injury) or edema in the interspinous region (interspinous ligament injury) on fluid-sensitive MR images.[8,17,42]

SURGERY: INDICATIONS, TIMING, TECHNIQUE, APPROACH, POSITIONS

Indications

There is no definitive Grade I or Grade II evidence for guiding the management of patients with T–L spine trauma. Usually, stable injuries without the potential for progressive deformity or neurologic injury are managed conservatively, eg, simple compression or stable burst fractures. Indications for an operative intervention can include:

- Neurologic instability (incomplete or progressive neurologic deficits, SC compression)
- Mechanical instability (disruption of PLC)
- Concomitant injuries that necessitate early mobilization

In general, severe flexion distraction injuries, unstable burst fractures, fracture dislocations, and translation/rotational injuries almost always require surgical stabilization.[7,10] The purpose of the surgery in patients with incomplete T–L SCI is to prevent further progression of the neurologic injury, facilitate maximal neurologic recovery, and allow early rehabilitation; hence, the surgery usually involves neural decompression and fracture reduction, followed by stabilization and fusion of the injured spinal segments.

Patients with complete SCI may also undergo surgery. Since they are unlikely to have any postoperative neurologic improvement, the surgery primarily facilitates early mobilization and is usually limited to restoration of spinal alignments and fracture stabilization; whether additional decompression should be performed remains controversial.[7,8,10]

Timing of surgery

Although the optimal timing is still not very clear, studies do suggest that early surgery performed within 24 hours of the injury is associated with better postoperative recovery.[43,44] Patients with progressive and/or incomplete neurologic deficits merit an urgent intervention because of the potential for neurologic recovery; they should be operated on once they are hemodynamically stable and don't have other severe injuries that might preclude surgery. Surgery in patients with a normal neurology or a complete neurologic deficit , is less urgent, and can be performed as soon as it is safe for the patient.[7]

Surgical approaches and techniques

T–L spine surgery can be performed through an anterior, posterior, or a combined anterior-posterior approach, via an open or a minimally invasive technique; the choice of a particular approach/ technique is generally determined by the type of injury, operative goal, presence of concomitant injuries, and familiarity of the surgeon with the approach/and or technique (Table 12.5).

ANTERIOR APPROACHES

These approaches are primarily indicated for unstable T–L burst fractures, which affect the anterior aspect of the spinal canal, and, in instances, where the spinal canal is compromised and cannot be adequately resolved by the posterior approach alone. They provide the most direct access for anterior neural decompression and reconstruction of the weight-bearing column; they provides superior mechanical stability, compared with the posterior-only approach (for unstable burst fractures); however, they are technically more difficult, less familiar to surgeons, and have significantly greater blood loss compared with the posterior approach.

The operative technique usually involves decompression (corpectomy and removal of retropulsed bone fragments in the spinal canal), deformity correction, and stabilization (anterior fixation screw-plate devices or rod-screw constructs), and fusion

(vertebral interbody cage/ autogenous bone graft) of the spine.

Thoracic spine: Transthoracic; retropleural; thoracoabdominal; transmanubrial (cervicothoracic junction)

Transthoracic approach (thoracotomy): T2–T12 level

This standard approach provides multilevel, bilateral access to the ventral thoracic spine (T2–T12), and is performed with the patient placed in the lateral decubitus position. Although either side can be used, a right-sided thoracotomy is preferred for T2–T9 vertebral injuries (to avoid manipulation of the aorta) and a left-sided approach for lower thoracic vertebral injuries (below T9, to prevent potential injury to the liver/vena cava). Since the exposure involves transpleural dissection and removal of a portion of a rib, a chest drain is inserted postoperatively. The surgical exposure can be improved in injuries at or above the T10 level, by allowing a collapse of the ipsilateral lung, with use of one lung ventilation (OLV).

This approach is associated with a high incidence of pulmonary complications, eg, pneumonia, lobar collapse, pleural effusion, and/or atelectasis; inadvertent injury to the Adamkiewicz artery can occur with the left-sided approach. The retropleural approach is an alternative approach, which prevents the morbidity associated with pleural cavity entry but provides limited exposure to multiple levels.

The anterior thoracoabdominal approach: T–L junction

This retroperitoneal approach allows multilevel exposure at the T–L junction and is performed in the lateral decubitus position. It involves a low, left-sided thoracotomy, along with division of the diaphragm; a chest tube is inserted postoperatively. The morbidity is high because both of the thoracic and abdominal cavities are manipulated; there is a potential risk of hemi-diaphragmatic palsy due to detachment of the diaphragm.

Lumbar spine: Retroperitoneal, transperitoneal approach

The retroperitoneal approach is performed in the lateral decubitus position (left side up); the exposure can be extended up to the diaphragm, and

Table 12.5 Thoracolumbar spine surgery: Approaches, positions, procedures

	Anterior approach	True posterior approach	Posterolateral approaches
Thoracic Spine			
Cervicothoracic junction **C7–T3** **T2–T12**	Transmanubrial approach (sternal splitting approach) **Position: Supine** Transthoracic approach for thoracotomy (T2–T12) Retropleural approach (T2–T10) Thoracoscopic approach (Endoscopic) **Position: Lateral decubitus**	Dorsal midline (laminectomy) Transpedicular **Position: Prone**	Costotransversectomy **Position: Prone or lateral decubitus** Lateral extracavitary approach **Position: Prone**
Lumbar Spine			
	Anterior Approach	**Posterior Approach**	
Thoracolumbar junction	Thoracoabdominal retroperito-neal approach **Position: Right Lateral decubitus**	Posterior midline approach **Position: Prone**	
L1–L5 vertebrae	Transperitoneal, transabdominal approach **Position: Supine** Retroperitoneal approach **Position: Lateral decubitus (usually left side up)** Endoscopic transperitoneal approach **Position: Supine**	Posterior midline approach; **Position: Prone**	
Surgery	OPEN: Decompression (corpectomy and removal of retropulsed bone fragments in the spinal canal), deformity correction, and stabilization (anterior fixation screw-plate devices or rod-screw constructs), and fusion (vertebral interbody cage/autogenous bone graft) ENDOSCOPIC Video-assisted thoracoscopy Minimal access surgery of the spine **Position: Lateral decubitus**	OPEN Canal decompression (laminectomy of fractured and overlying vertebra that covers the com-pressed part of the canal), spine reduction, and stabilization (three-column fixation with pedicle screw-rod); and spine fusion (autologous bone graft) ENDOSCOPIC Vertebroplasty Kyphoplasty **Position: Prone**	

allows mobilization of the kidney and, if required, the spleen and liver. Although there is a risk of renal and vascular injury (especially left iliac vein), it is lower than that with the transperitoneal approach; the peritoneal cavity is not opened but there is a risk of peritoneal injury.

The open transperitoneal approach, performed through a laparotomy, is relatively more complex and may require the services of a vascular surgeon. It involves mobilization of the abdominal viscera, branches of the aorta, inferior vena cava, and the iliac vessels. In addition to the risk of iatrogenic injury to these structures, the ureter and pelvic contents are also vulnerable to injury during exposure.

POSTERIOR APPROACHES: TRUE POSTERIOR, POSTEROLATERAL

These approaches are used for management of most of the T–L spine fractures (flexion distraction injuries, flexion dislocation fractures, unstable burst fractures with intact neurology). These approaches are performed with the patient placed in a prone position. They do not involve invasion of the thoracic and abdominal cavities; are technically easier to perform; and have fewer complications, especially lesser blood loss, when compared with the anterior approaches.

The surgery usually involves canal decompression (laminectomy of the fractured, overlying vertebra, which covers the compressed part of the canal); spine reduction and stabilization (three-column fixation with pedicle screw-rod); and spine fusion (autologous bone graft) (Figure 12.2). The stabilization may be performed with a short segment pedicle screw-rod (includes proximal and distal adjacent normal vertebrae), or it can be a multilevel spinal fixation (two to three segments above and below the injury) for grossly unstable injuries. Pedicle screw placement is associated with a risk of neural or vascular injury (if the cortical borders are breached); use of intraoperative neuroelectrophysiologic monitoring (IONM), especially triggered electromyography (tEMG), can help to reduce this risk.

True posterior approaches—Dorsal midline (laminectomy) and transpedicular approaches

These approaches provide access to the posterior spinal elements; in addition, the transpedicular approach also provides access to the lateral spine.

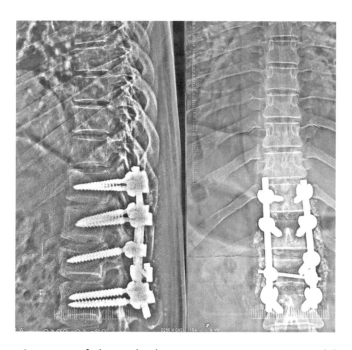

Figure 12.2 Postoperative x-ray of thoracolumbar spine: anteroposterior and lateral views, showing decompression of L1 vertebra and pedicle screw fixation at T12, L1, L2, and L3 vertebrae.

Posterolateral approaches— Costotransversectomy and lateral extracavitary Approach

These approaches have the advantage of providing simultaneous access to the anterior and posterior spine via a single dorsal incision without invading the pleural cavity. They are especially useful when combined anterior–posterior decompression is required.

Costotransversectomy involves removal of a portion of a rib and dissection of the trapezius, latissimus dorsi, and paraspinous muscles. The ventral exposure is relatively limited; however, the morbidity is also lower compared with a standard thoracotomy, which makes it a useful option for high-risk patients. Potential concerns about this approach include increased blood loss and pain due to extensive, soft tissue exposure; and the possibility of a pleural injury.

The lateral extracavitary approach is a modification of costotransversectomy; its advantages are superior visualization of the SC and combined anterior and posterior exposure; it is, however, technically more difficult, and also has a risk of pleural injury.

COMBINED ANTERIOR-POSTERIOR APPROACH

A combined anterior-posterior approach (eg, circumferential stabilization/360-degree instrumentation) may be required in selected patients who have highly unstable fractures (PLC disruption), with complete or partial preservation of neurologic function.[22,24] The surgery may be performed on the same day or as a staged procedure, depending on the medical condition and age of the patient. Needless to say, while this approach provides better mechanical stability, it is technically challenging and has greater morbidity in terms of a higher bleeding risk and a longer surgical time, compared with a posterior- or anterior-only approach.[7]

MINIMALLY INVASIVE SURGERIES (MIS)

Open surgical approaches require extensive exposure and often lead to significant blood loss, postoperative morbidity, and increased hospital stay. MIS are now being used in T–L spine trauma increasingly, in an effort to avoid the operative morbidity of open procedures. These procedures use smaller incisions and respect anatomic planes, and hence, cause less soft tissue dissection with less blood loss, significantly reduced postoperative pain, faster functional recovery, and a shorter hospital stay, while providing the same structural stability as the common open techniques. They are particularly useful in high-risk patients who cannot tolerate the morbidity of open procedures, eg, patients with polytrauma, compromised lung function, morbid obesity, and so on. Common MIS performed using the posterior approach include percutaneous posterior pedicle fixation and VB augmentation; video assisted thoracoscopic surgery (VATS) and minimal access spinal surgery (MASS) allow access to the ventral thoracic spine and T–L junction and may be used for an isolated anterior or a combined anterior/posterior approach to the T–L spine.[45,46]

VB augmentation: Kyphoplasty, vertebroplasty

In vertebroplasty, a cementing agent, for example polymethyl methacrylate, is injected into the collapsed VB (junction of anterior and middle third VB), through a percutaneously inserted, hollow-bore needle. The cement strengthens the structure of the VB and increases the stability of the spine. In kyphoplasty, the height of the collapsed VB is increased prior to injection of the cement; this involves inflation of a balloon that has been inserted through the needle. VB augmentation is also used in combination with posterior, short-segment pedicle-screw instrumentation (open/endoscopic), for treatment of acute unstable T–L burst fractures as an alternative to more lengthy reconstructions of the anterior column.[47]

POSITIONING

T–L spine surgeries are mostly performed in the prone or lateral decubitus positions; the supine position is required for the lumbar transperitoneal or thoracic transmanubrial approach. Positioning should be accomplished gradually (patients with NS poorly tolerate acute positional changes) and by carefully logrolling (head, body rotated in unison, maintaining a neutral neck position) the patient, to prevent further SCI. In addition, liberal padding of all pressure points helps prevent the development of decubitus ulcers (Table 12.5).

Prone position

Several positioning systems are available for prone positioning, for example, Wilson frame, Relton Hall frame, Jackson spine table, Andrews frame, or longitudinal chest rolls.[48] It is absolutely imperative that there is no compression of the chest wall or restriction of abdominal movements when patients are placed in the prone position. Compression of the abdomen in an improperly positioned patient can cause multiple problems: impaired ventilation (cephalad displacement of abdominal contents, restriction of diaphragmatic movements); reduced venous return (from pelvis, lower extremities) and decreased cardiac output; and increased surgical bleeding (due to engorgement of the valveless epidural venous plexuses).

The patient's head is placed in a horseshoe headrest or soft foam/gel pad with preconfigured cutouts; the neck is maintained in the neutral position. Eyes are closed and corneas are lubricated. There should be no external pressure on the eyes (to protect against postoperative visual loss), ears, nose, and face; slight reverse Trendelenburg position also helps to decrease venous congestion and dependent periorbital edema. Soft mouth guards are inserted to prevent a potential injury to the tongue and lips during intraoperative motor evoked potential (MEP) monitoring. Arms are placed on padded arm rests and "airplaned" (abducted at shoulder and elbow) to facilitate intraoperative fluoroscopy; knees are padded and flexed; feet are placed in the neutral position. The breasts are positioned medially and caudal to the supporting pads and direct pressure on the nipples is avoided, if possible; male genitalia are allowed to hang freely.

Lateral position

In this position, the patient's head rests on a padded doughnut; the back is placed close to the edge of the table, to facilitate surgical access. The position of the dependent arm merits special attention because of a potential risk of compression of the axillary artery and brachial plexus and development of compartment syndrome. The arm is placed on a low, padded-arm board, which is inserted between the table and head fixator and is positioned in a hanging or ventral position, with the shoulder abducted and the elbow flexed; an axillary roll (diameter of the upper arm) placed under the upper chest

(approximately 4 cm below the dependent axilla) takes the pressure off of the dependent shoulder.[48] The nondependent arm can be positioned on the "airplane" armrest or on a pillow placed anterior to the patient's body. The abdomen is kept as free as possible. The dependent knee is gently flexed; the common peroneal nerve is susceptible to pressure injury as it crosses the proximal portion of the fibula just distal to the knee; this area must, therefore, be amply padded and a pillow should be placed between the legs.

T–L SPINE TRAUMA: ROLE OF THE NEUROANESTHESIOLOGIST

Neuroanesthesiologists are actively involved in the management of patients with T–L spine trauma in the ED, operating room (OR), and in the neuro-intensive care unit. The concerns, and consequently the goals of management, change as the injury evolves from an acute, physiologically unstable phase, to a more stable but debilitating, chronic phase. The following sections describe the management of these patients in the ED and also delve into the principles of perioperative care when they present for urgent surgery in the acute phase or for a repeat spine-associated surgery in the chronic phase of SCI.

The initial postinjury period can be very difficult; besides the spinal instability, these patients can also have significant cardiorespiratory cerebral instability. At least 5% of the patients experience the onset of or worsening of neurologic symptoms, after admission to the ED, because of the worsening of secondary SCI. Hence, the goal in the acute phase of SCI is to protect the cord; limit the extent of secondary SCI by aggressive prevention and management of factors such as hypotension, hypoxemia, hypercapnia, anemia, hypothermia, acidosis, and hypo/hyperglycemia; and facilitate an early neural decompression and stabilization of the spine.

Management in the ED is based on the Advanced Trauma Life Support (ATLS®) protocol guidelines.[1] The initial "primary survey" includes spine immobilization, prompt resuscitation of vital functions, treatment of life-threatening injuries, and a preliminary neurologic assessment (Table 12.6). The subsequent "secondary survey" focuses on detection of specific injuries so that definitive care of these injuries can be initiated.

Table 12.6 Initial assessment in thoracolumbar spine trauma

Primary Survey

Immobilization of the Spine:

Cervical collar/cervical immobilization device/manual, inline immobilization

Neutral position: Place patient supine on a solid surface, eg, long spine board, without rotating or bending the spine (neutral position)

Logrolling of patient: Four people required for the procedure

One person to maintain manual inline immobilization of the patient's head and neck; one each for the torso, pelvis, and legs; and to direct the procedure and move the spine board

A: Airway Maintenance with Cervical Spine Protection

Assess and maintain patency of the airway

Establish a definitive airway, if required (while maintaining manual inline immobilization of the cervical spine)

B: Breathing—Ventilation and Oxygenation

Assessment: Rate, depth, and pattern of respiration; tracheal deviation, bilateral chest movement; chest percussion for dullness/or hyper-resonance; chest auscultation

Identify tension pneumothorax, open pneumothorax (sucking chest wound), flail chest and pulmonary contusion, massive hemothorax

Management:

Administration of high-concentration oxygen

Bag mask ventilation/endotracheal intubation (rapid sequence induction, under cervical spine immobilization) [if required]

Tension pneumothorax: Immediate needle decompression (second intercostal space in the midclavicular line of the affected hemithorax), followed by insertion of a chest tube (fifth intercostal space, just anterior to the midaxillary line)

Seal open pneumothorax: Close the defect with a sterile, occlusive dressing (large enough to overlap the wound's edges; taped securely on three sides in order to provide a flutter-type valve effect)

Small, asymptomatic pneumothorax: Observation and aspiration/placement of a chest tube

C: Circulation and Fluids

Assessment:

Blood pressure and peripheral circulation (radial, dorsalis pedis)

Peripheral pulse (rate, regularity, quality, paradox); skin pallor/temperature, blood pressure, pulse pressure; neck veins (distension in obstructive shock, cardiogenic shock; however, distension may be absent in patients with concomitant hypovolemia)

Identify source of hemorrhage (chest, retroperitoneal, abdominal injuries; pelvic and extremity fractures, laceration of the scalp vessels, vascular injury)

(Imaging: Plain radiographs of the chest and pelvis, in conjunction with a focused assessment sonography in trauma (FAST) to assess the presence of free fluid in the abdomen, pericardial, and intrapleural spaces)

Management:

Apply direct pressure to external bleeding site(s)

Insert two large-caliber IV catheters

Replace fluids for hypovolemia (1–2 L of warm Isotonic Saline/ Ringers Lactae,and blood if required), initiate vasopressors, if no response to fluids

Insert CVP line to guide fluid therapy

Insert a urinary catheter to monitor urinary output and prevent bladder distention

Perform a rectal examination before inserting the urinary catheter, assess for rectal sphincter tone and sensation (ability to perceive the examination, resting anal tone, the ability to voluntarily contract the external sphincter, presence/absence of bulbocavernous reflex)

(Continued)

Table 12.6 (Continued) Initial assessment in thoracolumbar spine trauma

Insert a gastric catheter, to prevent gastric distention and aspiration

Cardiac tamponade: Immediate pericardiocentesis (under ECG monitoring), followed by an exploratory thoracotomy

Massive hemothorax (>1500 mL blood): Simultaneous restoration of blood volume and decompression of the chest cavity, followed by exploratory laprotomy

Blunt cardiac trauma and great vessel injury: Urgent cardiothoracic surgical intervention

D: Disability—Brief Neurologic Examination:

Determine level of consciousness (GCS)

Assess pupils (size and reactivity)

Recognize paralysis/paresis

Spinal pain or tenderness

Motor assessment: Hand or foot weakness

Sensory assessment: Altered or absent sensation in the hands or feet

Priapism (in an unconscious or exposed male)

E: Exposure: Complete Examination

Prevent hypothermia

Secondary Survey: Neurologic and Systemic Assessment

Reassess level of consciousness (GCS score and pupils)

History

Type of trauma: High vs. low energy

Mechanism of injury: Automobile collisions: seat-belt use, steering-wheel deformation, direction of impact, damage to the automobile in terms of major deformation or intrusion into the passenger compartment and whether the patient was ejected from the vehicle. Fall: From what height

Symptoms: Pain in the back, weakness, inability to move, numbness, paresthesia or anesthesia below the injury level, urinary retention, bowel and bladder dysfunction

Medical history: Preexisting morbidities, allergies, medications

Assessment of the spine: (Carefully logroll the patient and assess the entire spine)

Inspection: Skin bruise/abrasion/open wound/contusions/lacerations/penetrating wounds over the spine; deformity, swelling/ecchymosis

Palpation: Pain, tenderness, deformity, local kyphosis, swelling, crepitations, palpable gap in between spinous processes

Neurologic assessment: (According to ASIA scale)

Sensory Examination: Test sensation to pinprick in all dermatomes and record the most caudal dermatome that feels the pinprick

Assess best motor function (determine level of paraplegia, nerve root level)

Determine complete/incomplete SCI

Determine ASIA impairment scale

Investigations:

Spine imaging (multidetector computerized tomography/spine radiographs), arterial blood gas measurements

Abbreviations: ASIA: American Spinal Injury Association; GCS: Glasgow Coma Scale.

Immobilization of the spine

There is approximately a 30% chance that a T–L spine injury may be missed during the initial evaluation, especially if the patient doesn't have any overt symptoms or has multiple distracting injuries, altered sensorium (concurrent head injury/ intoxication), and/or more pressing treatment priorities (life-threatening injuries); it is prudent to presume a spine injury in these situations and protect the SC by immobilizing the spine.[49] In fact, a full in-line spinal immobilization is essential in all patients with a known, presumed, or suspected spine injury (eg, polytrauma, high-energy mechanism of injury). This includes immobilization of the neck by a cervical collar/a cervical immobilization device, and placing the patient supine on a solid surface, eg, long spine board, without rotating or bending the spine (neutral position); no effort should be made to reduce any obvious deformity. Any movement of the patient, eg, for a clinical/radiologic examination, should be done by careful "logrolling," so that the neutral anatomic alignment of the entire VC is maintained at all times. Immobilization should be maintained until the VC fractures and SCI have been excluded by definitive clinical and/or radiologic imaging.

However, prolonged immobilization on a hard surface causes discomfort to the patient and also predisposes to the formation of decubitus ulcers; therefore, vulnerable areas should be well padded and the patient should be removed from the long spine board as soon as it is feasible. If this is not possible within 2 hours, "logrolling" the patient should be done every 2 hours, while maintaining the integrity of the spine.

Primary survey

AIRWAY AND BREATHING (MANAGEMENT OF AIRWAY, OXYGENATION, AND VENTILATION) WITH CERVICAL SPINE CONTROL

Patients with respiratory insufficiency and/or loss of airway reflexes (low Glasgow Coma Scale [GCS] due to concomitant head injury) require emergent control of the airway and/or breathing, to ensure adequate oxygenation (SaO$_2$ >95%) and ventilation; prevent risk of aspiration; and also to limit the extent of secondary SCI. Tracheal intubation may be required for definitive management and should be performed while maintaining manual inline stabilization (MILS) of the cervical spine; MILS should be continued during all phases of airway management.

Tension pneumothorax, flail chest with pulmonary contusion, massive hemothorax, and open pneumothorax require immediate intervention and should be identified; simple pneumothorax/hemothorax, fractured ribs, and pulmonary contusion can also compromise ventilation, although to a lesser degree.

CIRCULATION AND CONTROL OF HEMORRHAGE

As described in the previous sections, hemodynamic instability can occur due to hemorrhagic, neurogenic, obstructive and/or cardiogenic shock. The assessment includes a clinical evaluation and radiologic imaging to rapidly detect life-threatening injuries and potential sources of hemorrhage. (imaging: Plain radiographs of chest and pelvis, in conjunction with a focused assessment sonography in trauma [FAST] to assess the presence of free fluid in the abdomen, pericardial, and intrapleural spaces). The electrocardiogram (ECG) should be continually monitored in all patients with blunt thoracic trauma to detect occurrence of dysrhythmias.

A stepwise approach is followed for management of hypotension, by beginning with a trial of volume resuscitation (1–2 liters of warmed normal saline/Ringers lactate) and, if required, progressing to pharmacologic support (norepinephrine, dopamine, phenylephrine), ideally guided by CVP monitoring. Treatment goals include a MAP >85 mmHg and avoiding SBP of <90 mmHg. Cardiac tamponade, tension pneumothorax, and massive hemothorax are life-threatening conditions that require immediate intervention (needle decompression for tension pneumothorax; pericardiocentesis under ECG monitoring, for cardiac tamponade; chest drain for massive hemothorax; exploratory laparotomy for blunt cardiac trauma and great vessel injuries).

DISABILITY—BRIEF NEUROLOGIC EXAMINATION

The preliminary neurologic evaluation includes determination of the patient's level of consciousness (GCS); pupillary size and response; and recognition of paresis/paralysis. Evidence of paraplegia and/or a level of sensory loss on the chest or abdomen are highly suggestive of an unstable T–L spine injury.

EXPOSURE: COMPLETE EXAMINATION

Care should be taken to prevent hypothermia when undressing the patient for a complete evaluation of injuries. In addition, a gastric tube is inserted to reduce stomach distention, decrease the risk of aspiration, and detect an upper gastrointestinal bleed. The urinary bladder is catheterized to assess for hematuria (indicates a retroperitoneal etiology for the blood loss) and monitored for urinary output.

Secondary survey

The secondary survey begins after all life-threatening issues have been resolved and the patient is physiologically stable. Its aim is to evaluate the extent and severity of the spinal and systemic injuries; this includes a comprehensive history, detailed neurologic examination, complete systemic evaluation, and, if indicated, radiologic investigations, arterial blood gas (ABG) measurements, and laboratory studies.

Patients with a neurologic deficit undergo a detailed neurologic examination in the standardized format developed by the American Spinal Injury Association (ASIA).[50] This examination accurately evaluates and scores bilateral strength in 10 muscle groups and sensory testing in 28 dermatomes (for light touch and pinprick discrimination); it also includes an assessment of sacral sparing, to determine completeness of the injury. The severity of injury is graded from A–E, in a progressively decreasing order of severity (ASIA impairment scale). Grade A refers to complete loss of motor and sensory function, whilst ASIA grade E refers to intact motor and sensory function.

Pertinent features in the clinical evaluation, which are highly suggestive of a T–L spine injury, are:

Age 65 years or older and reported pain in the thoracic or lumbosacral spine, after a low impact fall.

High-energy mechanism of injury: high-speed automobile collision; ejection (partial or complete) from a motor vehicle; damage to the vehicle in terms of steering wheel deformation or intrusion onto the passenger's seat (roof: >12 inches/occupant site: >18 inches); rollover motor accident; lap belt restraint only; vehicle telemetry data consistent with high risk of injury; accidents involving motorized recreational vehicles; bicycle collision, horseback riding accidents, auto vs. pedestrian/bicyclist thrown, run over, or with significant (>20 mph) impact; fall from a height (>20 feet/6 meters in adults; 10 feet = 1 story) especially with a landing on feet or buttocks.[1,51]

- Midline or spinal pain (on coughing)
- Abnormal neurologic symptoms (paresthesia or weakness or numbness, urinary retention)
- Abnormal neurologic signs (motor or sensory deficit)
- New deformity or bony midline tenderness

The Eastern Association for the Surgery of Trauma (EAST) has provided evidence-based recommendations regarding the screening of T–L spine injuries in blunt trauma patients.[41] According to these recommendations, an image of the spine or further spine immobilization is not required in patients who are awake, alert, sober, have no complaints of neck or back pain, no tenderness to spine palpation, and no neurologic deficits (Level 2 evidence). T–L spine imaging is definitely indicated if any of the following features are present: back pain or midline tenderness; local signs of T–L spine injury, for example, bruising, neurologic deficits; cervical spine fracture; GCS <15; polytrauma, and alcohol or drug intoxication (level 2 evidence). Conventionally, spine radiographs have been the initial investigation for screening T–L spine injuries; more recently, however, multidetector CT is the preferred modality, if available. If an injury is identified, the entire spine should be screened to rule out other noncontiguous fractures.[41]

ANESTHETIC MANAGEMENT

Preoperative evaluation

The preoperative evaluation provides a comprehensive perspective of the perioperative concerns, and hence, facilitates the formulation of an optimal anesthesia plan. It includes a detailed evaluation of the T–L spine trauma; the proposed surgical procedure, concomitant injuries; systemic manifestations; co-existing morbidities; previous surgeries; and anesthetic exposures; allergies and current medications. Pertinent details regarding the preanesthetic evaluation are listed in Table 12.7.

Anesthesia plan

The anesthesia plan is formulated prior to the surgery and in consensus with the surgeon, on the basis of the information obtained during the initial evaluation (in the ED), and preanesthetic assessment of the patient.

In addition to the standard neuroanesthesia concerns, factors that merit particular attention in patients with acute SCI are: high thoracic complete SCI (spinal shock, autonomic dysfunction, NS, respiratory impairment); grossly unstable/multiple level fractures (careful positioning, prolonged procedures with extensive blood loss); anterior approach/combined approach surgeries (more blood loss, greater morbidity because of the risk of injury to thoracic/abdominal structures, possible need for OLV); coexisting thoracic and abdominal injuries that compromise the hemodynamic stability and pulmonary status; associated head injuries (raised intracranial pressure) and/or cervical spine injuries (airway concerns); complications pertaining to systemic manifestations of acute SCI, eg, risk of hypothermia, VTE, aspiration, pressure sores.

The chief concerns in patients with a chronic SCI are a debilitated general physical state because of anemia, chronic sepsis (recurrent pulmonary, urinary, renal infections) and multisystemic morbidities (involving the pulmonary, musculoskeletal, hemostatic, gastrointestinal, renal, and urinary systems); severe hypertensive episodes due to AH (in patients with high thoracic spine lesions); hypercalcemia; contractures; osteoporosis, and denervation hypersensitivity.

Anesthesia technique

Most surgeries for T-L spine trauma are performed under general anesthesia (GA) and controlled ventilation: monitored anesthesia care may be used occasionally for selected procedures, eg, VB augmentation procedures.

Anesthetic choices

Various inhalational and intravenous anesthetic agents have been used, however, there are no data to support the superiority of any specific technique, particularly in terms of providing neuroprotection or in influencing the surgical outcome. Hence, the anesthetic choices are largely driven by the perioperative requirements, eg, ability to provide an adequate anesthetic depth, amnesia, analgesia, and immobility; maintain hemodynamic stability; facilitate IONM, OVL; and, if indicated, allow a rapid postoperative awakening. Rather than individual drugs, it is more important to focus on providing conditions that maintain SC perfusion and prevent secondary SCI.

Monitoring

In addition to the standard monitoring, (ECG, heart rate, noninvasive BP, SaO_2, end tidal carbon

dioxide [$EtCO_2$], temperature, fluid intake and urine output), monitoring of arterial BP and CVP is highly recommended in patients with a labile cardiovascular status, especially if significant intraoperative blood loss is anticipated. An arterial line enables continuous monitoring of BP and also facilitates measurement of ABG, electrolytes, and glucose levels. The CVP line provides a reliable route for rapid transfusion of fluids, blood, and inotrope/vasopressor infusions; although the CVP may not accurately reflect the true preload in prone-position surgeries, but the CVP trend, over a period of time, provides meaningful inputs for guiding hemodynamic management. Temperature monitoring is important, especially in poikilothermic patients, during long surgeries, and for the correct interpretation of IONM. Monitoring of the depth of neuromuscular block is definitely indicated if MEP monitoring is planned; a depth of anesthesia monitor, for example, Bispectral Index, Patient State Index, enables a more precise titration of the anesthetic agent dosages.

Pre-induction

Acute SCI patients are at risk of profound hypotension during anesthetic induction because of the reduced sympathetic outflow and the concomitant vasodilatory effect of most anesthetic agents; this can be mitigated by obtaining a large bore intravenous access and preloading with 500 to 1000 mL of crystalloids.

The risk of aspiration (delayed gastric time; incompetence of the upper gastric sphincter due to the in situ gastric tube) is decreased by thorough aspiration of the gastric contents and by prophylactic administration of a proton pump inhibitor, eg omeprazole or a histamine 2 blocker, eg, rantidine; routine rapid sequence induction, is usually not performed but may be considered, if required.[36]

Measures for the prevention of hypothermia include use of forced air warming blankets, warm intravenous fluids, closed-circuit anesthesia, and an increase in ambient temperature; however, care should be taken regarding hyperthermia, because the lack of sweating below the level of injury increases the risk of iatrogenic hyperthermia from warming devices. Additionally, sequential mechanical compression devices are applied to lower extremities; a baseline ABG measurement is desirable in patients with respiratory dysfunction.

Table 12.7 Preoperative evaluation for thoracolumbar spine trauma

Patients's Age

Spine injury: Duration (acute, intermediate, chronic); level (high/low thoracic SC, conus medullaris, cauda equina); morphology; severity (complete/incomplete SCI); perceived extent of mechanical/ neurologic instability (ASIA impairment score, TLICS score); review of imaging studies (x-ray, CT scan, MRI)

Cardiovascular assessment: Baseline BP, heart rate, h/o postural hypotension, AH; review of ECG

Respiratory assessment: Respiratory Rate, pattern, chest auscultation; h/o repeated infections, tracheostomy in chronic SCI patients; review of vital capacity; chest radiograph; arterial blood gases

Assessment of associated injuries: Chest, abdomen, head, cervical spine, appendicular skeleton

Airway assessment: Especially associated cervical spine injury

Musculoskeletal system assessment: Pressure sores; contractures (in patients with chronic SCI), osteoporosis; review of metabolic panel

Assessment of aspiration risk: Last meal time (in acute SCI), presence/absence of a gastric tube in situ

Hematologic assessment: Hematocrit, total and differential leukocyte count; coagulation profile

Genitourinary system: h/o Repeated urinary tract infections, pyelonephritis, urinalysis, serum urea and creatinine levels.

VTE assessment: Calf tenderness; Doppler ultrasound of extremities

Basic metabolic panel: Liver function tests (in chronic SCI patients), previous surgeries, anesthetic exposures, preexisting comorbidities, allergies, and current medications (anticoagulants, baclofen, vasoactive drugs)

Assessment of surgical aspects: Surgical approach(anterior/posterior/combined; open/minimally invasive); surgical position, (prone/lateral/supine), intended surgical procedure; number of vertebral levels to be operated upon; significant procedural complications; anticipated surgical duration and blood loss, need for intraoperative neurophysiologic monitoring, postoperative ventilatory assistance, and timing of initiation of pharmacologic prophylaxis for VTE; need for specialist consultation and/or optimization of the patient's medical condition (within limitations of the surgical circumstances)

Abbreviations: AH: Autonomic hyper-reflexia; ASIA: American Spinal Injury Association; BP: blood pressure; CT: Computerized Tomography; ECG: electrocardiogram; h/o: history of; MRI: Magnetic Resonance Imaging; SC: spinal cord; SCI: spinal cord injury; TLICS: Thoracolumbar Injury Classification and Severity Score; VTE: venous thromboembolism.

Induction and maintenance

Anesthetic induction is usually achieved with carefully titrated doses of an intravenous opioid and a sedative–hypnotic drug, eg, propofol, thiopentone; ketamine or etomidate may be used if hemodynamic instability is a concern. A nondepolarizing muscle relaxant, eg, rocuronium, vecuronium, atracurium, facilitates tracheal intubation; succinyl-choline should be avoided between 3 days to 9 months following SCI, because of the potential risk of arrhythmias (severe hyperkalemia due to acute potassium efflux from extra-junctional acetylcholine receptors, following denervation hypersensitivity). A balanced technique is used for maintenance of anesthesia and usually includes opioids and muscle relaxants, in combination with intravenous sedative hypnotic drugs and/or inhalational agents; appropriate modifications are made if IONM is planned.

Perioperative management

Intraoperative measures to prevent further worsening of secondary SCI include optimizing SC perfusion and maintaining physiologic homeostasis by ensuring normal hemodynamic, ventilatory, hematologic, metabolic ,and hemostatic parameters; maintaining euvolemia and normothermia; carefully positioning the patient to avoid further injury to the neural/bony elements; efficiently managing perioperative complications, especially significant blood loss; and facilitating IONM. Use of high-dose methylprednisolone for neuroprotection has not shown any significant long-term benefit, although it may improve the short-term outcome, if given within 8 hours after the SCI; increased gastrointestinal bleeding has been reported with its use, in some observational studies.[29]

HEMODYNAMIC AND VENTILATORY MANAGEMENT

It is crucial to maintain adequate SC perfusion, but since it not feasible to monitor the SC blood flow, the focus is on ensuring normal systemic perfusion and gas exchange. As described in the previous sections, the target is to maintain a MAP of 85 to 90 mmHg and avoid a SBP of <90 mmHg. Furthermore, because CO_2 reactivity is usually normal in SCI, excessive hyperventilation may reduce blood flow to areas with inadequate perfusion; therefore, ventilation is adjusted to maintain normocapnia or mild hypocapnia.

The anesthesiologist should be attentive to all potential causes of cardiorespiratory compromise, including NS, surgical bleeding, and tension pneumothorax. In patients with NS, the loss of sympathetic tone can cause episodes of profound hypotension, and bradycardia or even asystole, especially during tracheal intubation, positioning, or tracheal suctioning. On the other hand, hypertension can increase the SC edema; epinephrine containing local anesthetic solutions should be avoided during skin infiltration due to higher sensitivity to catecholamines.[37] General anesthesia usually attenuates the severity of AH, hence, if it occurs in an anesthetized patient, it is usually brief and self-limiting. Management includes cessation of the stimulus, increasing the depth of anesthesia, and, if required, use of an antihypertensive drug.

A simple or occult pneumothorax is not uncommon in patients with thoracic spine injuries (usually managed conservatively); during GA and positive pressure ventilation, it can transition into tension pneumothorax, and cause sudden, severe, cardiorespiratory instability. It should be suspected if the patient develops acute hypotension in combination with an elevated airway pressure, unilaterally decreased breath sounds, distended neck veins, or a deviated trachea. It is managed by an immediate needle decompression in the second intercostal space, at the anterior axillary line. Both

the detection and management of tension pneumothorax can be rather difficult if the patient is in the prone position; the fifth intercostal space at the midaxillary line can be used as an alternative site for needle aspiration, in this situation; a preoperative thoracostomy might also be considered.[52]

Hyperglycemia is associated with poor neurologic outcomes after SCI and blood glucose >200 mg/dL must be treated aggressively.

FLUID AND BLOOD LOSS MANAGEMENT

Presently, there are no guidelines for optimal perioperative fluid administration in these patients. Typically, crystalloids, eg. normal saline, Ringers Lactate, are used as maintenance fluids; colloids (eg, Hetastarches) are administered to replace plasma deficits that exceed maintenance administration, eg, due to acute blood loss. Hypotonic crystalloids, eg, 5% dextrose in water, 0.45% normal saline, should be avoided as they may exacerbate SC swelling. Fluids should be cautiously administered; while under-transfusion is associated with hypovolemia, hypotension, and impaired SC perfusion, overzealous fluid administration can result in pulmonary edema (especially in patients with NS), and airway edema (in prolonged prone position surgeries).

Significant perioperative blood loss can occur during decompression and stabilization spine surgeries, especially if more than two vertebral levels are affected by the injury; excessive bleeding occurs from the highly vascularized decorticated VBs and the decompressed epidural veins. Appropriate preemptive measures include securing large bore intravenous access; invasive BP and CVP monitoring; serial ABGs with hemograms; careful assessment of blood losses; and prompt replacement of blood products (packed red blood cells, platelets, cryoprecipitate, coagulation factors, and/or fresh frozen plasma). Importantly, simple measures such as avoiding abdominal compression during prone position surgeries can help to decrease perioperative blood losses; relatively minor corrections in positioning on the Wilson frame have been reported to reduce blood loss per vertebral level by approximately 50%.[53]

Several strategies have been used to decrease intraoperative blood loss and transfusion requirements, eg, red blood cell salvage with cell saver, pharmacologic agents, eg, antifibrinolytics, desmopressin, and recombinant factor VII. Current evidence favors the use of antifibrinolytics, eg,

Tranexamic acid (loading dose 10 mg/kg IV, followed by infusion of 1 mg/kg/hr TXA) and epsilon aminocaproic acid (loading dose 100–150 mg/kg, IV infusion 10–15 mg/kg/hr).[54]

Viscoelastic point-of-care coagulation assays, for example, Sonoclot, Thromboelastogram TEG, Rotem, and the newer "Emergency Hemorrhage Panel," enable a rapid assessment of the coagulation system and may be useful for guiding the transfusion strategies in patients with anticipated major intraoperative blood loss.[53,55]

IONM

Intraoperatively, iatrogenic injury to the neural elements can occur for several reasons: surgical causes (excessive distraction/instrumentation resulting in nerve impingement or a decrease in blood supply; vascular injury); physiologic reasons (hypotension, anemia, hypoxia, hypothermia); impaired perfusion or nerve compression in an extremity due to abnormal positioning, edema or extrinsic compression, eg, by a BP cuff. IONM (somatosensory evoked potential [SSEPs], Transcranial MEPs, EMG) provides real time, subcontinuous feedback of the integrity of the SC/nerve roots and can help to decrease the incidence of these complications; it is particularly useful in patients who have a VC injury with a normal preoperative neurologic examination.[56]

SSEPs monitor the posterior cord (ascending sensory pathways) and can detect positioning-related problems; mechanical and physiologic insults. The recordings are obtained continuously throughout the case, (except when electrocautery is required) and signals are averaged with a 5-minute time lag.

Transcranial MEPs monitor the integrity of anterior SC (descending motor pathways) and are useful for detection of hypoperfusion-related cord injury, eg, due to hypotension, anemia, or blood vessel compression (the anterior spinal artery is the primary source of blood supply to these pathways and also of nearly 75% of the SC). However, the recordings are usually limited to above T11, as recordings from lumbar SC are not very reliable. MEPs are recorded intermittently (after each specific event that can compromise the cord integrity), because they require a train stimulation that forces the surgeon to interrupt the surgery for 15 to 30 seconds in order to obtain adequate readings; the results are obtained immediately after stimulation.

Spontaneous EMG records electrical potentials (EP) generated by muscle fibers and provides an immediate feedback of possible injury or irritation of nerve roots during surgery; it is widely used when the surgeon is working around the lumbar nerve roots (cauda equina). Triggered/evoked EMG (in response to active nerve stimulation) is very useful during pedicle screw placement, to reduce the risk of nerve injury due to misplaced pedicle screws; and in cauda equina surgery, to identify nerve roots to anal and urethral sphincters (S2–S4).[56,57]

Individually, these techniques have false-negative as well as false-positive results, however, their combined use significantly improves their sensitivity and specificity; Hence, "multimodality IONM" using SSEP, MEP, and EMG (rectus abdominis EMG) is the preferred approach for thoracic spine surgeries.[57,58] Usually, bilateral changes, especially in tests that use controls (eg, median nerve SSEPs in T–L spine surgery), are suggestive of anesthetic effects or physiologic changes (although they do not exclude the possibility of a surgical etiology); unilateral changes indicate a surgical event.[57]

Total intravenous anesthesia (TIVA) with propofol/dexmedetomidine-opioid infusion provides optimal monitoring conditions for both sensory and motor EP and is preferred over inhalational agents, though sensory recordings can also be obtained with <0.5 MAC (minimum inhalational concentration) doses of inhalational agents, especially if baseline EP waveforms are impaired because of spinal cord/nerve injury. TIVA without a muscle relaxant provides the ideal environment during MEP monitoring; partial NM blockade (of up to 50%), though acceptable, should preferably be avoided in patients with motor deficits. N_2O also suppresses EP (depresses the amplitude), and, therefore, is often excluded during IONM.

Bolus doses of anesthetic agents, hypotension, and hypothermia can confound the interpretation of EPs, and their perturbations should be avoided to eliminate any confusion in the interpretation of data.

OLV

Use of OLV allows a selective collapse of the lung on the operative side (nondependant lung) and facilitates exposure of the ventral spine in the anterior approach, open/MIS surgeries. It requires the use of a lung isolation device, such as a double lumen tube (DLT) or a bronchial blocker; a left-sided DLT is usually preferred. DLT allows rapid collapse and reinflation of either of the lungs and also enables selective application of continuous positive airway pressure (CPAP) to the collapsed lung; however, it is not suitable for postoperative ventilation and should be replaced by a conventional tracheal tube at the end of the surgery. A bronchial blocker is easier to position than DLT; it may be preferred in patients with a difficult airway and also if postoperative ventilation is indicated because it obviates the need for changing the tube at the end of the surgery. These devices tend to become displaced proximally during positioning, hence, it is prudent to reconfirm their final position by fiber-optic bronchoscopy prior to commencement of the surgery. Ventilation during OLV is maintained with low tidal volume (4–6 mL/kg, ideal body weight) and pressure-limited ventilation (plateau pressure <30 cm H_2O), along with the application of 5–10 cm of PEEP (positive end expiratory pressure) to the dependent lung.

Complications during OLV are usually a consequence of a traumatic insertion or improper placement of DLT/bronchial blocker or because of inappropriate management of OLV. Insertion-related injuries can range from minor, self-limiting tracheobronchial trauma, to serious glottic edema, and, rarely, to tracheal laceration and bronchial rupture. The selection of the appropriately sized lung isolation device and bronchoscopic confirmation of its final position, limiting cuff inflation and avoidance of N_2O, help to decrease the likelihood of these injuries. Malpositioning of the lung isolation device should be suspected if there is a sudden increase in peak inspiratory airway pressures despite the use of low tidal volumes for ventilation; it usually occurs because of proximal displacement of the bronchial cuff, blocker balloon, or the device itself into the trachea. In this situation, the cuff or the balloon is deflated, ventilation of both lungs is reestablished, and a fiber-optic evaluation is performed to reposition the device. Hypoxemia (SpO_2 <90%, with FiO_2 >0.5) can occur for various reasons—obstruction of the upper lobe of the ventilated lung (a malpositioned lung isolation device); transpulmonary shunting (perfusion of the collapsed, nonventilated lung); compression atelectasis of the dependent lung (downward movement of the mediastinal structures and upward displacement of the diaphragm by abdominal contents); or rarely, because of tension pneumothorax in the dependent ventilated hemithorax.[59] Management includes increasing the FiO_2, repositioning the device under fiber-optic guidance,

and improving the dependent lung ventilation (suctioning of secretions, increasing PEEP, performing lung recruitment maneuvers); simultaneously, possible causative factors are also explored. If the hypoxemia still persists, the surgeon should be informed and temporary ventilation of both lungs should be instituted.[59] Finally, serious thoracic injuries preclude the use of OLV.

Considerations for MIS

VB AUGMENTATION: KYPHOPLASTY, VERTEBROPLASTY

These procedures are performed under fluoroscopic guidance; the patient is placed in the prone position, with gentle hyperextension of the trunk (to help restore the anterior VB height). While monitored anesthesia care can be used, the patient may be uncomfortable in the prone position, which often necessitates a deeper level of sedation, which may cause respiratory depression and deterioration of an already-compromised pulmonary function; hence, GA is probably a safer option.

Since these are short, percutaneous procedures, standard monitoring and short-acting anesthetic agents are used in most cases; invasive BP may be monitored in patients with cardiorespiratory morbidities. Particular attention is given to proper positioning and liberal padding; rib fractures and skin lacerations due to improper positioning have also been reported. Hemodynamic stimulation can occur during injection of cement or inflation of the kyphoplasty balloon and is treated by titrating the anesthetic agent and opioid accordingly. Improper positioning of the needle or working cannula in the VB can result in severe complications, such as inadvertent vascular or cardiac dissection; neural injury; nerve compression; and paraplegia due to leakage of cement to the disc area. The most dreaded complication is intravascular injection of cement; an anaphylactic reaction, pulmonary embolism, severe hemodynamic instability, and even cardiovascular collapse can occur as a consequence. In this situation, the procedure is discontinued, the patient is turned supine, and prompt resuscitative measures are initiated.

VATS, MASS

These are performed with the patient placed in the lateral decubitus position; OLV is required for deflation of the nondependent lung; a chest tube is inserted postoperatively. N_2O should preferably be avoided if prolonged OLV is anticipated. Invasive monitoring and an arrangement of adequate blood products is recommended. Although considered to be minimally invasive, these techniques should not be considered equal in terms of lower perioperative risk. The average times for VATS and MASS are 224.5 ± 68.6 minutes, and 183.5 ± 33.2 minutes, respectively.[60] The median average estimated blood loss has been reported to be 585 mL (range: 310–1117 mL) with VATS, and 423 mL (range: 290–912 mL) with MASS.[60]

Perioperatively, the anesthesiologist should pay close attention to the procedural steps. Major hemodynamic perturbations can occur due to displacement of the major vessels and heart during the procedure; inadvertent damage to these structures can be disastrous and may necessitate a rapid conversion to an open thoracotomy. Other complications include pneumonia, pneumothorax, thromboembolism, Horner's syndrome, and intercostal neuralgia.[60]

Postoperative management

TRACHEAL EXTUBATION

The decision to extubate the trachea at the end of surgery is based on the preoperative status and the intraoperative course of the patient. Preoperative factors include: the spinal level and completeness of injury; respiratory status of the patient (preoperative baseline ABG, vital capacity); ability to generate an effective cough; presence of chest trauma and other significant concomitant injuries; extent of preexisting comorbidities; and a potentially difficult airway. Intraoperatively, duration and invasiveness of the surgery need to be considered; surgical approach and position; amount of intraoperative blood loss; and the perioperative hemodynamic status influence the timing of tracheal extubation.

In uncomplicated cases, tracheal extubation can be safely performed immediately after the surgery, as soon as the patient is conscious and demonstrates a purposeful response, adequate spontaneous respiratory efforts, muscle strength, and airway reflexes. On the other hand, it may be prudent to electively delay tracheal extubation in the following situations: poor preoperative status; difficult airway, turbulent intraoperative course (eg, significant blood loss, hemodynamic instability), major pulmonary insult after a thoracotomy; combined approach surgery; and/or due to airway edema after a prolonged

(>8 hours), multilevel surgery in the prone position (macroglossia, facial swelling, laryngeal and pharyngeal edema, especially if large volumes of fluid or blood have been transfused).[61,62] Fentanyl/midazolam or propofol/dexmedetomidine infusion can be used to provide sedation during this period.

Postoperative pain relief

Multimodal analgesia, using a combination of simple primary analgesics, opioids, and epidural analgesia, is recommended for postoperative pain relief. Commonly used parenteral drugs include opioids, acetaminophen, nonsteroidal anti-inflammatory drug (NSAIDs), and analgesic doses of ketamine, dexmedetomidine, clonidine, dexamethasone, gabapentin, and pregabalin. Epidural analgesia (single injection/continuous infusion by an epidural catheter) with opioids (morphine, fentanyl, sufentanyl, remifentanyl), provides superior pain relief with less opioid consumption and better patient satisfaction compared with parenteral drugs; the epidural catheter can be inserted by the surgeon at the end of the procedure. Epidural administration of local anesthetics (bupivacaine, ropivacaine) is controversial because it can potentially mask early symptoms of a spinal hematoma. A patient-controlled device can be used for both intravenous and epidural routes, to provide patient-controlled analgesia.

REFERENCES

1. American College of Surgeons Committee on Trauma. *Advanced Trauma Life Support. Manual*, 9th ed. Chicago, IL; 2012.
2. Wang H, Zhang Y, Xiang Q et al. Epidemiology of traumatic spinal fractures: Experience from medical university-affiliated hospitals in Chongqing, China, 2001-2010. *J Neurosurg Spine*. 2012;17(5):459-468.
3. Wang H, Liu X, Zhao Y et al. Incidence and pattern of traumatic spinal fractures and associated spinal cord injury resulting from motor vehicle collisions in China over 11 years: An observational study. *Medicine (Baltimore)*. 2016;95(43):(e5220).
4. Hu R, Mustard CA, Burns C. Epidemiology of incident spinal fracture in a complete population. *Spine (Phila Pa 1976)*. 1996;21(4):492-499.

5. Gertzbein SD. Scoliosis Research Society. Multicenter spine fracture study. *Spine (Phila Pa 1976)*. 1992;17(5):528-540.

6. Katsuura Y, Osborn JM, Cason GW. The epidemiology of thoracolumbar trauma: A meta-analysis. *J Orthop*. 2016;13(4):383-388.

7. Rajasekaran S, Kanna RM, Shetty AP. Management of thoracolumbar spine trauma: An overview. *Indian J Orthop*. 2015;49(1):72-82.

8. Kim BG, Dan JM, Shin DE. Treatment of thoracolumbar fracture. *Asian Spine J*. 2015;9 (1):133-146.

9. Hsu JM, Joseph T, Ellis AM. Thoracolumbar fracture in blunt trauma patients: Guidelines for diagnosis and imaging. *Injury*. 2003;34 (6):426-433.

10. Janicki R, Vaccaro AR, Kwon BK. Thoracolumbar trauma. In: Win HR ed. *Youmans Neurological Surgery*. 6th ed. Philadelphia, PA: Elsevier Saunders; 2011:3233-3249.

11. Marchan EM, Ghobrial GM, Harrop JS. Thoracolumbar spine fractures. In: Ellenbogen RG, Abdulrauf SI, Sekhar LN, eds. *Principles of Neurosurgery*. 3rd ed. Philadelphia, PA: Elsevier Saunders; 2012:413-420.

12. Saboe LA, Reid DC, Davis LA, Warren SA, Grace MG. Spine trauma and associated injuries. *J Trauma*. 1991;31(1):43-48.

13. Wood KB, Li W, Lebl DR, Ploumis A. Management of thoracolumbar spine fractures. *Spine J*. 2014;14(1):145-164.

14. Stevens RD, Bhardwaj A, Kirsch JR, Mirski MA. Critical care and perioperative management in traumatic spinal cord injury. *J Neurosurg Anesthesiol*. 2003;15(3):215-229.

15. Charles YP, Steib JP. Management of thoracolumbar spine fractures with neurologic disorder. *Orthop Traumatol Surg Res*. 2015;101(suppl 1):S31-S40.

16. White AA 3rd, Panjabi MM. The basic kinematics of the human spine. A review of past and current knowledge. *Spine (Phila Pa 1976)*. 1978;3(1):12-20.

17. Khurana B, Sheehan SE, Sodickson A, Bono CM, Harris MB. Traumatic thoracolumbar spine injuries: What the spine surgeon wants to know. *Radiographics*. 2013;33(7): 2031-2046.

18. Holdsworth F. Fractures, dislocations, and fracture-dislocations of the spine. *J Bone Joint Surg Am*. 1970;52(8):1534-1551.

19. Denis F. The three column spine and its significance in the classification of acute thoracolumbar spinal injuries. *Spine*. 1983;8(8):817-831.

20. McAfee PC, Yuan HA, Fredrickson BE, Lubicky JP. The value of computed tomography in thoracolumbar fractures. An analysis of one hundred consecutive cases and a new classification. *J Bone Joint Surg Am*. 1983;65 (4):461-473.

21. Magerl F, Aebi M, Gertzbein SD, Harms J, Nazarian S. A comprehensive classification of thoracic and lumbar injuries. *Eur Spine J*. 1994;3(4):184-201.

22. Vaccaro AR, Lehman RA Jr, Hurlbert RJ et al. A new classification of thoracolumbar injuries: The importance of injury morphology, the integrity of the posterior ligamentous complex, and neurologic status. *Spine (Phila Pa 1976)*. 2005;30(20):2325-2333.

23. Lee JY, Vaccaro AR, Lim MR et al. Thoracolumbar injury classification and severity score: A new paradigm for the treatment of thoracolumbar spine trauma. *J Orthop Sci*. 2005;10(6):671-675.

24. Rihn JA, Anderson DT, Harris E et al. A review of the TLICS system: A novel, userfriendly thoracolumbar trauma classification system. *Acta Orthop*. 2008;79(4):461-466.

25. Kim YH, Ha KY, Kim SI. Spinal cord injury and related clinical trials. *Clin Orthop Surg*. 2017;9(1):1-9.

26. Hurlbert RJ, Hadley MN, Walters BC et al. Pharmacological therapy for acute spinal cord injury. *Neurosurgery*. 2013;72(suppl 2):93-105.

27. Fehlings MG, Wilson JR, Cho N. Methylprednisolone for the treatment of acute spinal cord injury: Counterpoint. *Neurosurgery*. 2014;61(suppl 1):36-42.

28. Hansebout RR, Hansebout CR. Local cooling for traumatic spinal cord injury: Outcomes in 20 patients and review of the literature. *J Neurosurgery Spine*. 2014;20(5):550-561.

29. Evaniew N, Belley-Côté EP, Fallah N, Noonan VK, Rivers CS, Dvorak MF. Methylprednisolone for the treatment of patients with acute spinal cord injuries: A systematic review and meta-analysis. *J Neurotrauma*. 2016;33(5):468-481.

30. Ditunno JF, Little JW, Tessler A, Burns AS. Spinal shock revisited: A four-phase model. *Spinal Cord*. 2004;42(7):383-395.

31. Lindan R, Joiner E, Freehafer AA, Hazel C. Incidence and clinical features of autonomic dysreflexia in patients with spinal cord injury. *Paraplegia.* 1980;18(5):285-292.

32. Wilmot CB, Cope DN, Hall KM, Acker M. Occult head injury: Its incidence in spinal cord injury. *Arch Phys Med Rehabil.* 1985;66(4):227-231.

33. Ryken TC, Hurlbert RJ, Hadley MN et al. The acute cardiopulmonary management of patients with cervical spinal cord injuries. *Neurosurgery.* 2013;72(suppl 2):84-92.

34. Hawryluk G, Whetstone W, Saigal R et al. Mean arterial blood pressure correlates with neurological recovery after human spinal cord injury: Analysis of high frequency physiologic data. *J Neurotrauma.* 2015;32(24):1958-1967.

35. Veale P, Lamb J. Anaesthesia and acute spinal cord injury. *Br J Anaesthesia (CEPD Reviews).* 2002;2(5):139-143.

36. Bonner S, Smith C. Initial management of acute spinal cord injury. *Cont Ed Anaesth, Crit Care Pain.* 2013;13(6):224-231.

37. GS Umamaheswara Rao. Anaesthetic and intensive care management of traumatic cervical spine injury. *Indian Journal of Anaesthesia.* 2008;52(1):13-22.

38. Dhall SS, Hadley MN, Aarabi B et al. Deep venous thrombosis and thromboembolism in patients with cervical spinal cord injuries. *Neurosurgery.* 2013;72(suppl 2):244-254.

39. Gordon, RJ, Lombard FW. Perioperative venous thromboembolism: A review. *Anesth Analg.* 2017;125(2):403-412.

40. Mollinger LA, Spurr GB, el Ghatit AZ et al. Daily energy expenditure and basal metabolic rates of patients with spinal cord injury. *Arch Phys Med Rehabil.* 1985;66(7):420-426.

41. Sixta S, Moore FO, Ditillo MF et al. Screening for thoracolumbar spinal injuries in blunt trauma: An Eastern Association for the Surgery of Trauma practice management guideline. *J Trauma Acute Care Surg.* 2012;73(5 suppl 4):S326-S332.

42. Pizones J, Zúñiga L, Sánchez-Mariscal F, Alvarez P, Gómez-Rice A, Izquierdo E. MRI study of post-traumatic incompetence of posterior ligamentous complex: Importance of the supraspinous ligament. Prospective study of 74 traumatic fractures. *Eur Spine J.* 2012;21(11):2222–2231.

43. La Rosa G, Conti A, Cardali S, Cacciola F, Tomasello F. Does early decompression improve neurological outcome of spinal cord injured patients? Appraisal of the literature using a meta-analytical approach. *Spinal Cord.* 2004;42(9):503-512.

44. Liu JM, Long XH, Zhou Y, Peng HW, Liu ZL, Huang SH. Is urgent decompression superior to delayed surgery for traumatic spinal cord injury? A meta-analysis. *World Neurosurg.* 2016;87:124-131.

45. NarainAS, Hijji FY, Yom KH. Kudaravalli KT, Singh K. The role of minimally invasive techniques in the treatment of thoracolumbar trauma. *J Orthop Spine Trauma.* 2016;2(3):e10129.

46. Smith WD, Dakwar E, Le TV, Christian G, Serrano S, Uribe JS. Minimally invasive surgery for traumatic spinal pathologies: A mini-open, lateral approach in the thoracic and lumbar spine. *Spine (Phila Pa 1976).* 2010;35(26 suppl):S338–S346.

47. Marco RA, Kushwaha VP. Thoracolumbar burst fractures treated with posterior decompression and pedicle screw instrumentation supplemented with balloon-assisted vertebroplasty and calcium phosphate reconstruction. *J Bone Joint Surg Am.* 2009;91(1): 20-28.

48. Rozet I, Vavilala MS. Risks and benefits of patient positioning during neurosurgical care. *Anesthesiol Clin.* 2007;25(3):631-653.

49. Dai LY, Yao WF, Cui YM, Zhou Q. Thoracolumbar fractures in patients with multiple injuries: Diagnosis and treatment—A review of 147 cases. *J Trauma.* 2004;56(2):348-355.

50. Maynard FM, Jr., Bracken MB, Creasey G et al. International standards for neurological and functional classification of spinal cord injury. American Spinal Injury Association. *Spinal Cord.* 1997;35(5):266-274.

51. National Institute for Health and Care Excellence. Spinal injury: Assessment and initial management. Accessed February 2016. Available from: https://www.nice.org.uk

52. Rankin D, Mathew PS, Kurnutala LN, Soghomonyan S, Bergese SD. Tension pneumothorax during surgery for thoracic spine stabilization in prone position: A case report and review of literature. *J Investig Med High Impact Case Rep.* 2014;2(2):2324709614537233.

53. Dooney N, Dagal A. Anesthetic considerations in acute spinal cord trauma. *Int J Crit Illn Inj Sci.* 2011;1(1):36-43.

54. Egafy H, Bransford RJ, McGurie RA, Fischer D. Blood loss in major spine surgery: Are there effective measures to decrease massive hemorrhage in major spine fusion surgery? *Spine (Phila Pa 1976).* 2010;35(9):S47-S56.

55. Chandler WL, Ferrell C, Trimble S, Moody S. Development of a rapid emergency hemorrhage panel. *Transfusion.* 2010;50(12):2547-2552.

56. Park JH, Hyun SJ. Intraoperative neurophysiological monitoring in spinal surgery. *World J Clin Cases.* 2015;3(9):765-773.

57. Pajewski TN, Arlet V, Phillips LH. Current approach on spinal cord monitoring: The point of view of the neurologist, the anesthesiologist and the spine surgeon. *Eur Spine J.* 2007;16(suppl 2):S115-S129.

58. Gonzalez AA, Jeyanandarajan D, Hansen C, Zada G, Hsieh PC. Intraoperative neurophysiological monitoring during spine surgery: A review. *Neurosurg Focus.* 2009;27(4):E6.

59. Karzai W, Schwarzkopf K. Hypoxemia during one-lung ventilation: Prediction, prevention, and treatment. *Anesthesiology.* 2009;110 (6):1402-1411.

60. Lee CY, Wu MH, Li YY, Cheng CC, Lee CY, Huang TJ. Video-assisted thoracoscopic surgery and minimal access spinal surgery compared in anterior thoracic or thoracolumbar junctional spinal reconstruction: A case-control study and review of the literature. *BioMed Res Int.* 2016;2016:6808507.

61. Anastasian ZH, Gaudet JG, Levitt LC, Mergeche JL, Heyer EJ, Berman MF. Factors that correlate with the decision to delay extubation after multilevel prone spine surgery. *J Neurosurg Anesthesiol.* 2014;26 (2):167-171.

62. Li F, Gorji R, Tallarico R, Dodds C, Modes K, Mangat S, Yang ZJ. Risk factors for delayed extubation in thoracic and lumbar spine surgery: A retrospective analysis of 135 patients. *J Anesth.* 2014;28(2):161-166.

PART VI

Neuromonitoring

13

Monitoring in neurotrauma

FREDERICK A. ZEILER AND MAREK CZOSNYKA

INTRODUCTION

The management of moderate to severe traumatic brain injury (TBI) within the intensive care unit (ICU) is a complex task. Patient outcome is dependent on various factors, including: pre-hospital hemodynamic events, intracranial and extra-cranial injury burden, admission neurologic exam, secondary brain insults during ICU stay, development of complications and access to appropriate rehabilitation services.[1-3] Outcome models have been developed, in order to aid in the accuracy of clinician's ability to predict an individual patient's potential outcome,[1-3] with the International Mission on Prognosis and Analysis of Clinical Trials (IMPACT) model being one of the most widely referenced.[2] Despite these models, we are still left with area under the receiver operating curve (AUC) of up to ~0.80 in outcome prediction, taking into account various clinical and physiologic features of a given patient.[2,3] Thus, further work is required in order to improve on our understanding of cerebral pathophysiology post-TBI and our ability to predict patient outcome.

Imaging has played an important role in our ability to quantify injury burden. However, various intermittent imaging-based techniques for the assessment of cerebral physiology have been described with in TBI as a means of "monitoring."[4] To date, the application of computed tomography (CT), CT perfusion (CTP), Xenon enhanced CT (Xe-CT), positron emission tomography (PET), magnetic resonance imaging (MRI), and magnetic resonance angiography (MRA) have all been described within the TBI population.[4,5] Depending on the imaging modality employed, comments on CBF, cerebral blood volume (CBV), perfusion and cerebral metabolism may be made. There are, however, issues with these intermittent radiologic-based monitoring methods, including: time for data acquisition, transport of critically ill patients to scanners, post-acquisition processing of data, need for the manipulation of physiology during testing, potential need for contrast and radiotracers, and poor temporal resolution (ie, we only get a "snap-shot" of cerebral physiology, not continuous data).[4,5]

Thus, in an attempt to avoid the above limitations of intermittent radiologic "monitoring" techniques, continuous monitoring has been developed and employed within the ICU.[6-8] The goal of continuous monitoring of various aspects of cerebral physiology is to improve upon the prediction of secondary brain insults and implement therapies which may impact patient outcome.

To date, many institutions continuously monitor various aspects of cerebral and systemic physiology during a patient's ICU stay. Most commonly quoted physiologic variables monitored include: intracranial pressure (ICP), mean arterial pressure (MAP), and cerebral perfusion pressure (CPP). More recently, there has been a rapid expansion of multi-modal monitoring (MMM) techniques within TBI. In particular, we have seen the expansion of continuous and intermittent monitoring within the ICU to include: CPP optimum (CPPopt), brain oxygen status, cerebral autoregulation (CA), cerebrovascular reactivity (CVR), cerebral blood flow (CBF), cerebral microdialysis (CMD), autonomic monitoring, brain temperature (BT).[6-8] Many of these MMM devices have recently received support from international consensus statements on monitoring in TBI.[7,8]

Given the large number of potential modalities for cerebral monitoring in TBI, it can be difficult for the treating clinician to identify how to monitor various aspects of cerebral physiology, how this data is acquired, and the current data supporting its use. The goal of this chapter is to focus on MMM of the following physiologic variables in TBI: ICP, CPP, brain oxygenation, CA, CVR, CBF, cerebral metabolism, autonomic function, and brain temperature. Within, we outline the various techniques employed in the measurement of these physiologic variables (with a focus on continuous monitoring), commenting on advantages and disadvantages, and briefly outlining some of the supporting literature. A discussion of cerebrospinal fluid (CSF) or serum-based protein biomarkers is beyond the scope of this chapter, though it may be considered a form of "monitoring" in neurotrauma. Finally, we briefly touch on the potential future of MMM, including: integration of MMM in treatment, assessing signal-based entropy/stability of individual systems, and the use of computer modeling in order to classify patients and potentially predict "states."

MONITORED PHYSIOLOGIC VARIABLES IN TBI

Intracranial pressure (ICP)

INVASIVE ICP MONITORING

ICP monitoring was first described in 1783.[9] Clinically, it was initially adopted for the purpose of postoperative neurosurgical monitoring of cranial pressure during the era where CT and MRI were not available. The idea of monitoring cranial pressure focused on the notion that a dramatic increase within the postoperative period could potentially signal the accumulation of either an extra-axial or intra-axial hematoma, warranting early exploration. The application of ICP monitoring quickly expanded to routine monitoring in those with critical neurosurgical pathology,[10,11] in which a patient's neurological examination was poor or obscured secondary to pharmacologic interventions.

To date, invasive ICP monitoring is the mainstay of monitoring in TBI patients within the ICU. Since guidelines for the insertion of invasive ICP monitors have been suggested, with the Brain Trauma Foundation (BTF) guidelines as the most referenced example.[12] In general, a TBI patient with a poor neurological exam, abnormal CT of the brain and risk factors for secondary injury should be monitored. Many publications exist supporting the association between elevated ICP, and duration of ICP elevation, with poor patient outcome. Currently, both the BTF guidelines and MMM consensus statements support the use of invasive ICP monitoring in the care of TBI patients within the ICU.[7,8,12] The current thresholds for treatment of ICP is 22 mmHg, as suggested by the BTF guidelines.[12] This is based off of sequential chi-square analysis of ICP and various binary outcomes.[13]

It must be acknowledged, however, that despite a large body of evidence supporting the use of invasive ICP monitoring in TBI and treatment of elevated ICP,[7,8] there is some data to suggest that it may not make as dramatic of an impact on patient outcome as we think.[14] The Benchmark Evidence from South American Trials: Treatment of Intracranial Pressure (BEST-TRIP) trial is the best example of this, with randomized control trial evidence displaying no difference in outcome between ICP monitoring based ICP therapy compared to CT-based ICP qualitative ICP estimation followed by empiric treatment.[14] Critics say that the trial was underpowered and the measure of ICP as end-hour instant value was rather archaic and imprecise in an era of computer-supported monitoring. Despite the results of this trial, most modern ICUs and neurointensive care units (NICUs) employ invasive ICP monitoring as the standard of care for the monitoring of TBI patients in the ICU setting[15] (see examples in Figure 13.1).

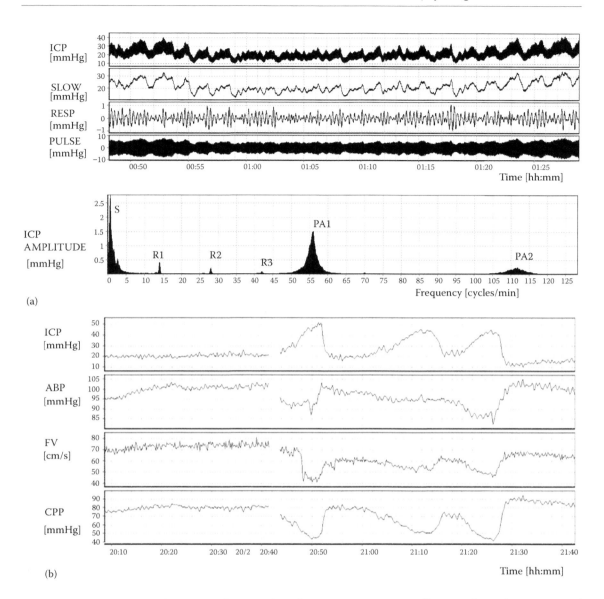

Figure 13.1 ICP is more than a number. In clinical practice we can usually record regular waves and irregular transients: (a) Regular waves of ICP. Upper panels show a recording of: unfiltered ICP waveform (ICP), filtered slow waves of ICP (SLOW) of frequency from 0.005 Hz to 0.05 Hz, respiratory wave-RESP (typically 12 to 25 breaths per minute in adults), and pulse wave of heart frequency and further harmonics-PULSE (meaningful up to sixth harmonics). In frequency domain (bottom panel), all components are separated along frequency axis (x): S—Slow waves. R1,R2,R3—fundamental and upper harmonics of respiratory waves. P1 and P2—fundamental and second harmonic of pulse wave. Of notice is a modulation of respiratory and pulse wave by SLOW component. (b) Example of three plateau waves of ICP. They are rather episodic transients, related to intrinsic maximal cerebral vasodilation. During plateau waves arterial pressure (ABP) changes minimally or does not change at all. Cerebral perfusion pressure (CPP) decreases always, and cerebral blood flow (here monitored as blood flow velocity [FV] with transcranial Doppler ultrasonography) also decreases. Plateau waves resolve spontaneously or to response to vasoconstrictory stimuli like hyperventilation or increase in ABP. (*Continued*)

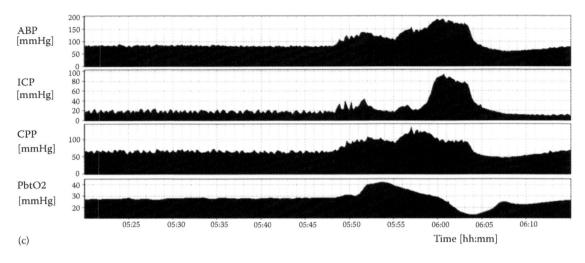

(c)

Time [hh:mm]

Figure 13.1 (Continued) ICP is more than a number. In clinical practice we can usually record regular waves and irregular transients: (c) Transients of ICP related to variation of arterial blood pressure. Two step-raises of ABP. Second raise, when upper limit of autoregulation was breached, resulted with increase in ICP and a decrease in brain tissue oxygenation (PbtO2).

Currently, invasive ICP monitoring is based on the measurement of either fluid or tissue pressure within the cranial cavity. Various catheters/monitors exist for the invasive assessment of ICP.[16] The most commonly utilized catheters/monitors include: (A) external ventricular drains (EVD), (B) strain gauge monitors, and (C) fiber-optic-based pressure sensors. Both the strain gauge and fiber-optic monitors can theoretically be placed anywhere within the cranial cavity, registering the pressure of that compartment. An EVD requires placement into the ventricular system, and thus involves a slightly higher degree of technical aptitude for placement. Complication rates are relatively low. A summary of common invasive ICP monitoring devices, with advantages/disadvantages, can be seen in Table 13.1.

NONINVASIVE ICP MONITORING

The noninvasive measurement of ICP has been a long-desired tool in the assessment of TBI patients. Given the invasive nature of standard ICP monitoring, and the requirement for specialized neurosurgical services for placement of these monitors, the objective measurement of ICP is limited to those centers with these services. However, there have been attempts to correlate noninvasive physiologic measures with ICP. To date, numerous physiologic measures have been compared to ICP, all resulting in relatively poor reliability for

accurate ICP estimation.[17,18] Thus, we will not get into too much detail regarding all of the noninvasive methods, and only focus on two: (A) optic nerve sheath diameter (ONSD) ultrasound, and (B) transcranial Doppler (TCD)-based methods.

ONSD

Ultrasound of the ONSD functions on the premise that the intracranial subarachnoid space communicates directly with the subarachnoid space surrounding the optic nerve.[19] Furthermore, any changes in intracranial pressure lead to direct changes in pressure within the optic nerve sheath. These pressure changes theoretically lead to a proportional change in the optic nerve sheath diameter, via stretching of the dural-based sheath. It is thought that measurement of the diameter of this sheath would correlate to ICP. Hence, given the availability of ultrasound in most emergency departments and ICUs, the application of ultrasound for this measurement has been recommended.[20]

There are some issues: (A) an individual's baseline non-pathologic ONSD varies from person to person, (B) to validate to the ONSD measurement with ICP we require invasive ICP monitoring, (C) the technique of ONSD ultrasound is operator dependent, and (D) large spikes in ICP may lead to irreversible stretching of the ONSD, not allowing it to return to "normal" even during resolution of elevated ICP episodes. Various studies suggest a

Table 13.1 Common invasive ICP monitoring devices and methods: Advantages/disadvantages

Invasive ICP monitoring device	Location of placement	Method of pressure assessment	Advantages	Disadvantages
Strain gauge	Parenchymal/CSF compartments/ subdural space	Piezoelectric strain gauge. Bending within the sensor related to ICP changes electrical resistance. This can be used to approximate ICP.	A. Ease of insertion relative to other invasive monitors. B. Can manipulate the wire without damaging the sensor.	A. Risk of hemorrhage B. Risk of infection C. Zero drift over lengthy recording periods significant D. Cannot re-zero once inserted
Fiber optic	Parenchymal	Light is continuously transmitted through fiber optics to the probe tip. ICP changes lead to the deflection of a mirror in the tip, leading to varying light intensity reflected. This is used to approximate ICP.	A. Ease of insertion relative to an EVD	A. Risk of hemorrhage B. Risk of infection C. Zero drift quite significant D. Cannot re-zero once inserted E. Fiber optics prone to damage with twisting/knotting
External ventricular drain (EVD)	Ventricular CSF compartment	Fluid pressure. Assessed with manometer or pressure transducer. Zero is typically at level of the foramen of Monro.	A. "Gold Standard" for ICP monitoring B. Can re-zero monitor in situ at any time C. Can be used for CSF sampling D. Can be used for therapeutic means during ICP treatment	A. Technique for insertion more demanding B. Risk of hemorrhage C. Risk of infection (though can mitigate with anti-microbial impregnated catheters)

Abbreviations: CSF: Cerebrospinal fluid; EVD: external ventricular drain; ICP: intracranial pressure.

"normal" range, based on patients with TBI, but normal ICP.[20,21] This is probably not the most accurate estimation of normal. Others have looked at ONSD in healthy volunteer populations, without invasive ICP to corroborate their findings.[22] Thus, "normal" values are not clear currently. Most quote a cutoff of ~5 mm or less for normal ONSD, with values above being pathologic. Some have quoted differences between males and females.[22] Furthermore, the learning curve associated with the ONSD ultrasound technique is of importance, with substantial between and within subject variability documented in novice operators.[23]

TCD-based measures

The use of TCD for the estimation of ICP has been described. Various techniques using TCD have been described. Three main methods have been outlined within the literature: (A) pulsatility index (PI)-based, (B) CPP estimation-based, and

(C) mathematical modeling methods.[18] To date, all have displayed varied reliability in ICP estimation in comparison with the gold standard invasive monitoring. Further investigation of this technique is required, prior to widespread application as a reliable method of noninvasive ICP.

CEREBRAL PERFUSION PRESSURE (CPP)

CPP, derived by the following relationship: CPP = MAP − ICP, is believed to represent the driving pressure for CBF. Numerous studies to date have highlighted the important association between CPP and patient outcome after TBI. The thought is that low CPP yields low CBF, which in the setting of TBI can lead to the deprivation of oxygen/nutrients to tissue, placing the parenchyma at risk for subsequent ischemia and potentially infarction.[24]

The gold standard of CPP measurement involves both invasive arterial blood pressure (ABP) and ICP recording, with CPP derived from the difference between MAP and ICP.[7,8,12] Various thresholds of CPP have been linked to poor outcome post-TBI. The recent version of the BTF guidelines highlights the main studies published to date.[12] Within the BTF guidelines, it is currently recommended that CPP be maintained between 60 and 70 mmHg.[12] Some literature suggests a threshold of 70 mmHg,

with those patients spending more time below 70 mmHg displaying worse outcomes.[13] Values below this range have been linked to worse clinical outcome, likely secondary to reduced CBF, cerebral ischemia, and potentially infarction. Values above this range have also been linked to poor clinical outcome, secondary to elevated precapillary arteriolar pressure, capillary bed filtration pressures, and cerebral edema. Furthermore, CPP values persistently above 70 mmHg have been linked to acute respiratory distress syndrome (ARDS) and subsequent poor outcomes.[12]

Noninvasive CPP estimation primarily stems from the application of TCD and TCD-based CPP measures.[18] Based on the inverse relationship between TCD PI and CPP, CPP can be estimated using TCD-based cerebral blood flow velocity (CBFV), as measured from the middle cerebral artery (MCA)[18,25] (see for example, Figure 13.2). Using continuous noninvasive blood pressure (NIBP) measurements, typically with fingertip-based cuffs, one could also derive CPP noninvasively using a noninvasive ICP measure, assuming reliability of the ICP measurement technique. To date, however, noninvasive CPP is still considered experimental, with much further work required to prove accuracy and reliability.[17,18]

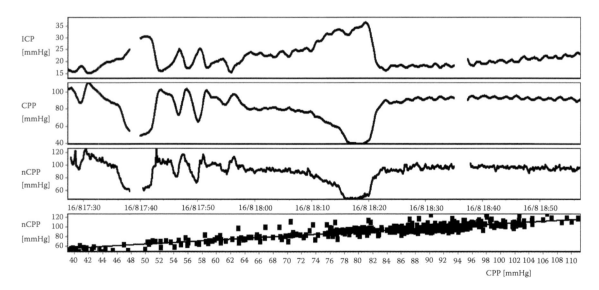

Figure 13.2 Example of TCD-based noninvasive monitoring of cerebral perfusion pressure (CPP). In this case, ICP was unstable, causing variations of CPP. Noninvasive estimator of CPP (nCPP) showed changes very well correlated with CPP (R = 0.903).

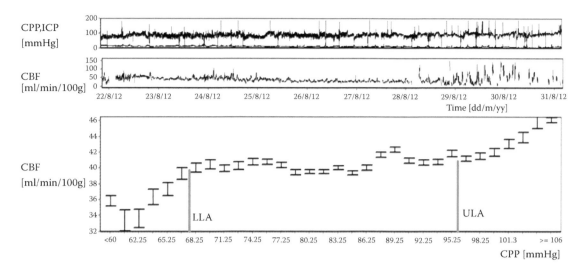

Figure 13.3 Relationship between ICP, CPP, and thermodilution CBF during 9 days monitoring after TBI. Even if time trends are not so obvious, plotting CBF versus CPP shows convergent Lassen autoregulatory curve with lower (LLA) und upper (ULA) thresholds of autoregulation clearly delineated.

CEREBRAL AUTOREGULATION (CA) MEASUREMENT

CA is defined as the brain's ability to maintain a relatively constant CBF over a wide range of systemic MAP. This initial description of CA was done by Lassen in 1959.[26] This work has formed the foundation for all further literature on the topic of CA, whether continuously or intermittently measured. Lassen defined normal CA to range between 50 mmHg (the lower limit of autoregulation) and 150 mmHg (the upper limit of autoregulation) of mean systemic arterial pressure,[26] or cerebral perfusion pressure—see the example in Figure 13.3. MAP values outside of this range lead to cerebral ischemia/infarction, in the case of being below the lower limit, or hyperperfusion/cerebral edema, in the case of MAP values above the upper limit.[24] This normal range for CA can be impacted by various chronic disease states, shifting the curve to the right or left, or even narrowing the normal CA range. The following subsections focus on different methods of CA measurement.

INVASIVE CONTINUOUS CA MEASURES

Most invasive and noninvasive continuous CA measures are derived from the same underlying concept of signal analysis within the time domain. Moving Pearson correlation coefficients are calculated between a surrogate measure of pulsatile CBV

or CBFV, such as ICP or TCD-based CBFV, and slow responses in the driving pressure for CBF, such as MAP or CPP.[6] These indices are typically calculated over a 5-minute window, utilizing 30 consecutive 10 second averaged values for the physiologic variables. The index calculations are then updated every minute. Variation in window length and update frequency have been described within the literature. The value for these indices range from −1 to +1; with negative values potentially indicating intact CA, and positive values indicating impaired autoregulatory capacity.[6] Both invasive and noninvasive continuous indices can be calculated during the baseline "passive" state of the patient, or during "dynamic" physiologic manipulations of CPP or MAP.

The main invasively derived continuous CA indices are: (A) ICP derived, (B) PbtO$_2$ derived, and (C) thermal diffusion (TD) CBF catheter derived.[6] Table 13.2 outlines the invasive continuous CA indices, methods of calculation and pros/cons of each.

ICP-derived indices

The commonly described ICP-derived indices include: pressure reactivity index (PRx)—correlation between ICP and MAP,[6,27] and pulse amplitude index (PAx)—correlation between pulse amplitude of ICP (AMP) and MAP.[28] Other "longer"

Table 13.2 Invasively obtained continuous indices of cerebral autoregulation—Methods and advantages/disadvantages

Invasive monitoring device	Signal recorded	Continuous CA indices derived	Method index derivation	Advantages	Disadvantages
Invasive ICP monitor	ICP – surrogate for pulsatile CBV	PRx and PAx	Moving Pearson correlation coefficient between: A. PRx – ICP and MAP B. PAx – AMP and MAP	PRx: A. Gives a "global" assessment of CA considering ICP is a global compartment signal B. Validated in animal model against the Lassen curve C. Ease of acquisition as ICP and MAP are both commonly recorded in ICU D. Significant correlations with patient outcome at 6 months[13] E. Critical thresholds for outcome are defined at: 0 for morbidity and +0.25 for mortality[13] F. Can be used for CPP optimum determination	PRx: A. Noisy signal B. Appears to be worse than PAx in outcome prediction for patients with low mean ICP PAx: A. Not validated in an animal model against the Lassen curve B. Some more calculation involved (ie, Fourier Transform of ICP signal for AMP) C. Critical thresholds related to outcome are not defined as of yet D. Use in CPP optimum assessment is unclear

(Continued)

Table 13.2 (Continued) Invasively obtained continuous indices of cerebral autoregulation—Methods and advantages/disadvantages

Invasive monitoring device	Signal recorded	Continuous CA indices derived	Method index derivation	Advantages	Disadvantages
				PAx: A. Similar global assessment B. Appears superior for outcome prediction in patients with low mean ICP	
Brain tissue oxygen	Regional Parenchymal PbtO$_2$ – Surrogate for pulsatile CBF/ CBV	ORx	Moving Pearson correlation coefficient between: A. ORx – PbtO$_2$ and CPP *NOTE: Calculation window length varies, but is typically 30 min or longer	A. May provide novel information surrounding oxygenated CBF and metabolism B. Has been used for CPP optimum estimation	A. PbtO$_2$ signal subject to both systemic, regional, and focal factors which impact oxygen carrying capacity, diffusion, uptake, and metabolism B. PbtO$_2$ signal is relatively "slowly" changing. Thus, window lengths for ORx calculations are longer than most other invasive/noninvasive indices C. Little literature to date to support its association with outcome and use in CPP optimum D. No critical thresholds defined E. Not validated in animal model (Continued)

Table 13.2 (Continued) Invasively obtained continuous indices of cerebral autoregulation—Methods and advantages/disadvantages

Invasive monitoring device	Signal recorded	Continuous CA indices derived	Method index derivation	Advantages	Disadvantages
Thermal diffusion (TD) catheter	Regional parenchymal CBF	CBFx and CBFx_a	Moving Pearson correlation coefficient between: A. CBFx – CBF and CPP B. CBFx_a – CBF and MAP	A. Utilizing a regional measure of CBF for the calculation of the index	A. Little literature on its use B. Recalibration of monitor device impedes continuous data stream for CBF measure, and may interrupt accurate CBFx measurement C. CBF signal can also be impacted by numerous systemic, regional, and focal factors related to CBF D. No critical thresholds E. Not validated in animal model

Abbreviations: AMP: Pulse amplitude of ICP; CBF: cerebral blood flow; CBFx: correlation between CBF and MAP; CBV: cerebral blood volume; CPP: cerebral perfusion pressure; ICP: intracranial pressure; PAx: pulse amplitude index (correlation between AMP and MAP); PRx: pressure reactivity index (correlation between ICP and MAP); ORx: oxygen reactivity index (correlation between PbtO$_2$ and CPP); TD: thermal diffusion.

versions of PRx exist, employing variations in window length for calculation.[29] PRx has been the index with the largest amount of literature in support of its application in NICU-based monitoring.[6] Literature supports its association with 6-month outcome, with critical thresholds for morbidity and mortality in TBI of 0 and +0.25, respectively.[6,13] Further to this, PRx is the only invasively-derived autoregulatory index which has been validated against the Lassen curve within animal models.[30] Permanently elevated PRx may be associated with refractory and terminal increase in ICP in those patients who die from brain stem herniation—see the example in Figure 13.4. PAx has recently emerged as an ICP-derived index with potentially improved predictive capacity in those with low mean ICPs.[28] Further work on PAx is required prior to widespread implementation as a continuous CA index.

PbtO$_2$-derived indices

PbtO$_2$-derived continuous indices include the oxygen reactivity index (ORx), which can be derived from varying lengths of data windows.[31,32] Given the slow response of the PbtO$_2$ signal to changes in cerebral physiology, both passive and dynamic, the calculation windows for ORx are typically 30 minutes or longer.[31] Thus, this index requires longer recording sessions for calculation. To date, limited literature exists on this index and its association with outcome. It hasn't been validated against the Lassen curve. Furthermore, the PbtO$_2$ signal is subject to numerous variables, including: blood–brain barrier oxygen diffusion, hemoglobin oxygen carrying capacity, anemia, CPP, MAP, pulmonary oxygen diffusion, and fractional inspired oxygen concentration (FiO$_2$).[33] Thus, it is currently unclear as to the exact relationship between ORx and CA. It should be considered experimental at this stage.

TD-derived indices

Finally, TD-based parenchymal CBF probes have been employed for the assessment of CA.[34] Using a dual thermistor probe inserted into brain parenchyma, the distal probe is heated to 2 degrees Celsius above tissue temperature, while the proximal probe records temperature outside of the distal probe heat field. The proximal probe is located approximately 5 mm proximal. The relative change in recorded temperature is believed to correlate to regional CBF. This CBF value can then be utilized within a moving correlation coefficient, using either MAP or CPP, to derive CBFx (correlation between TD-CBF and CPP) or CBFx_a (correlation between TD-CBF and MAP).[35] To date, very limited literature exists on TD-based CA measurement. The main issue with the technique is the constant recalibration and interruption of continuous data acquisition.[36] In addition, as with PbtO$_2$ monitoring, TD CBF may be influenced by numerous downstream factors. Thus, at this stage, TD-based CA measurements should also be considered experimental.

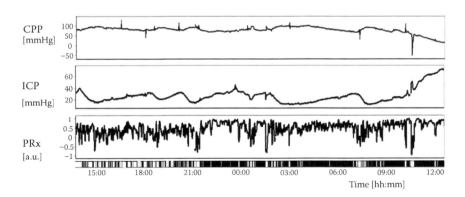

Figure 13.4 "Solid red line" effect in refractory intracranial hypertension. ICP and CPP monitored during 2 days after TBI. On day 1, ICP was not elevated. PRx was around 0. Summary "color plot" (bottom, here is white, gray, black) showed on average good reactivity (white or gray). Well before refractory rise in ICP on day 2, PRx increased (21:00, first day) to values above 0.3, with ICP still within a normal range and stable. Color plot of PRx showed "solid red line"—predominant black on the plot. It anticipated final rise of ICP leading to brainstem herniation by more than 12 hours.

NONINVASIVE CONTINUOUS CA MEASURES

As mentioned within the section on invasive continuous CA measures, noninvasive CA indices can be derived using the same concept of moving Pearson correlation coefficients.[4] The current monitoring modalities employed for the derivation of these noninvasive indices include: (A) TCD and (B) NIRS. Table 13.3 outlines the common continuous noninvasive CA measurements and the advantages/disadvantages of each.

TCD-derived indices

TCD-based indices have been readily referenced within the literature. Utilizing TCD-based CBFV, one can derive: mean flow velocity (FVm), systolic flow velocity (FVs), and diastolic flow velocity (FVd).[4,37,38] These derived flow velocities can then be utilized within a moving Pearson correlation coefficient with CPP (similar to the PRx calculation described above), to calculate: mean flow index (Mx), systolic flow index (Sx), and diastolic flow index (Dx). Similarly, if one wanted to use MAP in the coefficient calculation, this would produce: Mx_a, Sx_a, and Dx_a. Of note, only Mx_a/Sx_a/Dx_a are completely noninvasive, given that MAP can be obtained through continuous NIBP monitoring.[4] There is a potential to derive CPP noninvasively, using the TCD, derived techniques described above, however, these techniques require validation prior to clinical application. To date, Mx and Sx have displayed strong correlations with 6-month outcome, with Mx critical thresholds for morbidity and mortality in TBI defined as +0.05 and +0.30, respectively.[39] Mx appear to display stronger correlations to outcome, compared to Mx_a.[39] Furthermore, Mx displays moderate correlation to PRx.[37,38] The main issue with the TCD-derived technique is that TCD signal acquisition is labor intensive and usually yields short duration of recordings, producing a "semi-intermittent" method of CA estimation. In addition, TCD-based indices have not been validated against the Lassen curve.

NIRS-derived indices

NIRS has been applied in TBI for the assessment of oxygenated/deoxygenated hemoglobin. Through the application of frontal (typically bifrontal) emission and detector probes, near-infrared light is passed through the skin, skull, and dura, onto the cortical surface.[6] This light is absorbed in varying degrees, related to the hemoglobin content and oxygenation status of the hemoglobin in the blood located within the frontal lobes. The reflected signal recorded by the detector estimates the degree of oxygenated/deoxygenated hemoglobin concentrations.[6] The oxygenated concentration is believed to represent the arterial compartment, while the deoxygenated concentration is thought to reflect the venous side.[6]

Issues with signal contamination from the extracranial circulation exist, which has led to the development of "spatially resolved" NIRS.[6] This spatially resolved NIRS is based on proprietary algorithms and software which is employed to "scrub" the extracranial signal from the intracranial signal. Various signals are produced depending on the particular NIRS unit applied, including: (A) total oxygenation index (TOI) and (B) total hemoglobin index (THI).

Using TOI and THI, moving correlation coefficients can be calculated with MAP and CPP producing: TOx (also known as COx), TOx_a, THx, and THx_a. TOx has been validated against the Lassen curve in an animal model, leaving both TOx and PRx as the only two validated CA indices.[30] The literature on NIRS-based indices is limited, with some data to support an association with outcome.[6] The main limitations of the technique are: (A) labor intensity, (B) signal processing, and (C) cost of the device.

INTER-INDEX RELATIONSHIPS

Given the large number of continuous CA indices that can be generated from various MMM devices, it can get confusing to the clinician as to which index is the best, and what inter-index relationships exist. As previously mentioned, to date only PRx and TOx have been validated against the Lassen curve in an animal model.[30] PRx still poses the most robust continuous estimate at this time.[40]

In terms of the inter-index relationships, very little literature exists.[41] There are many studies correlating one index to another, in an isolated manner. However, this doesn't address the inter-index relationships across all MMM devices. The main limitation is that there are very few patient cohorts with all MMM devices concurrently recording signals, allowing for the assessment of all the indices simultaneously.

Table 13.3 Noninvasively obtained continuous indices of cerebral autoregulation—Methods and advantages/disadvantages

Invasive monitoring device	Signal recorded	Continuous CA indices derived	Method index derivation	Advantages	Disadvantages
TCD-based CBFV from MCA	MCA FVm, FVs, FVd – as surrogate measures of pulsatile CBF	A. Mx, Mx_a B. Sx, Sx_a C. Dx, Dx_a	Moving Pearson correlation coefficient between: A. Mx – FVm and CPP B. Mx_a – FVm and CPP C. Sx – FVs and CPP D. Sx_a – FVs and MAP E. Dx – FVd and CPP F. Dx_a – FVd and MAP	Mx/Mx_a: A. Gives a "Global/Regional" assessment of CA considering CBFV is a global/hemispheric signal B. Moderate correlation with PRx (r = 0.58)[37] C. Significant correlations with patient outcome at 6 months D. Critical thresholds of Mx for outcome are defined at: 0.05 for morbidity and +0.30 for mortality[39] E. Correlated to cortical CBF as per LDF in TBI patients[45] F. Mx_a is worse at outcome prediction[39] Sx/Sx_a: A. Similar global assessment B. Appears superior for outcome prediction compared to Mx[38]	For all TCD Indices: A. Noisy signal B. Not validated in animal model against the Lassen C. Labor intensive for signal acquisition D. Semi-intermittent in nature given nature of signal acquisition E. Length of recordings is usually limited For Sx/Sx_a/Dx/Dx_a A. Very little literature on these alternative ICP indices B. No critical thresholds for these indices

(Continued)

Table 13.3 (Continued) Noninvasively obtained continuous indices of cerebral autoregulation—Methods and advantages/disadvantages

Invasive monitoring device	Signal recorded	Continuous CA indices derived	Method index derivation	Advantages	Disadvantages
NIRS based	Regional (bifrontal) Cortical Oxy- and Deoxyhemoglobin Levels – Surrogate Measures of Pulsatile CBF *NOTE: Given contamination of extracranial blood flow signal with standard NIRS, we will only mention the spatially resolved NIRS measures (TOI and THI). Both of these have theoretically been "scrubbed" of this extracranial contamination.	A. TOx and TOx_a B. THx and THx_a	Moving Pearson correlation coefficient between: A. TOx – TOI and CPP B. TOx_a – TOI and MAP C. THx – THI and CPP D. THx_a – THI and MAP	A. Noninvasive B. Can remain attached for longer durations than TCD C. TOx has been validated against the Lassen curve in an animal model C. May be more correlated with PRx and PAx[41]	A. Use of non-spatially resolved NIRS measures leads to contamination with extracranial blood signal B. Proprietary algorithms used for spatially resolved measures are not disclosed by manufacturers. Thus, they remain "black box" C. Limited literature to date linking these indices to outcome D. No global assessments of CA given the regional nature of NIRS E. Labor intensive and expensive F. Potentially impacted by systemic factors related to oxygen diffusion and delivery

Abbreviations: CA: Cerebral autoregulation; CBF: cerebral blood flow; CFBV: cerebral blood flow velocity; CBV: cerebral blood volume; CPP: cerebral perfusion pressure; Dx: diastolic flow index (correlation between FVd and CPP); Dx_a: diastolic flow index based on MAP (correlation between FVd and MAP); ICP: intracranial pressure; LDF: laser Doppler flowmetry MCA: middle cerebral artery; Mx: mean flow index (correlation between FVm and CPP); Mx_a: mean flow index derived from MAP (correlation between FVm and MAP); NIRS: near infrared spectroscopy; Sx: systolic flow index (correlation between FVs and CPP); Sx_a: systolic flow index derived from MAP (correlation between FVs and MAP); TOI: total oxygen index; TOx: correlation between TOI and CPP; TOx_a: correlation between TOI and MAP; THI: total hemoglobin index; THx: correlation between THI and CPP; THx_a: correlation between THI and MAP.

To date, a single study has attempted to classify the inter-index relationships and co-variance in a cohort with various MMM devices.[41] Using cluster analysis techniques and basic machine learning, some interesting relationships were described. Mx/Mx_a/Dx/Dx_a appear to co-cluster away from all other MMM indices. $PbtO_2$-based ORx indices appear to not be related to any of the other indices derived from MMM. Finally, Sx/Sx_a appears more closely related to the ICP and NIRS-derived CA indices, compared to Mx/Mx_a/Dx/Dx_a. All of these relationships require further validation in a larger cohort.

OTHER INTERMITTENT/SEMI-INTERMITTENT METHODS

Despite the promising literature on continuous CA assessment in TBI, there are other techniques which deserve a quick mention, even though the focus of this chapter is on continuous monitoring.[4] Detailed description of the techniques and results can be found elsewhere.[4] Intermittent techniques for CA assessment include both imaging and non-imaging-based means.

Imaging-based assessments involve the use of CTP, Xe-CT, ^{15}O-PET, or MRA with dynamic manipulation of the patient's physiology during the testing. Typically, a baseline scan is obtained, followed by manipulation of CPP or MAP using vasopressor agents. Manipulation of systemic pressure can also occur via the thigh cuff deflation technique (TCDT). During the manipulation of systemic physiology, repeat imaging is conducted, allowing for comparison to baseline. Various post-acquisition processing of the data is required for quantitative assessment of CBF and CBV. The main limitations of these techniques are: (A) intermittent nature, (B) labor intensive, (C) transport of critically ill patients to the scanner, (D) requirement of manipulation of systemic physiology, and (E) post-acquisition signal processing. Literature for all of these techniques in TBI is limited, with MRI-based techniques rarely described in the TBI population.

Non-imaging-based assessments of CA in TBI have formed the foundation of autoregulation assessment, leading the development of the current continuous-based measures employed within the NICU. These techniques include TCD-based: transient hyperemic response testing (THRT), TCDT, orthostatic hypotension testing (OHT),

autoregulation index (ARI) estimation, and transfer function-ARI (TF-ARI). Finally, the use of jugular venous oxygen saturations ($SjvO_2$), comparing the arterial and venous differences in oxygen saturations ($AVDO_2$), have been employed as an invasive surrogate measure of CBF and CA, using: CBF ~ 1/$AVDO_2$; assuming a constant CMR of oxygen consumption ($CMRO_2$).[4] All of these methods produce intermittent evaluations of CA, and are labor intensive compared to the derivation of continuous measures.[4] Again, as with the imaging-based assessments, they rely on the concept of systemic physiologic manipulations. They do require mentioning, as most are noninvasive and may prove valuable in the assessment of CA in the subacute and chronic phase post-TBI.

OPTIMUM CEREBRAL PERFUSION PRESSURE (CPPOPT)

With the development of continuous indices of CA, such as PRx, there has been a desire to improve upon the relatively nebulous CPP-derived targets previously highlighted.[12] It's long been a belief that setting specific CPP targets/goals that are ubiquitously applied to all TBI patients is both incorrect and potentially harmful. Some patients may have their own individual "optimum" CPP, which should be targeted during their ICU course.[42]

Using continuous indices of autoregulation measurement, one can plot CPP versus the index. This distribution is typically parabolic in nature, with the minimum located at the point where the autoregulation index is the most negative (ie, indicating the "intact" CA).[42] The corresponding CPP at this minimum is termed CPPopt, and is patient specific. The most commonly utilized CA index for this purpose is PRx;[42] see the example in Figure 13.5. However, $PbtO_2$-based ORx has also be utilized.[43]

To date, there is an increasing literature base supporting two aspects of CPPopt: (A) that the larger the difference between actual CPP and CPPopt (delta CPP), the worse outcome, and (B) the longer duration spent with a CPP value different from CPPopt, the worse outcome at 6 months.[42] This is based on CPPopt measured via PRx. Similar comments regarding $PbtO_2$-based CPPopt determination cannot be made at this time. Future prospective trails comparing BTF-based CPP targets versus CPPopt are planned.

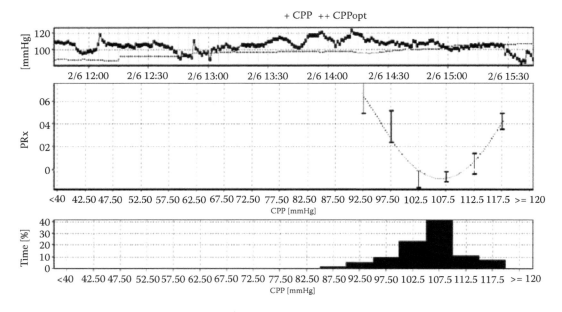

Figure 13.5 Five-hour plot of CPP and relationship between PRx and CPP showing U-shape curve. Optimal CPP was in this case 105 mmHg—much higher than it would result from the guidelines.

CEREBRAL BLOOD FLOW (CBF) MONITORING

Invasive continuous techniques

During the 1990s, cortically placed subdural laser Doppler flowmetry (LDF) probes were available for the assessment of cortical/pial CBF.[44,45] Various small cohort studies in TBI demonstrated a link between LDF CBF and patient outcome. CA indices were even derived from LDF data, with a moderate association between these indices and TCD-based Mx described in TBI patients.[45] Despite the promising early results, these devices are no longer available for clinical application.

Current continuous methods of CBF monitoring are limited to the invasive TD CBF catheter. As described within the TD subsection on CA measurement, this catheter is invasively placed within the parenchyma, yielding CBF values based on the impact of regional CBF on parenchymal temperature.[34] Aside from the derivation of CA indices, the core CBF value produced by these monitors has been evaluated as a predictor of outcome in TBI. A small number of publications, based on small cohorts of moderate to severe TBI patients, indicate some association between low TD-based CBF values and poor functional outcome.[6] These results do require validation.

The main limitation of TD is that the signal is interrupted by regular recalibration.[35] In addition, the CBF value produced is only regional, within the immediate area of the TD probe tip. Furthermore, the signal is subject to numerous systemic and location physiologic factors.[6,35] Thus, an abnormal CBF may not be entirely reflective of a regional CBF problem, but may be secondary to systemic pathology.

Invasive/noninvasive intermittent techniques

Given that the noninvasive techniques for CBF assessment are not continuous in nature, we will only briefly mention them, as the purpose of this chapter is to focus on continuous monitoring in cerebral neurotrauma. The main techniques for noninvasive CBF monitoring in TBI is based on imaging, $SjvO_2$-based $AVDO_2$ or TCD-based techniques.[4]

The imaging techniques involve the use of CTP, Xe-CT, ^{15}O-PET, or magnetic resonance perfusion (MRP).[4] These techniques still involve a degree of invasiveness as they typically require the administration of radiopaque contrast, inhaled xenon gas, or radiotracer. As more advanced arterial spin labeling (ASL) techniques are developed, potentially more accurate ASL-based MRP may be described, providing reliable quantitative data on CBV/CBF. All of the above-mentioned techniques rely on the transit of "labeled" blood through the cerebrovascular tree. The transit time, time to peak, and degree of filling are utilized to quantitatively estimate CBV and CBF. The issue with these techniques are: (A) administration of a contrast agent, (B) labor intensive nature, (C) intermittent nature, (D) post-acquisition processing, and (E) transport of critically ill patients to a scanner.[4] The literature on these techniques varies in size, depending on the modality. Most demonstrate the association between low CBF and poor patient outcome.

SjvO$_2$-based techniques for CBF estimation have been eluded to above in the CA section.[4] The concept revolves around measuring the difference between arterial oxygen saturation (SaO$_2$) and SjvO$_2$, the AVDO$_2$. Assuming a constant CMRO$_2$, CBF can be estimated by: CBF ~ 1/AVDO$_2$.[4,46] As mentioned in the CA section, SjvO$_2$-based estimation of CBF can be done during physiologic manipulations as well. The data on SjvO$_2$ is also limited, but points to impaired CBF, as indicated by elevated SjvO$_2$ levels, associated with poor patient outcomes.[4]

Finally, TCD-based noninvasive CBF estimates are based primarily on change in MCA CBFV and noninvasively derived CPP from TCD-based PI. Both methods of CBF estimation have limited literature, questioning the reliability of the values. Thus, this should be considered an experimental technique.

CEREBROVASCULAR REACTIVITY (CVR) TESTING

Aside from the classically defined pressure autoregulation, one can also assess the cerebrovascular systems responsiveness to metabolic changes, referred to as CVR. This requires either the manipulation of the partial pressure of carbon dioxide (pCO$_2$) or the administration of a carbonic anhydrase inhibitor. The quantification of CVR can be conducted through the use of continuous indices of CA (see above sections) or the intermittent assessment of CBV/CBF using with TCD,[47] SjvO$_2$-based AVDO$_2$ method or imaging-based techniques.[48] The use of continuous CA indices during CVR testing is attractive given the relative ease of calculation and the lack of need for transport to a scanner and the administration of a contrast agent.

To date, numerous publications exist linking impaired CVR responses to poor patient outcome in moderate to severe TBI. Furthermore, recent data in the mild traumatic brain injury cohort links impaired CVR during functional MRI (fMRI) blood oxygen level dependence (BOLD) signal measurements, to persistent postconcussive symptomatology during follow-up.[49]

One must be cautioned, however, that impaired CVR does not necessarily imply impaired pressure CA, as there is literature to suggested the impairment of one system and not the other is possible.[40] Thus, if one is commenting on CA, it is a pressure response phenomenon, not a metabolic one. Hence, CVR and CA are different entities.

BRAIN OXYGENATION

Various aspects of brain "oxygenation" can be assessed utilizing different methods of MMM. The main goals of monitoring cerebral oxygen are to ensure: (A) adequate delivery, (B) adequate diffusability, (C) adequate uptake, and (D) adequate metabolism. Imaging-based intermittent assessment of global oxygen metabolism will be addressed briefly in a later section.

SJVO$_2$

Though far from continuous, given the need for intermittent blood sampling, SjvO$_2$ measurements from jugular venous catheters require a brief mention. These catheters have been employed a long time with various degrees of acceptance within the NICU community. The concept is a shortened internal jugular catheter is inserted in a cranial direction, with the goal of having the catheter tip near the sigmoid sinus. This theoretically allows for sampling of only cerebral venous return.[46] Various analytes have been investigated, including oxygen[4,46] and lactate.[50] We have already mentioned the use of SjvO$_2$ for CBF assessment.[4,46] Jugular venous lactate will be touched upon briefly in a "Lactate" section to follow.

Numerous publications have emerged linking low SjvO$_2$ with poor patient outcome.[51,52] However, both extremes of SjvO$_2$ can be potentially attributed to concerning physiology. First, low SjvO$_2$ can signify excessive oxygen extraction and either impending or current metabolic crisis (see the example, Figure 13.6). Second, elevated SjvO$_2$ can signify metabolic failure with potential impaired oxygen extraction, utilization, and mitochondrial

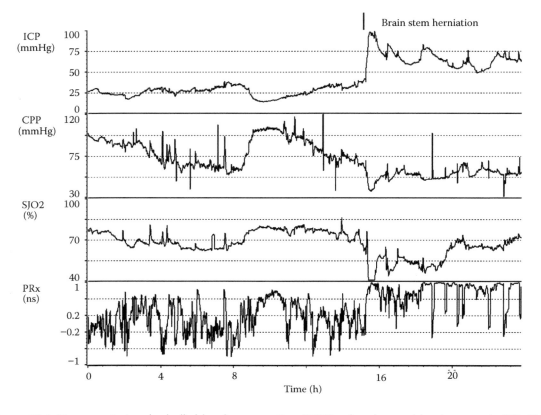

Figure 13.6 Decrease in jugular bulb blood oxygenation (SjO2) related to sudden increase in ICP. The decrease was below 40%–50%. It was associated with disturbance of pressure reactivity (PRx) and decrease in CPP.

dysfunction. The results of $SjvO_2$ need to be interpreted in combination with other MMM and the current clinical status. Normal values vary depending on the source, but 70% to 80% is believed to represent normality.[51,52] The main disadvantage is that $SjvO_2$ samples provide global information, as the venous blood collected is from the entire brain. Thus, the venous blood from the pathological regions is mixed with that from "normal" regions, muddying the interpretation of the results.

PARENCHYMAL BRAIN TISSUE OXYGEN (PBTO₂)

Placement of invasive parenchymal $PbtO_2$ monitors provide focal information about the extracellular partial pressure of oxygen near the catheter tip. Numerous studies to date support a link between low $PbtO_2$ and poor patient outcome in TBI.[53,54] Furthermore, low $PbtO_2$ has been associated with derangements in CMD analytes. Thresholds for normal are around 20 mmHg.

Elevated $PbtO_2$ levels can also signify concerns with impaired cellular uptake and potential focal mitochondrial dysfunction. $PbtO_2$ has also been utilized for both the assessment of CA and CPPopt, as previously outlined.

The main issue with this technique is that it is a very focal assessment and that the extracellular oxygen is influenced by numerous other factors. This was briefly outlined within the CA section. The exact utility of these focal $PbtO_2$ probes is not clear currently, with even less clear indications as to when to intervene for abnormal levels.

NEAR-INFRA-RED SPECTROSCOPY (NIRS)

We have outlined the technique of signal acquisition for NIRS within the CA section above.[6] NIRS provides focal, typically bifrontal, assessment of oxygenated and deoxygenated hemoglobin, with oxygenated and deoxygenated signals believed to represent the arterial and venous sides of the circulation, respectively. Aside from CA assessment, the raw values for TOx and THx have been associated with patient outcome.[55] The literature is limited to date.[6,56] The issue with interpreting these values is similar to $PbtO_2$, in that the oxygenated hemoglobin status can be influenced by numerous factors, as outlined in the CA section. The affinity to this type of monitoring is the ease of application and noninvasive nature.

CEREBRAL MICRODIALYSIS (CMD)—FOCAL CEREBRAL METABOLISM AND BIOMARKER ASSESSMENT

CMD involves the insertion of a parenchymal-based microdialysis catheter for the assessment of focal cerebral metabolism.[57,58] It is therefore an invasive technique. Exact procedural technique for CMD varies depending on country and individual institution. The catheter is typically placed in either normal or peri-lesional tissue for the assessment of metabolism in either "healthy" brain or the peri-lesional "at risk" tissue. Various catheters exist, with varying pore size. The typical CMD catheter pore size is between 20 to 100 kDa, which is sufficient for the "common analytes" mentioned below.[57] However, for the "uncommon" larger protein biomarkers, these pore sizes may be too small, hence the application of alternative catheters.[58,59] A perfusate is then infused, typically at 0.3 µl/minute, allowing for diffusion of these analytes of interest across the semipermeable CMD catheter membrane.[59] This fluid is then collected and sampled at various frequencies. The perfusate is commonly quoted as isotonic crystalloid based. However, in order to improve recovery of larger proteins, colloid-based solutions may need to be utilized.[59]

Numerous studies on the application of CMD in TBI have emerged over the past 15 to 20 years.[7,8,57] Most have focused on the association between various metabolic analytes and their associations with patient function outcome or other physiologic parameters. To cover all of the literature on this technique is out of the scope of this chapter.

Common CMD analytes in TBI

LACTATE, PYRUVATE, AND LACTATE: PYRUVATE RATIO (LPR)

CMD measurement of lactate, pyruvate, and the LPR is aimed at commenting on regional anaerobic metabolism and potential mitochondrial dysfunc-

tion. Various studies have demonstrated the association between high lactate/low pyruvate and poor outcome.[60] Thresholds for LPR have been described, with both >25 and 40 being described and those most associated with poor outcome.[57,58] Further to this, some have tried to further sub stratify types of LPR elevations into two main groups. Type I failure is considered to be classic the "ischemic" type, defined as elevated LPR in the setting of impaired $PbtO_2$, and even potentially elevated glycerol. Type II failure is considered to be a metabolic crisis, where there is elevated LPR in the setting of normal of high $PbtO_2$, signifying failure of energy metabolism and potentially mitochondrial dysfunction.

Elevated LPR has also been associated with increased ICP/low CPP, low $PbtO_2$, impaired PET-based oxygen and glucose metabolism, and low $SjvO_2$. In addition, elevated LPR has been linked to CA dysfunction. Finally, the degree and duration of LPR elevation has also been linked to cortical atrophy at 6 to 12 months post-TBI.

Glutamate

Glutamate levels are believed to represent the degree of excitotoxicity post-TBI. The extracellular CMD glutamate concentrations may reflect this. Hence, it is an analyte of interest for CMD sampling. Numerous studies have displayed the association between elevated CMD glutamate and poor 3- to 6-month functional outcome.[7,8,57] Thresholds for the association with poor outcome vary, with >20 umol/L. Elevated glutamate levels have also been found to be associated with elevated ICP/decreased CPP, low $SjvO_2$, low $PbtO_2$, and impaired CA.

Glycerol

Glycerol is believed to be an extracellular marker of cellular destruction and degradation. Thus, measuring this through CMD may provide insight into focal cellular viability. Elevated CMD glycerol levels have been associated with poor outcome at 3 to 6 months.[7,8,57] Thresholds are poorly defined. Mean CMD glycerol was also found to be associated with elevated ICP, low CPP, low $SjvO_2$, low $PbtO_2$, and impaired CA.

Glucose

Monitoring extracellular glucose provides insight into the diffusible concentrations of glucose, and the availability of this metabolic substrate during state of injury. CMD assessment of this analyte, not surprisingly, has displayed links between low glucose and poor outcome at 3 to 6 months.[7,8,57,58] Thresholds are poorly defined for "low CMD glucose." Low CMD glucose has also been associated with high ICP, low CPP, low $SjvO_2$, low $PbtO_2$, and impaired CA.

UNCOMMON CMD ANALYTES IN TBI

Electrolytes

Some consider the measurement of CMD electrolytes to be "uncommon" analytes. The literature to date is quite small on CMD-based electrolyte measurement. CMD potassium concentrations have been linked to poor outcome.[61] An issue with electrolyte recovery is the fact that most perfusates contain various concentrations of electrolytes, impeding interpretation of the recovered samples.

Pro-inflammatory cytokines

Pro-inflammatory cytokines have emerged in the literature as analytes of interest for CMD research. Immune system mediated injury post-TBI is a potential concern. CMD cytokines have been linked to poor clinical outcome, with preliminary data suggesting those cytokines associated with macrophage activation predominating in the acute phase post-TBI.[62] In particular, CMD levels of interleukin (IL)-1b, IL-1ra, IL-6, IL-8, IL-10, and tumor necrosis factor (TNF) have been linked to outcome in TBI.[63] In addition, a recent trial of a subcutaneous IL-1ra antagonist has displayed the ability to modulate CMD-based cytokine measures, potentially offering future therapeutic interventions.[64] Further research in this area is required.

Matrix metalloproteins

Matrix metalloproteinase (MMP) is an enzyme that has been linked to dysfunction of the blood–brain barrier during pathological states. Monitoring levels of MMPs post-TBI has recently emerged within the literature.[65,66] Data suggests various MMPs may be elevated post-TBI, particularly MMP-7 and MMP-9. These MMPs appear to peak during the first 72 hours postinjury. Furthermore, some preliminary data suggests an intimate link between CMD cytokine profiles and MMP expression, implicating the immune system in the MMP response seen post-TBI.[67] Further research is required as these results are based off of small studies.

Endothelial markers

This is an emerging area, with little literature in TBI regarding CMD endothelial markers. Potential exists to link markers of endothelial dysfunction with other physiologic parameters, such as CBF, CVR, and CA capacity. This is currently experimental work.

DISADVANTAGES OF CMD

The main disadvantage of CMD is the invasive and focal nature of the sampling. It is not clear that such focal metabolic sampling reflects larger regional or global metabolism. In addition, the technique is quite labor intensive, even for the measurement of common analytes. When interested in analyzing larger protein biomarkers, such as cytokines or MMPs, changes in catheter and perfusate are required.[58,59] Furthermore, the need for specialized biochemical analysis of the sample is required, in order to obtain reliable results for these biomarkers.[57,58] This adds the need for specialized personal and cost of processing. Thus, this technique may not be feasible in all institutions.

Global cerebral metabolism

Aside from CMD and $PbtO_2$, which provide a very focal assessment of cerebral metabolics at the catheter tips, most other methods of cerebral metabolism assessment focus on larger regions of interest (ROIs) or global assessments via imaging.[68-71] Within the imaging domain, PET can play an important role in the assessment of cerebral metabolics with the application of various radiotracers. The downside to all of these techniques, aside from CMD and $PbtO_2$, is that they provide an intermittent assessment of metabolic function, and do not provide continuously updating data streams. However, given the potential important information obtained from these studies, we felt it necessary to briefly mention some of the techniques despite the focus of this chapter being on continuous monitoring in neurotrauma. To date, numerous PET-based tracers have been developed to probe various aspects of cerebral metabolism.[68,69] A comprehensive outline of all of these tracers and techniques is beyond the scope of this chapter, thus we will only focus on the more commonly described ^{15}O and ^{18}F PET.

OXYGEN

Cerebral metabolic rate of oxygen consumption (CMRO$_2$) is typically commented on utilizing ^{15}O-PET. As mentioned within the CBF and CA sections above, PET can also be employed as a means of intermittent assessment of these aspects of cerebral physiology. The technique involves the administration of an ^{15}O radiolabeled tracer intravenously. Typically, ^{15}O labeled water is utilized for CBF assessment and labeled carbon monoxide (CO) is used for CBV assessments. Radiolabeled O$_2$ is also applied as a steady state inhalation. Then both an emission scan and spiral CT are obtained and subsequently co-registered. Maps of CBF, CBV, CMRO$_2$, and oxygen extraction fraction (OEF) are then created utilizing standard models and post processing. In theory, both low and high CMRO$_2$ in the setting of TBI can be of concern.[70,71] Extremely high CMRO$_2$ could be a sign of extreme metabolic stress and regional/global need for oxygen as a result of both initial injury severity and potentially ongoing secondary insult. Similarly, low CMRO$_2$ may indicate impaired oxygen metabolism, secondary to issues with delivery, diffusion, or mitochondrial dysfunction/failure.

Preliminary data within TBI supports an association between low CMRO$_2$ and impaired CA, as assessed via PRx.[70–72] Furthermore, changes in CPP seem to have corresponding alterations in PET-based CMRO$_2$. These studies are small however. The main disadvantages of this technique are: (A) labor intensive, (B) need for radiotracer administration, (C) significant data processing required, (D) transport of critically ill patients to the scanner, and (E) poor temporal resolution.

GLUCOSE

Outside of CMD assessment, glucose metabolism is also commonly assessed intermittently via PET. The use of ^{18}F radiolabeled tracers enables us to comment on the cerebral metabolic rate of glucose consumption (CMR$_{GLC}$) with the administration of labeled fluorodeoxyglucose (^{18}FDG).[69,73,74] The technique is similar to that described for oxygen metabolism, with the addition of multiple arterial blood samples taken during the course of FDG-PET scan acquisition. This allows for serum concentration input into a plasma input function. All of this information is utilized to reconstruct the CMR maps, which are co-registered to a spiral CT of the head. This information can be correlated with focal CMD assessments of parenchymal glucose and its metabolites in order to make more detailed comments on cerebral glucose metabolism.

Preliminary data suggests a strong correlation between FDG-PET-based low CMR$_{GLC}$ and elevated CMD lactate and pyruvate.[73,74] The association with LPR is not clear. All of this data is based on a small number of subjects and requires further validation. This technique suffers from the same limitation as other PET-based studies.

LACTATE

The assessment of cerebral lactate production has long been sought as a means of commenting on the degree of anaerobic metabolism in the brain. The use of jugular venous sampling of lactate, comparing to arterial lactate, can produce values for the arterial-venous difference in lactate (AVD$_{LAC}$).[50,75] Based on these values, gross/coarse comments on the anaerobic state of cerebral metabolism can be made. The issue with this is that we are left commenting on a "global" cerebral state with jugular lactate sampling.[76] Similar jugular venous sampling can be done for glucose, its intermediaries during glycolysis, or within the tricarboxylic acid (TCA) cycle, and other metabolites may be measured.

Application of magnetic resonance spectroscopy (MRS) also allows us to comment on focal cerebral metabolism. Lactate peaks can be identified within the spectra obtained through MRS. The data on the application of this technique is quite limited within TBI. The main issues are as follows: (A) long scan acquisition time, (B) small voxel-based assessment only (difficult to do whole brain maps), (C) labor intensive, and (D) transport of critically ill patients to an MRI for extended periods of time.

EMERGING TECHNIQUES

Emerging techniques for the global intermittent assessment of various aspects of cerebral metabolism show promise. Two paramagnetic isotopes require mentioning. In particular, the use of ^{13}carbon (^{13}C) labeled substrates within MRS.[69] The ability to label various metabolic substrates and intermediaries exists. This potentially allows for comment on various aspect, of cerebral glucose and lactate metabolism. In addition, ^{31}phosporus (^{31}P) labeled compounds allow us to potentially make comments on cerebral energy stores.[69] Both of these techniques are considered experimental.

AUTONOMICS

Given the association between autonomic dysfunction and poor outcomes within other areas of neuropathology,[77] and the potential involvement of the autonomic system with the regulation of numerous cerebral physiologic processes, (including CA), literature is emerging on the assessment of both heart rate variability (HRV) and baroreceptor reflex (BRS) in TBI.[78,79] Preliminary data links disordered HRV and BRS to poor patient outcome post-TBI.[79,80] The links between disordered HRV and BRS with other physiologic processes, such as CA, is not well understood at the moment. Further work is required to determine the association between injury patterns/burden with autonomic dysfunction, and the downstream associations between autonomic dysfunction with both cerebral physiologic events and tissue outcome.

BRAIN TEMPERATURE

Invasive brain temperature probes have recently been employed within the NICU, as another tool in the armamentarium of MMM post-TBI. The data to date is limited.[81,82] Conclusions surrounding the utility of this monitoring and its association with patient outcomes and other neurophysiologic events cannot be made at this time. There is some preliminary data that indicates an association between a rise in brain temperature during spreading depolarizations.[83] Further work is required in order to determine the utility of this monitoring device in TBI. Given the invasive nature of placement and the lack of literature surrounding its use, this modality should be considered experimental at this time.

CORTICAL ELECTROPHYSIOLOGY

Various aspects of cortical electrophysiology can be continuously monitored within TBI patients.[84–87] These aspects include, but are not limited to: (A) electroencephalography (EEG), (B) somatosensory evoked potentials (SSEP), and (C) motor evoked potentials (MEP). Other aspects of electrophysiology may be monitored, interrogating the cortical, subcortical, and brain stem structures. An extensive overview of both these cortical and sub-cortical electrophysiologic monitoring is beyond the scope of this review. We will only briefly focus on the above-mentioned commonly described aspects of cortical electrophysiologic monitoring in TBI.

CONTINUOUS EEG

Continuous electroencephalography (cEEG) is becoming more available as a potential monitoring device within the NICU. Both standard multi-channel and focal reduced channel versions of cEEG are available for application in the monitoring of TBI patients.[84] In addition, for those units in which regular epileptologist interpretation of the EEG results is not feasible, there are automatic signal detection algorithms available. cEEG has been employed in: (A) seizure detection, (B) prognostication post-TBI, (C) detection of ischemia, and (D) detection of spreading depolarizations. Signals for cEEG can be obtained cutaneously, via standard scalp electrodes, or invasively through the insertion of subdural paddles or parenchymal depth electrodes.

Seizures post moderate to severe TBI are not uncommon, and are a potentially important cause of secondary brain insult if not detected/treated early in their course. The application of cEEG post-TBI allows for this.[88]

Aside from the detection of post-traumatic epileptic events, cEEG monitoring has been utilized for outcome prediction within TBI, with detailed analysis of both regional and global electrical activity as it is associated with patient global outcome.[89] An ever-growing literature base in this area of outcome prediction with cEEG exists. This has been used as an adjunctive test in the assessment of brain death.[90,91]

Detection of ischemic potentials has also been described with cEEG, and thus adds to the benefit of this monitoring modality. This has been employed in the monitoring of other neuropathological processes, such as vasospasm post aneurysmal subarachnoid hemorrhage.[92] Potential exists for ischemia monitoring in TBI. Further research is required in this area to better understand the link between cEEG ischemic electrical potentials and cerebrovascular dysfunction, including impairment/failure of CA.

Finally, spreading cortical depolarizations (SCDs) post-TBI is an emerging area of the literature.

It is believed these SCDs may be associated with ischemia/infarction, metabolic dysfunction, and even disruption of CVR and/or CA.[83,87,93,94] The use of cEEG may aid in elucidating these relationships. The issue is that accurate detection of SCDs may not always be possible with cutaneous cEEG. Thus, there may be a future role for subdural paddle electrode or parenchymal depth electrode EGG monitoring. The majority of the literature to date is animal based, hence much work is needed with the clinical sphere in order to determine the utility of monitoring for SCDs.

SSEPs AND MEPs

The use of SSEPs and MEPs within the NICU has extended from their application within the operating room, as a means of injury detection. These modalities require a trained neurophysiologist to set up, monitor, and interpret the results. This, limits their current widespread use. Poor or absent signals have been attributed to poor neurologic outcome in TBI.[95] These aspects of electrophysiology have even been employed as adjunctive tests in the determination of brain death.[96]

SIGNAL ENTROPY

The degree of chaos (ie, entropy) within a given physiologic signal carries some potentially important information about the individual system from which the variable is derived. Recent analysis of signal entropy, using approximate entropy calculations, has linked reduced ICP and MAP entropy to worse functional outcome.[97] Further to this, reduced ICP signal entropy was inversely correlated to PRx values (r = −0.39, p < 0.000001).[97]

This is just preliminary data. However, the concept makes sense. The more ordered a particular system becomes (ie, less entropy), the more rigid and less able to respond to further insult. The assessment of multiple systems at once, including extracranial organ systems, has not been readily conducted. It is possible that a "holistic" multi-system-based signal analysis will provide more useful predictive information compared to any single system interrogated in isolation. The main limitation of this monitoring is the extensive post signal acquisition data processing that is required. Future work is required in this area of monitoring, and it should be considered experimental at this time.

Future of monitoring in cerebral neurotrauma

The future for MMM in cerebral neurotrauma is bright. As we have outlined, there are numerous aspects to monitoring cerebral physiology and metabolism post-TBI, employing various devices in the process. As technology advances and our understanding of pathophysiology after TBI improves, the number of monitoring devices and techniques will assuredly continue to increase. Thus, the biggest issue we face currently and in the future is that of information "overload." With data, both continuous and intermittent, streaming from various devices, how does the clinician integrate these findings into practice? When and how do we intervene on the information obtained? Which monitors provide useful information? Which provide unhelpful "noise?" All of these questions currently remain unanswered.

There is some potential for the application of computer-based algorithmic interpretation of the data.[98,99] Through application of basic machine learning techniques, and more advance-convolutional neural networks, we can potentially harness the power of automated interpretation of the data. This could allow us to impute missing data, generate more robust predictive models for outcome and secondary injury events, and provide comprehensive and detailed imaging analysis. More importantly, these techniques may allow us to more easily integrate all aspects of MMM in cerebral neurotrauma, creating the opportunity for ease of application of these techniques and clinician interpretation. Furthermore, as we learn from the data, so can computers; leading to ever improving analysis, interpretation, and prediction methods/models.

ACKNOWLEDGMENTS

FAZ—This work was made possible through salary support through the Cambridge Commonwealth Trust Scholarship, the Royal College of Surgeons of Canada—Harry S. Morton Travelling Fellowship in Surgery, the University of Manitoba Clinician Investigator Program, R. Samuel McLaughlin Research and Education Award, the Manitoba Medical Service Foundation, and the University of Manitoba Faculty of Medicine Dean's Fellowship Fund.

REFERENCES

1. Steyerberg EW, Mushkudiani N, Perel P et al. Predicting outcome after traumatic brain injury: Development and international validation of prognostic scores based on admission characteristics. *PLoS Med.* 2008;5:e165.
2. Lingsma H, Andriessen TM, Haitsema I et al. Prognosis in moderate and severe traumatic brain injury: External validation of the IMPACT models and the role of extracranial injuries. *J Trauma Acute Care Surg.* 2013;74:639-646.
3. Honeybul S, Ho KM. Predicting long-term neurological outcomes after severe traumatic brain injury requiring decompressive craniectomy: A comparison of the CRASH and IMPACT prognostic models. *Injury.* 2016;47:1886-1892.
4. Zeiler FA, Donnelly J, Calviello L, Smielewski P, Menon DK, Czosnyka M. Pressure Autoregulation Measurement Techniques in Adult TBI, Part I: A scoping review of intermittent methods. *J Neurotrauma.* 2017;34(23):3207-3223. doi:10.1089/neu.2017.5085.
5. Amyot F, Arciniegas DB, Brazaitis MP et al. A review of the effectiveness of neuroimaging modalities for the detection of traumatic brain injury. *J Neurotrauma.* 2015;32(22):1693-1721.
6. Zeiler FA, Donnelly J, Calviello L, Smielewski P, Menon DK, Czosnyka M. Pressure autoregulation measurement techniques in adult TBI, Part II: A scoping review of continuous methods. *J Neurotrauma.* 2017;34(23):3207-3223. doi:10.1089/neu.2017.5085.
7. Le Roux P, Menon DK, Citerio G et al. Consensus summary statement of the international multidisciplinary consensus conference on multimodality monitoring in neurocritical care: A statement for healthcare professionals from the Neurocritical Care Society and the European Society of Intensive Care Medicine. *Neurocrit Care.* 2014;21(2):S1-26.
8. Hutchinson PJ, Jalloh I, Helmy A et al. Consensus statement from the 2014 International Microdialysis Forum. *Intensive Care Med.* 2015;41(9):1517-1528.
9. Monro A. *Observations on Structure and Functions of the Nervous System.* Edinbourg, UK: Creech and Johnson; 1783.
10. Lundberg N, Troupp H, Lorin H. Continuous recording of the ventricular-fluid pressure in patients with severe acute traumatic brain injury. A preliminary report. *J Neurosurg.* 1965;22(6):581-590.
11. Kaufmann GE, Clark K. Continuous simultaneous monitoring of intraventricular and cervical subarachnoid cerebrospinal fluid pressure to indicate development of cerebral or tonsillar herniation. *J Neurosurg.* 1970;33(2):145-150.
12. Carney N, Totten AM, O'Reilly C et al. Guidelines for the Management of Severe Traumatic Brain Injury. 4th ed. *Neurosurgery.* 2017;80(1):6-15.
13. Sorrentino E, Diedler J, Kasprowicz M et al. Critical thresholds for cerebrovascular reactivity after traumatic brain injury. *Neurocrit Care.* 2012;16(2):258-266.
14. Chesnut RM, Temkin N, Carney N et al. Global Neurotrauma Research Group. A trial of intracranial-pressure monitoring in traumatic brain injury. *N Engl J Med.* 2012;367(26):2471-2481.
15. Härtl R, Stieg PE. Intracranial pressure is still number 1 despite BEST:TRIP study. *World Neurosurg.* 2013;79(5-6):599-600.
16. Raboel PH, Bartek J Jr, Andresen M, Bellander BM, Romner B. Intracranial pressure monitoring: Invasive versus non-invasive methods—A review. *Crit Care Res Pract.* 2012;2012:950393.
17. Khan MN, Shallwani H, Khan MU, Shamim MS. Noninvasive monitoring intracranial pressure—A review of available modalities. *Surg Neurol Int.* 2017;8:51.
18. Cardim D, Robba C, Bohdanowicz M et al. Non-invasive monitoring of intracranial pressure using transcranial doppler ultrasonography: Is it possible? *Neurocrit Care.* 2016;25(3):473-491.
19. Zeiler FA, Unger B, Kramer AH, Kirkpatrick AW, Gillman LM. A unique model for ultrasound assessment of optic nerve sheath diameter. *Can J Neurol Sci.* 2013;40(2):225-229.
20. Dubourg J, Javouhey E, Geeraerts T, Messerer M, Kassai B. Ultrasonography of optic nerve sheath diameter for detection of raised intracranial pressure: A systematic review and meta-analysis. *Intensive Care Med.* 2011;37(7):1059-1068.

21. Geeraerts T, Launey Y, Martin L et al. Ultra-sonography of the optic nerve sheath may be useful for detecting raised intracranial pressure after severe brain injury. *Intensive Care Med.* 2007;33(10):1704-1711.

22. Goeres P, Zeiler FA, Unger B, Karakitsos D, Gillman LM. Ultrasound assessment of optic nerve sheath diameter in healthy volunteers. *J Crit Care.* 2016;31(1):168-171.

23. Zeiler FA, Ziesmann MT, Goeres P et al. A unique method for estimating the reliability learning curve of optic nerve sheath diameter ultrasound measurement. *Crit Ultrasound J.* 2016;8(1):9.

24. Armstead WM. Cerebral blood flow autoregulation and dysautoregulation. *Anesthesiol Clin.* 2016;34(3):465-477.

25. Calviello LA, de Riva N, Donnelly J et al. Relationship between brain pulsatility and cerebral perfusion pressure: Replicated validation using different drivers of CPP change. *Neurocrit Care.* 2017;27(3):392-400. doi:10.1007/s12028-017-0404-9. [Epub ahead of print]

26. Lassen NA. Cerebral blood flow and oxygen consumption in man. *Physiol Rev.* 1959;39(2):183-238.

27. Czosnyka M, Smielewski P, Kirkpatrick P, Laing RJ, Menon D, Pickard JD. Continuous assessment of the cerebral vasomotor reactivity in head injury. *Neurosurgery.* 1997;41(1):11-17.

28. Aries MJ, Czosnyka M, Budohoski KP et al. Continuous monitoring of cerebrovascular reactivity using pulse waveform of intracranial pressure. *Neurocrit Care.* 2012;17(1):67-76.

29. Lang EW, Kasprowicz M, Smielewski P, Santos E, Pickard J, Czosnyka M. Short pressure reactivity index versus long pressure reactivity index in the management of traumatic brain injury. *J Neurosurg.* 2015;122(3):588-594.

30. Brady KM, Lee JK, Kibler KK, Easley RB, Koehler RC, Shaffner DH. Continuous measurement of autoregulation by spontaneous fluctuations in cerebral perfusion pressure: Comparison of 3 methods. *Stroke.* 2008;39:2531-2537.

31. Jaeger M, Schuhmann MU, Soehle M, Meixensberger J. Continuous assessment of cerebrovascular autoregulation after traumatic brain injury using brain tissue oxygen pressure reactivity. *Crit Care Med.* 2006;34:1783-1788.

32. Dias C, Silva MJ, Pereira E et al. Optimal cerebral perfusion pressure management at bedside: A single-center pilot study. *Neurocrit Care.* 2015; 23:92-102.

33. Ngwenya LB, Burke JF, Manley GT. Brain tissue oxygen monitoring and the intersection of brain and lung: A comprehensive review. *Respir Care.* 2016;61(9):1232-1244.

34. Vajkoczy P, Schomacher M, Czabanka M, Horn P. Monitoring cerebral blood flow in neurosurgical intensive care. *Eur Neurolog Dis.* 2007;1:8-10.

35. Rosenthal G, Sanchez-Mejia RO, Phan N, Hemphill JC 3rd, Martin C, Manley GT. Incorporating a parenchymal thermal diffusion cerebral blood flow probe in bedside assessment of cerebral autoregulation and vasoreactivity in patients with severe traumatic brain injury. *J Neurosurg.* 2011;114:62-70.

36. Oshorov A, Savin I, Popugaev K, Ptopov A. Influence of hyperthermia on the parameters of MAP, CPP and PRx in patients with severe TBI. *Brain Inj.* 2014;28:797.

37. Budohoski KP, Czosnyka M, de Riva N et al. The relationship between cerebral blood flow autoregulation and cerebrovascular pressure reactivity after traumatic brain injury. *Neurosurgery.* 2012;71(3):652-660.

38. Budohoski KP, Reinhard M, Aries MJ et al. Monitoring cerebral autoregulation after head injury. Which component of transcranial Doppler flow velocity is optimal? *Neurocrit Care.* 2012;17(2):211-218.

39. Sorrentino E, Budohoski KP, Kasprowicz M et al. Critical thresholds for transcranial Doppler indices of cerebral autoregulation in traumatic brain injury. *Neurocrit Care.* 2011;14(2):188-193.

40. Czosnyka M, Miller C. Participants in the International Multidisciplinary Consensus Conference on Multimodality Monitoring. Monitoring of cerebral autoregulation. *Neurocrit Care.* 2014;21(Suppl 2):S95-102.

41. Zeiler FA, Donnelly J, Menon D et al. Continuous autoregulatory indices derived from multi-modal monitoring: Each one is not like the other. *J Neurotrauma.* 2017;34(22):

3070-3080. doi:10.1089/neu.2017.5129. [Epub ahead of print]

42. Needham E, McFadyen C, Newcombe V, Synnot AJ, Czosnyka M, Menon D. Cerebral perfusion pressure targets individualized to pressure-reactivity index in moderate to severe traumatic brain injury: A systematic review. *J Neurotrauma*. 2017;34(5):963-970.

43. Dias C, Silva MJ, Pereira E et al. Optimal cerebral perfusion pressure management at bedside: A single-center pilot study. *Neurocrit Care*. 2015;23:92-102.

44. Kirkpatrick PJ, Smielewski P, Czosnyka M, Pickard JD. Continuous monitoring of cortical perfusion by laser Doppler flowmetry in ventilated patients with head injury. *J Neurol Neurosurg Psychiatry*. 1994;57(11):1382-1388.

45. Zweifel C, Czosnyka M, Lavinio A et al. A comparison study of cerebral autoregulation assessed with transcranial Doppler and cortical laser Doppler flowmetry. *Neurol Res*. 2010;32(4):425-428.

46. Sahuquillo J, Poca MA, Ausina A, Báguena M, Gracia RM, Rubio E. Arterio-jugular differences of oxygen (AVDO2) for bedside assessment of CO2-reactivity and autoregulation in the acute phase of severe head injury. *Acta Neurochir (Wien)*. 1996;138(4):435-444.

47. Steiner LA, Balestreri M, Johnston AJ et al. Effects of moderate hyperventilation on cerebrovascular pressure-reactivity after head injury. *Acta Neurochir Suppl*. 2005;95:17-20.

48. Puppo C, Fariña G, López FL Caragna E, Biestro A. Cerebral CO2 reactivity in severe head injury. A transcranial Doppler study. *Acta Neurochir Suppl*. 2008;102:171-175.

49. Mutch WA, Ellis MJ, Ryner LN et al. for The Canada North Concussion Network, and; for The University Health Network Cerebrovascular Reactivity Research Group. Brain magnetic resonance imaging CO2 stress testing in adolescent postconcussion syndrome. *J Neurosurg*. 2016;125(3):648-660.

50. Jalloh I, Helmy A, Shannon RJ et al. Lactate uptake by the injured human brain: Evidence from an arteriovenous gradient and cerebral microdialysis study. *J Neurotrauma*. 2013;30 (24):2031-2037.

51. White H, Baker A. Continuous jugular venous oximetry in the neurointensive care unit—A brief review. *Can J Anaesth*. 2002;49(6):623-629.

52. Schell RM, Cole DJ. Cerebral monitoring: Jugular venous oximetry. *Anesth Analg*. 2000;90(3):559-566.

53. Oddo M, Bösel J. Participants in the International Multidisciplinary Consensus Conference on Multimodality Monitoring. Monitoring of brain and systemic oxygenation in neurocritical care patients. *Neurocrit Care*. 2014;21(Suppl 2):S103-120.

54. Le Roux PD, Oddo M. Parenchymal brain oxygen monitoring in the neurocritical care unit. *Neurosurg Clin N Am*. 2013;24(3):427-439.

55. Zweifel C, Castellani G, Czosnyka M et al. Noninvasive monitoring of cerebrovascular reactivity with near infrared spectroscopy in head-injured patients. *J Neurotrauma*. 2010;27:1951-1958.

56. Weigl W, Milej D, Janusek D et al. Application of optical methods in the monitoring of traumatic brain injury: A review. *J Cereb Blood Flow Metab*. 2016;36(11):1825-1843.

57. Hutchinson PJ, Jalloh I, Helmy A et al. Consensus statement from the 2014 International Microdialysis Forum. *Intensive Care Med*. 2015;41(9):1517-1528.

58. Carpenter KL, Young AM, Hutchinson PJ. Advanced monitoring in traumatic brain injury: Microdialysis. *Curr Opin Crit Care*. 2017;23(2):103-109.

59. Helmy A, Carpenter KL, Skepper JN, Kirkpatrick PJ, Pickard JD, Hutchinson PJ. Microdialysis of cytokines: Methodological considerations, scanning electron microscopy, and determination of relative recovery. *J Neurotrauma*. 2009;26(4):549-561.

60. Timofeev I, Carpenter KLH, Nortje J et al. Cerebral extracellular chemistry and outcome following traumatic brain injury: A microdialysis study of 223 patients. *Brain*. 2011;134(Part 2):484-494.

61. Reinert M, Khaldi A, Zauner A, Doppenberg E, Choi S, Bullock R. High level of extracellular potassium and its correlates after severe head injury: Relationship to high intracranial pressure. *J Neurosurg*. 2000;93(5):800-807.

62. Helmy A, Guilfoyle MR, Carpenter KL, Pickard JD, Menon DK, Hutchinson PJ. Recombinant human interleukin-1 receptor antagonist promotes M1 microglia biased cytokines and chemokines following human traumatic brain injury. *J Cereb Blood Flow Metab.* 2016;36(8):1434-1448.

63. Zeiler FA, Thelin E, Helmy A, Czosnyka M, Hutchinson PJ, Menon DK. CSF and Microdialysis Cytokines in Severe TBI: A scoping systematic review. *Front Neurol.* 2017;8:331.

64. Helmy A, Guilfoyle MR, Carpenter KL, Pickard JD, Menon DK, Hutchinson PJ. Recombinant human interleukin-1 receptor antagonist in severe traumatic brain injury: A phase II randomized control trial. *J Cereb Blood Flow Metab.* 2014;34(5):845-851.

65. Guilfoyle MR, Carpenter KL, Helmy A, Pickard JD, Menon DK, Hutchinson PJ. Matrix metalloproteinase expression in contusional traumatic brain injury: A paired microdialysis study. *J Neurotrauma.* 2015;32(20):1553-1559.

66. Roberts DJ, Jenne CN, Léger C et al. A prospective evaluation of the temporal matrix metalloproteinase response after severe traumatic brain injury in humans. *J Neurotrauma.* 2013;30(20):1717-1726.

67. Roberts DJ, Jenne CN, Léger C et al. Association between the cerebral inflammatory and matrix metalloproteinase responses after severe traumatic brain injury in humans. *J Neurotrauma.* 2013; 30(20):1727-1736.

68. Carpenter KL, Czosnyka M, Jalloh I et al. Systemic, local, and imaging biomarkers of brain injury: More needed, and better use of those already established? *Front Neurol.* 2015;6:26.

69. Jalloh I, Carpenter KL, Helmy A, Carpenter TA, Menon DK, Hutchinson PJ. Glucose metabolism following human traumatic brain injury: Methods of assessment and pathophysiological findings. *Metab Brain Dis.* 2015;30(3):615-632.

70. Coles JP, Steiner LA, Johnston AJ et al. Does induced hypertension reduce cerebral ischaemia within the traumatized human brain? *Brain.* 2004;127(Pt 11):2479-2490.

71. Steiner LA, Coles JP, Johnston AJ et al. Responses of posttraumatic pericontusional cerebral blood flow and blood volume to an increase in cerebral perfusion pressure. *J. Cereb Blood Flow Metab.* 2003;23(11):1371-1377.

72. Steiner LA, Coles JP, Czosnyka M et al. Cerebrovascular pressure reactivity is related to global cerebral oxygen metabolism after head injury. *J Neurol Neurosurg Psychiatry.* 2003;74(6):765-770.

73. Hutchinson PJ, O'Connell MT, Seal A et al. A combined microdialysis and FDG-PET study of glucose metabolism in head injury. *Acta Neurochir.* 2009;151(1):51-61.

74. Vespa PM, McArthus D, O'Phelan K et al. Persistently low extracellular glucose correlates with poor outcome 6 months after human traumatic brain injury despite a lack of increased lactate: A microdialysis study. *J Cereb Blood Flow Metab.* 2003;23(7):865-877.

75. Chieregato A, Marchi M, Fainardi E, Targa L. Cerebral arterio-venous pCO2 difference, estimated respiratory quotient, and early posttraumatic outcome: Comparison with arterio-venous lactate and oxygen differences. *J Neurosurg Anesthesiol.* 2007;19(4):222-228.

76. Poca MA, Sahuquillo J, Vilalta A, Garnacho A. Lack of utility of arteriojugular venous differences of lactate as a reliable indicator of increased brain anaerobic metabolism in traumatic brain injury. *J Neurosurg.* 2007;106(4):530-537.

77. Tahsili-Fahadan P, Geocadin RG. Heart-brain axis: Effects of neurologic injury on cardiovascular function. *Circ Res.* 2017;120(3):559-572.

78. Takahashi C, Hinson HE, Baguley IJ. Autonomic dysfunction syndromes after acute brain injury. *Handb Clin Neurol.* 2015;128:539-551.

79. Sykora M, Czosnyka M, Liu X et al. Autonomic Impairment in severe traumatic brain injury: A multimodal neuromonitoring study. *Crit Care Med.* 2016;44(6):1173-1181.

80. Lavinio A, Ene-Iordache B, Nodari I et al. Cerebrovascular reactivity and autonomic drive following traumatic brain injury. *Acta Neurochir Suppl.* 2008;102:3-7.

81. Childs C, Wang L, Neoh BK et al. Multi-parameter brain tissue microsensor and interface systems: Calibration, reliability and user experiences of pressure and temperature sensors in the setting of neurointensive care. *J Med Eng Technol.* 2014;38(7):339-350.

82. Stewart C, Haitsma I, Zador Z et al. The new Licox combined brain tissue oxygen and brain temperature monitor: Assessment of in vitro accuracy and clinical experience in severe traumatic brain injury. *Neurosurgery.* 2008;63(6):1159-1164.

83. Schiefecker AJ, Kofler M, Gaasch M et al. Brain temperature but not core temperature increases during spreading depolarizations in patients with spontaneous intracerebral hemorrhage. *J Cereb Blood Flow Metab.* 2017:271678X17703940. doi: 10.1177/0271678 X17703940. [Epub ahead of print]

84. Schmitt S, Dichter MA. Electrophysiologic recordings in traumatic brain injury. *Handb Clin Neurol.* 2015;127:319-339.

85. Cohen AS, Pfister BJ, Schwarzbach E, Grady MS, Goforth PB, Satin LS. Injury-induced alterations in CNS electrophysiology. *Prog Brain Res.* 2007;161:143-169.

86. Wang JT, Young GB, Connolly JF. Prognostic value of evoked responses and event-related brain potentials in coma. *Can J Neurol Sci.* 2004;31(4):438-450.

87. Kramer DR, Fujii T, Ohiorhenuan I, Liu CY. Cortical spreading depolarization: Pathophysiology, implications, and future directions. *J Clin Neurosci.* 2016;24:22-27.

88. Vaewpanich J, Reuter-Rice K. Continuous electroencephalography in pediatric traumatic brain injury: Seizure characteristics and outcomes. *Epilepsy Behav.* 2016;62:225-230.

89. Stevens RD, Sutter R. Prognosis in severe brain injury. *Crit Care Med.* 2013;41(4):1104-1123.

90. Stecker MM, Sabau D, Sullivan L et al. American clinical neurophysiology society guideline 6: Minimum technical standards for EEG recording in suspected cerebral death. *J Clin Neurophysiol.* 2016;33(4):324-327.

91. Wijdicks EF, Varelas PN, Gronseth GS, Greer DM. American Academy of Neurology. Evidence-based guideline update: Determining brain death in adults: Report of the Quality Standards Subcommittee of the American Academy of Neurology. *Neurology.* 2010;74(23):1911-1198.

92. Vinciguerra L, Bösel J. Noninvasive neuromonitoring: Current utility in subarachnoid hemorrhage, traumatic brain injury, and stroke. *Neurocrit Care.* 2017;27(1):122-140. doi: 10.1007/s12028-016-0361-8. [Epub ahead of print]

93. Hartings JA, Watanabe T, Bullock MR et al. Co-Operative Study on Brain Injury Depolarizations. Spreading depolarizations have prolonged direct current shifts and are associated with poor outcome in brain trauma. *Brain.* 2011;134(Pt 5):1529-1540.

94. Hinzman JM, Andaluz N, Shutter LA et al. Inverse neurovascular coupling to cortical spreading depolarizations in severe brain trauma. *Brain.* 2014;137(Pt 11):2960-2972.

95. Bosco E, Zanatta P, Ponzin D et al. Prognostic value of somatosensory-evoked potentials and CT scan evaluation in acute traumatic brain injury. *J Neurosurg Anesthesiol.* 2014;26(4):299-305.

96. Erbengi A, Erbengi G, Cataltepe O, Topcu M, Erbas B, Aras T. Brain death: Determination with brain stem evoked potentials and radionuclide isotope studies. *Acta Neurochir (Wien).* 1991;112(3-4):118-125.

97. Gao L, Smielewski P, Czosnyka M, Ercole A. Cerebrovascular signal complexity six hours after intensive care unit admission correlates with outcome after severe traumatic brain injury. *J Neurotrauma.* 2016;33(22):2011-2018.

98. Jordan MI, Mitchell TM. Machine learning: Trends, perspectives, and prospects. *Science.* 2015;349(6245):255-260.

99. Lucas P. Bayesian analysis, pattern analysis, and data mining in health care. *Curr Opin Crit Care.* 2004;10(5):399-403.

PART VII

Neuroradiology

14

Neuroradiology in neurotrauma

ZAKIR HAJAT

INTRODUCTION

Traumatic brain injury (TBI) is relatively common and a potentially devastating event. It is the leading cause of death in North American males ages 1 through 45, and affects 235 per 100,000 Europeans. It disproportionality affects younger people, who suffer life-changing injuries that result in significant socioeconomic costs.[1,2]

The advent of computed tomography (CT) has revolutionized the detection and management of TBIs. Almost all level 1 trauma centers in the developed world employ the use of immediate plain (noncontrast-enhanced) CT scanning to identify gross abnormalities and mass effect, which helps the decision-making process to manage the injury conservatively or surgically. Magnetic resonance imaging (MRI) is not recommended as a first-line investigation in brain injury,[3] but its role in supplying detailed imagery for diagnosis and prognostication is important once the patient's initial stability has been achieved. Magnetic resonance (MR) scans are still time consuming, and in the context of time critical injuries the benefits of higher-resolution images do not outweigh the significant risk of exacerbating secondary brain injury. Plain x-ray films have been largely superseded by CT imaging and have no role in the immediate management of head trauma. Ultrasonography has been of limited use because of the attenuation of sound through the dense adult skull, but its use in the pediatric skull is well established. Research is ongoing in using basic ultrasound techniques through the thinnest segments of the adult skull to re-create three-dimensional images of the brain "in the field" to aid prehospital diagnosis.

COMPUTED TOMOGRAPHY

The invention of CT scanning in 1967 has revolutionized the management of trauma care and the practice of medicine altogether. The modern CT scanner emits, detects, and makes many measurements of attenuation of x-rays through tissues of differing density. A modern multi-slice scanner captures multiple cross-sectional slices of anatomy in a single acquisition, thereby avoiding superimposition of structures, a major benefit over conventional x-ray films. The x-ray "emitter" sits opposite multiple rows of "detectors" to form an array that rotates around a CT table at high velocity as the patient table moves through the scanner, resulting in a helical maneuver along the length of the patient table.[4] Radiation passes through air with ease and is attenuated greatly by water; this is represented on the Hounsfield unit (HU) scale. A graphical representation of this is displayed electronically with pixels graduated between black (air, –1000 HU) and white (water, 0 HU), and shades of gray to demonstrate the spectrum of densities between. Specific "windows" can be chosen such as "soft tissue" (50–300 HU) to better appreciate the densities in question.

The head CT takes slices of 5 to 10 mm at an angle parallel to the base of the skull. In the trauma setting, a plain film without enhancing contrast can highlight the presence of intra- and extra-axial blood within minutes, and the decision to intervene surgically can be made rapidly. The advantage of CT over MR studies is rapid acquisition (and therefore less movement artefact), which is particularly relevant in the confused patient who may not readily comply with instructions; superior bone detail (relevant in the trauma setting); and demonstration of calcifications.[5] The presence of ferromagnetic materials such as infusion pumps for sedation, and monitoring equipment for transfer of critical patients is of little consequence other than artefact for CT scanning equipment, but great care must be taken to keep such materials from the vicinity of the MR scanner.

MAGNETIC RESONANCE IMAGING

The CT scanner makes measurements of x-ray attenuation of tissue densities; the MRI is different in this regard by using a magnetic field and radiofrequency (RF) pulses to measure hydrogen (proton) density, tissue-relaxation times (T1, T2), and blood flows within tissue.[5] The presence of a magnetic field causes most hydrogen nuclei of tissue to align longitudinally along the field lines; the subsequent RF pulse disturbs the proton alignment into the transverse plane temporarily, and the protons relax to assume their previous alignment when the RF pulse is removed. The end result is a graphical image that displays differences in relaxation times. The hydrogen nuclei of fat-containing tissues relax rapidly; predominantly water-containing tissue relaxes slowly. The T1 signal refers to the relaxation time of nuclei from transverse to longitudinal alignment, with fatty tissue appearing bright and water-dense tissue appearing dark.[4]

As well as aligning with the magnetic field of the MR, the hydrogen nuclei in tissues spin on a natural axis. The presence of a magnetic field alters the "spin" to a specific frequency related to the energy of

the magnetic field. The RF pulse causes the "spin" to synchronize in phase; as the RF pulse is removed, the nuclei relax to their previous phase of "spin." T2 signal refers to this relaxation in phase (dephase); again hydrogen nuclei of water-dense tissue dephase slowly, although they appear bright on T2 weighted images, with fatty tissue appearing darker.[4,5]

With current technology, an MR scan takes considerably longer than CT to undertake and process, requiring patients to lie still for considerably longer periods. This becomes particularly relevant in non-compliant patients, those with learning disabilities and developmental delay who may not understand or comply with instructions, and the acutely confused. The anesthetist may be asked to provide conscious sedation or general anesthesia in the radiology environment; ideally, this should be conducted by senior staff trained in these surroundings with particular attention paid to MRI safety.

MRI SAFETY FOR ANESTHETISTS

The MR suite presents a unique set of problems for the anesthetist. An unfamiliar environment, anesthetic and MR equipment compatibility challenges, and restricted patient access make the provision of anesthesia particularly hazardous. The design of MR suites are subject to considerable planning; ideally, there should be the following:

- A suite reception where preliminary checks for MR safety are conducted by radiographers.
- A room fitted for the provision of volatile or intravenous anesthesia that is outside the scanner room (and therefore not necessarily MR compatible) where induction and stabilization of anesthesia occurs.
- MR-compatible anesthetic machines or infusion devices.
- MR-compatible monitoring equipment deemed safe for use within the inner controlled area.

Numerous manufacturers provide a variety of equipment for this purpose. A radiographer control room with good visibility into the inner controlled area of the patient is essential for continued monitoring by the anesthetist.[6]

Airway: Standard endotracheal tubes are satisfactory. Reinforced wire coil tubes are ill advised because of the heating effect. A pilot balloon containing metal springs is safe to use if adequately secured. Attention should be paid to adequately securing the endotracheal tube because the patient table will move longitudinally for the purpose of the scan, and reintubation with a ferromagnetic laryngoscope will not be possible. Face mask and MR-safe supraglottic airway devices should be kept in the controlled area in the event of accidental extubation.

Monitoring: Modern MR-safe equipment is increasingly wireless, with modules used within the inner control area that communicate wirelessly to a slave graphic display monitor in the radiographer's control room. Special electrocardiogram electrode stickers and fiber-optic cabling for saturations monitoring are required.

Anesthesia: Personal preferences will dictate the mode of anesthesia; both volatile and intravenous anesthesia or conscious sedation (if tolerable) are acceptable. The MR-compatible anesthetic machine may be located inside the inner controlled area or outside the controlled area with extended airway tubing. Consideration must be made for significant dead space in airway and intravenous tubing if located outside the inner controlled area. This will incur a delay in the delivery of intravenous drugs and inhaled volatile anesthesia, as well as a delay in capnography and gas sampling. It is good practice to prime and attach extra i.v. lumens with extended giving sets to allow the administration of vasopressors in the event of hemodynamic instability. Muscle relaxation is not usually necessary for the purpose of the scan.

Miscellaneous: Acoustic noise hazards should be minimized with ear protection and adequate padding of pressure areas to minimize tissue damage.

Recovery: A dedicated recovery area (or the anesthesia induction room) should be used for extubation or removal of any supraglottic airway, and postanesthesia care (PAC) should be delivered by trained PAC nursing staff. Depending on clinical requirements, some trauma patients will be transferred directly to the operating rooms, or critical care for a period of intubation or ventilation, and this area should be used to switch to conventional non-MR monitoring before transfer.

THE ROLE OF ANESTHESIA IN THE RADIOLOGY DEPARTMENT

Depending on local policies, the duty general anesthetist or subspecialty neuroanesthetist may be called on to attend the emergency department (ED) to perform or assist in the induction of anesthesia, and transfer of patients to the radiology suite for scanning and interventional procedures, transfer to theater for surgical intervention, and transfer to critical care thereafter.

The key areas of focus are:

- Induction of anesthesia
- Maintenance of anesthesia
- Airway protection (and control of CO_2)
- Hemodynamic stability
- Cervical spine immobility (for suspected spine injuries)
- Intracranial pressure (ICP) management (medical and pharmacological)

Induction: The induction of anesthesia in patients with critically increased ICP can be fraught with pitfalls. The conditions allowing intubation require a depth of anesthesia that is unresponsive to laryngoscopy, however, care has to be taken to maintain cerebral perfusion pressure in the context of raised intracranial pressure and minimizing secondary brain injury.

The induction agent of choice has been debated.[7] Etomidate has classically been used because of its favorable hemodynamic characteristics, but its use has fallen significantly in the last two decades over concerns of transient adrenal suppression from either a single dose or worse outcomes when it is used as a sedative in critical care.[8-16] Ketamine has historically been contraindicated, but this is based on weak evidence of raised ICP and concerns of hemodynamic stability; in fact, this has been labeled a "myth."[17-21] Some evidence even suggests ICP may be reduced by ketamine in adult and pediatric studies.[22,23] The debate has evolved, and there is a good argument for the use of ketamine in acute head injury with little evidence of worse outcomes.[24] Avoiding ketamine because of unproven theoretical concerns regarding raised ICP at the expense of hypotension caused by other agents (such as propofol) is ill-advised; in fact, ketamine should be considered the ideal agent.

Maintenance: The maintenance of anesthesia for the purpose of transfer to the radiology department and sedation during interventional procedures will depend entirely on the goals in mind. Volatile anesthesia is impractical, and nonscavenged vapor poses theoretical hazards for staff and is detrimental to the environment. If the purpose of sedation is to provide a completely still patient, then a combination of a hypnotic such as propofol or midazolam and opiate such as remifentanil or alfentanil to obtund stimulation is entirely appropriate and can be supplemented with muscle relaxant if necessary. Some radiologists will prefer a completely still patient to provide the best possible angiography images.

Surgical anesthesia is rarely necessary, and conscious sedation is considered much safer. Dexmedetomidine has been compared with propofol and remifentanil in a variety of surgical and interventional settings. It has been found to provide comparable sedation to propofol or remifentanil but with lower incidences of respiratory adverse events.[25] Dexmedetomidine is known to cause less respiratory depression[26,27] and is better suited to provide conscious sedation in the "awake" patient. Dexmedetomidine encourages natural sleep via endogenous sleep pathways,[28] producing a communicative patient compliant with operator requests. In time-critical procedures such as thrombectomy for cerebrovascular events, there may be insufficient time to deliver a loading dose of dexmedetomidine, a hybrid approach with propofol may be necessary.

Hemodynamic stability: The latest revision of the Brain Trauma Foundation guidelines[29] recommend maintaining systolic blood pressure >100 mmHg for patients ages 50 to 69, or >110 mmHg for patients ages 15 to 48 or over 70. The anesthetist may be asked to treat reactive vasospasm, which is covered elsewhere in this book.

CRITERIA FOR CT HEAD SCAN

Tools have been developed to apply evidence-based criteria to aid decision making in the ED. The most widely used and validated is the Canadian Head CT Rule (CCHR), which has also been adopted by the National Institute of Clinical Excellence UK in the 2014 best-practice guidance.[3] The CCHR investigated 3121 patients and identified five high-risk factors for neurological intervention and two additional medium-risk factors for clinically important brain injury on CT

scan, which were 100% and 98.4% sensitive, respectively, in patients who experienced a minor head injury. Patients who fulfill one of the following criteria should have a CT scan: witnessed loss of consciousness, definite amnesia, or witnessed disorientation in patients with a Glasgow Coma Scale (GCS) score of 13–15.[30]

High risk (for neurological intervention):

- GCS score <15 at 2 h after injury
- Suspected open or depressed skull fracture
- Any sign of basal skull fracture (hemotympanum, "racoon" eyes, cerebrospinal fluid otorrhea or rhinorrhea, Battle's sign)
- Two or more episodes of vomiting
- Age 65 years and older

Medium risk (for clinically important brain injury on CT):

- Amnesia before impact for more than 30 min, and
- Dangerous injury mechanism such as a pedestrian struck by a motor vehicle, a motor vehicle occupant ejected from the vehicle, or a fall from a height >3 feet or five stairsteps.

Patients with either two of the medium risk factors could have clinically important lesions that may be seen on CT but do not necessarily require surgical intervention.

The New Orleans Criteria (NOC) is another validated tool to aid decision making for CT head scans.[31] Recent studies have demonstrated that both the CCHR and NOC have comparable sensitivity (100%), although the CCHR has favorable specificity.[32–35] The NOC apply to patients with a GCS of 15 who fulfill one of the following criteria:

- Headache
- Vomiting
- Age >60
- Drugs or alcohol intoxication
- Persistent anterograde amnesia
- Visible trauma above the clavicle
- Seizure

Depending on local policy, the decision to perform scans will be taken jointly by ED physicians and radiologists. The role of the anesthetist is to safely facilitate these.

SUMMARY AND KEY POINTS

- The advent of CT and MRI technologies has revolutionized the management of traumatic brain injury.
- CT scanning is increasingly used as a routine diagnostic tool in the initial trauma survey, and anesthetists may be called upon to safely facilitate these investigations.
- MR scanning is rarely used in the acute trauma investigation series.
- General anaesthesia can be avoided with skilled sedation techniques.
- Multidisciplinary working with emergency department physicians, neurosurgeons, and radiologists is required to drive excellent patient outcomes.

REFERENCES

1. Alverson C, Browne D, Dunn K et al. *Traumatic brain injury in the United States: Centres for Disease Control and Prevention. A report to Congress*, Atlanta, GA; 1999.
2. Tagliaferri F, Compagnone C, Korsic M et al. A systematic review of brain injury epidemiology in Europe. *Acta Neurochir*. 2006;148:255.
3. NICE. Head injury: Assessment and early management. 2014. https://www.nice.org.uk/guidance/cg176/chapter/1-Recommendations#assessment-in-the-emergency-department-2.
4. Chowdhury R, Wilson I, Rofe C, Lloyd-Jones G. *Radiology at a Glance*. Chichester, UK: Blackwell Publishing; 2010.
5. Brant WE, Helms C. *Fundamentals of Diagnostic Radiology*. Philadelphia: Lippincot Williams & Wilkins, 2012.
6. Association of Anaesthetists of Great Britain and Ireland. Provision of anaesthetic services in magnetic resonance units. AAGBI May, 2002. https://www.aagbi.org/sites/default/files/mri02.pdf.
7. Upchurch CP, Grijalva CG, Russ S et al. Comparison of etomidate and ketamine for induction during rapid sequence intubation of adult trauma patients. *Ann Emerg Med*. 2017;69(1):24-33.
8. De Coster R, Helmers JH, Noorduin H. Effect of etomidate on cortisol biosynthesis: Site of action after induction of anaesthesia. *Eur J Endocrinol*. 1985;110(4):526-531.
9. Duthie DJ. Fraser R, Nimmo WS. Effect of induction of anaesthesia with etomidate on corticosteroid synthesis in man. *Br J Anaesth*. 1985;57(2):156-159.
10. Diago MC, Amado JA, Otero M, Lopez-Cordovilla JJ. Anti-adrenal action of a sub-anaesthetic dose of etomidate. *Anaesthesia*. 1988;43(8):644-645.
11. Vinclair M, Broux C, Faure P et al. Duration of adrenal inhibition following a single dose of etomidate in critically ill patients. *Intensive Care Med*. 2007;34(4):714-719.
12. Schenarts CL, Burton JH, Riker RR. Adreno-cortical dysfunction following etomidate induction in emergency department patients. *Acad Emerg Med*. 2001;8(1):1-7.
13. Absalom A, Pledger D, Kong A. Adrenocortical function in critically ill patients 24 H after a single dose of etomidate. *Anaesthesia*. 1999;54(9):861-867.
14. Ledingham I. Influence of sedation on mortality in critically ill multiple trauma patients. *Lancet*. 1983;321(8336):1270.
15. Watt I, Ledingham IM. Mortality amongst multiple trauma patients admitted to an intensive therapy unit. *Anaesthesia*. 1983;39(10):973-981.
16. Wagner RL, White PF, Kan PB, Rosenthal MH, Feldman D. Inhibition of adrenal steroidogenesis by the anesthetic etomidate. *N Engl J Med*. 1984;310(22):1415-1421.
17. Filanovsky, Y, Miller P, Kao J. Myth: Ketamine should not be used as an induction agent for intubation in patients with head injury. *CJEM*. 2010;12(2):154-157.
18. Pagel PS, Kampine JP, Schmeling WT, Warltier DC. Ketamine depresses myocardial contractility as evaluated by the preload recruitable stroke work relationship in chronically instrumented dogs with autonomic nervous system blockade. *Anesthesiology*. 1992;76(4):564-572.
19. Dewhirst E, Frazier WJ, Leder M, Fraser DD, Tobias JD. Cardiac arrest following ketamine administration for rapid sequence intubation. *J Intensive Care Med*. 2013;28(6):375-379.
20. Scherzer D, Leder M, Tobias JD. Pro-con debate: Etomidate or ketamine for rapid

sequence intubation in pediatric patients. *J Pediatr Pharmacol Ther*. 2012;17(2):142-149.

21. Cohen L, Athaide V, Wickham ME, Doyle-Waters MM, Rose NG, Hohl CM. The effect of ketamine on intracranial and cerebral perfusion pressure and health outcomes: A systematic review. *Ann Emerg Med*. 2015;65 (1):43-51.

22. Bar-Joseph G, Guilburd Y, Tamir A, Guilburd JN. Effectiveness of ketamine in decreasing intracranial pressure in children with intracranial hypertension. *J Neurosurg Pediatr*. 2009;4(1):40-46.

23. Himmelseher S, Durieux ME. Revising a dogma: Ketamine for patients with neurological injury? *Anesth Analg*. 2005;101 (2):524-534.

24. Bourgoin A, Albanèse J, Wereszczynski N, Charbit M, Vialet R, Martin C. Safety of sedation with ketamine in severe head injury patients: Comparison with sufentanil. *Crit Care Med*. 2003;31(3):711-717.

25. Goettel N, Bharadwaj S, Venkatraghavan L, Mehta J, Bernstein M, Manninen PH. Dexmedetomidine vs propofol-remifentanil conscious sedation for awake craniotomy: A prospective randomized controlled trial. *Br J Anaesth*. 2016;116(6):811-821.

26. Kamibayashi T, Maze M. Clinical uses of alpha^2-adrenergic agonists. *Anesthesiology*. 2000;93(5):1345-1349.

27. Hsu Y-W, Cortinez LI, Robertson KM et al. Dexmedetomidine pharmacodynamics: Part I. *Anesthesiology*. 2004;101(5):1066-1076.

28. Nelson LE, Lu J, Guo T, Saper CB, Franks NP, Maze M. The alpha^2-adrenoceptor agonist dexmedetomidine converges on an endogenous sleep-promoting pathway to exert its sedative effects. *Anesthesiology*. 2003;98 (2):428-436.

29. Brain Trauma Foundation. *Guidelines for the Management of Severe Traumatic Brain Injury* 4th Edition. September 2016. https://brain trauma.org/uploads/03/12/Guidelines_for _Management_of_Severe_TBI_4th_Edition .pdf.

30. Stiell IG, Wells GA, Vandemheen K et al. The Canadian CT head rule for patients with minor head injury. *Lancet*. 2001;357(9266):1391-1396.

31. Haydel MJ, Preston CA, Mills TJ, Luber S, Blaudeau E, DeBlieux PM. Indications for computed tomography in patients with minor head injury. *N Engl J Med*. 2000;343(2):100-105.

32. Valle Alonso J, Fonseca Del Pozo FJ, Vaquero Álvarez M, Lopera E, Garcia Segura M, García Arévalo R. Comparison of the Canadian CT head rule and the New Orleans criteria in patients with minor head injury in a Spanish hospital. *Med Clin (English Edition)*. 2016;147 (12):523-530.

33. Mata-Mbemba D, Mugikura S, Nakagawa A et al. Canadian CT head rule and new orleans criteria in mild traumatic brain injury: Comparison at a tertiary referral hospital in Japan. *Springerplus*. 2016;5(1):5-176.

34. Kavalci C, Aksel G, Salt O et al. Comparison of the Canadian CT head rule and the New Orleans criteria in patients with minor head injury. *World J Emerg Surg*. 2014;9(1): 31.

35. Stiell IG. Comparison of the Canadian CT head rule and the New Orleans criteria in patients with minor head injury. *JAMA*. 2005;294 (12):1511-1518.

PART VIII

Neurointensive care

15

Sedation and analgesia

PAOLA CRISTINA VOLPI, BARBARA CAMBIAGHI, AND GIUSEPPE CITERIO

INTRODUCTION

This chapter discusses the role of sedative and analgesic drugs in the management of critically ill patients with traumatic brain injury (TBI),[1] providing an overview of the main benefits from using sedatives on the brain metabolism in the intensive care unit (ICU). The main open questions remain whether to sedate and for how long. The use of sedatives should be carefully evaluated to prevent the patient from running into so-called oversedation. Deep sedation is in fact associated with increased mortality, prolonged mechanical ventilation, and hospitalization. In this context, TBI patients appear to be an exception requiring, in the more severe cases, deep sedation as neuroprotective strategy to lower intracranial pressure (ICP). An overview of the main sedatives and analgesics used in ICU is presented.

RATIONALE AND INDICATIONS FOR SEDATION AND ANALGESIA IN NEUROTRAUMA[2]

The management of critically ill patients in intensive care units (ICUs) benefits from the use of specific analgesic and sedative drugs.[3] Sedation aims to relieve anxiety, reduce pain and discomfort, promote sleep, and modulate the stress response. Other properties of the sedative drugs used specifically in the neurointensive care unit include the possibility of reducing intracranial hypertension, reducing cerebral energy metabolic demands, and controlling refractory epileptic seizures.[4]

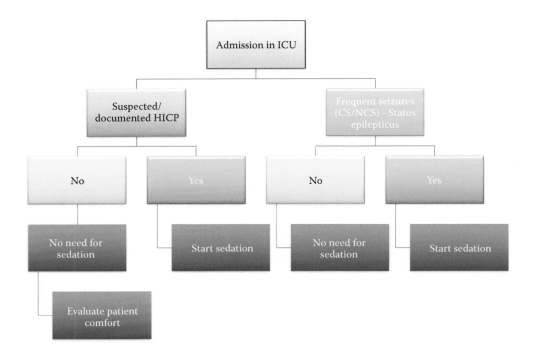

Deep sedation is responsible for prolonging ICU stays and hospitalization, worsening outcomes, and producing higher rates of delirium, muscle weakness, and death.[5–7] A light level of sedation should be sufficient and may avoid the potential harm caused by oversedation; minimal sedatives help reduce the duration of mechanical ventilation, improve short- and long-term mortality, and produce better long-term psychiatric outcomes with fewer post-traumatic stress disorders.[8,9]

In this background, the traumatic brain injured (TBI) patient appears to be a unique exception.[10]

In particular, sedatives play a major role in treating critically ill patients suffering from TBI because sedation exhibits a specific cerebral protective effect in reducing secondary damages. These agents are mainly used to reduce pain and handle discomfort and anxiety; in addition, they facilitate mechanical ventilation. But most of all, they control intracranial pressure.

In the case of a TBI, the brain suffers from major insults caused mainly by the potential mismatch between oxygen demand and delivery with a reduced tolerance to ischemia and other insults.[11,12]

Elevation of ICP after TBI is connected with brain edema, mass effects from hemorrhagic lesions, and disrupted pressure autoregulation. The treatments for ICP have focused on these pathophysiologic mechanisms, yet ICP often remains refractory to treatment and results in herniation and death. The mechanisms for persistently elevated ICP could be related to sustained hyperemia, excitotoxicity, and osmotic rebound.

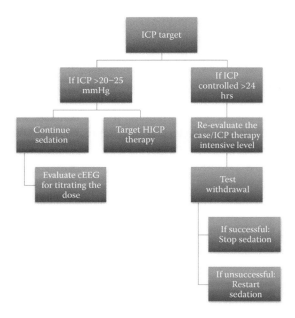

Goals for this regimen are several. Ideally, sedation and analgesia should decrease ICP and simultaneously sustain an adequate cerebral perfusion pressure and maintain cerebral autoregulation. In addition, $CMRO_2$ should be reduced, seizures avoided, and neuroprotection granted.

Sedation holds

Daily interruption of sedation (DIS) or a neurological wake-up test (NWT) is the most accurate way to detect neurological worsening, especially in the NICU, where the clinical exam remains the gold standard,[13] but this must be balanced with the risk that NWT can induce important ICP and CPP changes that may have negative effects on the injured brain.[14] Moreover, this could induce a biochemical stress response with increased levels of adrenocorticotropic hormone, cortisol, norepinephrine, and epinephrine,[15] even if it seems that it did not negatively alter focal neurochemistry or cerebral oxygenation.[16]

have been considered safe in medical and surgical ICU patients, but not for NICU patients, where a large number of trials had to be stopped because of safety issues and because only long-term benefits could be proven.[20]

In conclusion, DIS could be useful and considered together with definitive sedation interruption once the clinical picture and ICP, brain tissue PO_2, and cerebral physiology have normalized. While we are waiting for this moment, awakening should be replaced with multimodality monitoring and neuroimaging.[21]

Seizure suppression

In recent years, post-traumatic seizures have been documented as secondary events in addition to the already damaged brain because of the mismatch between oxygen delivery and metabolism. They have, in fact, been associated with increased ICP and increased metabolic requests with alterations of brain levels of glutamate and other excitatory

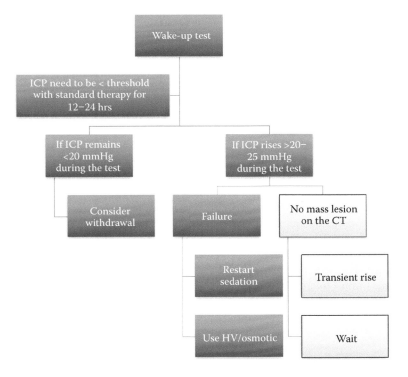

Benefits could be reducing the time of mechanical ventilation and the need for tracheostomy, shortening ICU and hospital stays, and reducing drug doses,[17–19] even if awakening trials

amino acids. Sedation serves as a therapeutic tool for high and persistent ICP. Moreover, sedation is well known to have a major role in the control of refractory *status* epilepticus, which occurs in a great number of primary and secondary forms of brain injury and requires the use of anesthetic agents followed by a slow reduction after at least 24 hours of effectiveness and the maintenance of anticonvulsants.[22] Convulsive and nonconvulsive seizures respond to 22% of neurological alterations after TBI.[23]

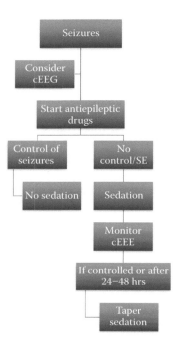

As for the mechanism underlying the development of status epilepticus, the alterations in the neurotransmitter compound have been found to be directly connected with so-called post-traumatic epilepsy (PTE). PTE is not an immediate manifestation following TBI but follows a latent period of epileptogenesis that depends on acute post-traumatic glutamate release and leads to immediate and delayed neuronal death and dysfunction.

In this context, the use of sedative agents is well known to improve the brain's tolerance to ischemia and augmented energetic requests, which thereby reduces the potential for epileptogenesis and its consequences.

Targeted temperature management

Sedation and analgesia help in the global management of TBI patients together with other strategies such as targeted temperature management. Even if mild hypothermia treatment is useful in decreasing ICP in TBI patients,[24] it is clear it does not improve outcome. Maintaining a normothermic TTM, on the other hand, does seem to be neuroprotective.[25–27]

TTM has become a standard treatment for TBI patients to reduce cerebral metabolism and control ICP and fever. It provides additional neuroprotective effects, but to reach a good result sedation itself is a challenging issue, mainly to avoid shivering and most important to blunt the endogenous stress response,[28] as already used after cardiac arrest.[29] Shivering is an impending phenomenon, starting from the masseter muscles and progressing to the neck muscles, the chest, and finally the extremities. It is normally assessed with a subjective tool called the Bedside Shivering Assessment Scale, which is correlated with indirect calorimetry and not used routinely. It therefore remains a pure research tool.

Different medications and doses have been proposed, yet we are still far from identifying the best approach. Prolonged sedative effects may confound neurological assessment and lead to erroneous decisions about a patient's prognosis. For this reason, new strategies have been analyzed to assess the depth of sedation.

Sedatives and analgesic agents and their effects are shown in Table 15.1.[30,31]

Propofol causes sedation and amnesia but has no analgesic activity. It is ideal for its characteristics and for daily reduction of sedation and neurologic examination of TBI patients. It increases the depth of sedation in a dose-dependent manner: at doses of ~4 mg/kg/h it preserves cerebrovascular reactivity and brain oxygenation and can be useful in neurologic injury because it reduces cerebral oxygen consumption and intracranial pressure. At higher doses, propofol may induce electroencephalogram (EEG) burst suppression, which can be used to treat status epilepticus.

Propofol may be related to a rare but fatal syndrome called propofol infusion syndrome (PRIS) (see the later section under "PRIS"). Another side effect is that propofol's vehicle is a lipid emulsion, and this can cause deep changes in albumin levels and disorders in fat metabolism that result in hypertriglyceridemia. For the same reason, the lipid emulsion in which propofol is carried includes additives containing soy proteins and egg yolk, which may provoke serious allergic reactions.

Dexmetomidine was introduced in 1999 as a light sedative that does not produce respiratory

Table 15.1 Major sedatives used in ICU, their pharmacology, and their effects on the CNS and adverse effects

Sedative	Mechanism	Characteristics	Onset	Elimination (after bolus)	CNS effects	Adverse effects
Propofol	Activate GABA Inhibit NMDA Modulate calcium influx	Highly lipophilic No active metabolites Eliminated by liver No impact on renal or hepatic function No drug interactions No analgesic properties No amnesia	1–2 min	10–15 min	Reduce ICP, $CMRO_2$, CBF Preserve CO_2 reactivity and cerebral autoregulation Reduce cerebral electrical activity	Tolerance and tachyphylaxis Vasodilatation and negative inotropic effect→ hypotension→ decrease in ICP Dose-dependent respiratory depression Bacterial contamination Allergic reactions (egg and soy proteins) Hypertriglyceridemia PRIS: propofol-related infusion syndrome
Dexmetomidine	α-2 agonist	Analgesic, hypnotic, and anxiolytic effects No respiratory depression Metabolism: CYP450 in liver, then kidney No active metabolites and no accumulation May reduce delirium by preserving focus and attention	15 min	2 hours	Little or no influence on ICP, CPP, $SjvO_2$, and $PbtO_2$	Bradycardia and hypotension after initial hypertension Careful in patients with renal and liver diseases
Benzodiazepines	Increase frequency of $GABA_a$ chloride channel opening in response to binding of GABA	Midazolam: accumulation of active metabolites but short duration of action (good for continuous infusion); highest lipid solubility; decrease dose also in renal failure.	1–5 min	1–2 hr	Reduce $CMRO_2$ and CBF Preserve CO_2 reactivity and cerebral autoregulation Antiepileptic effect	Tolerance and tachyphylaxis, with-drawal syndrome Dose-dependent respiratory depression

(Continued)

Table 15.1 (Continued) Major sedatives used in ICU, their pharmacology, and their effects on the CNS and adverse effects

Sedative	Mechanism	Characteristics	Onset	Elimination (after bolus)	CNS effects	Adverse effects
		Lorazepam: not for continuous infusion if rapid awakening is desired because of long elimination	5–20 min	2–6 hr	No analgesic properties	Careful in patients with renal and liver diseases ICU delirium
		Diazepam: not for continuous infusion for accumulation of active hepatic metabolites	2–5 min	2–4 hr		
Ketamine	NMDA-antagonist	Dissociative agent for brain function and electrophysiological dissociation Ensure analgesia and amnesia with hemodynamic and CPP stability No effects on respiratory drive or airway reflexes Bronchodilator activity Adjunct for refractory seizures or chronic pain management			Little or no influence on ICP, CPP, or $SjvO_2$	Hallucinations, dysphoria, blurred vision and diplopia, nystagmus Hypersalivation
Barbiturates	Increase duration of channel opening when stimulated by GABA Inhibit intracellular calcium influx Block glutamate receptors	Indications are limited to the treatment of refractory ICP and status epilepticus			Strongly reduce ICP, CBF, and $CMRO_2$ Preserve CO_2 reactivity and cerebral autoregulation	Hypotension and adrenal dysfunction Leucopoenia and immune suppression, increased risk of infections

depression and allows weaning from mechanical ventilation. In neurocritical care, it has shown promise because of its ability to allow patient arousal for neurologic examinations without interrupting the infusion. Adverse effects are hypotension and bradycardia; more important is the risk for agitation and "sympathetic rebound" following drug withdrawal. To minimize this risk dexmetomidine infusion should not be continued for longer than 24 hours.

In recent studies,[32,33] no significant differences have been demonstrated between the prevalence and severity of hypotension and bradycardia in both propofol and dexmetomidine when used with careful titration and no bolus dose.

Benzodiazepines are popular sedatives because they are generally safe in use and cause amnesia. They increase the seizure threshold and are useful anticonvulsants.[34] They are metabolized in the liver and excreted in the urine, so the dose needed for an adequate sedation is lower in elderly patients and patients with heart failure and hepatic insufficiency.

Ketamine does not alter systemic hemodynamic or respiratory drive, so it is better in hypotensive patients. The use of ketamine in TBI patients has been debated for a long time because of its effects on ICP, which have not been confirmed in the latest studies.[35]

The use of **barbiturates** is limited in NICU because of their adverse effects. They remain a second-line therapy for ICP control after propofol. Indications are limited to the treatment of refractory ICP and status epilepticus.

Volatile anesthetic agents have a long tradition of use in the operating room to provide general anesthesia. Since Kong et al.[36] demonstrated faster patient awakening and extubation times, interest in these anesthetics has increased. They are intrinsic vasodilators; they decrease $CMRO_2$ in a dose-dependent manner. Thereby, in the presence of intact flow metabolism, volatiles cause a coupled decrease in both $CMRO_2$ and cerebral blood flow (CBF). The decrease in CBF is opposed by the vasodilatory effect of these agents, ultimately resulting in either no change or small decreases in CBF at low minimum alveolar concentration (MAC). However, CBF increase with MAC after metabolic suppression is maximal.

At 0.5 MAC, for example, isoflurane, desflurane, and sevoflurane minimally delay but preserve the cerebral autoregulation, whereas at 1.5 MAC

autoregulation is considerably reduced by isoflurane and desflurane. Sevoflurane, in contrast, produces much less cerebral vasodilation and delays but preserves the autoregulatory response even at 1.5 MAC, making it the favored volatile agent during neuroanesthesia. However, the use of volatile agents requires specialized drug-delivery systems, gas scavenging, and education of nurses and intensivists with no anesthesia background. Adverse effects of these agents include nausea, vomiting, and possible fluoride-induced nephrotoxicity.

In a recent meta-analysis, the comparison between volatile agents and intravenous sedative drugs[37] showed no differences between the two modalities in adverse effects, death, and length of stay. Time to tracheal extubation is reduced with inhaled agents in comparison with standard intravenous sedatives, especially isoflurane with midazolam.

There are no studies comparing volatile agents and dexmetomidine; there is limited literature assessing safety and efficacy of these agents.

Opioids are the natural chemical derivatives of opium. They act as μ-opioid receptor agonists that produce a variety of effects, including analgesia, sedation, bradycardia, respiratory depression, nausea, and pruritus. They reinforce the effects of sedatives when used in combination, but do not cause amnesia when used alone.

Opioids could be used on boluses or continuous infusions, and individual dose requirements can vary widely. The effective dose of an opioid is determined by each patient's response, not by the numeric value of a dose.

In general, the *adverse effects* are similar in the different classes: a dose-dependent respiratory depression, centrally mediated, because of decreased respiratory rate and tidal volume, which can lead to hypercapnia (and thus increased ICP); chest wall rigidity; cardiovascular effects such as hypotension and bradycardia, especially in hypovolemic patients (and so increase in ICP, CPP, and CBF); nausea and vomiting via stimulation of the chemoreceptor trigger zone in the lower brainstem, gastrointestinal dysmotility; histamine release and so urticaria, flushing, and pruritus; and withdrawal symptoms if stopped suddenly after long infusions.

The most used classes of opioids in NICU are morphine, meperidine, fentanyl, and remifentanil.

- **Morphine** and **meperidine** have prolonged duration of action and can precipitate seizures, so they are not ideal for TBI patients. There is also accumulation in patients with renal diseases.

- **Fentanyl** is highly lipophilic and has a rapid onset (1–2 min) and short duration of action (30 min to 2 hours) after a single dose because of redistribution into peripheral tissues.

It is important to pay attention to prolonged administration because pharmacokinetics is altered and leads to accumulation and respiratory depression. Moreover, fentanyl is a CYP3A4 inducer, the same cytochrome used by phenytoin. This can be the reason for the variability of antiepileptic drugs in response to fentanyl administration.

- **Remifentanil**[38]: The rapid hydrolysis by non-specific esterase in plasma and tissues makes this opioid ideal for daily awakening for neurologic examination of patients. It has rapid blood–brain equilibration time (1–1.5 min), no accumulation in tissues, and ultrashort duration (half-time 3–10 min), so it requires continuous infusion. There is no problem using remifentanil in patients with renal or hepatic dysfunction. It can, however, cause bradycardia.

There are also **nonopioid** alternatives—NSAIDs—for providing analgesia via parenteral route, but they are less used in ICUs because of their adverse effects.

NEUROMONITORING FOR SEDATION AND ANALGESIA

Although sedation and analgesia remain important adjunct therapies for patients in ICU, they can mask changes in neurological examination. Clinical scales and new delivery technologies will help administering sedation become safer and more effective and help assess the appropriate level of depth of sedation and analgesia for each patient.[39]

Clinical Sedation Scales[40]

- The Ramsay Scale is used to describe the patient as "anxious," "calm," "reactive to orders," "reactive to pain or intense verbal stimuli," "minimal responsible," and "no answer."
- The Richmond Agitation-Sedation Scale (RASS)[41] is a more complete, logical, easy to administer, and readily recalled instrument. It goes from +4 (combative patient) to −5 (unarousable).

- The Riker Sedation Agitation Scale (SAS)[42] is a numeric scale from 7 to 1 with terms similar to RASS (dangerous agitation, very agitated, agitated, calm and cooperative, sedated, very sedated, unarousable).
- The Motor Activity Assessment Scale is the same as the SAS, with a score from 6 to 0.

All of these scales have reliability and validity in adult ICU patients. RASS and SAS are the most commonly reported, but neither is demonstrably superior.[7] The goal of sedation changes in different patients, ranging from calm and oriented to mildly sedated, depending on clinical conditions. No anxiety or panic should be present.

Clinical analgesia scales

- The Numeric Rating Scale (NRS) runs from 0, no pain, to 10, the worst pain ever experienced. It is used for patients who can communicate and self-report. The NRS target is ≤3.
- The Behavioral Pain Scale (BPS) from 3 to 12 evaluates some behavior of a patient who cannot communicate or who is ventilated. It takes into count "facial expression," "arm movements," and "ventilation compliance." The BPS target is <6.
- The Critical Care Pain Observation Tool (CCPOT)[43] is used to validate adults who are unable to reliably self-report. It has been deemed one of the most reliable behavioral pain-assessment tools. It takes into account and scores some indicators from 0 to 8: facial expression, body movements, muscle tension, compliance with ventilator in intubated patients, and vocalization in extubated patients. They seem to be the best behavioral and physiological indicators to recognize pain in these patients.
- The Nociception Coma Scale (NCS) is similar to CCPOT and has good validity with other scales used for noncommunicating patients. It is used especially in patients recovered from coma (vegetative state or minimally conscious state).

Assessment of pain is challenged by the patients' potential inability to report intensity of pain, especially severely brain-injured patients with disorders of consciousness. But "the inability to communicate verbally does not negate the possibility that an individual is experiencing pain" (International Association for the Study of Pain). Moreover,

TBI patients in NICU are known to experience more significant pain than initially presumed.

A diagnosis of coma, vegetative state, or minimally conscious state may affect pain perception by these patients and recognition by clinicians. The negative consequences of unrelieved pain are significant: insufficient sleep, post traumatic stress disorder (PTSD), and chronic pain.

Bispectral index monitoring

The Bispectral Index Monitor (BIS™, Covidien Inc., Boulder, CO, USA) came from processing the EEG signal with Fourier transformations, which produces a power-frequency spectrum used to monitor the depth of general anesthesia in patients without brain pathology. It provides a value from 0 to 100, with an awake patient scoring 90 or above and a patient under general anesthesia 40 to 60.

The bispectral index shows excellent correlations with the RASS and SAS scales in neurocritical care patients.[44] Brain injury may influence the bispectral array EEG algorithm because of EEG changes.

It could be used as an alternative to standard EEG for monitoring induction and maintenance of burst suppression instead of monitoring depth of sedation in neurotrauma patients.

EEG

An electroencephalographam is a graphical representation of voltage differences over certain areas of the cortex over time. Each EEG channel has two input electrodes to calculate a voltage difference, which could be negative or positive. If it is negative, the tracing goes upward; if it is positive, the tracing is deflected downward by convention.

This monitoring should be used to detect nonconvulsive seizure activity and to titrate medications to obtain burst suppression.

Focus

DELIRIUM

Delirium is an acute onset, but potentially reversible organic syndrome characterized by acute brain dysfunction, fluctuations in consciousness and cognition, inattention, disorganized thinking, and perceptual disturbances that develop over a brief period of time.[45] There may also be sleep disturbances, abnormal psychomotor activity, and emotional disturbances.

Patients may be agitated (hyperactive delirium), calm, or lethargic (hypoactive delirium). Delirium is a major public health problem, affecting 80% of mechanically ventilated adult ICU patients. The Confusion Assessment Method for the ICU[46] and the Intensive Care Delirium Screening Checklist[47] are the most valid delirium-monitoring tools.

Some risk factors must be known because delirium prevention is the best therapy: preexisting dementia, any history of hypertension or alcoholism, infections, metabolic disturbances, medications, elderly age, and coma. Noise reduction, hydration, and early mobilization can prevent delirium, but no medication.[48] It is important to recognize persisting sedation and underlying neurological issues as potential confounders.

There is no evidence that haloperidol can treat delirium (and it may increase the risk of seizures), whereas quetiapine and risperidone can be used.[49]

Propofol infusion syndrome

PRIS first appeared in pediatric literature by Bray in 1998. It described a clinical syndrome characterized by bradycardia and arrhythmias, cardiovascular collapse, and myocardial failure because of calcium channel blocking properties of propofol on the heart; metabolic lactic acidosis, hyperkalemia, rhabdomyolysis, and elevated creatine kinase because of muscle death; and then acute kidney injury and hepatomegaly.[50,51]

Pathophysiology consists in propofol-mediated defects in beta oxidation of fatty acids because acyl carnitine esters are impaired when entering the mitochondria, which produces failure in the mitochondrial respiratory chain. Fatty acids tend to accumulate in various organs.

Risk factors include high propofol dosage, prolonged use, young age, neurologic disease, catecholamine or glucocorticoid administration, mitochondrial disease, decreased carbohydrate store, and advanced stress. Moreover, all the conditions in which hepatic metabolism is reduced might aggravate the syndrome.

There is no specific treatment against PRIS.

CONCLUSION

Sedation and analgesia are fundamental tools in the management of TBI patients in the neurointensive care unit. Short-life sedatives (ie, propofol andremifentanil) should be preferred and deep sedation avoided, reserving it just when a neuroprotective strategy is required. Titration of drugs and suspension of sedatives should be considered when a patient's condition begins to improve; this will permit a global clinical evaluation and immediately detect any worsening of neurological conditions. Multimodal monitoring still remains the gold standard to individualize sedation when a patient's condition is not safe.

REFERENCES

1. Carney N, Totte AM, O'Reilly C et al. Guidelines for the Management of Severe Traumatic Brain Injury, 4th Edition. Neurosurgery. 2016.
2. Oddo M, Steiner LA. Sedation and analgesia in the neurocritical care unit. In: Oxford Textbook of Neurocritical Care. Oxford, UK: 2016.
3. Roberts DJ, Hall RI, Kramer AH, Robertson HL, Gallagher CN, Zygun DA. Sedation for critically ill adults with severe traumatic brain injury: A systematic review of randomized controlled trials. Crit Care Med. 2011;39: 2743-2751.
4. Oddo M, Crippa IA, Mehta S et al. Optimizing sedation in patients with acute brain injury. Crit Care. 2016;20:128.
5. Barr J, Fraser GL, Puntillo K, Ely EW, Gelinas C, Dasta JF. Clinical practice guidelines for the management of pain, agitation and delirium in adult patients in the intensive care unit. Crit Care Med. 2013;41:263-306.
6. Seder DB, Jagoda A, Riggs B. Emergency neurological life support: Airway, ventilation and sedation. Neurocrit Care. 2015;23:S5-S22.
7. Reade MC, Finfer S. Sedation and delirium in the intensive care unit. N Engl J Med. 2014;370:444-454.
8. Vincent J-L, Shehabi Y, Walsh TS et al. Comfort and patient centred care without excessive sedation: The eCASH concept. Intensive Care Med. 2016;42:962-971.
9. Gradwohl-Matis I, Mehta S, Dunser MW. What's new in sedation strategies? Intensive Care Med. 2015;41(9):1696-1699.
10. Citerio G, Cormio M. Sedation in neurointensive care: Advances in understanding and practice. Curr Opin Crit Care. 2003;9: 120-126.
11. Oertel M, Kelly DF, Lee JH. Metabolic suppressive therapy as a treatment for intracranial hypertension—Why it works and when it fails. Acta Neurochir Suppl. 2002;81: 69-70.
12. Robertson CS, Cormio M. Cerebral metabolic management. New Horiz. 1995;3:410-422.
13. Sharshar T, Citerio G, Andrews PJ, Chieregato A, Latronico N, Menon DK. Neurological examination of critically ill patients: A pragmatic approach. Report of an ESICM expert panel. Intensive Care Med. 2014;40:484-495.
14. Skoglund K, Enblad P, Marklund N. Effects of the neurological wake-up test on intracranial pressure and cerebral perfusion pressure in brain injured patients. Neurocrit Care. 2009;11:135-142.
15. Skoglund K, Enblad P, Hillered L, Marklund N. The neurological wake-up test increases stress hormone levels in patients with severe traumatic brain injury. Crit Care Med. 2012;40(1):216-222.
16. Skoglund K, Hillered L, Purins K et al. The neurological wake-up test does not alter cerebral energy metabolism and oxygenation in patients with severe traumatic brain injury. Neurocrit Care. 2014;20:413-426.
17. Brook AD, Ahrens TS, Schaiff R. Effect of a nursing-implemented sedation protocol on the duration of mechanical ventilation. Crit Care Med. 1999;27:2609-2615.
18. Kress JP, Pohlman AS O'Connor MF, Hall JB. Daily interruption of sedative infusions in critically ill patients undergoing mechanical ventilation. N Engl J Med. 2000;342:1471-1477.
19. Strøm T, Toft P. Time to wake up the patients in the ICU: A crazy idea or common sense? Minerva Anestesiol. 2011;77:59-63.
20. Helbok R, Kurtz P, Schmidt MJ et al. Effects of the neurological wake-up test on clinical examination, intracranial pressure, brain metabolism and brain tissue oxygenation in severely brain-injured patients. Crit Care. 2012;16(6):R226.
21. Prisco L, Citerio G. To wake-up, or not to wake-up: That is the Hamletic neurocritical care question! Crit Care. 2012;16:190.

22. Rossetti AO, Bleck TP. What's new in status epilepticus? *Intensive Care Med.* 2014;40: 1359-1362.

23. Vespa PM, Nuwer MR, Nenov V. Increased incidence and impact of nonconvulsive and convulsive seizures after traumatic brain injury as detected by continuous electroencephalographic monitoring. *J Neurosurg.* 1999;91:750-760.

24. Flynn LM, Rhodes J, Andrews PJ. Therapeutic hypothermia reduces intracranial pressure and partial brain oxygen tension in patients with severe traumatic brain injury: Preliminary data from the eurotherm 3235 trial. *Ther Hypothermia Temp Manag.* 2015;5(3):143-151.

25. Stein DM, Feather CBF, Napolitano LM. Traumatic brain injury advances. *Crit Care Clin.* 2017;33(1):1-13.

26. Dietrich WD, Bramlett HM. Therapeutic hypothermia and targeted temperature management in traumatic brain injury: Clinical challenges for successful translation. *Brain Res.* 1640:94-103.

27. Yokobori S, Yokota H. Targeted temperature management in traumatic brain injury. *J Intensive Care.* 2016;4:28.

28. Dell'Anna AM, Taccone FS, Halenarova K, Citerio G. Sedation after cardiac arrest and during therapeutic hypothermia. *Minerva Anestesiol,* 2014;80:954-962.

29. Riker RR, Gagnon DJ, May T, Seder DB, Fraser GL. Analgesia, sedation and neuromuscular blockade during targeted temperature management after cardiac arrest. *Best Pract Res Clin Anaesthesiol.* 2015;29(4):435-450.

30. DAS-Taskforce 2015. Evidence and consensus based guideline for the management of delirium, analgesia and sedation in intensive care medicine. Revision 2015 (DAS-Guideline 2015) - short version. *Ger Med Sci.* 2015.

31. Urwin SC, Menon DK. Comparative tolerability of sedative agents in head injured adults. *Drug Saf.* 2004;27:107-133.

32. Erdman MJ, Doepker BA, Gerlach AT, Phillips GS, Elijovich L, Jones GM. A comparison of severe hemodynamic disturbances between dexmetomidine and propofol for sedation in neurocritical care patients. *Crit Care Med.* 2014;42:1696-1702.

33. James ML, Olson DM, Graffagnino C. A pilot study of cerebral and haemodynamic physiological changes during sedation with dexmetomidine or propofol in patients with acute brain injury. *Anaesth Intensive Care.* 2012;40:949-957.

34. Hanley DF, Pozo M. Treatment of status epilepticus with midazolam in the critical care setting. *Int J Clin Pract.* 2000;54:30-35.

35. Himmelseher S, Durieux ME. Revising a dogma: Ketamine for patients with neurological injury? *Anaesth Analg.* 2005;101:524-534.

36. Kong KL, Willatts SM, Prys-Roberts C. Isoflurane compared with midazolam for sedation in the intensive care unit. *BMJ.* 1989;298:1277-1280.

37. Jerath A, Panckhurst J, Parotto M et al. Safety and efficacy of volatile anaesthetic agents compared with standard intravenous midazolam/propofol sedation in ventilated critical care patients. *Anesth Analg.* 2016; 1-10.

38. Fodale V, Schifilliti D, Pratico C, Santamaria LB. Remifentanil and the brain. *Acta Anaesthesiol Scand.* 2008;52:319-26.

39. Sheahan CG, Mathews DM. Monitoring and delivery of sedation. *Br J Anaesth.* 2014;113: ii37-ii47.

40. Riker RR, Fugate JE, Monitoring, Participants in the International Multi-disciplinary Consensus Conference on Multimodality. Clinical Monitoring scales in acute brain injury: Assessment of coma, pain, agitation and delirium. *Neurocrit Care.* 2014;21(suppl 2): S27-S37.

41. Sessler CN, Gosnell MS, Grap MJ. The Richmond Agitation-Sedation Scale: Validity and reliability in adult intensive care unit patients. *Am J Respir Crit Care Med.* 2002; 166:1338-1344.

42. Riker RR, Picard JT, Fraser GL. Prospective evaluation of the Sedation-Agitation Scale for adult critically ill patients. *Crit Care Med.* 1999;27:1325-1329.

43. Gélinas C, Fillion L, Puntillo KA, Viens C, Fortier, M. Validation of the Critical-Care Pain Observation Tool in Adult Patients. *Am J Crit Care.* 2006;15(4):420-427.

44. Deogaonkar A, Gupta R, DeGeorgia M et al. Bispectral index monitoring correlates with

sedation scales in brain injured patients. *Crit Care Med.* 2004;32:2403-2406.

45. *Diagnostic and statistical manual of mental disorders*, 4th ed. text rev.: DSM-IV-TR. American Psychiatric Association, Arlington, VA, 2011.

46. Ely EW, Inouye SK, Bernard GR. Delirium in mechanically ventilated patients: Validity and reliability of the Confusion Assessment Method for the Intensive Care Unit (CAM-ICU). *JAMA.* 2001;286:2703-2710.

47. Bergeron N, Dubois MJ, Dumont M, Dial S, Skrobik Y. Intensive Care Delirium Screening Checklist: Evaluation of a new screening tool. *Intensive Care Med.* 2001;27: 859-864.

48. Vidan MT, Sanchez E, Alonso M, Montero B, Ortiz J, Serra JA. An intervention integrated into daily clinical practice reduces the incidence of delirium during hospitalization in elderly patients. *J Am Geriatr Soc.* 2009; 57:2029-2036.

49. Brummel NE, Girard TD. Preventing delirium in the intensive care unit. *Crit Care Clin.* 2013;29:51-65.

50. Kang TM. Propofol infusion syndrome in critically ill patients. *Ann Pharmacother.* 2002;36(9):1453-1456.

51. Mirrakhimov AE, Voore P, Halytskyy O, Khan M, Ali AM. Propofol infusion syndrome in adults: A clinical update. *Crit Care Res Pract.* 2015;260385.

16

Nutrition and metabolic care

SWAGATA TRIPATHY

INTRODUCTION

Trauma is a leading cause of morbidity and mortality the world over. Affecting a productive population, it results in great monetary and social burdens on individuals, families, and healthcare systems. It includes traumatic brain injury (TBI) and spinal cord injury (SCI). Although both commonly occur together, they are different in how they affect the whole-body metabolism and the resultant nutritional requirements.

METABOLIC CHANGES IN NEUROTRAUMA

Trauma elicits a stress response in the body. The mechanism by which tissue injury affects the body physiology was first explained by Cuthbertson.[1] He classified the postinjury phase as that of a short "ebb" phase (characterized by decreases in cardiac output, oxygen consumption, body temperature, and metabolism) followed by a "flow" phase.

Increased circulating levels of stress hormones, breakdown of glycogen stores, and increased metabolic rates demarcate the flow phase. A period of anabolism may then follow this phase if the underlying pathology so allows.[2]

Metabolic response to traumatic brain injury

The brain is the primary gatekeeper of the metabolic activity of the whole body. Severe traumatic brain injury, therefore, predictably creates havoc in the metabolic milieu of the entire physiology.

Tissue damage results in changes in hormone and endocrine secretions. This results in severe catabolism, protein breakdown, and increased energy requirements. A proinflammatory cascade follows immediately after the trauma and is accompanied by the secretion of counter-regulatory hormones. Interleukins (IL-1, IL-6), tumor necrosis factor A, cortisol, catecholamine, and glucagon create a complex metabolic environment. A state of catabolism and altered immunity render the injured physiology susceptible to secondary infections and injury. As many as 75% of patients with TBI may suffer from infections, the most common complication in these patients.[3,4] Nuclear magnetic resonance spectroscopy using carbon 13 is used to investigate energy metabolism, neurotransmission, the intracellular redox state, and neuroglial compartmentation after TBI have revealed enhanced glycolytic production of lactate, pentose phosphate pathway activation, and alterations in neuronal and astrocyte oxidative metabolism that are dependent on injury severity.[5] The metabolic response to brain trauma can be of more than one type.

Differentiating between the two more common types of metabolic disturbances (the ischemic and the metabolic crisis) is important; treating for assumed ischemia may worsen a brain that is in metabolic crisis.

NORMAL PHYSIOLOGY

Pellerin and Magistretti's "neuron-astrocyte shuttle" model postulates that neuronal activity results in the release of glutamate at the neuronal clefts; when taken up by astrocytes, the glutamate stimulates the ion channels to allow the glucose in the vascular space to enter (the astrocyte).[6] This glucose is metabolized to lactate via the glycolytic pathway and is released into the extracellular space. The lactate then enters the neuron and is metabolized to pyruvate, which is used as energy substrate in the tricarboxylic acid (TCA) cycle. The astrocytes also convert glutamate into glutamine, which is converted back to glutamate in the neuronal cells.

METABOLIC DISTURBANCE IN ISCHEMIA

In ischemic conditions, the lack of oxygen and glucose at the level of the neurons causes decreased metabolism of pyruvate into glutamate via the TCA cycle. As pyruvate and glycogen continue to be converted to lactate in the astrocytes, the extracellular lactate levels increase, causing an elevated lactate pyruvate (LP) ratio. This is referred to as type 1 LP elevation and is associated with poor outcomes after TBI.[7]

METABOLIC CRISIS

A similar pattern of elevated LP ratio with increased extracellular glutamate may also occur in the absence of ischemia; this is called a type 2 LP elevation.

Vespa et al. postulated that mitochondrial dysfunction and increased metabolic demands in a background of traumatic brain injury may be the cause of this "metabolic crisis."[8] Following TBI, seizures and depolarization increase cerebral metabolism. The glycolytic pathway is inadequate to meet the increased demands, which leads to altered ion-channel activity, accumulation of Ca^{2+} ions in the cells, mitochondrial dysfunction, cell swelling, apoptosis, and death.[9]

Metabolic response to traumatic spinal cord injury

A period of intense hypercatabolism, urinary nitrogen, and whole-body protein loss follows acute spinal cord injury (SCI) as it does other injuries. Whereas in other trauma this phase stabilizes to a state of positive balance within 2 to 3 weeks, the stage of negative nitrogen balance continues for a long time in SCI patents. This results in muscle breakdown and dysimmunity despite adequate nutrition supplementation. Gut mucosal breakdown and sepsis are common occurrences. The cause of this resistant catabolic state is thought to be the result of widespread muscle denervation.[10]

Management of deranged metabolism

Multimodal monitoring of patients with TBIs frequently shows elevated LP ratios of >40. This may occur both with ischemia and in situations of metabolic crisis; the protocolized management in neurointensive care units (ICUs) with a focus on avoiding hypoxia and hypotension may be dealing with the former; the latter may be more difficult to detect and manage. A one-size-fits-all protocol management may be harmful in patients with "metabolic crises" because increased oxygen levels may worsen mitochondrial damage.

Currently, microdialysis and brain tissue oxygen monitoring values are being used to reach conclusions about the metabolic status of the brain. These modalities are neither used extensively nor are sufficiently sensitive or specific to enable changes in practice. There is a need to identify newer indicators of metabolic crisis in TBI patients that are easier to use and less expensive.

Nutrition and metabolism

Elevated extracellular lactate with normal $PtBO_2$ is common in patients with severe TBI, leading to the suggestion that lactate may be an effective energy substrate for the brain in these situations.[11] Clinical trial exploring the beneficial effects of exogenous infusion of lactates are currently ongoing.[12] As demonstrated in animal studies, a carbohydrate-free diet may result in lower lactate levels and better nitrogen balance in neurotrauma: ketones may provide energy more efficiently to the brain as compared to glucose.[13]

Neither adequate resuscitation after trauma nor complete enteral diets have been shown to reverse the metabolic derangements specific to neurotrauma.[2,3] It remains to be seen if any substrate-specific diet can improve outcomes for future neurotrauma patients. Until then, a strict adherence to good critical care feeding practices may avoid the common pitfalls in assessment, calculation, and delivery of nutrients to these patients in the ICU.

NUTRITIONAL CONSIDERATIONS IN NEUROTRAUMA

Timing of nutrition

Establishing nutrition supplementation by 48 hours has improved outcomes. Early supplementation of calories and proteins prevents loss of glycogen stores, improves immunity, and maintains gut integrity.[14] Despite problems with high residues, gastroparesis, and vomiting associated with neurotrauma, by the second day almost 50% of caloric requirement is tolerated by most patients. Lower volumes (trophic feeds) may be attempted in patients where this is not possible; this helps maintain blood flow to gastrointestinal mucosa and the integrity of the gut-associated lymphoid tissues. The Brain Trauma Foundation recommends that in these patients, 100% of the caloric goal should be reached at least by the fifth day and at most by the seventh day post-trauma (level IIa evidence).[15] Studies have suggested that early alimentation may improve mortality and endocrine response (thyroid and thyroid-stimulating hormone levels) after TBI.[16,17] It may also reduce early ventilator-associated pneumonia rates[18] and improve the Glasgow Coma Scale (GCS) score at 3 months after TBI.[19]

Route of nutrition

Patients with neurotrauma are at higher risk for swallowing difficulties, inability to protect the airway because of poor GCS, and high gastric residuals. The cause may be neurologic, cognitive-behavioral, or mechanical. Properly assessing swallowing reflexes is critically important.[20] If oral feeding is considered unsafe or inadequate, then enteral routes such as nasogastric, transpyloric (jejunal), or parenteral routes may be considered.

Naso- or orogastric tubes are unsuitable for long-term insertion and may result in trauma, sinusitis, strictures, and even tracheoesophageal fistulae. Percutaneous endoscopic gastrostomy (PEG) tubes are safe and well tolerated by these patients (Figure 16.1).

Evidence from one randomized control trial with TBI patients found that transpyloric feeding reduced gastric residual and incidence of ventilator-associated pneumonia as compared to gastric feeding, whereas other studies in ICU patients have found no difference between the simpler and more

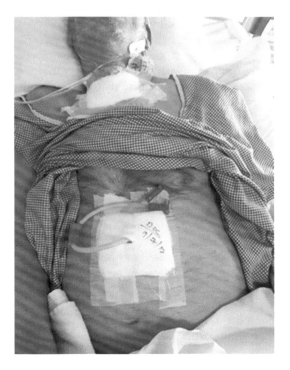

Figure 16.1 PEG tube in a patient to enable long-term enteral feeding.

cost-effective nasogastric tubes versus the PEG or nasojejunal feeding.[21-23]

For patients who do not tolerate enteral feeds or cannot achieve the caloric goals by the fifth to seventh day with only enteral feeds, parenteral nutrition may be beneficial by reducing the duration of mechanical ventilation and providing a better quality of life at 60 days.[24]

The incidence of swallowing difficulty may be as high as 61%, and the timing of the transition to oral diet is being debated. Usually by 4–6 weeks after initial injury, qualified speech and swallow therapists assess the patient for his or her ability to swallow. Clinical, fluoroscopic, or endoscopic evaluation enables the selection of the most nutritive and least restrictive diet.[25]

Calculating nutrition requirements

Indirect calorimetry is considered the gold standard for calculating caloric requirements. However, among patients with severe TBI, the frequent agitation, muscle movements, seizure, fever, and so on as well as the denervation of muscles in SCI patients may lead to errors in calorie calculation by the indirect calorimeter. Indirect calorimetry repeated over an ICU stay may be more accurate. Extrapolated values from a single indirect calorimetry may result in more erroneous calculations than using a predictive equation.[26]

An estimation of energy expenditure may also be made by using various equations. The accuracy of these calculated and formula-based derivations have been questioned.[27-30] Some of these equations were originally derived from normal volunteers (eg, the Harris–Benedict and Mifflin St. Jeor equations) or from hospitalized patients (the Ireton–Jones equation). These equations neither reflect nor account for the dynamic changes often seen in patients with neurotrauma.[26] None of these equations have been validated in neurotrauma patients. A recent comparison of predictive equations versus fixed-weight–based factors (25 calories/kg/day) showed only 40% accuracy: predicted energy expenditure from equations within 10% of measured resting energy expenditure (REE) by indirect calorimetry.[31]

In patients with acute isolated SCI, REE values are lower compared to the predicted values. Acute SCI patients have exaggerated nitrogen and 3-methylhistidine losses because of the atrophy of denervated muscle. The reduced metabolic activity may be attributed to the flaccidity of denervated muscles; as muscle loss and weight reduction progress, REE increases specially with return of muscle tone or power.[32]

In view of the absence of an accurate method of calculating calories, it has been recommended that each patient may be evaluated individually, considering not only his or her habitus and severity of trauma but also his or her preexisting nutrition status, severity of illness in ICU, degree of sedation or paralysis, sepsis, and so on. Where available, serial indirect calorimetry may be used as a guide for calculations.

Calculating protein requirements

Neurotrauma results in a state of severe catabolism and negative nitrogen metabolism. In TBI, this peaks at 2–3 weeks, whereas the peak appears later and lasts longer in SCI patients. Although provision of excess proteins in the diet is not found to promote assimilation, a minimum of 1.5–2 gm/kg of protein is recommended daily. The requirements may increase in conditions of sepsis and fever. Especially high doses of protein may lead to azotemia, however, and adequate free water must be supplemented.[27,33] The benefits of elemental, semi-elemental, and immune-modulating diet remain to be proved conclusively. Serum protein assessment to monitor nutrition status in a patient may be inaccurate because both serum albumin and prealbumin are acute-phase reactants, reflecting inflammation more than nutrition.

A previously healthy adult patient with TBI will need 25–30 nonprotein KCal/kg and 0.8–1.5 gm/kg per day of protein; requirements will increase in sepsis or seizures and decrease if the patient is paralyzed (because of injury or medication). Extra calories from intravenous fluids or propofol infusion (1.1 Kcal/mL) need to be included when calculating volume of feeds. Overfeeding will result in obesity and hepatic steatosis. Total fluid (30–35 mL/kg/day), vitamins, minerals, trace elements, and fibers will need to be supplemented, especially in patients on prolonged formula feeds.

An example for calculating or advising parenteral nutrition (PN) feed for the same patient follows is an example for initiating PN in the neurointensive care unit. Asking questions can help in decision making.

Q. Is PN necessary? If enteral feeding is deemed inadequate or impossible, what is the total caloric goal (ICU protocol based, HB equation, or indirect calorimetry)?

Q. Is there a risk of refeeding syndrome (eg, malnourished, chronic alcoholic, starving for last 4–5 days)? If yes, initiate at 50% of total requirement, with attention paid to serum electrolytes, minerals, and vitamins.

Q. Any comorbidities? For example, diabetes or renal or hepatic failure may need modification.

Q. Calculations to order PN?

- 25% dextrose 1000 mL = 250 gm dextrose = 850 kcal; (1 gm dextrose = 3.4 kcal) 20% lipid 200 mL = 40 gm lipid = 400 kcal; (1 gm lipid emulsion with glycerol = 10 kcal approximately)
- Protein requirements (1–2 gm/kg body weight) in gm × 4 = protein calories (1 gm protein = 4 Kcal)
- Osmolarity (mOsm/L) = dextrose/liter (gm) × 5 + proteins/liter (gm) × 10 + 350

For example, for a "normal" patient of 70 kg body weight with no comorbidity to supply approximately 1750 nonprotein calories and 70 gm protein (25 kcal/kg and 1.0 gm protein/kg) in 2500 mL fluid, 1500 mL 25% dextrose = 1275 kcal 250 mL/day 20% lipid = 500 kcal. Total = 1775 nonprotein kcal and 1750 mL fluids 10% AA 100 mL = 10 gm protein; 700 mL = 70 gm. Osmolarity of this prescription if given as a mixture = 250 × 5 + 10 × 10 + 350 = 1700 mOsm/L.

Medication and nutrition interactions in neurotrauma

Many commonly used drugs have a potential of interacting with enteral feeds resulting in poor delivery of the drug or nutrition (see Table 16.1).

CHALLENGES IN DELIVERING NUTRITION TO NEUROTRAUMA PATIENTS

Feed intolerance

In the early days after neurotrauma, increased gastric residues and the risk of aspiration may make delivery of adequate nutrients challenging. Ensuring elevation of the head end of the bed to 45°, introducing

Table 16.1 Nutrition and interaction with medications

Example	Effect of nutrition on drug
Phenytoin	Delayed absorption
Carbamazepine	Formation of rubbery precipitate
Ciprofloxacin	Chelation
Sucralfate	Obstruction of feeding tube
Example	**Effect of drug on nutrition**
Phenytoin	Decreased vitamin B
Carbamazepine	Hyponatremia
Loop diuretics	Decreased serum K, Mg, Ca, and Zn
Cyclosporine	Increased serum K and lipids; Decreased Mg
Penicillin	Increased K
Amphotericin B	Decreased K, Mg
Piperacillin or ticarcillin	Hyperglycemia
Steroids	Hypernatremia

calorie-dense low-volume feeds, delivering feeds as continuous drips instead of intermittent boluses,[34] or adding prokinetics such as erythromycin or metoclopramide may make it possible to achieve nutrition goals. Current guidelines accept 250–500 mL residues as normal. Feeding interruption for procedures common in the neurotrauma patient (CT scan, tracheostomy, MRI, etc.) must be kept to a minimum. Transpyloric feeding may improve absorption and decrease aspiration-related complications in patients with TBI.[35]

Glycemic control

Uncontrolled blood glucose levels can be detrimental to the recovery from neurotrauma, increasing infectious complications and decreasing wound healing.[36]

The stress response to trauma, infections, and ongoing vasopressors make adequate glycemic control a challenge. Evidence is divided over a tight glycemic control (serum level less than 110 mg%, which may improve neurologic outcome but increase episode of hypoglycemia) and a more relaxed regimen (<150 mg–180 mg%) is considered safer.[37–39]

Diarrhea

Neurotrauma patients frequently receive paralytic and anticholinergic agents that may decrease peristalsis. Constipation and straining can increase intracranial pressure, and current protocols usually include laxatives and stool softeners, which may result in loose, watery stools. Loose stools are often a deterrent to nutrition delivery in the neurotrauma patient. Drugs with high osmolarity, when administered enterally, can cause diarrhea—common examples being mannitol-, sorbitol-, and lactose-containing syrups. Infectious diarrhea or that due to *C. difficile* infection must be kept in mind with prompt laboratory investigations. If other causes are ruled out, then ensuring that the diet is lactose free, increasing the fiber content, and changing to a semi-elemental diet may be attempted.[40,41]

Electrolyte imbalance

Traumatic brain injury can result in electrolyte imbalance because of a variety of reasons: hormones, drugs, or nutrition. A patient's thirst mechanism may be impaired because of injury or as a result of sedation and mechanical ventilation. The amount of free water being provided enterally and through the intravenous route will need monitoring and titration according to serum electrolytes. Extra added salt in the diet and restricted free water in feeds, potassium syrup, and oral phosphate supplements can be tried if the patient is on an enteral feed.

Chronically, critically ill patients

Approximately 10% of all critically ill patients and a greater proportion of those with neurotrauma require long-term ventilation (>3 weeks).[42] They are prone to repeated infections and readmissions. These patients are termed "chronic critically ill" and require active metabolic and nutritional assessment and intervention.[43] It is suggested that professionals should perform early screening and intervention in the high-risk patient population with appropriate nutrition care instituted by a multidisciplinary team approach involving the neurointensivist, the endocrinologist, and the dietician or ICU nutritionist.[44]

CONCLUSION

Traumatic injuries of the brain and spinal cord result in severe hypercatabolism, although the estimation of basal energy requirements may be less than that predicted by equation in patients with spinal cord injuries because of muscle denervation. Indirect calorimetry to ascertain nutrition goals and early institution of nutrition supplement are desirable. The enteral path is preferred with full caloric goal attainment by 7 days. A multidisciplinary approach to nutrition in these patients will prevent dysimmunity and improve outcomes.

REFERENCES

1. Cuthbertson D, Tilstone WJ. Metabolism during the post injury period. *Adv Clin Chem.* 1969;12:1-55.
2. Charrueau C, Belabed L, Besson V, Chaumeil J-C, Cynober L, Moinard C. Metabolic response and nutritional support in traumatic brain injury: Evidence for resistance to renutrition. *J Neurotrauma.* 2009;26(11): 1911-1920.
3. Stein NR, McArthur DL, Etchepare M, Vespa PM. Early cerebral metabolic crisis after TBI influences outcome despite adequate hemodynamic resuscitation. *Neurocrit Care.* 2012;17 (1):49-57.
4. Boddie DE, Currie DG, Eremin O, Heys SD. Immune suppression and isolated severe head injury: A significant clinical problem. *Br J Neurosurg.* 2003;17:405-417.
5. Bartnik-Olson BL, Harris NG, Shijo K, Sutton RL. Insights into the metabolic response to traumatic brain injury as revealed by 13C NMR spectroscopy. *Front Neuroenergetics.* 2013;5:8.
6. Pellerin L, Magistretti PJ. Glutamate uptake into astrocytes stimulates aerobic glycolysis: A mechanism coupling neuronal activity to glucose utilization. *Proc Natl Acad Sci USA.* 1994;91:10625-10629.
7. Larach DB, Kofke WA, Le Roux P. Potential non-hypoxic/ischemic causes of increased cerebral interstitial fluid lactate/pyruvate ratio: A review of available literature. *Neurocrit Care.* 2011;15:609-622.

8. Vespa P, Bergneider M, Hattori N et al. Metabolic crisis without brain ischemia is common after traumatic brain injury: A combined microdialysis and positron emission tomography study. *J Cereb Blood Flow Metab.* 2005;25:763-774.

9. Sala N, Suys T, Zerlauth JB et al. Cerebral extracellular lactate increase is predominantly nonischemic in patients with severe traumatic brain injury. *J Cereb Blood Flow Metab.* 2013;33(11):1815-1822.

10. Rodriguez DJ, Benzel EC, Clevenger FW. The metabolic response to spinal cord injury. *Spinal Cord.* 1997;35(9):599-604.

11. Hillered L, Persson L, Nilsson P, Ronne-Engstrom E, Enblad P. Continuous monitoring of cerebral metabolism in traumatic brain injury: A focus on cerebral micro-dialysis. *Curr Opin Crit Care.* 2006;12:112-118.

12. Bouzat P, Sala N, Suys T et al. Cerebral metabolic effects of exogenous lactate supplementation on the injured human brain. *Intensive Care Med.* 2014;40(3):412-421.

13. White H, Venkatesh B. Clinical review: Aetones and brain injury. *Crit Care.* 2011;15:219.

14. Marik PE, Zaloga GP. Early enteral nutrition in acutely ill patients: A systematic review. *Crit Care Med.* 2001;29:2264-2270.

15. Carney N, Totten AM, O'reilly C et al. Guidelines for the management of severe traumatic brain injury. *Neurosurgery.* 2017;80(1):6-15.

16. Chourdakis M, Kraus MM, Tzellos T et al. Effect of early compared with delayed enteral nutrition on endocrine function in patients with traumatic brain injury: An open-labeled randomized trial. *J Parenter Enteral Nutr.* 2012;36 (1):108-116.

17. Hartl R, Gerber LM, Ni Q, Ghajar J. Effect of early nutrition on deaths due to severe traumatic brain injury. *J Neurosurg.* 2008;109(1): 50-56.

18. Taylor SJ, Fettes SB, Jewkes C, Nelson RJ. Prospective, randomized, controlled trial to determine the effect of early enhanced enteral nutrition on clinical outcome in mechanically ventilated patients suffering head injury. *Crit Care Med.* 1999;27(11):2525-2531.

19. Lepelletier D, Roquilly A, Demeuredit latte D et al. Retrospective analysis of the risk factors and pathogens associated with early-onset ventilator-associated pneumonia in surgical-ICU head-trauma patients. *J Neurosurg Anesthesiol.* 2010;22(1):32-37.

20. Howle AA, Baguley IJ, Brown L. Management of dysphagia following traumatic brain injury. *Curr Phys Med Rehabil Rep.* 2014;2:219.

21. Davies AR, Morrison SS, Bailey MJ et al. ENTERIC Study Investigators, ANZICS Clinical Trials Group. A multicenter, randomized controlled trial comparing early nasojejunal with nasogastric nutrition in critical illness. *Crit Care Med.* 2012;40:2342-2348.

22. Koc D, Gercek A, Gencosmanoglu R, Tozun N. Percutaneous endoscopic gastrostomy in the neurosurgical intensive care unit: Complications and outcome. *J Parenter Enteral Nutr.* 2007;31:517-520.

23. Acosta-Escribano J, Fernandez-Vivas M, Grau Carmona T et al. Gastric versus transpyloric feeding in severe traumatic brain injury: A prospective, randomized trial. *Intensive Care Med.* 2010;36(9):1532-1539.

24. Doig GS, Simpson F, Sweetman EA et al. Early PN Investigators of the ANZICS Clinical Trials Group. Early parenteral nutrition in critically ill patients with short-term relative contraindications to early enteral nutrition: A randomized controlled trial. *JAMA.* 2013;309:2130-2138.

25. Ward EC, Green K, Morton AL. Patterns and predictors of swallowing resolution following adult traumatic brain injury. *J Head Trauma Rehabil.* 2007;22:184-191.

26. McClave SA, Martindale RG, Kiraly L. The use of indirect calorimetry in the intensive care unit. *Curr Opin Clin Nutr Metab Care.* 2013;16:202-208.

27. Brain Trauma Foundation. Guidelines for the management of severe traumatic brain injury, 4th edition. https://braintrauma.org/uploads /03/12/Guidelines_for_Management_of _Severe_TBI_4th_Edition.pdf. 2016;1-244.

28. Frankenfield D, Smith JS, Cooney RN. Validation of 2 approaches to predicting resting metabolic rate in critically ill patients. *JPEN J Parenter Enteral Nutr.* 2004;28:259-264.

29. Frankenfield D, Hise M, Malone A, Russell M, Gradwell E, Compher C. Prediction of resting

metabolic rate in critically ill adult patients: Results of a systematic review of the evidence. *J Am Diet Assoc.* 2007;107:1552-1561.

30. Kolpek JH, Ott LG, Record KE et al. Comparison of urinary urea nitrogen excretion and measured energy expenditure in spinal cord injury and nonsteroid-treated severe head trauma patients. *JPEN J Parenter Enteral Nutr.* 1989;13:277-280.

31. Neelemaat F, van Bokhorst–de van der Schueren MA, Thijs A, Seidell JC, Weijs PJ. Resting energy expenditure in malnourished older patients at hospital admission and three months after discharge: Predictive equations versus measurements. *Clin Nutr.* 2012;31: 958-966.

32. Dhall SS, Hadley MN, Aarabi B et al. Nutritional support after spinal cord injury. *Neurosurgery.* 2013;72(suppl 3):255-259.

33. Bivins BA, Twyman DL, Young AB. Failure of nonprotein calories to mediate protein conservation in brain-injured patients. *J Trauma.* 1986;26:980-986.

34. Kattelmann KK, Hise M, Russell M, Charney P, Stokes M, Compher C. Preliminary evidence for a medical nutrition therapy protocol: Enteral feedings for critically ill patients. *J Am Diet Assoc.* 2006;106:1226-1241.

35. Rhoney DH, Parker DJ, Formea CM, Yap C, Coplin WM. Tolerability of bolus versus continuous gastric feeding in brain-injured patients. *Neurol Res.* 2002;24:613-620.

36. Lam AM, Winn HR, Cullen BF, Sundling N. Hyperglycemia and neurological outcome in

patients with head injury. *J Neurosurg.* 1991; 75(4):545-551.

37. Acosta-Escribano J, Fernandez-Vivas M, Grau Carmona T et al. Gastric versus transpyloric feeding in severe traumatic brain injury: A prospective, randomized trial. *Intensive Care Med.* 2010;36(9):1532-1539.

38. Bilotta F, Caramia R, Cernak I et al. Intensive insulin therapy after severe traumatic brain injury: A randomized clinical trial. *Neurocrit Care.* 2008;9(2):159-166.

39. Coester A, Neumann CR, Schmidt MI. Intensive insulin therapy in severe traumatic brain injury: A randomized trial. *J Trauma.* 2010;68(4):904-911.

40. Yang M, Guo Q, Zhang X et al. Intensive insulin therapy on infection rate, days in NICU, in-hospital mortality and neurological outcome in severe traumatic brain injury patients: A randomized controlled trial. *Int J Nurs Stud.* 2009;46(6):753-758.

41. Williams MS, Harper R, Magnuson B, Loan T, Kearney P. Diarrhea management in enterally fed patients. *Nutr Clin Pract.* 1998;13:225-229.

42. Schulman RC, Mechanick JI. Metabolic and nutrition support in the chronic critical illness syndrome. *Respir Care.* 2012;57:958-977.

43. Boniatti MM, Friedman G, Castilho RK, Vieira SR, Fialkow L. Characteristics of chronically critically ill patients: Comparing two definitions. *Clinics (Sao Paulo)* 2011;66:701-704.

44. Tripathy S. Nutrition in the neurocritical care unit. *J Neuroanaesthesiol Crit Care.* 2015;2: 88-96.

17

Role of antibiotics

MARTINA ORNAGHI, VALENTINA ORMAS, AND DANIELA FERLICCA

INTRODUCTION

Patients with traumatic brain injury (TBI) are a high-risk population for developing nosocomial infections compared with other critically ill and neurosurgical patients.

Ventilator-associated pneumonia (VAP) seems to be the most common infection in TBI patients. Other frequent infections are surgical site infections, urinary-tract infections, catheter-associated bacteremia, bloodstream infections, and meningitis and ventriculitis.[1] Central nervous system (CNS) infections represent only 4% of those experienced by trauma patients, but if cerebrospinal fluid (CSF) leakage exists, the incidence increases to 50%. Furthermore, the insertion of ventricular drains is associated with the development of both surgical-site infections and meningitis.[2,3] Infection-related mortality rate may be as high as 28%,[4] and intracranial infection such as those from meningitis, encephalitis, and brain abscesses is often related to poor neurologic prognosis and cognitive disorder.[2] Despite the significant financial burden and loss of life, few retrospective studies have investigated the risk factors for TBI patients to develop infections and the role of antibiotics in the prophylaxis of infectious complications.

This chapter will focus in particular on the management of prophylaxis, as well as CNS infections related to the presence of external ventricular drain (EVD). It will also provide an overview of the management of the most frequent infections according to recent guidelines.

ANTIBIOTIC PROPHYLAXIS

The efficacy of antibiotic prophylaxis in patients after TBI remains unclear. The risk of antibiotic use—including drug resistance, adverse reactions, and economic burden—require clinical assessments to antibiotic administration.[3]

Antibiotic prophylaxis in basilar skull fractures

A basilar skull fracture (BSF) is a serious injury resulting from a break in the bones of the skull base. Such fractures represent 7% to 15.8% of all skull fractures, with 2% to 20.8% of CSF leakage occurring.[5]

Clinical signs that may lead a physician to suspect a BSF include rhinorrhea, rhinorrhagia, periorbital ecchymosis, anosmia, otorrhea, otorrhagia, facial nerve palsy, hemotympanum or tympanic membrane perforation, retromastoid bruising (Battle's sign), hearing loss, evidence of vestibular dysfunction, and ipsilateral motor paralysis of the vocal cord.[6,7]

Basilar skull fractures may be missed at initial clinical evaluation, so detection of fractures at a computed tomography scan may require the need for close observation of patients for signs of complications from such fractures.[8]

One of these complications is post-traumatic meningitis. BSFs are often associated with dural tears that place the CNS in contact with bacteria from the paranasal sinuses, nasopharynx, and middle ear and may result in a cerebrospinal fluid fistula.[9] CSF leaks represent a corridor for bacteria to access the CSF space. In most cases of CSF leakage associated with basilar skull fractures, the leak spontaneously ceases within the first 10 to 12 days. Within this time frame, the risk of developing meningitis is rather low, but a greater associated risk has been reported when CSF leakage persists.[10] Antibiotic prophylaxis is often given, although its role in preventing post-traumatic bacterial meningitis remains controversial, and growing concern about the emergence of resistant bacteria discourages their use.[11]

A recently updated Cochrane Review does not support the use of antibiotic prophylaxis in basilar skull fractures.[12] The review examined five randomized controlled studies (RCTs) that divided 208 total participants with BSF into those who received antibiotic prophylaxis and those who did not to establish how many patients developed meningitis. All these studies were single center and conducted in South Africa, Iran, the United States, and Belgium and published between 1975 and 2004. The authors also identified 17 non-RCTs, comparing different types of preventive antibiotic therapy with placebos or no intervention in patients with BSF.

Most trials presented important methodologic limitations: the precise method of randomization was not explained in any trial. Only one study was double-blind, and only two studies reported the number of the patients leaving the trials and the reasons they left. Data were analyzed on a per-protocol basis in all trials. Missing data precluded several planned analyses in the systematic review.

The results from the studies were strikingly similar. The five RCTs showed no significant differences between antibiotic prophylaxis groups and control groups in terms of reduction of the frequency of meningitis, all-cause mortality, meningitis-related mortality, and the need for surgical correction in patients with CSF leakage. There were no reported adverse effects of antibiotic administration, although one of the five RCTs reported an induced change in the posterior nasopharyngeal flora toward organisms resistant to the antibiotics used in prophylaxis.

The authors also completed a meta-analysis of all the controlled non-RCTs (2168 total patients), which produced results comparable to data from RCTs.

In conclusion, currently available evidence does not prove the effectiveness of antibiotic prophylaxis for preventing meningitis in patients with BSF, with or without CSF leakage.

Future large and appropriately designed RCTs are needed to establish whether or not there is a clear benefit from preventive antibiotic therapy in BSF.

Antibiotic prophylaxis for penetrating brain injuries

Penetrating brain injuries (PBIs) are less common than blunt TBI but are associated with worse prognoses, with only 9% survival reported.[13] Primary injuries can be the result of scalp lesions, cranial fractures, intracranial bleeding, and cerebral lacerations. Brain injuries can occur along the path of a projectile, as well as in more distant locations because of pressure waves and coup and contrecoup lesions. High-energy PBIs are often followed by harmful increases in intracranial pressure.[10] Penetrating brain injuries are most commonly from firearms, which account for 12% of all TBIs. The incidence of penetrating brain injuries has increased since the 1990s, primarily because of increases in gun violence, which have resulted in 32,000 to 35,000 civilian deaths annually in the United States.[14] In civilian settings, the majority of PBIs are caused by a low-velocity gunshot wound to the head (GSWH). Approximately 70% of patients with GSWHs die before reaching the hospital, and another 12% die within 3 hours of injury.[15,16] However, survivors often experience a favorable outcome, with 74% having a good recovery or moderate disability.[17] Shrapnel, and not low-velocity gunshot, is the major cause of PBIs in military conflicts. The military prehospital and hospital management are highly effective, and the overall mortality rate are therefore lower (around 20%).[18]

PBI patients show an extensive list of delayed complications such as cerebral vasospasm, traumatic intracranial aneurysm formation, CSF leaks, post-traumatic epilepsy, and infections. The risk of infectious complications increases following the first week postinjury, with recent postsurgical infectious complications occurring at a rate of 5% to 23%.[19] The risk of intracranial infection is high because of the presence of contaminated foreign objects, skin, hair and bone fragments driven into the brain along the missile track.[20] The presence of air sinus wounds or CSF fistulas may further increase the risk of infection.[14]

Relatively few published studies have reported the results of bacteriologic analysis of removed fragments or the causative agents of infection in PBIs. The main microbiologic studies were conducted on samples cultured during the Vietnam War and the Iran–Iraq War. Most of the contaminating organisms were skin flora such as *Staphylococcus epidermidis*, but *Staphylococcus aureus* and gram-negative bacilli were also common pathogens, as reported in Table 17.1. Nevertheless most of these studies do not describe the results of anaerobic cultures and do not differentiate between colonization and infection. Furthermore, the quality of the microbiology did not equal modern standards, so most isolates cannot be considered to have been conclusively identified.[21]

Effective debridement can actually reduce the risk of infection from such contaminants.[14] Debriding both entrance and exit wounds; removing necrotic tissue, hematomas, bone, and metal fragments where these are accessible; removing foreign material, including hair and clothing; and closing the dura with reconstruction, if necessary, represent standard validated management in use today.[22]

Table 17.1 Typical microorganisms causing infection in penetrating brain injury

Staphylococcus epidermidis

Staphylococcus aureus

Gram-negative bacilli

Anaerobic bacteria

Besides the importance of surgery, antibiotic prophylaxis was introduced in World War II. The infection rate in the preantibiotoic period during World War I was reported to be 58.8%. In World War II, the reported infection rate with local application of sulfa powder or parenteral sulfonamide therapy was 21% to 31%. When penicillin was added to this regimen, the clinical infection rate dropped to 6%–13%.[21]

Considerable variability exists in the literature regarding prophylactic antibiotics following PBIs.[14] Bayston et al. performed a systematic review of prophylactic antibiotics for penetrating craniocerebral trauma and found only retrospective and anecdotal studies and no controlled trials.[22] A working party was instituted by the British Society for Antimicrobial Chemotherapy to investigate and produce recommendations for the appropriate use of antibiotics in various areas of neurosurgical practice. The microbiologic and neurosurgical members of this council recommend that, for both military and civilian PBIs, antimicrobial prophylaxis should be started as soon as possible after injury and consist of amoxicillin or clavulanic acid, orcefuroxime, and metronidazole. Administration should be continued for 5 days postoperatively.[22] Broad-spectrum antibiotic cover is also recommended in the PBI guidelines.[21] Lin et al. suggest antimicrobial prophylaxis with vancomycin, gentamycin, and metronidazole for 48–72 hours.[3] Nevertheless, recent U.S. military guidelines warn against the association between broad-spectrum antibiotic coverage and the increase of multidrug-resistant microorganism, particularly *Acinetobacter*. Therefore, the current recommendation of the U.S. military guidelines is cephazolin for 5–7 days.[23]

In conclusion, preventing infection through extensive debridement of all contaminated, macerated, or ischemic tissues represents a basic and universally recognized step in treating PBIs.[24] Prophylactic antibiotic use should be determined on an individual basis and strongly consider the patient's overall risk for infection and an infectious disease consult. In general, broad-spectrum antibiotics that cover *Staphylococci* and gram-negative bacilli are appropriate. If dirt, debris, or clothing contaminates the wound, expansion to anaerobic coverage with metronidazole is also recommended.[14] Table 17.2 presents an overview of the different prophylactic antibiotic regimens suggested in current literature.

Table 17.2 Prophylactic antibiotic regimens suggested in penetrating brain injury: An overview of current literature

Article title	Authors, publication year	Suggested empiric antibiotic regimen	Duration of therapy
Use of antibiotics in penetrating craniocerebral injuries. "Infection in Neurosurgery." Working Party of British Society for Antimicrobial Chemotherapy.[22]	Bayston R, de Louvois J, Brown EM, Johnston RA, Lees P, Pople IK Year 2000	Amoxicillin or clavulanic acid or cefuroxime + metronidazole	5 days
Analysis on the risk factors of intracranial infection secondary to traumatic brain injury.[3]	Lin C, Zhao X, Sun H Year 2015	Vancomycin + gentamycin + metronidazole	2–3 days
United States Army Institute of Surgical Research Joint Theater Trauma System. Clinical Practice Guideline (Management of Patients with Severe Head Trauma).[23]	U.S. Army Institute of Surgical Research Year 2012	Cephazolin	5–7 days
Penetrating Traumatic Brain Injury: A Review of Current Evaluation and Management Concepts.[14]	Van Wyck DW, Grant GA Year 2015	Broad-spectrum antibiotics that cover Staphylococci and gram-negative bacilli + metronidazole in case of wound contamination with dirt, debris, or clothing	

Antibiotic prophylaxis in patients with external ventricular drains

An EVD is often used after a closed head injury; this temporary device permits therapeutic CSF drainage and monitoring of intracranial pressure. Like any external device, an EVD carries a risk of infection—in particular, ventriculomeningitis. The exact incidence of ventriculomeningitis is not known, and its rate in the literature varies from 1% to 24%; such variability depends on the definition of infection used and the characteristics of the study population.

A large meta-analysis of 23 major studies comprising 5733 EVD insertions among 5261 patients found a cumulative rate of positive CSF cultures of 8.8% per patient or 8.1% per EVD placement.[25] A recent meta-analysis of 35 observational studies has estimated a higher ventriculostomy-related infection (VRI) incidence rate of 11.4 per 1000 catheter days—that is, one VRI per 88 catheter days.[26]

Recognizing risk factors is important to prevent infections. Unfortunately, risk factors for VRIs are not currently clearly identified and vary among different studies; elements of main importance are reported in Table 17.3.

Traditionally considered risk factors include the indication for placement (because the presence of hemorrhage poses more risk), duration of catheterization, differences in placement technique, antimicrobial use, and frequency of manipulation and

Table 17.3 Risk factors for VRIs

Presence of intraventricular or subarachnoidal hemorrhage

Duration of catheterization

Antimicrobial use

Frequency of manipulation and sampling

Presence of extracranial infections

Device placement outside the operating room

sampling.[27] Moreover, an Italian study found that extracranial infections and placement of the device outside the operating room were also risk factors.[28]

The duration of EVD placement is positively associated with the risk of infection, but it is not clear if the risk is linear. Although evidence suggests increasing risk in the first week after placement, studies are conflicting after the first seven days: some suggest that the risk still increases,[29–31] while others show no association[32] and find that the daily infection rate reaches a peak at day 10 and late infections are less frequent. This finding suggests that the insertion procedure is responsible for the major part of infections, and delayed contamination associated with EVD care is less important than thought.[27] Cleansing the insertion site using an antimicrobial agent at the time of the surgical procedure and using clean dressing are good practices.

Available data suggest that EVDs should be removed as early as the clinical situation allows, and this constitutes the safest approach.[33]

If continued EVD use is necessary, there is a strong recommendation against routinely prophylactic removal and reinsertion because it has not proved to be beneficial.[33–35]

The most commonly found pathogens in ventriculomeningitis-related EVDs have traditionally been skin flora, and empiric antibiotics are frequently selected on this basis, but gram-negative pathogens are gaining increasing importance. The meta-analysis by Ramanan et al.[26] found that 64% of positive culture infections were caused by gram-positive bacteria, predominantly coagulase negative Staphylococci, including S. epidermidis (39%) and S. aureus (15%). The 35% of infections were by gram-negative bacteria, including Acinetobacter spp.

(9.3%), Pseudomonas spp. (6%), and enteric organisms; in 1% of positive cultures, Candida spp. were isolated. Table 17.4 summarizes the epidemiology.

Common practice is to administer antimicrobial prophylaxis to prevent EVD infection. Prophylaxis regimen can be exclusively periprocedural (before or during EVD insertion) or continue for the entire duration that the EVD is in place. A small trial[36] and two retrospective studies[37,38] compared periprocedural and duration use (respectively of cefazolin in the first two studies and Cefuroxime in the last one) and found no significant difference in infection rates between the two groups. One study[37] found an increased rate of Clostridium difficile colitis in patients receiving antimicrobials for the duration of EVD placement. Therefore, one dose of antimicrobials is recommended before EVD insertion and not for the duration of EVD placement. There is insufficient evidence to recommend a specific antimicrobial for periprocedural prophylaxis; the choice should be guided by local antibiograms.[33]

Another issue to consider in clinical practice is whether to use antimicrobial coated catheters. Currently, EVD catheters impregnated with clindamycin–rifampicin, minocycline–rifampicin, and silver are commercially available. Various studies have demonstrated that they can potentially reduce VRI rates.

In 2003, Zabramski et al.[39] performed a randomized controlled trial comparing an antimicrobial-impregnated catheter (with minocycline–rifampicin) with a standard silicone catheter and demonstrated a reduction of positive cultures from 9.4% in the control group to 1.3% in the intervention group. This study was followed by other RCTs and observational

Table 17.4 Typical microorganisms causing ventricular catheter-associated infections

Microorganism		Isolation percentage
Gram-positive bacteria	Coagulase-negative *Staphylococci*, *Staphylococcus aureus*, *Propionibacterium* acnes	64
Gram-negative bacteria	Enterobacteriaceae, *Pseudomonas aeruginosa*, *Acinetobacter*	35
Anarobes	*Bacteroides* spp.	Rare
Candida species	*Candida* spp.	1

studies, but in general all the studies demonstrated that antimicrobial-impregnated catheters were superior to standard catheters in lowering the rate of VRIs, especially in case of coagulase-negative *Staphylococci*. Furthermore, a significantly decreased rate of catheter bacterial colonization was noticed for antimicrobial-impregnated catheters. Silver-impregnated catheters also appear effective in reducing VRI rates.[40] Silver-impregnated catheters should obviate two concerns regarding antimicrobial impregnated catheters: the fact that a CSF culture drawn through a coated catheter could be falsely negative and concerns about the development of resistance to drugs (at the moment not demonstrated).[27] At the moment, there is insufficient evidence to compare the efficacy of antibiotic versus silver-impregnated catheters; the choice should be made on the basis of local availability and cost, although the use of an impregnated catheter is recommended.[33]

MANAGEMENT OF EVD-RELATED INFECTIONS

Diagnosis

The most frequently used definition of acquired meningoventriculitis is the one proposed by the Centers for Disease Control and Prevention (CDC). To diagnose infection, at least one of the following criteria must be present:

1. The patient has one or more organisms identified from cerebrospinal fluid by a culture- or nonculture-based microbiologic testing method that is performed for purposes of clinical diagnosis or treatment.
2. The patient has at least two of the following:
   a. Fever (>38.0°C) or headache (*Note*: Elements of "a" alone may not be used to meet the two required elements)
   b. Meningeal sign(s)
   c. Cranial nerve sign(s)
   And at least one of the following:
   a. Increased white cells, elevated protein, and decreased glucose in CSF (per reporting laboratory's reference range)
   b. Organism(s) seen on gram stains of CSF (reference CDC and National Health Service [NHS] surveillance definition, January 2017)

c. Organism(s) identified from blood by a culture- or nonculture-based microbiologic testing method that is performed for purposes of clinical diagnosis
d. Diagnostic single-antibody titer (IgM) or fourfold increase in paired sera (IgG) for organism

This definition can lead to confusion in practice. The presence of a positive culture does not distinguish between infection, colonization, or contamination and may lead to overtreatment. Clinical features defined by the second criterion are also controversial: patients with recent neurosurgical interventions frequently show fever, headache, stiff neck, or meningeal signs, which can be difficult to assess in ICU patients who are often sedated and intubated.[27]

For this reason, Lozier and colleagues[25] proposed a different diagnostic method that differentiates between contamination, colonization, and infection (as shown in Table 17.5):

- Contamination—An isolated positive CSF culture (or gram stain) with CSF glucose, protein, and cell count in the expected range
- Colonization—Repeated positive CSF culture or gram stain with normal CSF glucose, protein, and cell count without clinical symptoms

Table 17.5 Definitions of ventricular catheter contamination, colonization, and infection

Contamination	An isolated positive CSF culture or gram stain, with CSF glucose, protein, and cell count in the expected range
Colonization	Repeated positive CSF culture or gram stain, with normal CSF glucose, protein, and cell count without clinical symptoms
Infection	Progressive decline in CSF glucose and increase of CSF protein and CSF pleocytosis with one or more positive CSF cultures or gram stains

- Infection—Progressive decline in CSF glucose and increase of CSF protein and CSF pleocytosis with one or more positive CSF culture or gram stains

Defining what constitutes an abnormal CSF finding in patients with a disease of CNS is not easy because of variability in CSF profiles from physiologic inflammation after neurosurgery or chemical meningitis induced by blood degradation products.

Treatment

Few controlled trials have evaluated appropriate treatment strategies for VRIs. It is important, however, to establish an early and appropriate antimicrobial therapy and to choose an agent that is active against the most likely organisms encountered based on local trends and ensure it achieves adequate concentration in the CNS.

For high rates of staphylococcal infections, vancomycin is often the first-line empiric agent chosen. Its CNS penetration, however, is not guaranteed. Linezolid is an alternative agent for patients with allergy to vancomycin, significant comorbidities or pathogens known to be vancomycin-resistant. A good achievement of linezolid concentration above minimum inhibitory concentration (MIC) in CSF has been demonstrated.[41] Daptomycin cannot cross the blood–brain barrier.

Because gram-negative infections are also common, an antipseudomonal cephalosporin or carbapenem should be used in the empiric initial management of a suspected VRI along with vancomycin. The decision to use a carbapenem should be based on local rates of β-lactamase–producing organisms. Aminoglycosides do not cross the blood–brain barrier; aztreonam and colistin have not been well studied.

The best regimen for fungal infection has not been established, although fluconazole and voriconazole achieve the best levels in the CSF.[27]

Intraventricular antimicrobials might be considered in the setting of severe ventriculitis with persistently positive CSF cultures that fail to respond to intravenous antimicrobials or in case of multidrug-resistant pathogens requiring a specific antimicrobial that does not reach adequate CSF concentrations or when patients have serious comorbidities limiting systemic administration of antimicrobials. Their use is not supported by any reliable clinical data, and no agent has been approved by the U.S. Food and Drug Administration for intraventricular use. The most commonly used agents are vancomycin, aminoglycosides, and colistin, for which pharmacokinetics and safety have been studied.[27,33]

VENTILATOR-ASSOCIATED PNEUMONIA

Pneumonia is the most common nosocomial infection and has an extremely negative impact on patient outcomes: mortality of ventilation-associated pneumonia was estimated at approximately 13% in a recent meta-analysis,[42] and it undoubtedly prolongs the length of mechanical ventilation and hospitalization.

Pneumonia is defined as the presence of new lung infiltrate plus clinical evidence that the infiltrate is of an infectious origin, which may include evidence such as a fever of new onset, purulent sputum, leukocytosis, or a decline in oxygenation. VAP is pneumonia occurring >48 hours after endotracheal intubation, a definition that has remained unchanged in the 2005 and 2016 Clinical Practice Guidelines developed by the Infectious Diseases Society of America and the American Thoracic Society.[43]

Prevention of pneumonia targets modifiable risk factors; numerous interventions have been investigated, often finding conflicting evidence on their benefits.[44–46]

Specific VAP-related measures include avoiding intubation or reintubation whenever feasible as well as keeping intubation time as short as possible, daily lightening sedation and limiting paralytic agents to limit cough depression, maintaining endotracheal tube cuff pressure greater than 20 cm H_2O, carefully managing ventilator circuits (with prevention of condensate inhalation and use of closed endotracheal suction systems and humidification), and keeping patients in the semirecumbent position to prevent aspiration. Other well-established measures are enteral nutrition to prevent villous atrophy of the intestinal mucosa, which may increase the risk of bacterial translocation; conservative transfusional strategies to avoid the possible immunosuppressive effect of allogeneic blood products; and aggressive hyperglicemia management.

Stress bleeding prophylaxis with sucralfate was associated with reduced VAP incidence but higher gastric-bleeding rates compared with proton pump inhibitors and histamine 2 receptor antagonists; both strategies are deemed acceptable. Oral decontamination with chlorhexidine was shown to reduce VAP occurrence in patients undergoing cardiac surgery, but results are still unclear in other populations. Selective digestive decontamination (SDD) with oral antibiotics has helped contain outbreaks of VAP but is not currently recommended for routine use; a recent systematic review[47] found SDD with systemic antibiotics results in lower mortality, underlying the need for further research on this issue.

Establishing a microbiologic diagnosis with cultures of respiratory secretions is desirable in every patient with suspected VAP because identifying causative organisms makes it possible to adjust the initial empiric antibiotic regimen. Noninvasive sampling is suggested with semiquantitative cultures to diagnose VAP rather than invasive sampling such as bronchoscopic techniques or blind bronchial sampling.

Early-onset VAP, which occurs during the first four days of mechanical ventilation, is likely to be caused by pathogens that originate in the oropharyngeal cavity: *Staphylococcus aureus*, *Streptococcus pneumoniae*, and *Haemophilus influenzae*. Late-onset VAP can occur five or more days after starting mechanical ventilation and is more likely to be caused by gram-negative bacilli such as *Pseudomonas aeruginosa* or *Acinetobacter* spp., with less frequent involvement of gram-positives such as *S. aureus*. All of these organisms are more likely to be multiresistant to antimicrobials and therefore difficult to treat.

However, even if time of onset is an informative epidemiologic factor, the most recent American Thoracic Society guidelines consider it a less pivotal element of decision making for the initial empiric treatment regime. The choice of the antimicrobial agents should be based on the presence of patient-linked multidrug resistance (MDR) risk factors as well as on the local distribution of potentially involved pathogens and their antimicrobial susceptibilities.

Risk factors for VAP caused by any MDR organism include previous intravenous antibiotic use within 90 days, septic shock at time of VAP, acute respiratory distress syndrome (ARDS) preceding VAP, five or more days of hospitalization before VAP,

and acute renal replacement therapy before VAP onset. Mainstay concepts regarding the epidemiology of VAP are presented in Tables 17.6 and 17.7.

The empiric antibiotic regimen should include an agent active against methicillin-resistant staphylococcus aureus (MRSA)—either vancomycin or linezolid—if the patient presents a risk factor for antimicrobial resistance or when the rates of MRSA in the considered care unit are >10% to 20% (or not known). Otherwise, for MSSA coverage piperacillin-tazobactam, cefepime, levofloxacin, imipenem, or meropenem can be considered.

For *Pseudomonas* coverage, it is deemed preferable to add two antipseudomonal antibiotics from different classes in patients with a risk factor for antimicrobial resistance or in care units where >10% of gram-negative isolates are resistant to an agent being considered for monotherapy (or when local antimicrobial susceptibility rates are not available).

Combination therapy is usually achieved through a β-lactamic agent plus a non–β-lactamic one. Suitable β-lactam-based agents are antipseudomonal penicillins (piperacillin-tazobactam),

Table 17.6 Epidemiology of early and late VAP

Early-onset VAP	In the first 4 days of hospitalization Better prognosis Often non-MDR bacteria: *Staphylococcus aureus*, *Staphylococcus pneumoniae*, *Haemophilus influenzae*
Late-onset VAP	After fifth day of hospitalization Increased morbidity and mortality Often MDR bacteria: gram-like *Pseudomonas aeruginosa*, *Acinetobacter* spp.; less often *S. aureus*

Table 17.7 Risk factors for MDR VAP

Prior intravenous antibiotic use within 90 days

Septic shock at time of VAP

ARDS preceding VAP

Five or more days of hospitalization before occurrence of VAP

Acute renal replacement therapy before VAP onset

cephalosporins (cefepime, ceftazidime), carbapenems (imipenem, meropenem), or monobactams (aztreonam). Non β-Lactamic agents include the classes of fluoroquinolones (ciprofloxacin, levofloxacin), aminoglycosides (amikacin, gentamicin, tobramycin), and polymyxins (colistin, polymyxin B).

Monotherapy with one of the aforementioned medications is indicated for a patient with no MDR risk factors who is admitted to a care unit with <10% of resistant gram-negative isolates.

A recent Cochrane Review[48] attempting to evaluate the best antibiotic choice for VAP could not reach definitive conclusions because of a lack of studies, but the review did suggest that carbapenems as a class may result in better clinical cure than other tested antibiotics. It should be noted that the 2016 American Thoracic Society Giudelines[43] suggest avoiding aminoglycosides if alternative agents with adequate gram-negative activity are available because of poor lung penetration, increased risk of nephrotoxicity and ototoxicity, and possible poorer clinical response.

A key element of a correct antibiotic therapy is the necessity to deescalate from broad-spectrum empiric regimen whenever possible to limit the emergence of resistance.

The optimal duration of therapy has been debated. The 2016 American Thoracic Society Guidelines[43] found evidence in favor of a short-course antibiotic that decreases antibiotic exposure and antibiotic resistance and reduces costs and side effects.

The recommended duration of therapy is seven days; the decision to interrupt antibiotics in a patient with clinical signs of resolving VAP can be strengthened by assessing PCT levels.

REFERENCES

1. Kourbeti IS, Vakis AF, Papadakis JA et al. Infections in traumatic brain injury patients. *Clin Microbiol Infect.* 2012;18(4):359-364.
2. Boque MC, Bodi M, Rello J. Trauma, head injury, and neurosurgery infections. *Semin Respir Infect.* 2000;15(4):280-286.
3. Lin C, Zhao X, Sun H. Analysis on the risk factors of intracranial infection secondary to traumatic brain injury. *Chin J Traumatol.* 2015;18(2):81-83.
4. Harrison-Felix C, Whiteneck G, Devivo MJ, Hammond FM, Jha A. Causes of death following 1 year postinjury among individuals with traumatic brain injury. *J Head Trauma Rehabil.* 2006;21(1):22-33.
5. Buchanan RJ, Brant A, Marshall LR. Traumatic cerebrospinal fluid fistulas. In: Winn H, ed. *Youmans Neurological Surgery.* 5th ed. Philadelphia, PA: Saunders; 2004:5265-5272.
6. Lloyd KM, DelGaudio JM, Hudgins PA. Imaging of skull base cerebrospinal fluid leaks in adults. *Radiology.* 2008;248(3):725-736.
7. Hsu K-C, Wang A-C, Chen S-J. Mastoid bone fracture presenting as unusual delayed onset of facial nerve palsy. *Am J Emerg Med.* 2008;26(3):386.e1-386.e2.
8. Olabinri EO, Ogbole GI, Adeleye AO, Dairo DM, Malomo AO, Ogunseyinde AO. Comparative analysis of clinical and computed tomography features of basal skull fractures in head injury in southwestern Nigeria. *J Neurosci Rural Pract.* 2015;6(2):139-144.
9. Phang SY, Whitehouse K, Lee L, Khalil H, McArdle P, Whitfield PC. Management of CSF leak in base of skull fractures in adults. *Br J Neurosurg.* 2016;30(6):596-604.
10. Sundstrom T, Grande P-O, Juul N, Kock-Jensen C, Romner B, Wester K. *Management of Severe Traumatic Brain Injury.* Berlin Heidelberg: Springer; 2012:109-111.
11. Chang WT, Badjatia N. Neurotrauma. *Emerg Med Clin North Am.* 2014;32(4):889-905.
12. Ratilal B, Costa J, Sampaio C. Antibiotic prophylaxis for preventing meningitis in patients with basilar skull fractures. *Cochrane Library.* 2006;(1).
13. Aarabi B, Tofighi B, Kufera JA et al. Predictors of outcome in civilian gunshot wounds to the head. *J Neurosurg.* 2014;120(5):1138-1146.
14. Van Wyck DW, Grant GA. Penetrating traumatic brain injury: A review of current evaluation and management concepts. *J Neurol Neurophysiol.* 2015;6:(6).
15. Siccardi D, Cavaliere R, Pau A, Lubinu F, Turtas S, Viale GL. Penetrating craniocerebral missile injuries in civilians: A retrospective analysis of 314 cases. *Surg Neurol.* 1991;35(6):455-460.
16. Joseph B, Aziz H, Pandit V et al. Improving survival rates after civilian gunshot wounds to the brain. *J Am Coll Surg.* 2014;218(1):58-65.

17. Levi L, Linn S, Feinsod M. Penetrating cranicerebral injuries in civilians. *Br J Neurosurg.* 1991;5(3):241-247.

18. Potapov AA, Shahinian GG, Kravtchouk AD. Surgical management of penetrating brain injury. *J Trauma.* 2001;51(2):16-25.

19. Aarabi B, Mossop C, Aarabi JA. Surgical management of civilian gunshot wounds to the head. *Handb Clin Neurol.* 2015;127:181-193.

20. Alvis-Miranda H, Rubiano A, Agrawal A et al. Craniocerebral gunshot injuries; A review of the current literature. *Bull Emerg Trauma.* 2016;4(2):65-74.

21. Antibiotic prophylaxis for penetrating brain injury. *J Trauma.* 2001;51suppl:S34–S40.

22. Bayston R, de Louvois J, Brown EM, Johnston RA, Lees P, Pople IK. Use of antibiotics in penetrating craniocerebral injuries. "Infection in Neurosurgery" Working Party of British Society for Antimicrobial Chemotherapy. *Lancet.* 2000;355(9217):1813-1817.

23. United States Army Institute of Surgical Research Joint Theater Trauma System Clinical Practice Guideline (Management of Patients with Severe Head Trauma). 2012.

24. Vakil MT, Singh AK. A review of penetrating brain trauma: Epidemiology, pathophysiology, imaging assessment, complications, and treatment. *Emerg Radiol.* 2016;4(2):65-74.

25. Lozier AP, Sciacca RR, Romagnoli MF, Connolly ES Jr. Ventriculostomy-related infections: A critical review of the literature. *Neurosurgery.* 2002;51(1):170-181.

26. Ramanan M, Lipman J, Shorr A, Shankar A. A meta-analysis of ventriculostomy-associated cerebrospinal fluid infections. *BMC Infect Dis.* 2015;15(1):3.

27. Stenehjem E, Armstrong WS. Central nervous system device infections. *Infect Dis Clin North Am.* 2012;26(1):89-110.

28. Citerio G, Signorini L, Bronco A, Vargiolu A, Rota M, Latronico N. External ventricular and lumbar drain device infections in ICU patients. *Crit Care Med.* 2015;43(8):1630-1637.

29. Lyke KE, Obasanjo OO, Williams MA, O'Brien M, Chotani R, Perl TM. Ventriculitis complicating use of intraventricular catheters in adult neurosurgical patients. *Clin Infect Dis.* 2001;15;33(12):2028-2033.

30. Mayhall CG, Archer NH, Lamb VA et al. Ventriculostomy-related infections. A prospective epidemiologic study. *N Engl J Med.* 1984;310(9):553-559.

31. Kim J-H, Desai NS, Ricci J et al. Factors contributing to ventriculostomy infection. *World Neurosurg.* 2012;77(1):135-140.

32. Winfield JA, Rosenthal P, Kanter RK, Casella G. Duration of intracranial pressure monitoring does not predict daily risk of infectious complications. *Neurosurgery.* 1993;33(3):424-430.

33. Fried HI, Nathan BR, Rowe AS et al. The insertion and management of external ventricular drains: An evidence-based consensus statement. *Neurocrit Care.* 2016;24(1):61-81.

34. Holloway KL, Barnes T, Choi S et al. Ventriculostomy infections: The effect of monitoring duration and catheter exchange in 584 patients. *J Neurosurg.* 1996;85(3):419-424.

35. Lo CH, Spelman D, Bailey M, Cooper DJ, Rosenfeld JV, Brecknell JE. External ventricular drain infections are independent of drain duration: An argument against elective revision. *J Neurosurg.* 2007;106(3):378-383.

36. Saini NS, Dewan Y, Grewal SS. Efficacy of periprocedural vs extended use of antibiotics in patients with external ventricular drains— A randomized trial. *Indian J Neurotrauma.* 2012;9(1):30-32.

37. Dellit TH, Chan JD, Fulton C et al. Reduction in *Clostridium difficile* infections among neurosurgical patients associated with discontinuation of antimicrobial prophylaxis for the duration of external ventricular drain placement. *Infect Control Hosp Epidemiol.* 2014;35(5):589-590.

38. Alleyne CH Jr, Hassan M, Zabramski JM. The efficacy and cost of prophylactic and perioprocedural antibiotics in patients with external ventricular drains. *Neurosurgery.* 2000;47(5):1124-1127.

39. Zabramski JM, Whiting D, Darouiche RO et al. Efficacy of antimicrobial-impregnated external ventricular drain catheters: A prospective, randomized, controlled trial. *J Neurosurg.* 2003;98(4):725-730.

40. Wang X, Dong Y, Qi X-Q, Li Y-M, Huang C-G, Hou L-J. Clinical review: Efficacy of antimicrobial-impregnated catheters in external ventricular drainage—A systematic

review and meta-analysis. *Crit Care*. 2013;17 (4):234.

41. Beer R, Engelhardt KW, Pfausler B et al. Pharmacokinetics of intravenous linezolid in cerebrospinal fluid and plasma in neuro-intensive care patients with staphylococcal ventriculitis associated with external ventricular drains. *Antimicrob Agents Chemother*. 2007;51(1):379-382.

42. Melsen WG, Rovers MM, Groenwold RHH et al. Attributable mortality of ventilator-associated pneumonia: A meta-analysis of individual patient data from randomised prevention studies. *Lancet Infect Dis*. 2013;13(8):665-671.

43. Kalil AC, Metersky ML, Klompas M et al. Management of adults with hospital-acquired and ventilator-associated pneumonia: 2016 clinical practice guidelines by the infectious diseases society of america and the american thoracic society. *Clin Infect Dis*. 2016;63(5):e61-111.

44. Tablan OC, Anderson LJ, Besser R et al. Guidelines for preventing health-care–associated pneumonia, 2003: Recommendations of CDC and the healthcare infection control practices advisory committee. *MMWR Recomm Rep*. 2004;53(RR-3):1-36.

45. Dodek P, Keenan S, Cook D et al. Clinical guidelines. Evidence-based clinical practice guideline for the prevention of ventilator-associated pneumonia. *Ann Intern Med*. 2004;141(4):305-313.

46. Focaccia R, Gomes Da Conceicao OJ. Guidelines for the management of adults with hospital-acquired, ventilator-associated, and healthcare-associated Pneumonia. *Am J Respir Crit Care Med*. 2005;171(4):388-416.

47. Roquilly A, Marret E, Abraham E, Asehnoune K. Pneumonia prevention to decrease mortality in intensive care unit: A systematic review and meta-analysis. *Clin Infect Dis*. 2015;60(1):64-75.

48. Arthur LE, Kizor RS, Selim AG, van Driel ML, Seoane L. Antibiotics for ventilator-associated pneumonia. *Cochrane Database Syst Rev*. 2016;10:CD004267.

18

Mechanical ventilation and respiratory care

BASTIA LUCA, MAGNI FEDERICO, POZZI MATTEO, AND GIUSEPPE CITERIO

INTRODUCTION

Several pulmonary disorders may occur after brain injury and several mechanisms are involved in their pathophysiology. Unfortunately, these complications are very common in neurologically critically ill patients and are associated with longer length of stay in intensive care units and with a poor outcome.

Trauma-related complications

The injury mechanism that leads to the development of a traumatic brain injury (TBI) can simultaneously produce other non-neurological injuries such as pneumo- or hemothorax, pulmonary contusions, rib fractures, and flail chest. A patient full assessment is mandatory in order to diagnose and treat these complications.[1] Physical examination is the primary tool for diagnosing thoracic trauma, but signs of significant thoracic injury may be subtle or even absent. Serial examinations and use of diagnostic adjuncts are important. Chest x-ray remains the standard initial evaluation of chest trauma and should be performed in the emergency department in all hemodynamically unstable chest-trauma patients to exclude conditions that require lifesaving surgical intervention. In recent years, lung ultrasound has been widely used to evaluate pneumothorax, pleural effusion, and lung consolidation. A computed tomography (CT) scan is the most reliable exam and should be adopted in hemodynamically stable patients for any clinical suspicion of major chest trauma. For more details on primary and secondary surveys of thoracic trauma patients, refer to the Advanced Trauma Life Support (ATLS) guidelines.[2] The most common disorder related to chest trauma will be briefly summarized.

A pneumothorax occurs when air leaks into the pleural space and induces a collapse of the lung.

It can result both from both penetrating and nonpenetrating thoracic injuries. A pneumothorax can be:

- Simple (or closed)—When there is no communication with the external environment and no mediastinal shift
- Open—When a communication exists (direct or through a fistula) between external space and pleural space
- Tension—Characterized by a progressive buildup of air within the pleural space (through a one-way-valve effect) that produces a positive intra-thoracic pressure that pushes the mediastinum to the opposite side and impairs venous return, thus causing a considerable hemodynamic effect

Hemothorax is defined by the presence of blood in the pleural space. When the amount of blood exceeds 1000 mL (or a chest tube output is more than 200 mL/h), we talk about massive hemothorax.[3]

Pulmonary contusion is an injury to lung parenchyma, leading to edema and blood collecting in alveolar spaces and loss of normal lung structure and function. This usually develops over 24 h and reaches its peak at 72 h after injury and can impair gas exchange, increase pulmonary vascular resistance, and decrease lung compliance. A CT scan is highly sensitive in finding the contusion and can help determine its degree of severity.[4,5]

Rib fractures are usually extremely painful. For that reason, an impaired breathing pattern becomes more rapid and shallow. This alteration can induce atelectasis in both lungs. A flail chest occurs when three or more adjacent ribs are fractured at two different points causing a separation between the injured segment (that becomes free) and the rest of the thoracic cage. It is almost always associated with a severe lung contusion and high mortality rate (10%–20%). Optimal analgesia (via epidural catheter) and chest physiotherapy should be started as soon as possible.[5]

Lung infections

As many as 60% of neurointensive care unit (ICU) patients develop pneumonia. Aspiration pneumonia is a common finding in critically ill patients after using the inhalation of either oropharyngeal or gastric contents into the lower airways. All neurological patients are at higher risk of aspiration pneumonia because of their inability to protect their airways because of swallowing dysfunction (neurogenic dysphagia). Moreover, a high incidence of aspiration pneumonia is reported also in tracheostomized patients (aspiration in adults with tracheostomies is reported to be 30%–50%).[6] After discharge, TBI victims were 79 times more likely to die from aspiration pneumonia than the general population.[7]

The critically ill neurologic patient has prolonged intubation and mechanical ventilation. Thus, the risk of ventilator-associated pneumonia (VAP)—defined as a pneumonia that develops after at least 48 hours of mechanical ventilation[8]—is high. Other risk factors include decreased level of consciousness and deep sedation, diabetes, immuno-compromised status, polytransfusion, age, and obesity.[9–11] The incidence of VAP in TBI patients ranges from 21% to 60%, and the most common pathogen encountered is methicillin-susceptible Staphylococcus aureus.[12] VAP is associated in these patients with a threefold increase in in-hospital mortality and a longer length of stay.[1]

Neurogenic pulmonary edema

Neurogenic pulmonary edema (NPE) is a well-documented complication that arises acutely a few hours after a central nervous system (CNS) injury; it is characterized by a protein-rich fluid into the lung parenchyma.[13] The pathophysiology is complex and not well understood, but it seems that the adrenergic discharge occurring after a rise in intracranial pressure (ICP) leads to a sudden increase in systemic vascular resistance. The higher afterload and increase of myocardial work set by catecholamine release can reduce the pump efficiency. Furthermore, the adrenergic discharge also increases venous return to the right heart. The global effect is a strong hydrostatic pressure augmentation in the pulmonary capillary that causes interstitial edema formation.[14] Endothelial damage called "pulmonary venule adrenergic hypersensitivity" that persists even when the blood pressure is back to normal values contributes to protein leakage.[15,16] The entire mechanism that causes NPE is called "blast injury theory." The incidence of NPE changes with different CNS injuries; in TBI patients, it ranges from 32% to 50%.[17] This is normally an exclusion diagnosis and must be ruled out like other complications such as pneumonia, lung contusion, and heart failure.

Pulmonary embolism

A pulmonary embolism (PE) causes a sudden rise in pulmonary dead space (a dramatic decrease in alveolar perfusion that leads to a pathologic increase in the ventilation/perfusion ratio) with a net reduction of alveolar ventilation (tidal volume/dead space). To ensure a normal alveolar ventilation, the patient (or the ventilator) must increase minute ventilation. Often the origin of that complication comes from a venous thromboembolism (VTE), especially from a deep vein thrombosis. A TBI seems to carry a higher risk of VTE, probably because of the type of trauma and some delay in pharmacological prophylaxis. Approximately 20% of TBI patients develop VTE, most within 3 days of admission. Common risk factors for VTEs are obesity, injury severity, age, and LOS in the ICU. A fat embolism (FE) is less likely than a VTE, but is common in trauma patients, especially in those with bilateral femur fractures and multiple lower-extremity fractures. The incidence of post-traumatic FE has been reported to be as low as 0.25% or as high as 35%.[18] FE should be suspected in every trauma patient who develops respiratory failure and confirmed with a normal chest x-ray.

Acute respiratory distress syndrome

Acute respiratory distress syndrome (ARDS) is, according to the latest definition, "an acute diffuse, inflammatory lung injury, leading to increased pulmonary vascular permeability, increased lung weight, and loss of aerated lung tissue . . . with hypoxemia and bilateral radiographic opacities, associated with increased venous admixture, increased physiological dead space and decreased lung compliance." It can be diagnosed following the Berlin criteria (see Table 18.1).[19] TBI is an independent risk factor for ARDS, with a prevalence ranging from 20% to 25%.[20,21] The severity of neurological injury—classified by the Glasgow Coma Scale (GCS)—seems to be the most accurate predictor for the development of ARDS in this kind of patient. Other conditions are associated with the development of ARDS in TBI patients: male gender, younger age, white ethnicity, congestive heart failure, hypertension, chronic obstructive

Table 18.1 ARDS Berlin criteria

Timing	Within 1 week of a known clinical insult or new or worsening respiratory symptoms
Chest imaging	Bilateral opacities: not fully explained by effusion, lobar or lung collapse, or nodules
Origin of edema	Respiratory failure not fully explained by cardiac failure or fluid overload
Oxygenation	
Mild	200 mmHg $<PaO_2$–FiO_2 ≤300 mmHg with PEEP or CPAP ≥5
Moderate	100 mmHg $<PaO_2$–FiO_2 ≤200 mmHg with PEEP ≥5
Severe	PaO_2–FiO_2 ≤100 mmHg with PEEP ≥5

pulmonary disease, chronic renal and liver failure, sepsis, and multiorgan dysfunction.[1,12,22] A survey found a significant association between the early need of balanced crystalloid resuscitation or platelets transfusion and development of ARDS.[23] In all reports, the length of stay of these patients is higher than the control group without lung injury. A significant majority of studies defined ARDS post-TBI as an independent predictor of mortality (ranging from 28%–30%) and worse outcomes. Only one study did not confirm this finding.[20,21,24]

Pathophysiology of respiratory failure after TBI

A link between TBI (or brain injuries in general) and a subsequent lung injury has been advocated. In some items reported in the previous section, the relationship is linear and easy to understand because there is a single mechanism that impairs the lung physiology (such as PE, trauma, or aspiration pneumonia). Conversely, the development of ARDS post-TBI is a multistep process that leads to a decrease in gas exchange (PaO_2–FiO_2 ratio <300) and increases lung weight rapidly (<96 h from trauma) even in the absence of pneumonia on chest x-ray or direct lung injury. The first step is the blast injury theory mentioned for NPE formation: a sudden rise in lung capillaries' hydrostatic pressure shifts liquids and proteins in the interstitial space. This mechanism is certainly the fastest but not the only one; recently, new evidence underlines the importance of systemic inflammation, opening the way to the development of a "double-hit model."[25] After an injury, the brain releases into systemic circulation proinflammatory cytokines (IL-6, IL-1β, and TNFα) and proinflammatory mediators produced probably by microglia and astrocytes.[26–31] Moreover, the cholinergic pathway has an anti-inflammatory role, but during the blast injury stage, the adrenergic discharge (and the inhibition of vagus tone) reduces this effect. Finally, we must consider the acute secondary adrenal insufficiency that takes place after TBI in 25% to 50% of patients and is associated with worse neurological and global outcomes.[32] Hence, in the first hour after brain injury there is a strong pro-inflammatory cascade, and the lung is the most susceptible organ to this insult. Some experimental models found 24 hours postinjury elevated cytokines and increased migration of neutrophils and macrophages into the airways combined with a damage in type II pneumocytes.[33,34] The blast injury and the inflammation (and their related alterations at the lung level) represent the first hit in the double-hit model that makes the lung vulnerable to other different insults. Once weakened, the system is prone to be seriously damaged by a second hit such as high pressures or high volumes during mechanical ventilation, infections, surgical procedures, related alterations, or transfusions.[25] The global effect is an ARDS-pattern development and a sustained systemic inflammation that can lead to multiple organ failure and more negative long term outcomes.

MECHANICAL VENTILATION IN TBIs

Mechanical ventilation (MV) in neurocritical patients should be targeted not only to provide acceptable gas exchange but also to protect the brain and the lung from additional insults.[35,36] Clinicians should be aware of the interactions of positive pressure ventilation with brain compliance, intracranial circulation, and cerebral autoregulatory reserve to avoid intracranial pressure increase and allow adequate brain tissue oxygenation. In the following section, the pathophysiology of lung–brain interaction will be briefly revisited and practical suggestions about setting the ventilator will be provided.

Setting positive end-expiratory pressure

Clinicians should be aware that high positive end-expiratory pressure (PEEP) may worsen or trigger intracranial hypertension. Studies addressing the relationship between airway pressure and ICP have shown conflicting results.[37–39] A Starling resistor effect acting between dural sinus and cerebral veins (that damp the effect of intrathoracic pressure on cerebral vessels) has been advocated to explain these conflicting data. For these reasons, continuous ICP monitoring is mandatory in brain injury patients who suffer extracranial disorders and may profit from a higher PEEP. From a pathophysiological point of view, the effect of positive pressure on ICP depends on volemic status and lung compliance. Hypovolemic patients may suffer from cardiac output drop when higher PEEP is applied to the lung, leading to a fall in cerebral perfusion pressure. Moreover, the rates of cerebrospinal fluid absorption and cerebral venous return may be hampered, increasing ICP. These effects should be magnified in patients with high respiratory system compliance because the high intrathoracic pressure is more transmitted to the vessels and impairs venous return.

Setting tidal volume

Tidal volume (TV) in brain injury patients undergoing mechanical ventilation should be set to 6–8 mL/kg of ideal body weight. This suggestion comes from the evidence that low TV ventilation improves mortality in ARDS patients.[40] Moreover, recent studies have identified the use of large tidal volumes as a major risk factor for the development of lung injury and pulmonary complications in mechanically ventilated patients without acute respiratory failure.[41,42] When hyperventilation is required to control intracranial pressure, clinicians should be aware of the detrimental effect of high tidal volume (>8 mL/kg) in mechanically ventilated patients. Hence, it seems reasonable to increase respiratory rate rather than tidal volume when hypocapnia is required to lower ICP.

Setting fraction of oxygen

There is no evidence to support the use of eubarichyperoxia or hyperbaric oxygen[43–45] in TBI patients. Increasing oxygen tension at cellular level can be beneficial in ischemic regions, where oxygen is lacking. Few papers analyze cerebral regional metabolism through microdialysis showing a reduced lactate production and possibly an improvement of regional oxygen delivery and oxidative metabolism. However, mitochondrial dysfunctions usually occur in TBI lesions even in the presence of an adequate regional oxygen tension, sparing the effect of therapy that aims to increase oxygen availability.

ARDS IN TBI PATIENTS

Management of ARDS in neurologically critically ill patients should be double protective for the lung and the brain.[35] In this scenario, the historical "brain-directed" ventilation strategy (optimized oxygen delivery, tight pCO_2 control, minimized effect of positive pressure) should coexist with the lung protective strategy (low tidal volume, high PEEP to avoid atelectrauma and volutrauma, permissive hypercapnia). Adjustment of ventilator settings should be dictated mainly to avoid hypoxemia and protect cerebral perfusion. Tight pCO_2 control should be a concern only if the patient has a very low intracranial compliance and cannot tolerate normocarbia.

HYPERVENTILATION IN ACUTE BRAIN INJURY

It is well known by classical physiology that carbon dioxide exerts a remarkable effect in controlling vasoregulation of intracranial circulation.[46] Thus, tight carbon dioxide control is a priority in patients with acute brain injuries. Hyperventilation lowers ICP by inducting vessel vasoconstriction with a subsequent decrease in cerebral blood volume. Extreme cerebral vasoconstriction may supposedly reduce brain regional blood flow to a level near the ischemic threshold, fostering the development of ischemic lesions. The real impact of this event in the clinical practice is not known and has yet to be determined. There is no evidence to support recommendation for this specific topic. Balancing the risk–benefit ratio, it would appear reasonable to exploit the hyperventilation only in patients who present clinical signs of high ICP (anisocoria or neurological deterioration) or with raised ICP measured through an intracranial device (intraparenchymal catheter or external

ventricular drain). Anyhow, the clinicians should use different degrees of hyperventilation in a tailored way and under continuous monitoring. Prolonged prophylactic hyperventilation with partial pressure of carbon dioxide ($PaCO_2$) in arterial blood of 25 mmHg or less is not recommended.[47] In neurocritical patients suffering from high intracranial pressure in which hyperventilation is used, some authors suggest routine measurements of cerebral oxygenation (eg, $PbtO_2$) through an intraparenchymal catheter to minimize the risk of hyperventilation-induced ischemic damage. Others advise measuring oxygenation in the jugular bulb (eg, SjO_2). Both approaches have limitations. $PbtO_2$ reveals the oxygen pressure of a specific region but neglects the effect in the whole parenchyma. Conversely, SjO_2 monitoring reflects the balance between the global cerebral blood flow and global cerebral metabolic rate.

Common pitfalls: Intrinsic PEEP and dynamic hyperinflation

When a patient exhales (or the ventilator open expiratory valve at the end of the inspiratory time), the lung passively deflates to the end-expiratory lung volume that approximates relaxation volume—that is the volume where the opposite elastic recoils of lung and chest wall are equal. Whether spontaneously breathing or mechanically ventilated, patient expiration is normally a passive process. Incomplete emptying of the lungs at the end of expiration increases alveolar pressure relative to opening pressure, a condition called auto-positive end-expiratory pressure or autoPEEP or intrinsic PEEP. Many conditions predispose to autoPEEP. In the absence of flow limitation or increased airway resistance, a short expiratory time, caused by high respiratory rate, is frequently associated with incomplete expiratory alveolar emptying. Although the presence of autoPEEP can be suspected on the basis of persistent expiratory flow at the end of expiratory time, it can be feasibly measured during an expiratory hold maneuver: if the expiratory valve is closed at the end of expiration, gas trapped in the alveoli during the previous breath, which represent the "volume" gain accomplished for the increased end-expiratory alveolar pressure, have enough time to move from the distal airway to mount opening, causing a proportional increase of PEEP. AutoPEEP has detrimental effects on cardiovascular function, reducing cardiac output and arterial pressure.[48] AutoPEEP can be suspected in any mechanically ventilated patient with persistent expiratory flow at the end of expiration and can be calculated according to the end-expiratory occlusion method. Briefly, an end-expiratory occlusion maneuver of at least 4 seconds is performed. The amount of gas trapped in the airway at end-expiration will have time enough to leave distal airways, and this "plus" of expiratory flow will increase airway pressure at mount opening. The difference between pre-occlusion PEEP and end-occlusion PEEP is the autoPEEP.

Airway management

ENDOTRACHEAL INTUBATION

Airway management has a pivotal role in the early phase of resuscitation of brain-injured patients. Indeed, if the neurological injury often affects airway patency, inadequate oxygenation and ventilation in the earliest phase of resuscitation accounts for a significant burden of secondary brain injury. The goals of airway management in brain-injured patients are to prevent aspiration and ensure adequate oxygenation and ventilation. The decision to intubate a brain-injured patient always involves a comprehensive evaluation of different physiological, clinical, and environmental variables. Patients with impending respiratory arrest or vomiting without protecting airways should be intubated without delay. On the other side, intubation itself can represent a life-threatening procedure because its hemodynamic effects or unanticipated difficulties can worsen brain injury as well as prevent neurological assessment during the following period, which is always critical. The need for inter- or intrahospital transfer, imaging, or invasive procedure must be considered. Emergency Neurological Life Support (ENLS) suggests an algorithm for initial airway management.[49] For summary purposes, the most commonly accepted indication to emergency tracheal intubation (ETI) are:

1. Failure to oxygenate
2. Failure to ventilate
3. Anticipated clinical deterioration or need for transportation or invasive procedures
4. Failure to protect the airway

Although pulse oximetry, blood-gas analysis, or clinical examination can help the clinician recognize the first conditions, to decide whether a patient defends his airways is not always easy. It is generally agreed that depressed mental status is a risk factor for the inability to protect the airway. Brain Trauma Foundation guidelines recommend ETI for patients with severe traumatic brain injury, a depressed mental status, and a Glasgow Coma Scale <9.[50] Although this value represents a reasonable threshold, note that it comes from a single retrospective case-control study of a patient with severe traumatic brain injury with a GCS <9 who showed a higher survival rate than those who underwent prehospital intubation.[51] Above this class III recommendation, the choice to intubate a patient leans on a fine evaluation about bulbar functions, quantity of secretions, strength of cough reflex, and other variables such as anticipated neurological decline and need for transportation. When the clinician decides for ETI, a rapid sequence intubation (RSI) protocol should be used because it protects against a rise in ICP because of reflex response to laryngoscopy[52]; blood pressure, oxygenation, and end tidal CO_2 ($ETCO_2$) should be carefully monitored to avoid further neurological injury. In particular, postintubation $ETCO_2$ should be maintained within normal values (35–40 mmHg), and hyperventilation ($ETCO_2$ <35 mmHg) should be avoided unless a patient shows signs of cerebral herniation.[50]

Before intubation, the patient should be evaluated for a potential difficult airway because unanticipated difficult intubation is associated with negative patient outcome.[53] If this is true in the anesthesia and emergency department settings, one can imagine what a catastrophic physiological effect an unexpected difficult intubation would have on a brain-injured patient. The anticipation of difficult intubation or ventilation will help prepare appropriate skilled individuals and devices. Current bedside tests for airway assessment have low predicted value; their performance is heterogeneous among different populations, and trauma patients have not been specifically studied. ENLS guidelines propose the mnemonic LEMON—look, evaluate mouth opening and airway position, Mallampati score, obstruction, neck mobility—as an operative checklist to predict difficult intubation.[49]

Note that all patients with severe TBI should be treated as if they had spinal fractures until proved otherwise. If the likelihood of a cervical spine fracture is 2% to 7% in this population, then the clinician must keep in mind that a significant portion of all post-traumatic spinal cord injuries are indeed iatrogenic, occurring during the early resuscitation and transportation phase. If a patient requires ETI, it should be performed providing inline cervical spine immobilization according to ATLS standards.

LIBERATION FROM MECHANICAL VENTILATION

Liberation from mechanical ventilation involves two separate steps: weaning from a ventilator and extubation. A successful extubation requires the patient to meet criteria for both requirements. The American College of Chest Physicians, the Society of Critical Care Medicine, and the American Association of Respiratory Care have endorsed evidence-based guidelines[54] whose principles are summarized in Table 18.2. Unlike a general ICU population, brain-injured patients are usually intubated solely for airway management. General rules may not fulfill the needs of this special population: extubation failure, for example, may be related to reduced level of consciousness or bulbar palsy, leading to an inability to protect the airways or else respiratory failure because of respiratory center dysfunction and spinal or peripheral neuropathy but not just pulmonary pathology. If both extubation delay or extubation failure (ie, the need of a new intubation or a tracheostomy after extubation) can worsen patient outcome until increasing mortality, then it is critically important to recognize the right time to extubate the patient. Many indices have been extensively studied relative to their capacity to predict extubation readiness in the neurocritical care setting. Because of the noted peculiarity of this population, most studies focused on the level of consciousness, measures with the Glasgow Coma Scale or a Full Outline of Unresponsiveness score, although patients with low GCS were safely extubated in a large retrospective study,[55] or the ability to follow commands. A recent systematic review found that pneumonia, atelectasis, a mechanical ventilation lasting for more than 24 hours, low GCS score, inability to follow commands (especially to close the eyes), thick secretion, and impaired gag reflex significantly predict extubation failure.[56]

Table 18.2 Criteria for successful extubation

Recommendation from ACCP/ATS American College of Chest Physicians/American Thoracic Society (ACCP/ATS) for liberation from mechanical ventilation

For acutely hospitalized patients ventilated more than 24 h, initial SBT should be conducted with inspiratory pressure augmentation (5–8 cm H_2O) rather than without (T-piece or CPAP).

For acutely hospitalized patients ventilated for more than 24 h, protocols attempting to minimize sedation should be applied.

For patients at high risk for extubation failure who have been receiving mechanical ventilation for more than 24 h and who have passed an SBT, they should be extubated to preventative noninvasive ventilation (NIV).

For acutely hospitalized adults who have been mechanically ventilated for >24 h, protocolized rehabilitation directed toward early mobilization should be applied.

Acutely hospitalized adults who have been mechanically ventilated for >24 h should be managed with a ventilator liberation protocol.

A cuff leak test (CLT) should be performed in mechanically ventilated adults who meet extubation criteria and are deemed high risk for postextubation stridor.

Adults who have failed a CLT but are otherwise ready for extubation should be premedicated with systemic steroids at least 4 h before extubation; a repeated CLT is not required.

Tracheostomy

A tracheostomy has several anticipated advantages over ETI in terms of oral care, patient tolerability and sedation request, feeding route, and airway resistance.[57] Current recommendations suggest that in a general population tracheostomy is preferred when there is an anticipated need of an artificial airway for more than 21 days. The effect of early tracheostomy (generally defined as performed within 10 days of intubation) failed to show significant benefits in mixed critical care population.[58]

Differently, a recent systematic review, although taking into account a small number of trials, found that an early tracheostomy, compared with a late tracheostomy or a prolonged intubation, may lower ICU and long-term mortality in the neurocritical care population.[59] To perform a tracheostomy on a recently brain-injured patient raised some safety concerns in terms of effect on ICP of peri-procedural head positioning and unwanted hypoventilation. Many clinical observations seem to indicate that this procedure, also if performed early in the clinical course, is safe and does not cause clinically significant changes in brain hemodynamics.[60–63]

Special considerations for patients with spinal cord injuries

Less than 10% of patients with TBIs suffer a coex-isting cervical spinal fracture[64,65] with a variable prevalence of high spinal cord injury (SCI). Approximately two-thirds of patients with SCI suffer from respiratory complications such as atel-ectasis, pneumonia, and respiratory failure requiring prolonged MV. Respiratory mechanical impair-ment depends on the lesion level and severity[66]: the higher the lesion, the more significant the respira-tory muscles involvement. Briefly, the inspiration involves contraction of the diaphragm and external intercostal muscles, which expand the chest wall. When inspiratory effort increases, accessory muscles (such as the sternocleidalmastoid) can be recruited to participate to this process.[67] Expiration is generally passive but can become active with the contraction of abdominal muscles. Table 18.3 summarizes the innervation of respiratory muscles. Lesions occurring above C3 result in paralysis of the diaphragm and the intercostal and abdominal muscles and require immediate ventilatory support and long-term MV. High incomplete lesions (C2–C4) or lesions below C5 can produce weakness or spasticity in the muscles used for forced inspiration, but they leave neural control of the diaphragm intact. However, in these patients, usually quad-riplegics, respiratory function is severely compro-mised and respiratory failure requiring MV develops. Lesions above C5 require intubation in most cases. It is worth noting that lower thoracic spinal lesions are also frequently associated with a high risk of pulmonary complication.[68]

The main clinical consequence of expiratory muscles dysfunction is an impaired cough. Although cough reflex may be intact even in complete spinal section, as the afferent branch of the reflex bypass spinal cord running through vagal nerves, expiratory muscles paralysis or weakness causes ineffective cough with secretions accumulation.[69] At the same time, spinal-cord–injured patients frequently develop abundant and tenacious secretions, perhaps because of the unopposed parasympathetic vagal activity by the disrupted thoracic orthosypathetic plexus on bronchial mucosa. This parasympathetic imbalance also causes bronchial spasm, vascular congestion, and decreased mucociliary activity, which causes pneumonia, atelectasis and respiratory failure.[69]

No evidence-based recommendations exist on how to ventilate these patients with normal lungs but who are at high risk of respiratory failure. If the patient needs controlled mechanical ventilation, has

Table 18.3 Innervation and action of the main inspiratory and expiratory muscles

Muscle	Nerve	Origin	Action
Inspiratory Muscles			
Diaphragm	Phrenic nerve	C3–C5	Enlarge rib cage
External intercostal	Intercostal nerves	T2–T6	Elevate the ribs
Accessory Muscles			
Scalenes	Spinal nerves	C2–C7	Elevate the first rib
Sternocleidalmastoid	Accessory nerve (XI)	XI nerve nuclei	Elevate the first ribs and sternum
Upper trapezious	Accessory nerve (XI)	XI nerve nuclei	Elevate the ribs
Expiratory Muscles			
Internal intercostal	Spinal nerves	T1–T6	Reduce rib cage
Rectus abdominis	Spinal nerves	T5–L1	Increase abdominal pressure

"normal lungs," and pCO_2 does not matter, our practice is to set the ventilator according to the so-called lung-protective ventilation strategy, with a tidal volume of 6–8 mL/kg, and the use of PEEP with or without recruiting maneuvers. Such a strategy is associated with better pulmonary outcome in terms of ARDS and pulmonary infections incidence.[42] If the patients fit the criteria for spontaneous breathing, our goal is to maintain an adequate but nonexcessive level of patient effort tailoring ventilatory support with any of the available monitoring tool of muscular activity (electrical activity of the diaphragm, esophageal pressure, P 0.1).[70] This monitoring also allows clinicians to recognize and minimize patient–ventilator asynchronies and diaphragmatic dysfunction. Such a strategy—called "muscle-protective ventilation"—although not already assessed in large randomized clinical trial, is a new challenge to the field of mechanical ventilation.[71]

REFERENCES

1. Lee K, Rincon F. Pulmonary complications in patients with severe brain injury. *Crit Care Res Pract.* 2012;2012:1-8.
2. ATLS Subcommittee, American College of Surgeons' Committee on Trauma, International ATLS working group. Advanced trauma life support (ATLS®): 9th ed. *J Trauma Acute Care Surg.* 2013;74(5):1363-1366.
3. Kortbeek JB, Al Turki SA, Ali J et al. Advanced trauma life support, 8th edition: The evidence for change. *J Trauma.* 2008;64 (6):1638-1650.
4. Cohn SM, Dubose JJ. Pulmonary contusion: An update on recent advances in clinical management. *World J Surg.* 2010;34 (8):1959-1970.
5. Bastos R, Calhoon JH, Baisden CE. Flail chest and pulmonary contusion. *Semin Thorac Cardiovasc Surg.* 2008;20(1):39-45.
6. Kang Y, Chun MH, Lee SJ. Evaluation of salivary aspiration in brain-injured patients with tracheostomy. *Ann Rehabil Med.* 2013;37 (1):96-102.
7. Howle AA, Nott MT, Baguley IJ. Aspiration pneumonia following severe traumatic brain injury: Prevalence and risk factors for long-term mortality. *Brain Impairment.* 2011;12 (3):179-186.
8. Muscedere J, Dodek P, Keenan S, Fowler R, Cook D, Heyland D. Comprehensive evidence-based clinical practice guidelines for ventilator-associated pneumonia: Prevention. *J Crit Care.* 2008;23(1):126-137.
9. Kollef MH, Morrow LE, Niederman MS et al. Clinical characteristics and treatment patterns among patients with ventilator-associated pneumonia. *Chest.* 2006;129(5): 1210-1218.
10. Bronchard R, Albaladejo P, Brezac G et al. Early onset pneumonia: Risk factors and consequences in head trauma patients. *Anesthesiology.* 2004;100(2):234-239.
11. Dirnagl U, Klehmet J, Braun JS et al. Stroke-induced immunodepression: Experimental evidence and clinical relevance. *Stroke.* 2007;38(Suppl 2):770-773.
12. Mrozek S, Constantin J-M, Geeraerts T. Brain-lung crosstalk: Implications for neuro-critical care patients. *World J Crit Care Med.* 2015;4(3):163-178.
13. Theodore J, Robin ED. Speculations on neurogenic pulmonary edema (NPE). *Am Rev Respir Dis.* 1976;113(4):405-411.
14. Busl KM, Bleck TP. Neurogenic pulmonary edema. *Crit Care Med.* 2015;43(8):1710-1715.
15. Melon E, Bonnet F, Lepresle E et al. Altered capillary permeability in neurogenic pulmonary oedema. *Intensive Care Med.* 1985;11 (6):323-325.
16. McClellan MD, Dauber IM, Weil JV. Elevated intracranial pressure increases pulmonary vascular permeability to protein. *J Appl Physiol.* 1989;67(3):1185-1191.
17. Rogers FB, Shackford SR, Trevisani GT, Davis JW, Mackersie RC, Hoyt DB. Neurogenic pulmonary edema in fatal and nonfatal head injuries. *J Trauma.* 1995;39(5):860-868.
18. Akhtar S. Fat embolism. *Anesthesiol Clin.* 2009;27(3):533-550.
19. The ARDS Definition Task Force. The Berlin definition of acute respiratory distress syndrome. *JAMA J Am Med Assoc.* 2012;307 (23):2526-2533.
20. Holland MC, Mackersie RC, Morabito D et al. The development of acute lung injury is associated with worse neurologic outcome in patients with severe traumatic brain injury. *J Trauma.* 2003;55(1):106-111.

21. Aisiku IP, Yamal J-M, Doshi P et al. The incidence of ARDS and associated mortality in severe TBI using the Berlin definition. *J Trauma Acute Care Surg.* 2016;80(2):308-312.

22. Rincon F, Ghosh S, Dey S et al. Impact of acute lung injury and acute respiratory distress syndrome after traumatic brain injury in the United States. *Neurosurgery.* 2012;71(4):795-803.

23. Hendrickson CM, Howard BM, Kornblith LZ et al. The acute respiratory distress syndrome following isolated severe traumatic brain injury. *J Trauma Acute Care Surg.* 2016;80(6):989-997.

24. Salim A, Martin M, Brown C et al. The presence of the adult respiratory distress syndrome does not worsen mortality or discharge disability in blunt trauma patients with severe traumatic brain injury. *Injury.* 2008;39(1):30-35.

25. Mascia L. Acute lung injury in patients with severe brain injury: A double hit model. *Neurocritical Care.* 2009;11(3):417-426.

26. Koutsoukou A, Katsiari M, Orfanos SE et al. Respiratory mechanics in brain injury: A review. *World J Crit Care Med.* 2016;5(1):65-73.

27. McKeating EG, Andrews PJ, Signorini DF, Mascia L. Transcranial cytokine gradients in patients requiring intensive care after acute brain injury. *Br J Anaesth.* 1997;78(5):520-523.

28. Hutchinson PJ, O'Connell MT, Rothwell NJ et al. Inflammation in human brain injury: Intracerebral concentrations of IL-1alpha, IL-1beta, and their endogenous inhibitor IL-1ra. *J Neurotrauma.* 2007;24(10):1545-1557.

29. López-Aguilar J, Villagrá A, Bernabé F et al. Massive brain injury enhances lung damage in an isolated lung model of ventilator-induced lung injury*. *Crit Care Med.* 2005;33(5):1077-1083.

30. Ott L, McClain CJ, Gillespie M, Young B. Cytokines and metabolic dysfunction after severe head injury. *J Neurotrauma.* 1994;11(5):447-472.

31. Fisher AJ, Donnelly SC, Hirani N et al. Enhanced pulmonary inflammation in organ donors following fatal non-traumatic brain injury. *Lancet.* 1999;353(9162):1412-1413.

32. Dimopoulou I, Tsagarakis S, Theodorakopoulou M et al. Endocrine abnormalities in critical care patients with moderate-to-severe head trauma: Incidence, pattern and predisposing factors. *Intensive Care Med.* 2004;30(6):1051-1057.

33. Yildirim E, Kaptanoglu E, Ozisik K et al. Ultrastructural changes in pneumocyte type II cells following traumatic brain injury in rats. *Eur J Cardiothorac Surg.* 2004;25(4):523-529.

34. Kalsotra A, Zhao J, Anakk S, Dash PK, Strobel HW. Brain trauma leads to enhanced lung inflammation and injury: Evidence for role of P4504Fs in resolution. *J Cereb Blood Flow Metab.* 2007;27(5):963-974.

35. Oddo M, Citerio G. ARDS in the brain-injured patient: What's different? *Intensive Care Med.* 2016;42(5):790-793.

36. Mascia L. Acute lung injury in patients with severe brain injury: A double hit model. *Neurocrit Care.* 2009;11(3):417-426.

37. Caricato A, Conti G, Della Corte F et al. Effects of PEEP on the intracranial system of patients with head injury and subarachnoid hemorrhage: The role of respiratory system compliance. *J Trauma.* 2005;58(3):571-576.

38. Burchiel KJ, Steege TD, Wyler AR. Intracranial pressure changes in brain-injured patients requiring positive end-expiratory pressure ventilation. *Neurosurgery.* 1981;8(4):443-449.

39. Frost EA. Effects of positive end-expiratory pressure on intracranial pressure and compliance in brain-injured patients. *J Neurosurg.* 1977;47(2):195-200.

40. The Acute Respiratory Distress Syndrome Network. Ventilation with lower tidal volumes as compared with traditional tidal volumes for acute lung injury and the acute respiratory distress syndrome. The Acute Respiratory Distress Syndrome Network. *N Engl J Med.* 2000;342(18):1301-1308.

41. Guay J, Ochroch EA. Intraoperative use of low volume ventilation to decrease postoperative mortality, mechanical ventilation, lengths of stay and lung injury in patients without acute lung injury. In: Guay J, ed. *Cochrane Database of Systematic Reviews.* Chichester, UK: John Wiley & Sons, Ltd.; 2015.

42. Neto AS, Simonis FD, Barbas CS et al. Lung-protective ventilation with low tidal volumes and the occurrence of pulmonary complications in patients without acute respiratory distress syndrome: A systematic review and individual patient data analysis. *Crit Care Med.* 2015;43(10):2155-2163.

43. Longhi L, Stocchetti N. Hyperoxia in head injury: Therapeutic tool? *Curr Opin Crit Care.* 2004;10(2):105-109.

44. Diringer MN. Hyperoxia: Good or bad for the injured brain? *Curr Opin Crit Care.* 2008;14 (2):167-171.

45. Figaji AA, Zwane E, Graham Fieggen A, Argent AC, Le Roux PD, Peter JC. The effect of increased inspired fraction of oxygen on brain tissue oxygen tension in children with severe traumatic brain injury. *Neurocrit Care.* 2010;12(3):430-437.

46. Stocchetti N, Maas AIR, Chieregato A, van der Plas AA. Hyperventilation in head injury. *Chest.* 2005;127(5):1812-1827.

47. Carney N, Totten AM, Hawryluk GWJ et al. *Guidelines for the Management of Severe Traumatic Brain Injury* 4th Edition. 2016;6–15

48. Laghi F, Goyal A. Auto-PEEP in respiratory failure. *Minerva Anestesiol.* 2012;78(2):201-221.

49. Seder DB, Jagoda A, Riggs B. Emergency neurological life support: Airway, ventilation, and sedation. *Neurocritical Care.* 2015; 23:5-22.

50. Surgeons. BTFAA of NSC of N. Guidelines for the Management of Severe Traumatic Brain Injury 3rd Edition. *J Neurosurg.* 2007;24(Suppl 212):S1-106.

51. Winchell RJ, Hoyt DB. Endotracheal intubation in the field improves survival in patients with severe head injury. *Arch Surg.* 1997;132:592-597.

52. Walls RM. Rapid-sequence intubation in head trauma. *Ann Emerg Med.* 1993;22 (6):1008-1013.

53. Caplan RA, Posner KL, Ward RJ, Cheney FW. Adverse respiratory events in anesthesia: A closed claims analysis. *Anesthesiology.* 1990;72(5):828-833.

54. Schmidt GA, Girard TD, Kress JP et al. Official executive summary of an American thoracic society/American college of chest physicians clinical practice guideline: Liberation from mechanical ventilation in critically ill adults. *Am J Respir Crit Care Med.* 2017;195(1): 115-119.

55. Coplin WM, Pierson DJ, Cooley KD, Newell DW, Rubenfeld GD. Implications of extubation delay in brain-injured patients meeting standard weaning criteria. *Am J Respir Crit Care Med.* 2000;161(5):1530-1536.

56. Wang S, Zhang L, Huang K, Lin Z, Qiao W, Pan S. Predictors of extubation failure in neurocritical patients identified by a systematic review and meta-analysis. *PLoS One.* 2014;9(12):e112198.

57. Terragni P, Faggiano C, Martin EL, Ranieri VM. Tracheostomy in mechanical ventilation. *Semin Respir Crit Care Med.* 2014;35(4):482-491.

58. Gomes Silva BN, Andriolo RB, Saconato H, Atallah AN, Valente O. Early versus late tracheostomy for critically ill patients. *Cochrane Database Syst Rev.* 2012;3(3):CD007271.

59. McCredie VA, Alali AS, Scales DC et al. Effect of early versus late tracheostomy or prolonged intubation in critically Ill patients with acute brain injury: A systematic review and meta-analysis. *Neurocrit Care.* 2017;26(1)14-25.

60. Milanchi S, Magner D, Wilson MT, Mirocha J, Margulies DR. Percutaneous tracheostomy in neurosurgical patients with intracranial pressure monitoring is safe. *J Trauma.* 2008;65 (1):73-79.

61. Imperiale C, Magni G, Favaro R, Rosa G. Intracranial pressure monitoring during percutaneous tracheostomy percutwist in critically Ill neurosurgery patients. *Anesth Analg.* 2009;108(2):588-592.

62. Kocaeli H, Korfali E, Taşkapilioğlu O, Ozcan T. Analysis of intracranial pressure changes during early versus late percutaneous tracheostomy in a neuro-intensive care unit. *Acta Neurochir (Wien).* 2008;150(12):1263-1267; discussion 1267.

63. Kleffmann J, Pahl R, Deinsberger W, Ferbert A, Roth C. Effect of percutaneous tracheostomy on intracerebral pressure and perfusion pressure in patients with acute cerebral dysfunction (TIP Trial): An observational study. *Neurocrit Care.* 2012;17(1):85-89.

64. Clayton JL, Harris MB, Weintraub SL et al. Risk factors for cervical spine injury. *Injury.* 2012;43(4):431-435.

65. Holly LT, Kelly DF, Counelis GJ, Blinman T, McArthur DL, Cryer HG. Cervical spine trauma associated with moderate and severe head injury: Incidence, risk factors, and injury characteristics. *J Neurosurg.* 2002;96(suppl 3):285-291.

66. Como JJ, Sutton ERH, McCunn M et al. Characterizing the need for mechanical ventilation following cervical spinal cord injury with neurologic deficit. *J Trauma.* 2005;59 (4):912-916; discussion 916.

67. Butler JE. Drive to the human respiratory muscles. *Respir Physiol Neurobiol.* 2007;159 (2):115-126.

68. Cotton BA, Pryor JP, Chinwalla I, Wiebe DJ, Reilly PM, Schwab CW. Respiratory compli-cations and mortality risk associated with thoracic spine injury. *J Trauma.* 2005;59 (6):1400-1407.

69. de Paleville DGLT, McKay WB, Folz RJ, Ovechkin AV. Respiratory motor control disrupted by spinal cord injury: Mechanisms, evaluation, and restoration. *Transl Stroke Res.* 2011;2(4):463-473.

70. Bellani G, Pesenti A. Assessing effort and work of breathing. *Curr Opin Crit Care.* 2014;20(3):352-358.

71. Goligher EC, Ferguson ND, Brochard LJ. Clinical challenges in mechanical ventilation. *Lancet.* 2016;387(10030):1856-1866.

19

Cardiovascular care

JOVANY CRUZ NAVARRO, VIBHA MAHENDRA, AND ANDREW W. KOFKE

INTRODUCTION

Neurotrauma is a leading cause of death and disability in the world.[1] Estimates indicate that more than 2 million people per year suffer from some degree of traumatic brain injury (TBI) in the United States alone, and approximately 10% of these require extensive care in the Neurocritical Care Unit (Neuro-ICU).[2] Managing TBI and spinal cord injury (SCI) poses a distinctive set of additional challenges for the neurocritical care and neuroanesthesia practitioner. In addition to general ICU resuscitation, the intensivist must always be aware of the potential deleterious effects of secondary insults that would further worsen a neurologic outcome. Cardiovascular complications account for a wide spectrum of secondary insults, including but not limited to, hypotension or hypertension, arrhythmias, stunned/contused myocardium, and cardiac biomarkers elevation. Fortunately, most of these events are usually reversible and managing them should be always guided by considering the primary brain or spine injury. Current evidence–based guidelines are effective in reducing the impact of secondary insults and improving overall outcomes.[3,4] However, outcome improvement has also been reported just by quality improvement techniques.[5] By the end of this chapter, the practitioner should have a general sense of how to address cardiovascular complications in the Neuro-ICU.

CARDIOVASCULAR CONSIDERATIONS FOR PATIENTS WITH SEVERE TRAUMATIC BRAIN INJURY

Initial assessment

Before arriving at the ICU, patients with severe TBI are usually received, resuscitated, and stabilized in the emergency department or operating room. This initial assessment is crucial in determining both treatment and potential prognostication in neurotrauma. Every patient should be approached according to the basic Advanced Trauma Life Support principles, which include airway, breathing, circulation, disability (including Glasgow Coma Scale, GCS) and exposure assessment. Particular attention must be paid to blood pressure and oxygenation when there is a strong suspicion of brain and/or spinal cord injury. Once the severely head-injured patient has been transferred to the ICU, management consists of providing high quality general intensive care and using different strategies aimed at maintaining hemostasis as well as preventing intracranial hypertension, maintaining an adequate and stable cerebral perfusion pressure (CPP), avoiding systemic secondary brain insults, and optimizing cerebral hemodynamic and oxygenation. For purposes of this chapter we will focus on cardiovascular care in the Neuro-ICU, but framed to support management of the traumatically injured brain and spinal cord.

Hemodynamics—Arterial hypotension

Blood pressure management in TBI is of utmost importance, since systolic blood pressure <90 mmHg has been associated with increased mortality by approximately 150%, as well as being an independent outcome predictor of severe TBI.[6-8] Evidence from the Traumatic Coma Data Bank shows that up to 73% of patients have at least one episode of hypotension during their ICU stay.[9] Fortunately, among all predictors of outcome in TBI, hypotension is usually preventable and should be avoided and/or aggressively treated when established. In neurotrauma patients, neurogenic and hypovolemic shock represent the most common causes of hypotension. However, diagnosing hypovolemia can sometimes be complicated because hypovolemic hypotension can be masked by the hypertensive Cushing response from increased ICP, which in turn maintains cerebral perfusion pressure (CPP). Nonetheless, it is very unlikely that an isolated head trauma will cause severe hypotension unless there is an existing spinal cord injury or brain death. Therefore, other causes of hypotension should be ruled out; these include associated injuries such as intrathoracic or intraabdominal trauma, long bone fractures, scalp lacerations, and neck vessel injury.

Additionally, anesthetic drugs used during endotracheal intubation can predispose a patient to transient hypotension.[10] Current guidelines suggest systolic blood pressure goals of ≥100 mmHg for patients 50 to 69 years old, or ≥110 mmHg or above for patients 15 to 49 or >70 years old to decrease mortality and improve outcomes.[11] The recommended target CPP value for survival and favorable outcomes is between 60 and 70 mmHg. Whether 60 or 70 mmHg is the minimum optimal CPP threshold is unclear and may depend upon the autoregulatory status of the patient.[11] Notably, the location of the arterial transducer, heart or brain, can have significant effects on CPP determination.[12,13] In 2013 Kosty et al. surveyed practices used at U.S. Neuro-ICUs regarding arterial transducer location to determine CPP[13] and a wide variation in practice was found. Moreover, they further evaluated methods used in foundational studies underlying recommendations for managing TBI, and found that these also had widely varying methodologies.

When considering pharmacologic therapy to increase blood pressure, for hypotension management, its need must be seriously considered. Excessive increases in blood pressure can exacerbate cerebral edema.[14-18] This presumably occurs in brain areas with dysautoregulation and blood–brain barrier (BBB) disruption, and increasing blood pressure, rather than producing vasoconstriction and no change in regional cerebral blood flow (rCBF), can cause vascular distention, increased rCBF, and transudation of fluid across the damaged BBB. This in turn can impede cerebral venous drainage, leading to a positive feedback cycle and further exacerbation of brain edema.[19] Additionally, this can lead to increases in blood pressure risk producing or exacerbating intracranial hemorrhage, further contributing to the venous outflow problem.

Normally, exogenously administered catecholamines do not cross the BBB and have no effect on CBF or metabolism.[20] However, it has been demonstrated that catecholamine infusion in the presence of BBB disruption leads to increased blood flow and metabolism.[21] An unintended pharmacologic increase in metabolic rate is theoretically deleterious for outcome or local tissue viability, but this has not been tested.

In general, norepinephrine produces more consistent improvement in cerebral perfusion than dopamine and therefore is typically recommended.[22] Some evidence suggests that phenylephrine use is associated with a higher CPP compared with nor-epinephrine and dopamine,[23] although arguably dose correction should be a straightforward adjustment for such concerns. Overall, vasopressor use should be individualized based on a patient's specific hemodynamic and cerebrovascular status and pre-existing medical conditions (Table 19.1).

Hemodynamics—Arterial hypertension

Hypertension, defined as Systolic Blood Pressure (SBP) >160 mmHg or Mean Arterial Pressure (MAP) >110 mmHg, has been shown to be a secondary insult that can worsen intracranial hypertension and cerebral edema. However, systemic hypertension should not be treated until brain imaging has clearly demonstrated the absence of intracranial mass lesions. Lowering an increased blood pressure that is acting as a compensatory mechanism for increased ICP can worsen cerebral ischemia. Once the absence of an intracranial mass has been ruled out, and an ICP monitor or other monitors have been placed, MAP management should be guided by the CPP and neurophysiologic indicators of nutritive cerebral perfusion (eg, PbO_2, microdialysis assessment of lactate/pyruvate ratio, glucose, and glutamate; oxygen extraction fraction).

Multiple medications are currently available to treat arterial hypertension, and among these, calcium channel antagonists may have brain protective side effects. Nimodipine and nicardipine, which were developed specifically for brain protection purposes, have been assessed in numerous studies and there are several reports of their conferring protection versus vasospasm and ischemic brain damage.[24–29] However, one must consider that they are vasodilators and can modestly increase ICP,[30,31] either through direct vasodilation or reflex autoregulatory vasodilation in response to a blood pressure decrement.

Peripheral vasodilators such as nitroprusside, nitroglycerin, and hydralazine all have the potential to induce cerebral vasodilatation (directly or indirectly as previously noted) and thus cause hyperemic intracranial hypertension.[32–35] Additionally, they are associated with a compensatory increase in peripheral catecholamines and renin,[36] factors which theoretically may worsen ischemic brain injury.[37,38]

If such a drug is chosen and the patient is at risk for neurologic deterioration from cerebral ischemia or high ICP, close clinical observation is needed.

Any deterioration would mandate discontinuation of the drug. These concerns are critical for deciding which of these three drugs should be used. Although hydralazine is convenient, it cannot be reversed at the receptor and its effects can last for hours. Therefore, it may be preferable to use nitroprusside, nitroglycerin, or nicardipine in such situations, since adverse effects can be treated quickly and simply by discontinuing the infusion.

The choice of antihypertensive agent in a patient at risk of cerebral ischemia is not straightforward. Therapeutic urgency, sympatholytic and brain protective side effects, and the potential to increase ICP are all important considerations in choosing an antihypertensive drug.

Blood pressure effects on ICP—Plateau waves and determination of blood pressure optimum

In 1960 Lundberg monitored ICP in hundreds of patients, identifying characteristic pressure waves.[39] One of these waves has been identified as a plateau wave and is known to be associated with increased cerebral blood volume.[40] These waves occur when the ICP abruptly increases to nearly systemic levels for about 15 to 30 minutes, occasionally accompanied by neurologic deterioration. Rosner has observed and synthesized the data which convincingly suggests that intracranial blood volume dysautoregulation is responsible for plateau waves,[41] or perhaps for normal blood volume regulation in less severely injured or normal areas of the heterogeneously injured brain.

Cerebral blood volume (CBV) in normally autoregulating brain tissue increases due to vasodilation with decreasing blood pressure. There is an exponential increase in CBV as blood pressure decreases below 80 mmHg.[12] A small decrease in blood pressure, although in the normotensive range, produces exponential increases in CBV in a setting of abnormal intracranial compliance with the ICP at the elbow of the ICP-intracranial volume relation. Thus, a small decrease in blood pressure introduces an exponential CBV change on an exponential ICP relation such that ICP will increase abruptly and significantly (Figure 19.1).

Conversely, systemic hypertension can also increase ICP. Typically, within the normal auto-regulatory range and normal ICP, changes in blood

Table 19.1 Common vasopressors and inotropic agents used in the Neuro-ICU

Drug type	Receptor activated	Indications	Comments	Initial dosage
Inotropic Agent				
Dobutamine	α, β_1, β_2	Acute decompensated heart failure, cardiogenic shock, septic shock with depressed cardiac function	Can decrease SVR and provoke hypotension Tolerance may occur with prolonged administration	2.5–10 µg/kg/min
Milrinone	Phosphodiesterase III inhibitor	Increase CO in decompensated heart failure	Reduce dose if low CrCl Adverse effects: hypotension, arrhythmias, thrombocytopenia	0.25–0.75 µg/kg/min
Vasopressors				
Epinephrine	α, β_1, β_2	First-line agent in septic shock, anaphylactic shock	Risk of dysrhythmias and myocardial ischemia Adverse effects: Tachyarrhythmias, hyperglycemia, lactic acidosis, hypokalemia	2–5 µg/kg/min Children: 0.03–2 µg/kg/min
Norepinephrine	α, β_1	First-line agent in septic shock with low SVR	May increase oxygen consumption, risk of dysrhythmias and myocardial ischemia, may decrease intestinal perfusion and increase lactate levels	2–5 µg/min OR 0.02–0.06 µg/kg/min
Phenylephrine		Rapid MAP increases ↓ outflow tract gradient in patients with obstructive hypertrophic cardiomyopathy	May decrease CO, may cause reflex bradycardia, not indicated for septic shock, no β effect, therefore, less arrhythmogenic	10–100 µg/min 0.1–1 µg/kg/min Children: 0.03–0.1 µg/kg/min
Ephedrine	α, β_1, β_2	IV: Postanesthesia-induced hypotension	Can stimulate release of endogenous norepinephrine	IV: 5–25 mg slow IV push, may repeat after 5–10 min
Vasopressin	V_1	Refractory hypotension in septic shock, diabetes insipidus	Not first-line agent in shock, may decrease splanchnic perfusion and increase gut ischemia	0.04 units/min Children: 0.3–2 milliunits/kg/min
Dopamine	Dopa, α, β_1 variable			Dopa: 1–3 µg/kg/min α: 3–10 µg/kg/min β: 10–20 µg/kg/min

Abbreviations: CO: Cardiac output; CrCl: creatinine clearance, MAP: mean arterial pressure.; SVR: systemic vascular resistance

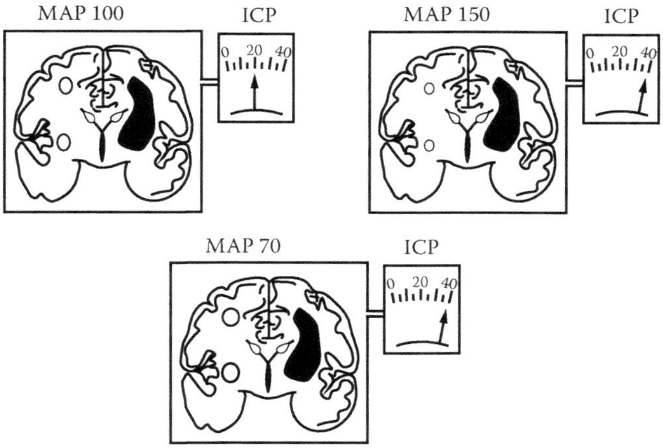

Figure 19.1 In the setting of heterogenous autoregulation in the brain, conditions may predispose to CBV-mediated increases in ICP with either increases or decreases in blood pressure.

pressure have no effect on ICP. However, brain injury and associated vasoparalysis blood pressure increases are thought to mechanically produce cerebral vasodilation that increase ICP.[42] This observation forms the basis for the detailed notion of using such ICP variations to quantitate autoregulation.[43]

Nemoto[44] and Nakagawa[45] have also observed that cerebral venous pressure tends to be consistently higher than the ICP. Thus, the increased cerebral venous pressure promotes and exacerbates brain edema. As previously mentioned, this then leads to a positive feedback cycle wherein increased ICP increases cerebral venous pressure, which then increases ICP.[19,44] Therefore, any other factors which may promote brain edema or otherwise increase ICP in this tenuous situation (eg, high extraventricular drain, systemic hypertension,[46] or hypoosmolarity) may initiate or contribute to such a positive feedback process.

It also appears that both increasing and decreasing blood pressure can increase ICP, suggesting the presence of a CPP optimum for ICP. In the absence of any patient-specific physiologic information this is probably about 80–100 mmHg.

These considerations underlie a current controversy regarding blood pressure management in the context of elevated ICP. One argument is that blood pressure should be maintained high to ensure adequate CBF and minimize the probability of plateau waves. The contrary argument is for ample fluids and low blood pressure to primarily promote CBF rather than pressure. It is this authors' opinion

that the preferred approach would be to induce the lowest blood pressure that allows sufficient CBF as indicated by repeated (preferably bedside) measurement of CBF and its adequacy.

Recent advances in transcranial Doppler ultrasonograpy have allowed insights into dynamic, nearly instantaneous, assessment of cerebral autoregulation in critically ill patients. This approach determines the correlation coefficient in real time to make inferences regarding autoregulation. A high correlation of blood flow velocity with ICP suggests poor autoregulation whereas no correlation is normal.

The ICP pressure-reactivity index (PRx) is a described quantitation of the aforementioned description of abnormal dynamic correlation of ICP changes with ABP changes and is another means to dynamically evaluate autoregulation,[43,47–49] with reports indicating that PRx correlates well with other autoregulation indices.[47,48,50,51] Steiner reported on the use of PRx monitoring in TBI patients to determine the optimal CPP.[43] Patients with better autoregulation in this optimal range as defined by PRx had better restrospectively determined outcomes. Moreover, patients with dysautoregulation related to higher ABP with corresponding ICP elevation also had worse outcomes, suggesting that autoregulation monitoring, to ensure adherence to an individual's optimal CPP, may be an outcome-altering ICU measure. Notably, PRx, as with TCD-based autoregulation studies, also appears to undergo a U-shaped curvilinear relationship with variations in CPP, with it being abnormally high (ie, ICP varies with ABP) at low (ischemic) and high (hyperemic)

CPP in TBI patients. This is underscored by reports of a significant ischemic burden in TBI patients[52–55] suggesting a delicate balance between hypotension-associated hypoperfusion and hypertension-associated edema/ICP exacerbation, both of which will worsen regional ischemia. All in all, these auto-regulation studies introduce the hypothesis that there is an individualized ABP optimum in TBI patients[48] that should be a therapeutic goal. This is an attractive notion but has yet to undergo prospective validation.

BEDSIDE CARDIOVASCULAR MONITORING AND FLUID ADMINISTRATION

Volume resuscitation should be implemented early during the process of TBI management. In order to achieve this, adequate intravenous access must be obtained including at least two large bore peripheral intravenous lines (14–16G). A radial or femoral arterial cannulation should be obtained for contin-uous blood pressure monitoring and blood sam-pling. Also, pulse pressure variation, stroke volume, cardiac index and output can be calculated by using noninvasive monitors such as NiCOM, EV1000, and so on. Femoral/subclavian central cannulas should be placed when possible to administer vasoactive medications and fluids. Of note, internal jugular vein cannulation should be avoided when there is concern for cervical spine injury or intracranial hypertension. Central venous pressure (CVP) should no longer be used as a marker of fluid res-ponsiveness, since tremendous amount of evidence shows that a given value of CVP does not predict fluid responsiveness.[56,57] Occasionally, the place-ment of a pulmonary artery catheter should be considered if the patient shows an inappropriate response to common measures of resuscitation, demonstrating hemodynamic instability or evidence of cardiac compromise. A Foley catheter should also be placed to help guide fluid administration.

Normal saline is the resuscitation fluid of choice for neurotrauma. Hypotonic solutions or dextrose-containing solutions should be avoided since they may decrease plasma osmolality and increase the possibility of cerebral edema. Moreover, colloids have been associated with more adverse outcomes and should be avoided as possible in TBI patients.[58] Although hypertonic saline solutions have been associated with the rapid restoration of blood pressure and the improvement of intracranial hypertension, no survival benefit has been shown and its use is not recommended during the acute period of resuscitation.[59] Additionally, it is very important for the NICU practitioner to be familiar with the composition of resuscitation fluids (Table 19.2), since many times the fluid of choice is dependent on an individual's hemodynamic, renal, and electrolyte profile.

Fluid overload after active resuscitation remains a routine problem, both in the intensive care unit and after major surgical interventions. Recent evidence supports this association with adverse outcomes since it is related to multi-organ complications including poor wound healing, gastrointestinal malabsorption, ileus, cholestasis, pulmonary edema,

Table 19.2 Composition of most common fluids used in the Neuro-ICU

| Fluid | Osm | mEq/L | | | | g/L | |
		Na	Cl	K	Ca	Lactate	Dextrose
Normal saline—0/9% NaCl	308	154	154				
Lactated Ringer's solution	275	130	109	4	3	28	
5% Dextrose in water	278						50
0.45% NaCl	154	77	77				
3.0% NaCl	1026	513	513				
5.0% NaCl	1710	855	855				
5% Dextrose in Lactated Ringer	525	130	109	4	3		50
5% Dextrose in normal saline	561	154	154				50
5% Dextrose in 0.45% NaCL	405	77	77				50

ARDS, prolonged mechanical ventilation, decreased lung compliance, delirium, renal interstitial edema leading to reduced renal blood flow, and glomerular filtration rate.[60,61] Therefore, it is essential for the ICU provider to understand some basic concepts of fluid responsiveness tests in order to guide adequate resuscitation.[62]

Dynamic tests of fluid responsiveness

Several predictors of fluid responsiveness have been developed over the last two decades including the passive leg raise test, pulse pressure/stroke volume variations, inferior/superior vena cava diameter variations, end-expiratory occlusion test, and the "fluid challenge." The main concept behind these fluid response dynamic tests is based on the principle of inducing short-term changes in cardiac preload, with the subsequent monitoring of the net effect on cardiac output. Of these, pulse pressure and stroke volume variations were first developed, but they are reliable only under strict conditions. The variations in vena cava diameters share many limitations of pulse pressure variations. Unlike the traditional fluid challenge, these dynamic tests do not lead to fluid overload. For purposes of this chapter, we will only review some basic concepts.

Pulse pressure and stroke volume variation (PPV/SVV) tests

The principle behind SVV use states that during mechanical ventilation, positive pressure during insufflation reduces preload to the right ventricle, with a subsequent decrease in preload to the left ventricle. If the LV stroke volume is diminished, this indicates that both ventricles are preload dependent. SVV is then calculated from the difference between the maximum and minimum stroke volumes divided by the average of the minimum and maximum SV over one entire ventilatory cycle.[63] A stroke volume variability ≥9.5% predicts an increase in SV of at least 5% in response to a 100-mL volume loading test.[64] SVV and PPV depend on tidal volume; at lower tidal volumes SV variability is decreased.[65] The reliability of such assessments, however, are likely altered in a continuum fashion with progressively decreased pulmonary compliance. For example, in severe Acute Respiratory Distress Syndrome (ARDS) no variation in pulse pressure or even pulmonary artery pressure may be observed.

Large evidence has been accumulated over the past decade that favors using PPV as a reliable marker of fluid responsiveness.[56,66–68] This is calculated as the difference of the maximum and minimum pulse pressure divided by its mean value during one respiratory cycle and subsequently averaged over 3 to 5 cycles (Figure 19.2). PPV >13% is an indicator of fluid responsiveness with a sensitivity of 94% and a specificity of 96%. Thus, the higher the PPV, the greater the increase in cardiac index will be after fluid administration.[66] PPV depends on several factors including the tidal volume used, respiratory frequency, Positive End-Expiratory Pressure (PEEP), driving pressure (plateau pressure—PEEP), and lung compliance.[69,70] PPV has been shown to predict fluid responsiveness only when tidal volumes >8 ml/kg are used in compliant lungs.[71] Different clinical situations can affect the interpretation and utility of PPV and SVV. In patients with right ventricular heart failure and pulmonary hypertension, or left ventricle EF <30%, PPV does not predict hypovolemic status.[72,73]

Limitations where the use of PPV/SSV becomes unreliable is very well documented. These limitations include, but are not limited to, spontaneous breathing or CPAP during mechanical ventilation, cardiac arrhythmias, use of low tidal volumes during ARDS,[69] intra-abdominal hypertension,[74,75] right ventricular failure,[72] and thoracic surgery with an open chest.[76]

Other dynamic tests

Passive leg raising (PLR) is a reversible preload challenge of around 300 ml of pooled blood in the lower extremities that induces significant changes in both right and left cardiac preload.[77,78] PLR can be used in spontaneously breathing patients, cardiac arrhythmias, low tidal volumes, and poor lung compliance.[69] Additionally, it does not lead to fluid overload.

The end expiratory occlusion test is used in patients who are undergoing mechanical ventilation. The rationale for its use is that with each inspiratory cycle, cardiac preload tends to decrease impeding venous return. If mechanical ventilation is paused (no less than 15 seconds), venous return improves, leading to a transient increase in preload. If cardiac output increases after this pause, the test is predictive of fluid responsiveness. The main disadvantage of this test is that it can't be used in

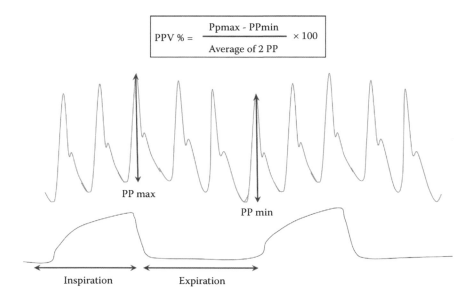

$$PPV \% = \frac{Ppmax - PPmin}{Average\ of\ 2\ PP} \times 100$$

Figure 19.2 Pulse pressure variation is calculated as the difference of the maximum and minimum pulse pressure divided by its mean value during one respiratory cycle and subsequently averaged over 3 to 5 cycles.

patients who are not intubated, and/or cannot tolerate at least a 15-second ventilatory pause.

MISCELLANEOUS

Blood products transfusion

Patients with severe traumatic brain injury commonly develop anemia and/or require emergent blood products administration. For patients with neurological injury, anemia can be a potential cause of secondary injury. Transfusions of packed red blood cells do restore hematocrit levels, but have been linked to a diverse set of complications including an increased risk of infection, multi-organ failure (including acute lung injury, thromboembolic events, etc.). Multiple studies have shown that there is no advantage to maintaining a relatively high hemoglobin concentration.[79,80] Current evidence suggests a worse overall outcome when hemoglobin is maintained above 10 g/dL.[81] However, there is strong physiologic support in preclinical studies and human data to recognize the patient's cerebrovascular reserve in making transfusion decisions. Thus, despite these recommendations, the practitioner should make a personalized decision regarding

blood transfusion, which should be based on each patient's hemodynamic profile.

Neurogenic stunned myocardium (NSM)

NSM, also known as Takotsubo Cardiomyopathy, stress-induce cardiomyopathy, or "broken heart syndrome," is most commonly seen after subarachnoid hemorrhage, but it can occur in the setting of acute traumatic brain injury. Prompt recognition and early management are key factors that can improve outcomes.

NSM is a reversible condition in the absence of coronary arterial disease. Its pathophysiology relates to an excessive release of catecholamines at the time of primary injury, resulting in a syndrome similar to that of an acute myocardial infarction. Acute stress stimulates autonomic centers of the brain such as the amygdala, the hypothalamus, and the insula, resulting in an exaggerated sympathetic outflow.[82-84] The catecholamine release induces excessive calcium influx and production of free radicals leading to a reduced ventricular function.[85] However, some believe the pathogenesis is more complicated than a simple catecholamine effect, given the infrequency with which it is seen in other contexts requiring high catecholamine administration.

Stress-induced cardiomyopathy is a diagnosis of exclusion, and acute myocardial infarction, cardiac contusion, and pericardial tamponade must be ruled out based on EKG, cardiac markers, and echocardiography. The diagnosis also requires an inciting stressful event, with evidence of reversible ventricular wall motion dysfunction. In NSM, dilated apical or mid-apical LV segments with hypokinesis or akinesis usually involves multiple coronary artery distribution without underlying coronary artery obstruction. These echocardiographic changes are partially or completely reversed within weeks. Additionally, a cardiac catheterization should be considered to rule out coronary atherosclerotic disease.

The foundation of management includes treating the underlying condition, hemodynamic support with vasopressors, and general ICU care. Initial therapy should try to minimize the primary neurologic injury. Aggressive treatment of intracranial hypertension must be performed according to the current guidelines. NSM can be complicated by severe LV dysfunction, acute heart failure, and pulmonary edema (which may itself have multifactorial contributors). Administering inotropes should be guided with advanced bedside monitoring including the use of a Swan-Ganz catheter when possible.[86,87] In more severe cases, an intra-aortic balloon pump can be considered.[88] Extracorporeal support can be considered as a final option but in the context of TBI this is fraught with multiple severe complications, largely related to the need for anticoagulation and locations of cannula placement.

ECG abnormalities and cardiac arrhythmias

Brain injury-related electrocardiographic abnormalities are a very well-known phenomenon and are particularly common after aneurysmal subarachnoid hemorrhage (aSAH). They can also be seen after a TBI. The most common findings are ST segment elevation/depression, U waves, flat or inverted T waves, and QT prolongation.[89] Although neurogenic ECG changes are not related to coronary hypoperfusion, manifestations are clinically undistinguishable from true myocardial infarction. Therefore, extensive cardiac workup must be performed to rule out active cardiac disease.

Coronary angiography is the definitive test that can rule out true coronary disease, however, it is rarely performed in this subset of patients. Neurogenic ECG changes usually reverse after 8 weeks.

Cardiac arrhythmias are common after a TBI and usually occur within the first week after an injury. These include sinus tachycardia, AV dissociation, and premature atrial and ventricular contractions.[89] Most neurogenic arrhythmias are benign and up to 35% of patients with SAH experience some type of cardiac arrhythmia, with 5%–8% being life threatening.[90] Drugs related to prolongation of QT segment should be avoided. A 12-lead EKG should be performed on admission and at 24-hours intervals to monitor for resolution. Monitoring and correcting electrolyte abnormalities is also recommended. Overall, treatment of the underlying neurologic condition will eventually lead to resolution of ECG abnormalities. Rarely, arrhythmias associated with ventricular dysfunction may require specific treatment with inotropic and vasopressor support.

Propofol infusion syndrome (PRIS)

PRIS is a collection of clinical and laboratory findings that develop after propofol infusion and are characterized by metabolic acidosis, elevated CK, hyperkalemia, elevated liver enzymes, rhabdomyolysis, triglyceride elevation, and acute renal failure.[91] PRIS is more frequently seen after long-term (>48 hrs) or high-dose infusion >4 mg/kg/hr or 67 mcg/kg/minute. PRIS incidence is around 17% in patients receiving at least 5 mg/kg/hour and around 31% in patients receiving more than 6 mg/kg/hour.[92] The exact etiology is not clearly understood, but there seem to exist impaired mitochondrial utilization of fatty acids.

Treatment includes immediate discontinuation if there is a high clinical suspicion. Practitioners should not use propofol infusion for more than 48 hours or at doses higher than 64 mcg/kg/minute. If sedation longer than 48 hours is needed, another sedative agent should be considered. Metabolic acidosis should be managed according to hospital protocol and in some cases renal replacement therapy may be needed. Patients with hyperkalemia and rhabdomyolysis should receive aggressive hydration if medical conditions allow it. Calcium administration, insulin with dextrose, beta-2 agonists, and potassium binding resins can be considered.

Cardiac dysfunction and arrhythmias are a major cause of mortality among patients who develop PRIS. Cardiogenic shock should be managed with inotropic and vasopressor support, and mechanical devices and extracorporeal support in refractory cases.[93,94] Although its clinical significance is not well described, some evidence suggests a potential association between QT prolongation and the use of propofol infusions in the ICU.[95] Physicians need to be aware that propofol pharmacology includes the blockade of calcium channels and beta-blocking properties, potentially making the effect of vasopressors less efficacious.[96]

In conclusion, PRIS is a rare but life-threatening condition. Thus, optimum management is prevention based on attention to risk factors and vigilant monitoring for early warning signs such as lactic acidosis, elevated CPK, and elevated triglyceride levels. When established, cardiac, metabolic, and/or renal complications should be aggressively treated.

CARDIOVASCULAR CONSIDERATIONS FOR PATIENTS WITH SPINAL CORD INJURY

Spinal cord injury (SCI) is a life-threatening condition that is associated with severe long-term disability and psychologic impairment. According to the National SCI Statistical Center, motor vehicle accidents, sports-related injuries, falls, and violence account for most SCI cases. The cervical spine is the most commonly injured area (51%) followed by the thoracic (35%) and the lumbosacral (11%).[97] The sudden loss of motor, sensorial, and autonomic functions predisposes the patient to dramatic hemodynamic, respiratory, and vasomotor changes. The prompt assessing and managing of these changes is crucial to improve short- and long-term outcomes. As with intracranial injury, secondary insults must be treated and/or prevented whenever possible. Adequate understanding and managing cardiovascular complications is crucial since these are among the most common causes of death in patients who suffer a SCI.

Understanding the pathophysiology involved in a SCI is critical to plan for the best protective management. Primary injury is caused by the direct trauma and/or lack of perfusion to the spinal cord. While there is no current effective acute therapy to treat primary injury, it is extremely important to recognize that secondary insults can be not only prevented, but potentially treated. Secondary injury resulting from hypoperfusion and hypoxia can occur within minutes of the primary injury, since potential watershed perfusion areas exist along its anterior and posterior blood supply distribution (Figure 19.3). Spinal cord blood flow has been estimated to be around 60 ml/100g/min.[98] Autoregulation mimics what occurs in the brain, with optimal blood flow occurring with MAP between 60–120 mmHg.[99] Also, an identical vascular response to hyper- and hypocarbia has been demonstrated. After trauma, the spinal cord exhibits impaired autoregulation; therefore, unidentified or untreated hypotension and hypoxia can cause further damage to the spinal cord.[100] Consequently, it is imperative to maintain hemodynamics, ventilation, and oxygenation within optimal range during the active phase of resuscitation and Neuro-ICU stay.

A SCI has a profound effect on the cardiovascular system and this effect can vary depending on the severity and cord level affected. Immediately after injury, there is an intense sympathetic discharge that causes transient marked hypertension

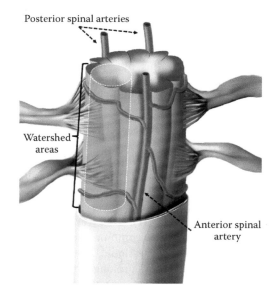

Figure 19.3 Secondary injury resulting from hypoperfusion and hypoxia can occur within minutes of the primary injury, as watershed perfusion areas exist along its anterior and posterior blood supply distribution.

that has been observed in both animal models of a SCI[101] and in human subjects.[102] This period of sympathetic discharge is followed by neurogenic shock which, by current definitions, consists of four stages that develop over weeks to months (Table 19.3)[103] In this chapter we will focus on the phase 1 of areflexia or hyporeflexia during the management of spinal shock.

Phase 1 of spinal or neurogenic shock is seen in 60% to 70% of patients who have a complete transection of the spinal cord[104] and it is characterized by profound hypotension associated with vasodilatation and decreased vasoconstrictive response, reduced cardiac output, and hypovolemia. Severity of hemodynamic alterations correlates with the area of spinal cord affected. The more cephalad the injury, the more severe the hemodynamic compromise. Bradycardia is seen in virtually all patients with complete cervical spine injury, resulting from the injured and/or impaired regulation of cardio-accelerator fibers at the T1–T4 level. Bradycardia occurs much less frequently if the thoracolumbar spine is involved. Therefore, preserving stroke volume is extremely important in order to maintain CO in the absence of a compensatory increase in heart rate. Currently, the proper blood pressure level that should be achieved after a SCI has not been established, but evidence recommends maintaining MAPs above 85 mmHg during the first week after an injury.[105–107] Treatment of hypotension should initially include crystalloids administration, followed by vasopressors if MAP goals are not achieved with the use of fluids only. Combined therapy with fluids and vasopressors has been associated with improved outcomes.[107]

Fluid management

Intravascular volume after a SCI, in the context of uncontrolled vasodilation, is insufficient to maintain adequate blood pressure, so active intravenous fluid resuscitation must be a priority. Isotonic crystalloid is the initial fluid of choice during a SCI resuscitation. However, experimental preclinical studies have shown hypertonic saline to be useful in decreasing spinal cord edema and inflammation.[106] Fluid resuscitation should be guided with invasive monitoring such as an arterial line, and possibly a pulmonary artery catheter in cases where significant pulmonary edema and hemodynamic impairment are suspected.[108] Careful fluid administration should be considered in order to avoid further cardiorespiratory damage in patients with neurogenic pulmonary edema resulting from the initial sympathetic discharge and/or myocardial dysfunction.

Vasopressors

The use of vasopressors should be accompanied with invasive hemodynamic monitoring including arterial cannula and central venous access as needed. The goal should be to achieve MAP levels of at least 85 mmHg during the first 7 days for neurologic outcome improvement. The vasopressor of choice should be a potent α-agonist such as norepinephrine or phenylephrine. However, the ideal vasopressor must be chosen and adjusted (as needed) based on the patient's overall hemodynamic profile and pre-existing cardiac function, as sudden increases in SVR and afterload can precipitate left ventricle failure. If the goal is to achieve a certain MAP level quickly, norepinephrine is likely the agent of choice as it has mild to no beta-2 agonism activity, thereby decreasing the possibility of peripheral vasodilation. If the decision to use a pure α-agonist such as phenylephrine is made, the practitioner should be aware of the risk of reflex bradycardia that can further worsen preexisting bradycardia in patients with high-level cervical injury. Epinephrine has some pro-arrhythmic activity and should be avoided unless physiologic and echocardiographic evidence indicate that the patient would benefit from its added inotropic support.

Table 19.3 Four-phase spinal shock model

Phase I	Day 1	Areflexia due to the loss of excitatory input
Phase II	Day 1–3	Return of spinal reflexes when nerve endings develop supersensitivity
Phase III	Day 3 to 1 month	Hyper-reflexia
Phase IV	1 month to 1 year	Progressive spasticity Classic autonomic dysreflexia develops during this phase

Miscellaneous

Cardiac dysrhythmias are frequently observed after a SCI because of an unopposed vagal activity. Bradycardia is the most common arrhythmia secondary to the loss of cardioaccelerator fibers at the T1–T4 level. Therefore, it is recommended to have atropine available at the patient's bedside during the acute phase of a SCI. Occasionally, a temporary pacemaker may be needed when severe hemodynamic instability exists. In 1987, Lehmann found that the incidence of bradycardia is higher with cervical spine injuries and is most commonly seen around day 4 after the injury, with complete resolution of cardiac electric abnormalities after 4 to 6 weeks.[103]

In patients with a SCI above T5–T7, splanchnic innervation is intact. Thus, distended intra-abdominal hollow viscera can cause excessive sympathetic outflow. This phenomenon is called autonomic dysreflexia, and is most commonly seen in patients with chronic spinal cord injury, but can be seen as early as 2 weeks after a SCI. It is characterized by reflex vasoconstriction below the lesion and vasodilation above, followed by baroreceptor reflex bradycardia. Symptoms include paroxysmal hypertension, bradycardia, headache, and diaphoresis. It can be quite severe, leading to myocardial infarction, seizures, and intracerebral hemorrhage. Hypertension should be managed with the use of quick onset intravenous agents such as labetalol, nitrates, or calcium channel blockers like nicardipine.

CONCLUSION

Acute traumatic brain injury and SCI are life-threatening conditions with lifetime morbidity. Cardiovascular complications represent a major problem in the Neuro-ICU and must be addressed in a timely manner to potentially improve outcomes. The Neuro-ICU practitioner has a very unique challenge in treating neurologic trauma patients, since they must consider the cerebral and spinal cord physiologic status before making any treatment decisions.

REFERENCES

1. Faul M, Xu L, Wald MM, Coronado VG. Traumatic Brain Injury in the United States: Emergency Department Visits, Hospitalizations and Deaths 2002–2006. Atlanta (GA): Centers for Disease Control and Prevention, National Center for Injury Prevention and Control; 2010.
2. Waxweiler RJ, Thurman D, Sniezek J, Sosin D, O'Neil J. Monitoring the impact of traumatic brain injury: A review and update. J Neurotrauma. 1995;12(4):509-516.
3. Le Roux P, Menon DK, Citerio G et al. Consensus summary statement of the International multidisciplinary consensus conference on multimodality monitoring in neurocritical care: A statement for healthcare professionals from the neurocritical care society and the European society of intensive care medicine. Neurocrit Care. 2014;21(Suppl 2): S1-S26.
4. Griesdale DEG, Örtenwall V, Norena M et al. Adherence to guidelines for management of cerebral perfusion pressure and outcome in patients who have severe traumatic brain injury. J Crit Care. 2015;30 (1):111-115.
5. Penn-Barwell JG, Roberts SA, Midwinter MJ, Bishop JR. Improved survival in UK combat casualties from Iraq and Afghanistan: 2003-2012. J Trauma Acute Care Surg. 2015;78(5):1014-1020.
6. Chesnut RM, Marshall LF, Klauber MR et al. The role of secondary brain injury in determining outcome from severe head injury. J Trauma. 1993;34(2):216-222.
7. Manley G, Knudson MM, Morabito D, Damron S, Erickson V, Pitts L et al. Hypotension, hypoxia, and head injury: Frequency, duration, and consequences. Arch Surg. 2001;136(10):1118-1123.
8. Marmarou A, Ward JD, Young HF et al. Impact of ICP instability and hypotension on outcome in patients with severe head trauma. J Neurosurg. 1991;75(Suppl):S59-S66.
9. Chesnut RM, Marshall SB, Piek J, Blunt BA, Klauber MR, Marshall LF. Early and late systemic hypotension as a frequent and fundamental source of cerebral ischemia following severe brain injury in the traumatic coma data bank. Acta Neurochir Suppl (Wien). 1993;59:121-125.

10. Schulz-Stübner S. Sedation in traumatic brain injury: Avoid etomidate. *Crit Care Med*. 2005;33(11):2723.

11. Carney N, Totten AM, O'Reilly C et al. Guidelines for the management of severe traumatic brain injury, fourth edition. *Neurosurgery*. 2017;80(1):6-15.

12. Rosner M, Becker D. The etiology of plateau waves: A theoretical model and experimental observations. In: Ishii S, Nagai H, Brock M, eds. *Intracranial Pressure*. New York: Springer-Verlag; 1983:301-306.

13. Kosty JA, Leroux PD, Levine J et al. Brief report: A comparison of clinical and research practices in measuring cerebral perfusion pressure: A literature review and practitioner survey. *Anesth Analg*. 2013;117:694-698.

14. Meinig G, Reulen H, Hadjidimos A, Siemon C, Bartko D, Schurmann K. Induction of filtration edema by extreme reduction of cerebrovascular resistance associated with hypertension. *Eur Neuro*. 1972;8(1):97-103.

15. Langfitt T, Marshall W, Kassell N, Schutta H. The pathophysiology of brain swelling produced by mechanical trauma and hypertension. *Scand J Clin Lab Invest –Suppl*. 1968;102(XIV):B.

16. Marshall WJ, Jackson JL, Langfitt TW. Brain swelling caused by trauma and arterial hypertension. *Hemodynamic aspects. Arch Neuro*. 1969;21(5):545-553.

17. Schutta HS, Kassell NF, Langfitt TW. Brain swelling produced by injury and aggravated by arterial hypertension. *A light and electron microscopic study. Brain*. 1968;91(2):281-294.

18. Marshall WJ, Weinstein JD, Langfitt TW. The pathophysiology of brain swelling produced by mechanical trauma and hypertension. *Surg Forum*. 1968;19:431-432.

19. Grande P, Asgeirsson B, Nordstrom C. Volume-targeted therapy of increased intracranial pressure: The Lund concept unifies surgical and non-surgical treatments. *Acta Anaesth Scand*. 2002;46:929-941.

20. Olesen J. The effect of intracarotid epinephrine, norepinephrine, and angiotensin on the regional CBF in man. *Neurology*. 1972;22:978-987.

21. MacKenzie ET, McCulloch J, Harper AM. Influence of endogenous norepinephrine on CBF and metabolism. *Am J Physiol*. 1976;231(2):489-494.

22. Steiner LA, Johnston AJ, Czosnyka M et al. Direct comparison of cerebrovascular effects of norepinephrine and dopamine in head-injured patients. *Crit Care Med*. 2004;32(4):1049-1054.

23. Sookplung P, Siriussawakul A, Malakouti A et al. Vasopressor use and effect on blood pressure after severe adult traumatic brain injury. *Neurocrit Care*. 2011;15(1):46-54.

24. Kakarieka A, Schakel EH, Fritze J. Clinical experiences with nimodipine in cerebral ischemia. [Review]. *J Neural Trans Suppl*. 1994;43:13-21.

25. Rosenbaum D, Zabramski J, Frey J et al. Early treatment of ischemic stroke with a calcium antagonis. *Stroke*. 1991;22(2):437-441.

26. Pickard JD, Murray GD, Illingworth R et al. Effect of oral nimodipine on cerebral infarction and outcome after subarachnoid haemorrhage: British aneurysm nimodipine trial. *BMJ*. 1989;298(6674):636-642.

27. Kucharczyk J, Chew W, Derugin N et al. Nicardipine reduces ischemic brain injury. Magnetic resonance imaging/spectroscopy study in cats. *Stroke*. 1989;20(2):268-274.

28. Alps BJ, Calder C, Hass WK, Wilson AD. Comparative protective effects of nicardipine, flunarizine, lidoflazine and nimodipine against ischaemic injury in the hippocampus of the Mongolian gerbil. *Br J Pharmacology*. 1988;93(4):877-883.

29. Grotta J, Spydell J, Pettigrew C, Ostrow P, Hunter D. The effect of nicardipine on neuronal function following ischemia. *Stroke*. 1986;17(2):213-219.

30. Bedford RF, Dacey R, Winn HR, Lynch CD 3rd. Adverse impact of a calcium entry-blocker (verapamil) on intracranial pressure in patients with brain tumors. *J Neurosurg*. 1983;59(5):800-802.

31. Hayashi M, Kobayashi H, Kawano H, Handa Y, Hirose S. Treatment of systemic hypertension and intracranial hypertension and intracranial hypertension in cases of brain hemorrhage. *Stroke*. 1988;19:314-321.

32. Overgaard J, Skinhoj E. A paradoxical cerebral hemodynamic effect of hydralazine. *Stroke.* 1975;6(4):402-410.

33. Griswold WR, Roznik V, Mendoza SA. Nitroprusside induced intracranial hypertension. *JAMA.* 1981;246(23):2679-2680.

34. Marsh ML, Shapiro HM, Smith RW, Marshall LF. Changes in neurologic status and intracranial pressure associated with sodium nitroprusside administration. *Anesthesiology.* 1979;51(4):336-338.

35. Dohi S, Matsumoto M, Takahashi K. The effects of nitroglycerin on cerebrospinal fluid pressure in awake and anesthetized humans. *Anesthesiology.* 1981;54(6):511-514.

36. Stanek B, Zimpfer M, Fitzal S, Raberger G. Plasma catecholamines, plasma renin activity and haemodynamics during sodium nitroprusside-induced hypotension and additional beta-blockage with bunitrolol. *Eur J Clin Pharmacol.* 1981;19(5):317-322.

37. Werner C, Hoffman WE, Thomas C, Miletich DJ, Albrecht RF. Ganglionic blockade improves neurologic outcome from incomplete ischemia in rats: Partial reversal by exogenous catecholamines. *Anesthesiology.* 1990;73:923-929.

38. Busto R, Harik SI, Yoshida S, Scheinberg P, Ginsberg MD. Cerebral norepinephrine depletion enhances recovery after brain ischemia. *Ann Neurol.* 1985;18(3):329-336.

39. Lundberg N. Continuous recording and control of ventricular fluid pressure in neurosurgical practice. *Acta Psychiatr Neurol Scand.* 1960;36 (Suppl 149): 1-193.

40. Risberg J, Lundberg N, Ingvar DH. Regional cerebral blood volume during acute rises in the intracranial pressure(plateau waves). *J Neurosurg.* 1969;31(3):303-310.

41. Rosner M, Becker D. Origin and evolution of plateau waves. Experimental observations and a theoretical model. *J Neurosurg.* 1984;50:312-324.

42. Matakas F, Von Waechter R, Knupling R, Potolicchio SJ Jr. Increase in cerebral perfusion pressure by arterial hypertension in brain swelling. A mathematical model of the volume-pressure relationship. *J Neurosurg.* 1975;42(3):282-289.

43. Steiner LA, Czosnyka M, Piechnik SK et al. Continuous monitoring of cerebrovascular pressure reactivity allows determination of optimal cerebral perfusion pressure in patients with traumatic brain injury. *Crit Care Med.* 2002;30:733-738.

44. Nemoto EM. Dynamics of cerebral venous and intracranial pressures. *Acta Neurochir Suppl.* 2006;96:435-437.

45. Nakagawa Y, Tsuru M, Yada K. Site and mechanism for compression of the venous system during experimental intracranial hypertension. *J Neurosurg.* 1974;41:427-434.

46. Kongstad L, Grande PO. Arterial hypertension increases intracranial pressure in cat after opening of the blood–brain barrier. *J Trauma.* 2001;51:490-496.

47. Czosnyka M, Brady K, Reinhard M, Smielewski P, Steiner LA. Monitoring of cerebrovascular autoregulation: Facts, myths, and missing links. *Neurocrit Care.* 2009;10:373-386.

48. Zweifel C, Lavinio A, Steiner LA et al. Continuous monitoring of cerebrovascular pressure reactivity in patients with head injury. *Neurosurg Focus.* 2008;25(4):E2.

49. Czosnyka M, Pickard JD. Monitoring and interpretation of intracranial pressure. *J Neurol Neurosurg Psychiatry.* 2004;75: 813-821.

50. Czosnyka M, Smielewski P, Kirkpatrick P, Laing RJ, Menon D, Pickard JD. Continuous assessment of the cerebral vasomotor reactivity in head injury. *Neurosurgery.* 1997;41:11-17.

51. Lang EW, Lagopoulos J, Griffith J et al. Cerebral vasomotor reactivity testing in head injury: The link between pressure and flow. *J Neurol Neurosurg Psychiatry.* 2003;74:1053-1059.

52. Coles J, Minhas P, Fryer T et al. Effect of hyperventilation on cerebral blood flow in traumatic head injury: Clinical relevance and monitoring correlates. *Crit Care Clin.* 2002;30(9):1950-1959.

53. Coles JP, Fryer TD, Smielewski P et al. Incidence and mechanisms of cerebral ischemia in early clinical head injury. *J Cereb Blood Flow Metab.* 2004;24:202-211.

54. Coles JP, Fryer TD, Smielewski P et al. Defining ischemic burden after traumatic brain injury using 15O PET imaging of cerebral physiology. *J Cereb Blood Flow Metab*. 2004;24:191-201.

55. Menon DK, Coles JP, Gupta AK et al. Diffusion limited oxygen delivery following head injury. *Crit Care Med*. 2004;32:1384-1390.

56. Bentzer P, Griesdale DE, Boyd J, MacLean K, Sirounis D, Ayas NT. Will this hemodynamically unstable patient respond to a bolus of intravenous fluids? *JAMA*. 2016;316:1298-1309.

57. Marik PE, Cavallazzi R. Does the central venous pressure predict fluid responsiveness? An updated meta-analysis and a plea for some common sense. *Crit Care Med*. 2013;41:1774–1781.

58. Van Aken HK, Kampmeier TG, Ertmer C, Westphal M. Fluid resuscitation in patients with traumatic brain injury: What is a SAFE approach? *Curr Opin Anaesthesiol*. 2012;25 (5):563-565.

59. Strandvik GF. Hypertonic saline in critical care: A review of the literature and guidelines for use in hypotensive states and raised intracranial pressure. *Anaesthesia*. 2009;64(9):990-1003.

60. Bouchard J, Soroko SB, Chertow GM et al. Fluid accumulation, survival and recovery of kidney function in critically ill patients with acute kidney injury. *Kidney Int*. 2009;76 (4):422-427.

61. Claure-Del Granado R, Mehta RL. Fluid overload in the ICU: Evaluation and management. *BMC Nephrol*. 2016;17(1):109. doi:10.1186/s12882-016-0323-6.

62. Mehta RL, Bouchard J. Controversies in acute kidney injury: Effects of fluid overload on outcome. *Contrib Nephrol*. 2011;174: 200-211.

63. Guinot PG, de Broca B, Abou Arab O et al. Ability of stroke volume variation measured by esophageal Doppler monitoring to predict fluid responsiveness during surgery. *Br J Anaesth*. 2013;110:28-33.

64. Berkenstadt H, Margalit N, Hadani M et al. Stroke volume variation as a predictor of fluid responsiveness in patients undergoing brain surgery. *Anesth Analg*. 2001;92 (4):984-989.

65. Reuter D, Bayerlein J, Goepfert MSG et al. Influence of tidal volume on left ventricular stroke volume variation measured by pulse contour analysis in mechanically ventilated patients. *Intensive Care Med*. 2003;29 (3):476-480.

66. Michard F, Boussat S, Chemla D et al. Relation between respiratory changes in arterial pulse pressure and fluid responsiveness in septic patients with acute circulatory failure. *Am J Respir Crit Care Med*. 2000;162:134-138.

67. Yang X, Du B. Does pulse pressure variation predict fluid responsiveness in critically ill patients? A systematic review and meta-analysis. *Crit Care*. 2014;18(6):650.

68. Marik PE, Cavallazzi R, Vasu T, Hirani A. Dynamic changes in arterial waveform derived variables and fluid responsiveness in mechanically ventilated patients: A systematic review of the literature. *Crit Care Med*. 2009;37:2642-2647.

69. Monnet X, Bleibtreu A, Ferré A et al. Passive leg-raising and end-expiratory occlusion tests perform better than pulse pressure variation in patients with low respiratory system compliance. *Crit Care Med*. 2012;40(1):152-157.

70. Michard F, Chemla D, Richard C et al. Clinical use of respiratory changes in arterial pulse pressure to monitor the hemodynamic effects of PEEP. *Am J Respir Crit Care Med*. 1999;159(3):935-939.

71. De Backer D, Heenen S, Piagnerelli M, Koch M, Vincent J-L. Pulse pressure variations to predict fluid responsiveness: Influence of tidal volume. *Intensive Care Med*. 2005;31 (4):517-523.

72. Mahjoub Y, Pila C, Friggeri A et al. Assessing fluid responsive-ness in critically ill patients: False-positive pulse pressure variation is detected by doppler echocardiographic evaluation of the right ventricle. *Crit Care Med*. 2009;37(9):2570-2575.

73. Wyler von Ballmoos M, Takala J, Roeck M et al. Pulse-pressure variation and hemodynamic response in patients with elevated pulmonary artery pressure: A clinical study. *Crit Care*. 2010;14(3):R111.

74. Diaz F, Erranz B, Donoso A, Salomon T, Cruces P. Influence of tidal volume on pulse pressure variation and stroke volume variation during experimental intraabdominal hypertension. *BMC Anesthesiol.* 2015;15:127.

75. Jacques D, Bendjelid K, Duperret S, Colling J, Piriou V, Viale JP. Pulse pressure variation and stroke volume variation during increased intra-abdominal pressure: An experimental study. *Crit Care.* 2011;15:R33.

76. Jeong DM, Ahn HJ, Park HW, Yang M, Kim JA, Park J. Stroke volume variation and pulse pressure variation are not useful for predicting fluid responsiveness in thoracic surgery. *Anesth Analg.* 2017;125(4):1158-1165.

77. Jabot J, Teboul JL, Richard C, Monnet X. Passive leg raising for predicting fluid responsiveness: Importance of the postural change. *Intensive Care Med.* 2009; 35:85-90.

78. Boulain T, Achard JM, Teboul JL, Richard C, Perrotin D, Ginies G. Changes in BP induced by passive leg raising predict response to fluid loading in critically ill patients. *Chest.* 2002;121:1245-1252.

79. Hajjar LA, Vincent JL, Galas FR et al. Transfusion requirements after cardiac surgery: The TRACS randomized controlled trial. *JAMA.* 2010;304(14):1559-1567.

80. Hébert PC, Wells G, Blajchman MA et al. Transfusion Requirements in Critical Care Investigators; Canadian Critical Care Trials Group. A multicenter, randomized, controlled clinical trial of transfusion requirements in critical care. *N Engl J Med.* 1999;340(6):409-417.

81. Robertson CS, Hannay HJ, Yamal JM et al. Effect of erythropoietin and transfusion threshold on neurological recovery after traumatic brain injury: A randomized clinical trial. *JAMA.* 2014;312(1):36-47. doi:10.1001/jama.2014.6490.

82. Cheung RT, Hachinski V. The insula and cerebrogenic sudden death. *Arch Neurol.* 2000;57(12):1685-1688.

83. Masuda T, Sato K, Yamamoto S et al. Sympathetic nervous activity and myocardial damage immediately after subarachnoid hemorrhage in a unique animal model. *Stroke.* 2002;33(6):1671-1676.

84. Nguyen H, Zaroff JG. Neurogenic stunned myocardium. *Curr Neurol Neurosci Rep.* 2009;9(6):486-491.

85. Bolli R, Marban E. Molecular and cellular mechanisms of myocardial stunning. *Physiol Rev.* 1999;79(2):609-634.

86. Naidech A, Du Y, Kreiter KT et al. Dobutamine versus milrinone after subarachnoid hemorrhage. *Neurosurgery.* 2005;56(1):21-61 [discussion: 26-7].

87. Lazaridis C, Pradilla G, Nyquist PA, Tamargo RJ. Intra-aortic balloon pump counterpulsation in the setting of subarachnoid hemorrhage, cerebral vasospasm, and neurogenic stress cardiomyopathy. *Case report and review of the literature. Neurocrit Care.* 2010;13(1):101-108.

88. Apostolides PJ, Greene KA, Zabramski JM, Fitzgerald JW, Spetzler RF. Intra-aortic balloon pump counterpulsation in the management of concomitant cerebral vasospasm and cardiac failure after subarachnoid hemorrhage: Technical case report. *Neurosurgery.* 1996;38 (5):1056-1059 [discussion: 1059-60].

89. Grunsfeld A, Fletcher JJ, Nathan BR. Cardiopulmonary complications of brain injury. *Curr Neurol Neurosci Rep.* 2005;5: 488-493.

90. Bruder N, Rabinstein A. Cardiovascular and pulmonary complications of aneurysmal subarachnoid hemorrhage. *Neurocrit Care.* 2011;15:257-269.

91. Otterspoor LC, Kalkman CJ, Cremer OL. Update on the propofol infusion syndrome in ICU management of patients with head injury. *Curr Opin Anaesthesiol.* 2008;21: 544-551.

92. Hwang WS, Gwak HM, Seo D. Propofol infusion syndrome in refractory status epilepticus. *J Epilepsy Res.* 2013;3(1):21-27.

93. Cooper HA, Panza JA. Cardiogenic shock. *Cardiol Clin.* 2013;31(4):567-580.

94. Khan M, Corbett B, Hollenberg S. Mechanical circulatory support in acute cardiogenic shock. *F1000Prime Rep.* 2014;6:91.

95. Scalese MJ, Herring HR, Rathbun RC, Skrepnek GH, Ripley TL. Propofol associated QTc prolongation. *Ther Adv Drug Saf.* 2016;7(3):68-78.

96. Zhou W, Fontenot HJ, Liu S, Kennedy RH. Modulation of cardiac calcium channels by

propofol. *Anesthesiology*. 1997;86(3):670-675.

97. Macias MY, Maiman DJ. Spinal cord injury. In: Torbey MT, ed. *Neurocritical Care*. New York: Cambridge University Press; 2010:283-293.

98. Sandler AN, Tator CH. Effect of acute spinal cord compression injury on regional spinal cord blood flow in primates. *J Neurosurg*. 1976;45:660-676.

99. Hickey R, Albin MS, Bunegin L, Gelineau J. Autoregulation of spinal cord blood flow: Is the cord a microcosm of the brain? *Stroke*. 1986;17(6):1183-1189.

100. Guha A, Tator CH, Rochon J. Spinal cord blood flow and systemic blood pressure after experimental spinal cord injury in rats. *Stroke*. 1989;20:372-377.

101. Eidelberg EE. Cardiovascular response to experimental spinal cord compression. *J Neurosurg*. 1973;38:326-331.

102. Piepmeier JM, Lehmann KB, Lane JG. Cardiovascular instability following acute cervical spinal cord trauma. *Cent Nerv Syst Trauma*. 1985;2:153-160.

103. Ditunno JF, Little JW, Tessler A, Burns AS. Spinal shock revisited: A four-phase model. *Spinal Cord*. 2004;42:383-395.

104. Lehmann KG, Lane JG, Piepmeier JM, Batsford WP. Cardiovascular abnormalities accompanying acute spinal cord injury in humans: Incidence, time course, and severity. *J Am Coll Cardiol*. 1987;10:46-52.

105. Hedley MN, Walters BC, Grabb PA et al. Blood pressure management after acute spinal cord injury. *Neurosurgery*. 2002;50 (suppl 3):S58-S62.

106. Nout YS, Mihai G, Tovar CA, Schmalbrock P, Bresnahan JC, Beattie MS. Hypertonic saline attenuates cord swelling and edema in experimental spinal cord injury: A study utilizing magnetic resonance imaging. *Crit Care Med*. 2009;37:2160-2166. PMID: 19487936.

107. Vale FL, Burns J, Jackson AB, Hadley MN. Combined medical and surgical treatment after acute spinal cord injury: Results of a prospective pilot study to assess the merits of aggressive medical resuscitation and blood pressure measurement. *J Neurosurg*. 1997;87:239-246.

108. Mackenzie CF, Shin B, Krishnaprasad D, McCormack F, Illingworth W. Assessment of cardiac and respiratory function during surgery on patients with acute quadriplegia. *J Neurosurg*. 1985;62:843-849.

20

Neurologic care

MARIA CHIARA CASADIO, PAOLA CRISTINA VOLPI, AND GIUSEPPE CITERIO

INTRODUCTION

Neurotrauma or traumatic brain injury (TBI) is an acute brain dysfunction that is caused by an external mechanical force (direct impact, penetrating trauma, acceleration, deceleration, or blast wave). This chapter focuses on the current standards of ICU neurologic care for neurotrauma. The aim of this treatment is to restore and preserve cerebral homeostasis, thereby preventing additional brain injury.

Some pathophysiological and monitoring aspects are briefly discussed in order to clarify the ICU management of neurotrauma, but please refer to previous chapters for more extensive treatment of these topics.

CLASSIFICATION

Neurotrauma can be classified by several different systems. These systems are based on:

- Injury severity with the Glasgow Coma Scale (GCS): A 3–8 score is classified as a severe TBI, a score of 9–13 is considered a moderate TBI, and a score of 14–15 is classified as a mild TBI[1]

- Pathophysiology of damage including parenchyma contusions, diffuse axonal injury, hematomas, subarachnoid hemorrhage, and petechiae
- Radiologic assessment (CT scan) through the Marshall scoring system[2] or the Rotterdam Scale[3]

PATHOPHYSIOLOGY

Neurotrauma includes a sequence of pathophysiological processes that have different characteristics and effects on cerebral function. We can identify a primary injury, due to the impact of the external mechanical forces, and a secondary injury that develops minutes, hours, or days after the trauma, that amplifies the initial damage. This phase is characterized by glutamate accumulation, production of oxygen radicals, mitochondrial dysfunction, alteration of axonal transport, and intracellular calcium accumulation. Vasogenic and cytotoxic cerebral edema, eventually worsened by impaired autoregulation, can increase intracranial pressure (ICP) and alter cerebral blood flow (CBF). All these pathophysiological events lead to cell necrosis or apoptosis and every process that increases cerebral metabolism may worsen energy dysfunction.

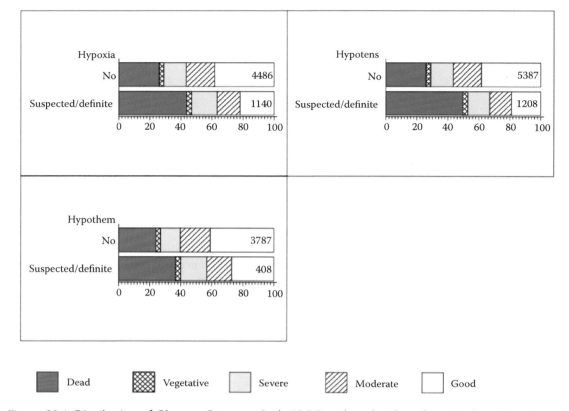

Figure 20.1 Distribution of Glasgow Outcome Scale (GOS) with and without hypoxia, hypothermia, and hypotension.

Additionally, a TBI triggers an inflammatory response. Acute neuroinflammation is an important response that can act as a neuroprotective process or can exacerbate a secondary injury. Potential triggers are changes caused by the primary injury or/and autoimmunization against neural epitopes.[4]

In this context, it's essential to avoid the deleterious effect of hypoxia (paO$_2$ <60 mmHg) and hypotension (systolic blood pressure <90 mmHg) that are independently associated with increased morbidity and mortality in TBI patients (Figure 20.1).[5]

ICU MANAGEMENT OF NEUROTRAUMA

ICU management of severe TBI consists of two pillars:

- General intensive interventions (hemodynamic optimization, respiratory care, infection control, nutrition); the goal of these treatments is to preserve a systemic physiological homeostasis in terms of normoxia, normocapnia, normoglycemia and electrolytes balance, thereby avoiding anemia and coagulopathy (Table 20.1).
- Specialized neurologic care; the goal is to address specific neurologic issues, such as intracranial volume control, optimization of cerebral oxygen supply and demand, and maintenance of cerebral homeostasis.

Neuromonitoring

The term TBI better describes a syndrome rather than a single pathological entity, including several lesions characterized by different pathophysiological processes that require different therapeutic goals and management approaches. Therefore, it's essential to target every therapeutic intervention to the specific mechanisms of brain injury. From this perspective, neuromonitoring is the most useful tool to tailor treatment.

Table 20.1 Goals of treatment

Pulse oximetry ≥95%	ICP 20–25 mmHg	Serum Sodium 135–145 mEq/L
PaO_2 ≥100 mmHg	$PbtO_2$ ≥15 mmHg	INR ≤1.4
$PaCO_2$ 35–45 mmHg	CPP ≥60 mmHg	Platelets ≥75 × 10^3/mm^3
Systolic pressure ≥100 mmHg	Temperature 36.0°C–38°C	Hemoglobin ≥7g/dL
pH 7.35–7.45	Glucose 80–180 mg/dL	

Abbreviations: CPP: Cerebral perfusion pressure; ICP: intracranial pressure; $PaCO_2$: arterial carbon dioxide partial pressure; PaO_2: arterial oxygen partial pressure; $PbtO_2$: brain tissue oxygen partial pressure.

PRINCIPAL

The principal aims of neuromonitoring are[6]:

1. Identifying any worsening of neurologic function and any secondary cerebral damage
2. Tailoring therapies to patient-specific pathophysiology rather than to predefined thresholds
3. Assisting with prognostication

Given the complexity of TBI pathophysiology, a single monitoring system seems insufficient to adequately explore brain physiology and guide critical care. Multimodal monitoring is defined as the simultaneous collection of data from multiple sources, with the ability to view the data in an integrated manner[7] and it's the most suitable monitoring approach for the complexity of neurotrauma.[8] One key purpose of multimodal monitoring is to anticipate any neuroworsening which is defined as (1) a decrease of two points of the GCS motor component, or (2) the loss of pupillary reactivity or asymmetry, or (3) a deterioration in neurological or CT status that is sufficient to warrant immediate medical or surgical intervention.[9]

In neurotrauma patients, a neuroworsening is often related to an increase of ICP due to an expanding lesion that can require an emergent surgical intervention, and it's often associated with a poor outcome.[10,11]

CLINICAL NEUROLOGIC ASSESSMENT

The first and most fundamental component of patient evaluation is the clinical neurologic examination. It should include assessing the level of consciousness by using the GCS[1] or the Full Outline of UnResponsiveness (FOUR) score,[12] which provides additional information on brainstem reflexes and respiratory drive. Pupil size and pupillary light reflex should be assessed with an automated pupilometer, which provides greater accuracy than a clinical pupil examination.[13]

Several recent studies showed that the combination between GCS, arterial blood pressure, age, and pupillary reactions[14] is highly predictive of patient outcome.[15]

The clinical neurologic evaluation of a patient is the most accurate way to detect neuroworsening and it should be done without sedatives and repeated several times a day. Assessment can be impaired by the presence of an altered mental status or by therapeutic intervention (endotracheal intubation, sedatives, analgesics, and neuromuscular blocking agents). Furthermore, the sedation hold (wake-up test) could be a risk for patients with a recent TBI because of possible effects on ICP and CPP and, consequently, on cerebral metabolism.[16] In a low compliance system, a wake-up test can be dangerous and interrupting continuous sedation should be excluded in conditions with critical ICP, low brain-tissue oxygenation, and hemodynamic instability. Multimodal monitoring can help to distinguish situations where interrupting continuous sedation can be useful or hamful[17,18] (Please also see the chapter "Sedation and Analgesia").

Radiologic monitoring

After classifying the primary lesion at the time of hospital admission, by using the Marshall scoring system, it's essential to pursue the radiological monitoring of severe neurotrauma. It has been demonstrated that a high prevalence of severe TBIs has a radiological evolution of hours and days after the initial injury.[19] The following actions are suggested for radiological monitoring:

- If the CT scan doesn't show any cerebral lesion when the patient is first admitted to the hospital, the exam can then be repeated after 24 hours. It has to be repeated after 12 hours in case of systemic hypotension or coagulopathy.

- If the CT scan shows a cerebral lesion when the patient is first admitted to the hospital, the exam can be repeated after 24 hours if the first one was performed 6 hours after the neurotrauma and in the absence of risk factors. It has to be repeated after 12 hours if the first one was performed 3–6 hours after the neurotrauma.

Any detection of neuroworsening or increasing ICP is an appropriate reason to perform an additional imaging test.[19]

ICP monitoring and intracranial volume control

Intracranial volume control is often a pathophysiological problem of neurotrauma that is due to either expanding hematomas or the secondary evolution of primary lesions such as intraparenchymal contusions.[20]

Since intracranial hypertension is harmful for cerebral function, ICP monitoring is usually considered essential after a severe TBI in order to prevent secondary injury,[21,22] even though a recent multicenter trial showed that ICP-based treatment was not superior to care based on imaging and clinical evaluation.[23]

The latest guidelines of the Brain Trauma Foundation (BTF)[24] suggest that managing of a severe TBI with ICP monitoring reduces in-hospital and 2 weeks postinjury mortality (level of evidence IIB); in the previous edition of BTF's guidelines.[25] ICP monitoring was recommended in the following conditions:

- Severe TBI (GCS 3–8 postresuscitation) and abnormal CT scan (hematomas, contusions, swelling, herniation, compressed basal cisterns)
- Severe TBI (GCS 3–8 postresuscitation) with normal CT scan if two or more of the following features are present: age >40 years, unilateral or bilateral motor posturing, systolic blood pressure >90 mmHg

In the latest guidelines, the suggested ICP threshold is 22 mmHg (level IIB),[24] but this value has been questioned, in favor of a more individualized ICP target, selected through a multimodal monitoring approach, which takes into account other patients' characteristics, such as CPP and cerebral metabolism.[8] The duration of increased ICP episodes has an important impact on neurologic outcome, and a recent trial demonstrated that high ICP can only be tolerated for short periods of time.[26]

Invasive devices (intra-ventricular or intra-parenchymal transducers) are the most accurate and utilized methods for ICP monitoring. Less accurate, noninvasive techniques include transcranial Doppler (through the determination of the pulsatility index)[27] or optic nerve sonography.[28] Both are limited in determining the correct ICP value. Regarding the optic nerve sonography, optic nerve sheath diameter (ONSD) determination has a high specificity of 93% and a sensibility of 88% for detecting ICP greater than 20 cmH_2O.[29] However, the technique has several pitfalls: ONSD measurement cannot be performed in patients with severe ocular trauma and many pathologies can stretch the optic nerve sheath, such as optic neuritis, arachnoid cyst, anterior orbital masses and others.

Intracranial volume control and consequently treating elevations of ICP follow several stepwise approaches. In case of intracranial hypertension, the first thing to do is to look for expanding mass lesions that can be surgically treated. Prompt evacuation has to be performed in these situations.[30]

- Extradural hematomas with a volume greater than 30 cm^3 and a midline shift greater than 5 mm or a clot thickness less than 15 mm
- Acute subdural hematomas with a midline shift greater than 5 mm or a clot thickness less than 10 mm

Immediate evacuation should be considered also for intraparenchymal lesions associated with raising ICP or neurological deterioration.

If the presence of a surgically treatable expanding mass is excluded, first-line therapeutic strategies for ICP control include (Figure 20.2):

- Analgesia and sedation. Anesthetics, analgesics and sedatives are useful tools as neuroprotective agents in suppressing cerebral metabolism and oxygen consumption. In addition, they decrease CBF and consequently cerebral blood volume and ICP by reducing metabolic demand. Attention should be paid to the impact of these agents on CPP and on a patient's hemodynamics.[31]

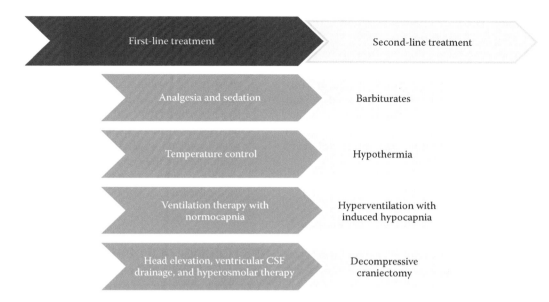

First-line treatment	Second-line treatment
Analgesia and sedation	Barbiturates
Temperature control	Hypothermia
Ventilation therapy with normocapnia	Hyperventilation with induced hypocapnia
Head elevation, ventricular CSF drainage, and hyperosmolar therapy	Decompressive craniectomy

Figure 20.2 Therapeutic strategies for ICP control.

Moreover, the use of sedation precludes the possibility of clinical assessment of a patient's level of consciousness.

- Ventilation therapy. Mechanical ventilation and airway protection are often necessary in severe TBI as a consequence of the neurotrauma itself or from the need for sedation. Since $paCO_2$ is the most determinant of CBF, normocapnia ($paCO_2$ 35–45 mmHg) is the therapeutic goal of mechanical ventilation, in the absence of impending cerebral herniation.
- Head elevation. This maneuver facilitates the cerebral venous outflow.
- Avoiding hyperpyrexia and other causes of cerebral vasodilatation. Cerebral oxygen metabolism strictly depends on brain temperature; an increase of 1°C in temperature causes a consequent increase of 6% to 7% in brain oxygen metabolism rate. Every condition that increases cerebral metabolism also increases CBF and intracranial blood volume, raising ICP in a low compliance compartment; all these conditions have to be avoided. Additionally, pyrexia determines glutamate release, raises oxygen radical production, and augments the permeability of the blood–brain barrier. Neurotrauma is a noninfective cause of pyrexia that occurs in 20% to 50% of TBI patients. Fever has to be controlled with oral Paracetamol and low doses of continuous Diclofenac infusion (75 mg/day), followed by body cooling devices.

- Cerebrospinal fluid (CSF) drainage. Even in the absence of hydrocephalus, external ventricular drainage can help lower intracranial hypertension by quickly removing intracranial volume (the procedure is possible only if a ventricular catheter is in place). Possible complications of this maneuver are hemorrhage, increase of contralateral expansive process if the drainage is abruptly performed, and infections.
- Hyperosmolar therapy. The hyperosmolar agents routinely employed are mannitol and hypertonic saline.
  - Mannitol is a polyalcohol that has a reologic and osmotic effect. Its hemodynamic effects are volemia expansion, blood viscosity reduction, an increase in cardiac output and systemic blood pressure, an increase of CPP and CBF, and finally a decrease of ICP by reactive vasoconstriction to increased CBF. Its osmotic effect decreases cerebral edema by reabsorping water through the osmotic pressure gradient in the region of intact blood-brain barrier. Conversely, in the region where this barrier is damaged, mannitol diffuses and worsens intracranial hypertension. This event is more common in case of continuous infusion. Side effects of mannitol use are serum hyperosmolarity (that has to be <320 mOsm), electrolyte imbalance, hypervolemia followed by blood volume depletion, and acute renal

failure. The dose of administration is 0.25 to 1 g/kg in 15 to 20 minutes.

- Hypertonic saline, ranging from 1.7% to 7% of NaCl concentration, reduces ICP through an osmotic pressure gradient in the undamaged cerebral tissue. Attention should be paid to serum electrolytes after hypertonic saline administration, avoiding abrupt increases in sodium concentration (maximum tolerated increase: 8 mEq/24 h).

Second-line treatments include:

- *Hyperventilation.* As mentioned before, $paCO_2$ heavily influences CBF and consequently cerebral blood volume; therefore hyperventilation can be used as a therapeutic intervention to decrease ICP, attaining levels of hypocapnia ($paCO_2$ <25 mmHg). The latest BTF guidelines recommend the use of hyperventilation with $paCO_2$ <25 mmHg only as a temporizing measure to reduce intracranial hypertension (level IIB).[24] Given the risk for cerebral ischemia carried by prolonged hypocapnia,[32] monitoring of brain tissue oxygenation through jugular venous oxygen saturation (SjO_2), or brain tissue oxygen, partial pressure ($PbtO_2$) measurements should be performed during hyperventilation.[8]
  - *Barbiturates.* These anesthetic agents decrease ICP by suppressing cerebral metabolism until burst suppression. However, their administration as a prophylaxis against intracranial hypertension is not recommended (level IIB), and their use is limited to treatment of refractory elevated ICP.[24] Side effects of barbiturates include: hemodynamic instability, hepatic enzymes induction, increase of sepsis incidence, and electrolyte imbalance.[33]
- *Hypothermia.* Moderate hypothermia (32–34°C) reduces cerebral basal metabolism and decreases ICP by reducing CBF. Additionally, hypothermia inhibits glutamate-related damage, post-traumatic inflammatory response, and calcium-related neuronal toxicity. However, hypothermia as an early treatment for intracranial hypertension in TBI hasn't shown benefits or potential harm[34] and current BTF guidelines do not recommend using prophylactic hypothermia to improve outcomes in TBI patients (level IIB).[24] Risks relative to hypothermia are coagulopathy, immunosuppression, and cardiac dysrhythmia.

- *Decompressive craniectomy (DC).* This surgical intervention has been proposed to relieve intracranial hypertension and has been shown to be beneficial in specific situations.[35,36] The most recent randomized control trial on DC and severe TBI with refractory intracranial hypertension (ICP >25 mmHg) showed a decrease in 6-month mortality, but a higher prevalence of vegetative state and severe disability in the group treated with DC compared with patients treated with only medical care.[37]

RESTORING AND PRESERVATION OF CEREBRAL HOMEOSTASIS

Cerebral blood flow and autoregulation

Monitoring CBF is crucial after severe neurotrauma; in the vast majority of TBI patients CBF is decreased early after the first cerebral insult and it can approach the ischemic threshold (15–17 mL/100 g of cerebral tissue/min). CBF can be monitored indirectly with TCD or with the thermal diffusion flowmetry through an intra-parenchymal thermistor (Hemedex®).

Cerebral pressure perfusion (calculated as the difference between mean arterial pressure, MAP, and ICP) is often interpreted as a surrogate for CBF, and it's therefore used to evaluate the adequacy of the CBF supply and demand.[8,38] The latest BTF guidelines recommend management of severe TBI using CPP monitoring in order to decrease 2-week mortality; the target value for survival and favorable outcome is between 60 and 70 mmHg (level IIB).[24]

In conditions of normal cerebral autoregulation, CBF is kept constant over a wide range of CPP values (usually 50–150 mmHg), through variations in cerebral vascular resistances.[39] Several pathologic processes, such as neurotrauma, can affect cerebral vasoreactivity, causing a linear increase in ICP consequent to MAP increase; in some patients autoregulation is preserved, but in a different range of CPP. However, testing vasoreactivity is essential in TBI patients. Autoregulation can be described by the pressure reactivity index (PRx); this index is provided by the analysis of the MAP and ICP curves through a statistical correlation model.

It identifies the optimal CPP for each patient, avoiding hypoperfusion or excessive CBF.[40] To better individualize the best cerebral perfusion threshold, data on brain oxygenation and metabolism should be integrated into the PRx. Once this target is determined, the therapeutic interventions are focused on modifying ICP (see above) and MAP through vasopressors, in order to reach the optimal CPP, paying attention to possible cardiopulmonary complications.

Cerebral metabolism

Cerebral oxygen metabolism rate ($CMRO_2$; normal value: 3.4 mL/100g of cerebral tissue/min) is very high compared with other organs: the brain represents 2% of total body weight, but is responsible for 20% of the oxygen consumption for the entire body. Pathological processes involved in neurotrauma can limit oxygen and glucose delivery to brain tissue, causing cerebral metabolism failure. Advanced monitoring of $CMRO_2$ includes jugular venous bulb oximetry (SjO_2) and measuring the brain oxygen tissue tension ($PbtO_2$). The first method allows the determination of the arterojugular oxygen content difference ($AJDO_2$; normal value 6.5 mL/dL); the probable SjO_2 threshold to avoid is 50% (level III).[24] $PbtO_2$ measures oxygen content through a parenchymal polar electrode and the threshold for cerebral hypoxia is 15 to 20 mmHg.[41] Other instruments that are used to monitor brain oxygen are the positron emission tomography (PET), the magnetic resonance spectroscopy (MRS), and the near-infrared spectroscopy (NIRS).

Microdialysis allows the evaluation of brain metabolism by measuring the metabolites (glucose, lactate, pyruvate, and glutamate) in the extracellular fluid; a lactate/pyruvate ratio >25 is highly suggestive of anaerobic metabolism[42] and it's an independent risk factor for mortality in TBI patients.[43]

The goal of neurologic care is the optimization of cerebral oxygen supply and demand. $CMRO_2$ depends on:

- **CBF.** All processes that cause the uncoupling of $CMRO_2$ and CBF lead to cerebral energy dysfunction. The CBF threshold for ischemia and treatments that improve CBF were discussed previously.

- **Systemic oxygenation and oxyphoretic power.** These variables can be modulated by varying the inspired oxygen fraction (FiO_2) in order to maintain arterial oxygen tension (paO_2) above 60 mmHg, eventually achieving levels of hyperoxia[44]; blood transfusion, if necessary; and optimization of the hemodynamic status of the patient.

- **Oxygen diffusion and brain tissue extraction ability.** This can be altered by endothelial swelling, microvascular collapse, perivascular edema or mitochondrial dysfunction; the resolution of these processes is the only option to increase brain oxygen extraction and utilization.[45]

Several preliminary clinical trials are currently exploring alternative treatments for restoring homeostasis in TBI. One of them showed an improvement in glucose metabolism through the infusion of hypertonic sodium lactate.[46] Exogenous lactate supplementation on the brain has a glucose sparing effect, because systemic lactate passes the blood–brain barrier, is converted into pyruvate, and acts as preferential substrate.[47]

NEUROPROTECTIVE AGENTS

Several clinical trials have been conducted on neuroprotective agents, however, at present, the effects on neurologic outcome are still lacking. The most relevant ones concern progesterone,[48,49] erythropoietin,[50,51] synthetic cannabinoid,[52] cyclosporine,[53] and other molecules. Even the use of steroids (such as methylprednisolone), that were proposed for their anti-inflammatory action, has been determined to be deleterious[54] and current BTF guidelines do not recommend their use (level I) in TBI patients.[24] The reason for these failures probably should be researched in the enrollment criteria of these trials, to ensure that they didn't target a specific mechanism of injury.[55] At present, there are no effective drug treatments for neurotrauma.

CONCLUSION

Neurotrauma is a complex syndrome that is characterized by different pathophysiological processes and requires different therapeutic goals and management approaches. Current standards of ICU neurologic care of neurotrauma have to take into account this complexity and target every therapeutic intervention for patient specific pathophysiology rather than for predefined thresholds. Multimodal monitoring is the most suitable monitoring approach for the complexity of neurotrauma.

REFERENCES

1. Teasdale G, Maas A, Lecky F, Manley G, Stocchetti N, Murray G. The Glasgow Coma Scale at 40 years: Standing the test of time. *Lancet Neurol*. 2014;13(August):844-854.

2. Marshall LF, Marshall SB, Klauber MR et al. The diagnosis of head injury requires a classification based on computed axial tomography. *J Neurotrauma*. 1992;9(1):S287-S292.

3. Mass AI, Hukkelhoven CW, Marshall LF, Steyerberg EW. Prediction of outcome in traumatic brain injury with computed tomographic characteristics: A comparison between the computed tomographic classification and combinations of computed tomographic predictors. *Neurosurgery*. 2006;57(6):1173-1182.

4. Simon DW, McGeachy MJ, Bayir H, Clark SB, Loane DJ, Kochanek PM. The far-reaching scope of neuroinflammation after traumatic brain injury. *Nat Rev Neurol*. 2017;13:171-191.

5. McHugh GS, Engel DC, Butcher I et al. Prognostic value of secondary insults in traumatic brain injury: Results from the IMPACT study. *J Neurotrauma*. 2007;24:287-293.

6. Stocchetti N, Le Roux P, Vespa P et al. Clinical review: Neuromonitoring—An update. *Crit Care*. 2013;17(1):201.

7. Lazaridis C, Robertson CS. The role of multimodal invasive monitoring in acute traumatic brain injury. *Neurosurg Clin NA [Internet]*. 2016;27(4):509-517. Available from: http://dx.doi.org/10.1016/j.nec.2016.05.010.

8. Le Roux P, Menon DK, Citerio G et al. Consensus summary statement of the international multidisciplinary consensus conference on multimodality monitoring in neurocritical care: A statement for healthcare professionals from the neurocritical care society and the european society of intensive C. *Intensive Care Med*. 2014;40:1189-1209.

9. Roozenbeek B, Maas AI, Menon DK. Changing patterns in the epidemiology of traumatic brain injury. *Nat Rev Neurol*. 2013; 9:231-236.

10. Morris GF, Juul N, Marshall SB, Benedict B, Marshall LF. Neurological deterioration as a potential alternative endpoint in human clinical trials of experimental pharmacological agents for treatment of severe traumatic brain injuries. Executive committee of the international selfotel trial. *Neurosurgery*. 1998;43:1369-1374.

11. Juul N, Morris GF, Marshall SB, Marshall LF. Intracranial hypertension and cerebral perfusion pressure: Influence on neurological deterioration and outcome in severe head injury. The executive committee of the international selfotel trial. *J Neurosurg*. 2000;92:1-6.

12. Wijdicks EFM, Bamlet WR, Maramattom BV, Manno EM, Mcclelland RL. Validation of a new coma scale: The FOUR score. *Ann Neurol*. 2005;58:585-593.

13. Larson MD, Behrends M. Portable infrared pupillometry: A review. *Anesth Analg*. 2015; 120:1242-1253.

14. MRC CRASH TRIAL, Collaborators. Predicting outcome after traumatic brain injury: Practical prognostic models based on large cohort of international patients. *BMJ*. 2008; 366:425-429.

15. Utomo WK, Gabbe BJ, Simpson PM, Cameron P. Predictors of in-hospital mortality and 6-month functional outcomes in older adults after moderate to severe traumatic brain injury. *Injury*. 2009;40(9):973-977.

16. Skoglund K, Enblad P, Marklund N. Effects of the neurological wake-up test on intracranial pressure and cerebral perfusion pressure in brain injured patients. *Neurocrit Care*. 2009; 11:135-142.

17. Helbok R, Kurtz P, Schmidt MJ et al. Effects of the neurological wake-up test on clinical examination, intracranial pressure, brain metabolism and brain tissue oxygenation in severely brain-injured patients. *Crit Care [Internet]*. 2012;16(6):R226. Available from: http://ccforum.com/content/16/6/R226.

18. Prisco L, Citerio G. To wake-up, or not to wake-up: That is the Hamletic neurocritical care question! *Crit Care*. 2012;16:190.

19. Brown CV, Zada G, Salim A et al. Indications for routine repeat head computed tomography (CT) stratified by severity of traumatic brain injury. *J Trauma.* 2007;62:1339-1345.

20. Iaccarino C, Schiavi P, Picetti E et al. Patients with brain contusions: Predictors of outcome and relationship between radiological and clinical evolution. *J Neurosurg.* 2014;120: 908-918.

21. Fowler RA, Mainprize TG, Scales DC et al. Intracranial pressure monitoring in severe traumatic brain injury: Results from the American College of Surgeons. *J Neurotrauma.* 2013; 30(20):1737-1746.

22. Farahvar A, Gerber LM, Chiu YL, Carney N, Hartl R, Ghajar J. Increased mortality in patients with severe traumatic brain injury treated without intracranial pressure monitoring. *J Neurosurg.* 2012;117(4):729-734.

23. Chesnut RM, Temkin N, Carney N et al. A trial of intracranial-pressure monitoring in traumatic brain injury. *N Eng J Med.* 2012; 367:2471-2481.

24. Carney N, Totten AM, Reilly CO et al. Guidelines for the Management of Severe Traumatic Brain Injury, 4th Edition. *Neurosurgery.* 2016.

25. Bratton SL, Chestnut RM, Ghajar J et al. Guidelines for the management of severe traumatic brain injury. *J Neurotrauma.* 2007; 24(1):1-106.

26. Guiza F, Depreitere B, Piper I et al. Visualizing the pressure and time burden of intracranial hypertension in adult and paediatric traumatic brain injury. *Intensive Care Med.* 2015;41(6):1067-1076.

27. Wakerley BR, Kusuma Y, Yeo LLL et al. Usefulness of transcranial Doppler-derived cerebral hemodynamic parameters in the noninvasive assessment of intracranial pressure. *J Neuroimaging.* 2015;25:111-116.

28. Geeraerts T, Launey Y, Martin L et al. Ultrasonography of the optic nerve sheath may be useful for detecting raised intracranial pressure after severe brain injury. *Intensive Care Med.* 2007;33(10):1704-1711.

29. Kimberly HH, Shah S, Marill K, Noble V. Correlation of optic nerve sheath diameter pressure. *Acad Emerg Med.* 2008;15(2):201-204.

30. Bullock MR, Chestnut RM, Ghajar J et al. Surgical management of acute epidural hematomas. *Neurosurgery.* 2006;58:S7-S15.

31. Roberts DJ, Hall RI, Kramer AH, Robertson HL, Gallagher CN, Zygun DA. Sedation for critically ill adults with severe traumatic brain injury: Systematic review of randomized controlled trials. *Crit Care Med.* 2011;39 (12):2743-2751.

32. Coles JP, Fryer TD, Coleman MR et al. Hyperventilation following head injury: Effect on ischemic burden and cerebral oxidative metabolism. *Crit Care Med.* 2007;35:568-578.

33. Schalén W, Messeter K, Nordström CH. Complication and side effects during thiopentone therapy in patients with severe head injuries. *Acta Anaesthesiol Scand.* 1992;36: 369-377.

34. Andrews PJ, Sinclair HL, Rodriguez A et al. Hypothermia for intracranial hypertension after traumatic brain injury. *N Engl J Med.* 2015;373:2403-2412.

35. Bor-Seng-Shu E, Figuiredo EG, Amorim RLO et al. Decompressive craniectomy: A meta-analysis of influences on intracranial pressure and cerebral perfusion pressure in the treatment of traumatic brain injury. *J Neurosurg.* 2012;117(3):589-596.

36. Eberle BM, Schnuriger B, Inaba K, Gruen JP, Demetriades D, Belzberg H. Decompressive craniectomy: Surgical control of traumatic intracranial hypertension may improve outcome. *Injury.* 2010;41(9):894-898.

37. Hutchinson PJ, Kolias AG, Timofeev IS et al. Trial of decompressive craniectomy for traumatic intracranial hypertension. *N Engl J Med.* 2016;375:1119-1130.

38. Wagner EM, Traystman RJ. Hydrostatic determinants of cerebral perfusion. *Crit Care Med.* 1986;14(5):484-490.

39. Heistad DD, Kontos H. *Handbook of physiology, The Cardiovascular System, Peripheral Circulation and Organ Blood Flow.* 1983;137-182.

40. Aries MJ, Czosnyka M, Budohoski KP et al. Continuous determination of optimal cerebral perfusion pressure in traumatic brain injury. *Crit Care Med.* 2012;40:2456-2463.

41. Doppenberg EM, Zauner A, Watson JC et al. Determination of the ischemic threshold for

brain oxygen tension. *Acta Neurochir Suppl.* 1998;71:166-169.

42. Hutchinson PJ, Carpenter KLH, Chen JW et al. Consensus statement from the 2014 international microdialysis forum. *Intensive Care Med.* 2015;41:1517-1528.

43. Nordström CH, Nielsen TH, Schalén W, Reinstrup P, Ungerstedt U. Biochemical indications of cerebral ischaemia and mitochondrial dysfunction in severe brain trauma analysed with regard to type of lesion. *Acta Neurochir.* 2016;158:1231-1240.

44. Nortje J, Coles JP, Timofeev I et al. Effect of hyperoxia on regional oxygenation and metabolism after severe traumatic brain injury: Preliminary findings. *Crit Care Med.* 2008;36:273-281.

45. Menon DK, Coles JP, Gupta AK et al. Diffusion limited oxygen delivery following head injury. *Crit Care Med.* 2004;32:1384-1390.

46. Quintard H, Patet C, Zerlauth JB et al. Improvement of neuroenergetics by hypertonic lactate therapy in patients with traumatic brain injury is dependent on baseline cerebral lactate/pyruvate ratio. *Neurotrauma.* 2015;33:681-687.

47. Bouzat P, Sala N, Suys T et al. Cerebral metabolic effects of exogenous lactate supplementation on the injured human brain. *Intensive Care Med.* 2014;40:412-421.

48. Wright DW, Yeatts SD, Silbergleit R et al. Very early administration of progesterone for acute traumatic brain injury. *NEJM.* 2014;371:2457-2466.

49. Skolnick BE, Maas AI, Narayan RK et al. A clinical trial of progesterone for severe traumatic brain injury. *NEJM.* 2014;371:2467-2476.

50. Robertson CS, Hannay HJ, Yamal JM et al. Effect of erythropoietin and transfusion threshold on neurological recovery after traumatic brain injury: A randomized clinical trial. *JAMA.* 2014;312:36-47.

51. Nichol A, French C, Little L et al. Erythropoietin in traumatic brain injury (EPO-TBI): A double-blind randomised controlled trial. *Lancet.* 2015;386:2499-2506.

52. Maas AI, Murray G, Henney H 3rd et al. Efficacy and safety of dexanabinol in severe traumatic brain injury: Results of a phase III randomized, placebo-controlled, clinical trial. *Lancet Neurol.* 2006;5(1):38-45.

53. Mazzeo AT, Alves OL, Gilman CB et al. Brain metabolic and hemodynamic effects of cyclosporine A after human severe traumatic brain injury: A microdialysis study. *Acta Neurochir Wien.* 2008;150(10):1019-1031.

54. Roberts I, Yates D, Sandercock P et al. Effect of intravenous corticosteroids on death within 14 days in 10008 adults with clinically significant head injury (MRC CRASH trial): Randomized placebo-control trial. *Lancet.* 2004;364:1321-1328.

55. Stocchetti N, Taccone FS, Citerio G et al. Neuroprotection in acute brain injury: An up-to-date review. *Intensive Care Med.* 2015;19:186.

21

Electrolyte disturbances and endocrinal care

RAFFAELE DI FENZA AND GIUSEPPE CITERIO

INTRODUCTION

Human cells, and especially neurons, need very tight regulation of extracellular sodium in order to be protected from hypertonic and hypotonic stress.[1] Most recurring electrolyte disorders in the neuro-critical care unit (NCCU) involve sodium and water homeostasis. Serum sodium disturbances have a peculiar physiopathology and clinical aspects in patients who suffer from any type of acute brain injury (ABI), causing increased morbidity and mortality in these patients.[2] An aware and effective approach to these disorders requires some basic knowledge of water and sodium physiology. The reader is invited to check the references for further information. Electrolyte disturbances other than dysnatremias can occur in the clinical management of these patients and will be briefly discussed later in this chapter.

SODIUM AND BODY WATER PHYSIOLOGY

Total body water and its distribution

Water is the main constituent of the human body and is the ceaseless medium in which human cells live and operate. The distribution of total body water (TBW) is a function of tissue composition, age, gender, and body weight. Traditionally, TBW has been esteemed to be 60% of body weight in men and 50% in women, with a reduction of 5% in elderly patients. Accumulated evidence suggests that these ratios are quite correct in average. TBW can be divided into two domains: intracellular fluid (ICF), which includes on average 57% of TBW in men and 53% in women, and extracellular fluid (ECF). Human cells do not have walls, instead, they have aquaporins making their membranes semipermeable, so that water movement between ECF and ICF is influenced by the osmotic activity of these solutions and not only by their difference in osmotic pressure.[3]

Plasma tonicity and its determinants: The role of plasma sodium

Tonicity refers to the effective osmotic activity in vivo. It is the property of a solution to allow the movement of water between two compartments through a semipermeable membrane, like the cell lipid bilayer.[4] Solutes that determine an effective osmotic activity are called effective osmoles and must have a high reflection coefficient, which is the ratio between the observed osmotic pressure gradient that they can generate and the osmotic pressure gradient caused by an ideal solute that cannot pass the semipermeable membrane. In other words, effective osmoles have limited diffusion and tend to remain on one side of the membrane.[3] If two fluid compartments are not isotonic, there is a net movement of water from the hypotonic solution to the hypertonic solution.[4] If the environment is hypertonic, water will leave the cells through aquaporins until intracellular fluid (ICF) becomes isotonic with ECF; but if ECF is hypotonic, water will enter the cells until their ICF becomes isotonic.[1] Being the main electrolyte in the ECF and having a high refraction coefficient (cells are almost impermeable), sodium is the main determinant of plasma tonicity, and if its blood level decreases or increases by a sufficient quantity and within a sufficiently short time, it can expose cells to hypotonic or hypertonic stress.[1,3] The osmotic activity of ECF can be described by plasma osmolality (Posm), which is the number of osmotically active moles of solute in a kilogram or liter of water (plasma is 93% water). This number can be measured by

the freezing point depression method or calculated using the following formula:

$$Posm = 2^*[Na] + [Glu]/18 + [BUN]/2.8$$

where Na is the sodium concentration in mEq/L, Glu and BUN are respectively glycemia (mg/dL) and blood urea nitrogen (mg/dL) divided by a correction factor (which converts deciliters to liters and divides by the molecular weight). Plasma osmolality is normally within a narrow range of 285–295 mOsm/KgH$_2$O. Sodium makes by far the highest contribution and its concentration can be doubled in the calculation to include chloride activity.[5] Chloride is the main anion in the ECF and is involved in many physiological processes (including maintenance of acid-base equilibrium), yet the electrochemical gradient between ECF and ICF is minimized by passive chloride channels so that its concentration can be tightly regulated at the cellular level[6] and consequently, it is not an effective osmole. Glucose is the second most important determinant of ECF tonicity after sodium, yet its contribution is limited unless severe hyperglycemia occurs.[5] A sudden decrease of blood urea nitrogen (BUN) may cause hypotonic stress in specific situations. Sodium readily crosses through endothelial cells of systemic capillaries so that in most tissues, sodium concentration in ECF is in equilibrium with that of plasma, with a small interference caused by albumin.[1] The second most effective osmole in the human body is potassium. It is used intracellularly together with large and fixed or poorly permeable anions. These help create a constant entry of water through aquaporins, which is counteracted by Na$^+$/K$^+$ ATPase that actively extrudes sodium in order to maintain osmotic equilibrium, passively followed by chloride to preserve electroneutrality.[3] Total body water may be considered a continuous solution where sodium in the ECF is directly proportional to the sum of exchangeable body sodium (eNa) plus potassium (eK) and indirectly proportional to TBW, so that:

$$pNa = [eNa + eK]/TBW$$

This is the simplified Edelman's equation; a useful approximation that does not consider total body sodium and potassium. Sodium especially is mostly contained in proteoglycans forming connective tissues (especially bones and cartilages) and the kinetics of this compartment as a sodium reservoir are too slow and not interesting in the critical care setting of acute dysnatremias.[1]

Plasma tonicity and the blood–brain barrier

The blood–brain barrier (BBB) makes brain capillaries impermeable to sodium, but not to water, which is the opposite of systemic capillaries. As a consequence, the whole brain tissue is affected by plasma tonicity of plasma tonicity and, given its anatomical structure and the limited volume excursion allowed by the skull, only a limited degree of swelling and shrinkage can occur without causing severe damage.[1,3] In vivo, BUN levels do not change fast enough to cause hypo- or hyperosmolar stress, with one main exception. Urea has a high enough reflection coefficient at the BBB so that an over rapid correction of BUN (more than 50 mg/dL/hour) during hemodialysis may cause cerebral interstitial edema and must be carefully avoided.[3] Neurosurgical patients, in which neuroanatomical integrity is not preserved, are particularly vulnerable to plasma hypertonicity and/or hypotonicity and their related water shifts.[2]

Regulation of total body water and plasma sodium

Humans can modify their sodium and water content either from oral intake or from modulating the quantity of urine and the concentration of sodium excreted in urine. The main regulatory pathway has three inputs: hypothalamic tonicity receptors, low pressure baroceptors located in the right atrium and the great veins, and carotid sinus high pressure baroceptors. Stimuli from both plasma tonicity and intravascular fullness lead to finely tuned activation or inhibition of two regulators: thirst and secretion of antidiuretic hormone/arginine vasopressin (ADH/AVP).[7] ADH/AVP is synthetized at the supraoptic and paraventricular nuclei, and then transferred to the posterior hypophysis for storage and release.[8] Secretion and thirst are normally inhibited when plasma sodium concentration (pNa) is lower than 135 mmol/l. With no circulating ADH/AVP, the renal collecting duct is set to yield maximally diluted urine (50 mOsm/kg). At increasing plasma concentrations, both thirst and ADH/AVP release increase. The

activation of V2 ADH/AVP receptors leads to the insertion of specific aquaporin channels in the renal collecting duct that increase permeability to water and its reabsorption, which is driven by the high tonicity of medullary ECF. A pNa of 145 mmol/l is usually sufficient to yield maximum concentrated (hypertonic) urine at 1200 mOsm/kg.[1] It is not urine osmolarity, rather its solute content which determines more directly the concentration of plasmatic electrolytes.[3] In general, secretion of sodium responds to intracellular volume: volume expansion cause natriuresis while volume depletion inhibits it.[1] Sodium is freely filtered at the glomerulus with the majority of it being rapidly reabsorbed. Natriuresis is the result of an interplay involving the central nervous system (CNS) through sympathetic nerves and the natriuretic peptides that control glomerular filtration and sodium reabsorption at the proximal tubule. Bone natriuretic peptide (BNP) is also involved in the inhibition of sodium transportation in the medullary duct (leading to decreased urine sodium content) and of the renin-angiotensin-aldosterone (RAA) system.[9] The activation of the RAA system plays an important backup function when hypovolemia and hypotonicity are both present. These occur in settings like gastrointestinal or renal disorders, and lead to contraction of diuresis despite hypotonicity.[10] Also, consider that hypovolemia shifts the threshold for ADH/AVP release to the left: the more severe the hypovolemia, the more ADH/AVP is released despite low plasma tonicity.[11]

Laboratory measures for plasma and serum sodium concentration

Point-of-care (POC) analyzers perform direct ion-specific electrode (ISE) assays on fresh plasma which yield a stat measure of pNa. Biochemistry assays in central laboratories, instead, are indirect ISE assays with a sample predilution of plasma or serum to measure pNa or serum sodium concentration (sNa). The yielded results are based on the assumption that the fluid phase is 93% water and 7% lipid and proteins. Any condition that rises or decreases the circulating levels of these substances will cause, respectively, underestimation or overestimation of sodium concentration. In the critical care setting, pNa should thereby be measured only by POC analyzers in order to diagnose and treat dysnatremias. If POC analyzers are unavailable, the dosage of sNa/pNa should be requested together with serum total protein (sTP) dosage: for every 0.7 g/l increase or decrease in sTP, 1 mmol/l should be added to the pNa/sNa value.[12] Unfortunately, many available studies on dysnatremias are based on classic biochemistry assays.

HYPERNATREMIA

Hypernatremia is defined as a sNa exceeding 145 mmol/l. The reported incidence on intensive care unit (ICU) admission can be 6% and up to 26% of ICU patients develop hypernatremia during their stay. Any sodium level over 145 mmol/l has an independent negative effect on outcome in all ICU patients.[13] Various thresholds for definition of "severe hypernatremia" are reported, such as a pNa of 150 mmol/l[1,14] or a sNa of 160 mmol/l.[7,15] Available measuring methods of pNa and sNa have specific technical issues and their results may be inaccurate (see previous paragraph). Mortality rates between 30% and 48% have been observed in patients with sNa of over 150 mmol/l.[13] In the NCCU, hypernatremia is more often caused by central diabetes insipidus (CDI) following posterior pituitary dysfunction that leads to insufficient ADH/AVP secretion and the excessive renal loss of free water.[15] In this setting, hypernatremia is commonly associated with severe traumatic brain injury (TBI) with an incidence of 26% in the acute phase and of 6.9% in survivors.[16] Other common causes in the NCCU are pituitary surgery or apoplexy and brain death. When secondary to CDI, hypernatremia is an independent risk factor for poor outcome. It is associated with elevated mortality in TBI patients (20.6%, 42.4%, 86.8% in stratified groups with sNa between 150 and 155, 155 and 160, and over 60%, respectively, with odds ratio for mortality of 9.50, 4.34, and 29.35, respectively).[15]

Physiopathology

Hypernatremia is always a hypertonic condition whether it is caused by a relative sodium accumulation in the ECF compared with TBW, or by a relative loss of TBW compared with sodium content that leads to decreased sodium concentration in the ECF.[1,3,13] A third and rare mechanism

characterizes overt physical exercise and muscle cell swelling due to the accumulation of osmolytes from glycogen catabolism which causes a relative hypernatremia.[4] Causes of hypernatremia are listed in Table 21.1 and may coexist in the critical care setting.[1,4,13] If the hypothalamus and posterior pituitary gland are preserved, hypertonicity causes the secretion of ADH/AVP and activates the thirst mechanism. If this reflex is intact and the patient has access to water, CDI does not generally cause hypernatremia, because the patient drinks enough free water to sustain a maximally dilute urine output (about 750 mL/h if consuming a Western diet).[1] Unfortunately, many factors can impair thirst in the neurocritical patient, such as unconsciousness and/or sedation, focal lesions., and advanced age, if present.[13] Aquaresis (from untreated CDI, treatment with vaptans or spontaneous recovery from hyponatremia) increases the plasma sodium concentration of 2.5 mmol/l/h. In the absence of urinary flux, 3% saline at 1 ml/kg/h increases a plasma sodium concentration of 1 mmol/l. Consequently, aquaresis has the same effect of an ongoing infusion of 2.5 ml/kg/h of 3% saline.[1] When extracellular sodium reaches a critical concentration, cells suffer from hypertonic stress causing a net loss of intracellular water and, in the CNS, brain volume. Generation of osmotically active intracellular solutes like glutamate, myo-inositol and taurine gradually restores cell and brain volume within two days.[1] Cell shrinkage damages the membrane and the cytoskeleton leading to a global metabolic malfunction.[17] In case of extreme and hyperacute hypertonicity, cell necrosis from membrane rupture has been described. When this phenomenon involves brain vascular cells, there is an increased risk for vessel damage and subarachnoid hemorrhage (SAH).[1] Moreover, cerebral demyelination has been observed in fast onset hypernatremia, more frequently in patients with end-stage liver disease.[13] Hypertonicity affects all tissues, yet muscles and the CNS are the most impaired in a clinically relevant way because of metabolic impairment.

Clinical features

Symptoms may appear and differ in seriousness at a different pNa in each patient depending on the speed of onset and the patient's comorbidities.[7,13] Hypertonicity causes derangements in cell

Table 21.1 Causes of hypernatremia

Relative free water deficit in the ECF
Extrarenal loss of hypotonic fluid exceeding free water intake (Dehydration)

Urine volume × [1–(uNa + uK)/pNa] <0

Loss of thirst
    Advanced age
    Sedation
    Coma
    Focal lesions
    ABI
Insensible losses (14 mL/kg/d + 3.5 mL/kg/d for every degree >37°C)
Diarrhea *prior to onset of hyponatremia*
Vomiting
Nasogastric suction/drain
Surgical drains
Hyperhidrosis
Burns
Hyperventilation

Renal loss of hypotonic fluid exceeding free water intake

Urine volume x [1–(uNa + uK)/pNa] >0

Diabetes insipidus (↑pNa + polyuria >2.5 L/d and uOsm < pOsm)
    Central diabetes insipidus
    Nephrogenic diabetes insipidus
      Hereditary
      Drug induced
        Lithium
        Foscarnet
        Amphotericin B
        Ifosfamide
Osmotic diuresis (↑pNa + polyuria >2.5 L/d and uOsm > pOsm)
    Glycosuria (urinary glucose >250 mmol/L)
    Urea diuresis (urinary urea >250 mmol/L)
AKI or CRF ("hyposthenuria")
Hypokalemia
Chronic hypercalcemia
Loop diuretics *administered prior to hypernatremia*

(Continued)

metabolism that appear more clearly at a neurological level.[13] Patients may show irritability and restlessness, ataxia, seizures, and an increasing level of sedation ranging from confusion and lethargy to coma.[7] Cerebral demyelination and SAH from a sudden vascular injury can complicate severe hypernatremia,[13] especially when the onset is within minutes (eg, from massive ingestion of salt, excessive infusion of hypertonic solutions, and dialysis errors).[1] Muscle weakness and cramps may be present because of muscular metabolic distress. Furthermore, left ventricular dysfunction leading to cardiac failure has been reported in hypernatremic patients while rhabdomyolysis leading to acute kidney failure (AKI) has been correlated with severe hypernatremia.[13] In CDI-related hypernatremia, polyuria is usually evident while thirst may be absent; other electrolyte disturbances may occur like hypokalemia and hypomagnesemia. Hypophosphatemia may be present as well.[15]

Table 21.1 (Continued) Causes of hypernatremia

Relative sodium excess in the ECF

$$(iNa + iK) - (uNa + uK) > 0$$

Iatrogenic infusion therapy
    Normal saline (Na 154 mmol/l)
    Hypertonic solution in osmotherapy (3%: Na 513 mmol/l; 10%: Na 1711 mmol/l)
    Sodium bicarbonate (Na 1000 mmol/l)
    Intravenous agents with high sodium content (ciprofloxacine, fluconazole, voriconazole)
Oral salt ingestion
    Prescribed salt tablets
    Accidental or intentional massive salt ingestion
Mineralocorticoid action
    Primary hyperaldosteronism (Conn's syndrome)
    Secondary hyperaldosteronism—stimulation of RAA axis during
        Hepatic failure
        Renal failure
        Cardiac failure
    Cushing (excess of glucocorticoids endowed with some mineralocorticoid activity)
    Exogenous administration

Sources: Wright WL, *Curr Neurol Neurosci Rep.* 2012;12(4):466-473; Lindner G, Funk GC, *J Crit Care.* 2013;28 (2):216.e11-220; Sterns RH, *N Engl J Med.* 2015;372(1):55-65.

Diagnosis

In a patient with TBI or a recent pituitary surgery, CDI should be promptly included or excluded. CDI is suggested by the presence of polyuria (urine output of more than 2.5 L or 40 mL/kg in 24 hours), polydipsia (in the awake patient) and of a urine osmolarity which is lower than expected when compared with plasma osmolality. The administration of synthetic ADH/AVP (see the section Management) serves both as a treatment start and as a differential with nephrogenic diabetes insipidus (NDI). Urine osmolality should increase to more than 600 mOsm/kg, indicating the absence of circulating native hormone, while no changes in this value indicate a peripheral resistance to the hormone. During an ICU-NCCU stay, both sodium gain and water loss may happen at the same time and with many ongoing mechanisms. Hypernatremia can develop anytime and, if it is ongoing since admission, many factors can contribute to its persistence or worsening. Diagnostic assessment (Figure 21.1) should be continuous, and recognizing and limiting all alterations in sodium and water homeostasis in order to favor treatment success.

Calculating electrolyte free water clearance discriminates between renal and extrarenal losses. It is mandatory to monitor all sources of water and sodium intake (including nutrition and medications) and all fluid losses.[13] Remembering that only urine can be hypertonic.[13] In the absence of CDI in TBI, a large and unreplaced loss of electrolyte free water due to aquaresis is most commonly caused by glycosuria.[1] Sodium excretion is difficult to measure because not all fluid losses are measurable as diuresis, but if the calculated sodium intake is less than urinary sodium (uNa), sodium accumulation can be firmly excluded.[13] Iatrogenic hypernatremia is a common consequence of osmotherapy in the treatment of cerebral edema due to TBI. The use of hypertonic saline is efficient in decreasing the intracranial brain pressure (ICP) and, compared with mannitol, is more effective in maintaining adequate cerebral blood flow. However, there is no sufficient evidence to indicate that this strategy is as safe as mannitol therapy.[17] A recent retrospective study indicates that if mild hypernatremia is allowed, ICP can be significantly decreased by careful administration of hypertonic solution without any increase in hospital mortality.[18]

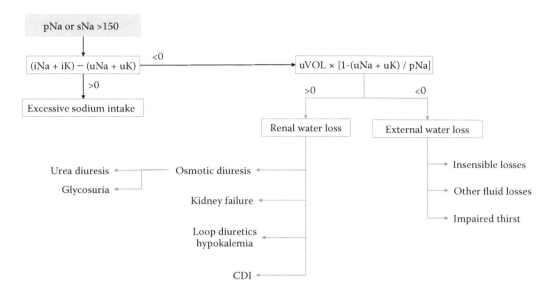

Figure 21.1 Flowchart showing diagnostic assessments in hypernatremia.

Management

In any form of dysnatremia, frequent measures of pNa and reassessments of fluid status are essential for patient management.[1,7,13] To date, there are no evidence-based protocols for treating hypernatremia in any type of ABI and current indications are expert recommendations. Acute hypernatremia is defined by documented onset within 48 hours and it should always be treated if symptomatic. Hypotension and/or hypovolemia should be assessed and corrected before starting an infusion for correcting hypernatremia. When free water loss is the cause (eg, CDI/NDI, glycosuria), the correction should be administered with hypotonic infusions.[13] If the patient is awake and able to drink safely or if a nasogastric tube is in place and absorption is adequate, enteral water administration is a feasible correction. Assuming no urine output, 3 ml/kg of free water decrease pNa by 1 mmol/l. Titration may be optimized starting from this dosage and by the careful monitoring of all water losses.[13] If central venous line is unavailable, 5% dextrose is preferable to minimize the risk for hemolysis.[13,7] Although 0.45% hypotonic saline, may be administered as well,[7] the, infusion should be titrated to decrease pNa by no more than 2 mmol/l/hour and 12 mmol/l/day.[7,13] This daily threshold is historically derived from multiplying

the indications on correcting chronic hypernatremia, that especially in children should not exceed 0.5 mmol/l/hour. Calculations are available on the internet and smartphones that estimate total water content and its fractions from body weight in order to establish the infusion rate according to pNa and the composition of selected fluid. Overcorrection should be avoided because of reported cases of cerebral edema with seizures, coma, and even death, especially after 48 hours since onset, when compensatory mechanisms have already developed.[13] Fear of overcorrection is a leading cause of undertreatment, while it is debatable whether overcorrection of acute severe hypernatremia is of any harm.[1] One exception is acute brain injury with raised ICP. In this setting, a decreased plasma tonicity can evolve into cerebral edema and increase damage.[7] In fact, many clinicians tolerate a mild degree of hypernatremia by osmotherapy in order to contain ICP when treating patients with TBI.[19] If CDI is diagnosed, hormonal therapy with vasopressin 5–10 U SC q6h or desmopressin acetate 0.125–2 μg SC/IV q8–12h may be started.[7] Desmopressin may cause a significant hyponatremic rebound and overcorrection should be avoided.[20] Instead, if sodium excess is the documented main cause, diuretic therapy may be started in order to promote natriuresis together with a titrated IV infusion or oral water in order to avoid hypovolemia.[13] In hyperacute hypernatremia presenting in minutes to hours (caused by salt ingestion, iatrogenic administration of hypertonic saline, dialysis errors), rapid infusion with 5% dextrose in water and emergency dialysis should be considered. In this particular setting, overcorrection is not discouraged.[1] Continuous renal replacement therapy (CRRT) has not been addressed by large clinical trials for treating hypernatremia, but it has proven useful, allowing for constant correction of the disorder.[13]

HYPONATREMIA

Hyponatremia is classically defined as a sNa of less than 135 mmol/l.[2,7,10] Values between 131 and 135 mmol/l are considered of no clinical significance and thresholds for severe hyponatremia of 130[21] or 120 mmol/l have been reported.[1] It is the most common electrolyte disturbance encountered in clinical medicine and it increases mortality in a variety of clinical settings, both as dependent and independent factors.[2] In the ICU, hypernatremia of any severity increases mortality with a relative risk (RR) of 2.6.[22] The incidence is particularly high in NCCU patients, especially in those who suffer from ABI[10], and it is associated with increased morbidity and mortality.[2] Hyponatremia is found in 9% of all patients who have suffered from TBI. Over 56% of patients with SAH of any etiology develop hyponatremia and more than 19% of these have a pNa of less than 130 mmol/l.[21] When SAH is caused by a ruptured aneurysm, 30% of patients develop hyponatremia, which constitutes an additional risk factor for stroke in those with high grade hemorrhage (WFNS 4-5).[23] Hyponatremia in SAH is associated with worse functional outcomes.[24] Fatal brain swelling is a rare complication reported in hyponatremic patients with intracranial disease or in cases of postoperative hyponatremia or water intoxication.[1]

Physiopathology

Common causes of hyponatremia are listed in Table 21.2.[1,10,25,26] Hyponatremia is most often a hypotonic condition, especially in the NCCU, although non-hypotonic hyponatremia can occur (eg, in hyperglycemia for every 100 mg/dL of excess blood glucose there is a decrease in pNa of 1.6 mmol/l with an increase of 2 mOsm/kg of pOsm). Hypotonic hyponatremia is related to an impairment of water excretion with the exception of psychogenic polydipsia, in which there is an exaggerated intake of hypotonic fluid (oral water).[26] In the general medical population, hyponatremia reflects a situation where proper urine dilution is impaired by continuous ADH/AVP agonism. This is caused by hypovolemia and by a stress-response-activated RAA system. This is typical in heart failure, liver cirrhosis, nephrogenic edema, stress, chronic pain, cortisol deficiency, and drugs like diuretics altering sodium transportation in renal diluting sites.[1] The main mechanisms leading to hyponatremia in the NCCU are the inappropriate secretion of antidiuretic hormone syndrome (SIADH) and cerebral salt wasting syndrome (CSWS).[10] Less frequently, brain injury can cause acute hypocortisolemia[27]. Both SIADH and CSWS cause hypotonic hyponatremia with increased natriuresis.[26] In SIADH, hyponatremia is a consequence of hemodilution and is a normo- or hypervolemic condition.[10] In the NCCU, SIADH generally complicates the clinical course of patients affected by TBI, SAH, intracranial infections, and brain tumors. In these patients there is a (not fully understood) release of ADH/AVP which is "inappropriate," that is, happening in the absence of its physiological stimuli, which are plasma hypertonicity and low intravascular volume.[26] Continuous hypertonic diuresis leads to the expansion of intravascular volume which increases natriuresis (to decrease intravascular volume) despite hyponatremia (leading to worsening of hyponatremia).[1] CSWS, instead, is a hypovolemic hyponatremia caused by primary natriuresis and associated water loss, whose etiology and pathogenesis are not completely understood.[28] This condition can complicate any type of ABI, although it does not seem involved in cases of nontraumatic SAH.[29] CSWS is likely related to secretion of natriuretic factors like ANP and BNP as much as reduced sympathetic tone to the kidney.[28] Independently from the onset mechanism, plasma hypotonicity leads to an inwards shift of water through the BBB causing cerebral edema.[7] Extreme hypotonicity alters the cytoskeleton leading to chromosome damage and, thereby, apoptosis. If the onset of hyponatremia is abrupt, the resulting brain swelling may cause an increase in intracranial pressure with an impairment of cerebral blood flow and, in some cases, herniation.[1] A first defense mechanism is

Table 21.2 Causes of hyponatremia

Hypovolemic hyponatremia (decreased TBW with more decreased exchangeable sodium)
    Renal sodium loss
        CSWS
        Diuretics
        Ketonuria (from T1DM or prolonged starvation)
        Mineralocorticoid insufficiency
    Extrarenal sodium loss
        Gastrointestinal losses: Diarrhea, vomiting
        Skin losses: Sweating, burns
        Internal losses: Hemorrhage, pancreatitis
    Iatrogenic
        Insufficient volume correction with hypotonic solutions
Euvolemic hyponatremia (increased amount of TBW with normal or reduced exchangeable sodium)
    SIADH
        CNS
            SAH/TBI
            Stroke
            Infection/inflammatory disorders/demyelination
        Drugs – Iatrogenic SIADH
            Desmopressin/vasopressin
            Oxytocin
            MDMA
            CBZ/oxcarbazepine/lamotrigine
            Phenothiazines/TCA
            SSRIs/SNRIs
            Chlorpropamide
            Clofibrate
            Narcotics
            NSAIDs
            Cyclophosphamide/vincristine
        Pulmonary diseases: infections, asthma, ALI
        Malignancies: CNS, lung, gastrointestinal, genitourinary
    Iatrogenic
        Irrigation during gynecologic or urologic surgery
        Adequate volume correction with hypotonic solutions
    Psychogenic
        Polydipsia
    Renal electrolyte loss
        Thiazide diuretics
        Glucocorticoid insufficiency
        Hypothyroidism
        Stress/pain/nausea
    Extrarenal electrolyte loss
        Exercise-associated hyponatremia

(Continued)

Table 21.2 (Continued) Causes of hyponatremia

Hypervolemic hyponatremia (TBW more increased than exchangeable sodium)
    CHF
    Cirrhosis/liver insufficiency
    Nephrotic syndrome
    AKI and chronic renal failure
    Iatrogenic
        Volume overcorrection with hypotonic solutions

Sources: Mewasingh L et al., *Lancet.* 2000;356(9230):656; Rabinstein AA, Wijdicks EF, *Neurologist.* 2003;9(6):290-300; Tisdall M et al., *J Neurosurg Anesthesiol.* 2006;18(1):57-63; Sterns RH, *N Engl J Med.* 2015;372(1):55-65; Buffington MA, Abreo K, *J Intensive Care Med.* 2016;31(4):223-236.

purely hydrostatic and consists of a shift of water to the cerebrospinal fluid (CBF) and hence to systemic circulation.[28] If hyponatremia develops slowly, activating the adaptive cellular mechanism can minimize edema, even if very low levels of pNa are reached and despite the persistence of a hypotonic state.[26] In the presence of a hypotonic environment, brain cells release osmolytes in a biphasic process that occurs in the first 3 hours after the onset of acute hyponatremia with active release of electrolytes that cause an extracellular outflow of water. Within 48 hours, organic osmolytes (myo-inositol, taurine, glutamate, creatine) are generated within the cytoplasm and released in order to maintain the extracellular flow of water and counterbalance persisting or worsening plasma hypotonicity.[7,28] The adaptive release of glutamate to reach an isotonic environment may help reduce the epileptic threshold and explain the increased incidence of seizures in these patients.[1] In the acute setting, astrocytes release taurine to neurons through a cell-to-cell interaction and swell, allowing neurons to maintain their volume. Within 24 hours, astrocytes regain their volume by losing organic osmolytes.[1] The correction of hyponatremia reverses these processes, but once accumulating transporters for organic osmolytes have been downregulated (within 48 hours since onset), re-entry of these molecules is slowed down since a too quick correction of hyponatremia may cause hypertonicity. Possible consequences are cell apoptosis with BBB destruction and, eventually, demyelination.[1]

Clinical presentation

Symptoms usually appear at a pNa of 120–125 mmol/l but their appearance depends on individual susceptibility and speed of onset. Patients may suffer from headache, nausea and/or vomiting, and may be agitated and irritable. Vigilance may be impaired ranging from confusion to sedation. Muscle weakness and/or cramps occur, similarly with hypernatremia and metabolic impairment of muscle tissue. If pNa is lower (<115 mmol/l) or at higher concentration if the onset is acute (<48 hours) vigilance impairment may be worse, ranging from drowsiness to overt coma. Seizures are possible, reflexes may be depressed, and brain stem herniation should be suspected and excluded.[11]

Diagnosis

A useful chart for diagnostic workout is shown in Figure 21.2. Overhydration with hypotonic solutions should always be considered as a potential cause of hyponatremia, including postoperative hydration and irrigation during urologic and gynecologic surgery. It is fundamental to recognize a true hypotonic hyponatremia. Hyperglycemia and/or administration of IV sugar alcohols (eg, mannitol or sorbitol) or sucrose (contained in many preparations like IV immunoglobulins) cause plasma hypertonicity because these substances are effective osmolytes. As a consequence, water freely moves out of cells diluting plasma and possibly causing low pNa/sNa values. An initial evaluation of hyponatremia should therefore always include a Posm measurement, remembering that a high value does not immediately exclude hypotonicity: alcohol and high BUN increase pOsm, yet those substances are not effective osmolytes. If pNa or sNa are measured with indirect ISE assays (central lab biochemistry), a change in the ratio between

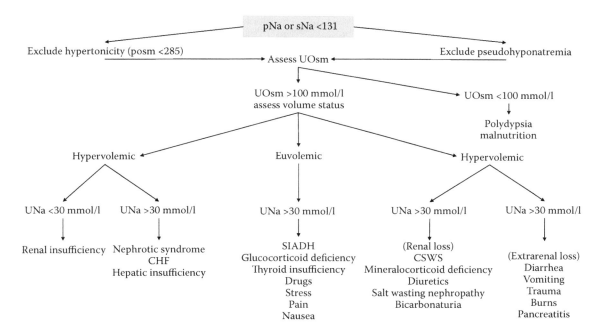

Figure 21.2 Flowchart showing diagnostic assessments in hyponatremia.

liquid and non-liquid component of blood caused by hypertriglyceridemia (eg, sedation with propofol) and/or hyperproteinemia (eg, parenteral nutrition, myeloma, macroglobulinemia) may cause a false positive (pseudohyponatremia). Instead, if pNa is measured with direct potentiometry (POC) on fresh plasma, the yielded value is not influenced by this ratio. The second step is assessing urine osmolality (UOsm) to verify ongoing dilution of urine in response to hypotonicity. If UOsm is less than 100 mmol/l diluting capacity is intact, so the patient is responding to whether an excess of free water intake or a low solute intake. If UOsm is more than 100 mmol/l patient volume status should be assessed.[11] Any available source of information should be sought including anthropometric measures (to estimate TBW and ECF), vitals, clinical examination, hematocrit, BUN, echocardiography, central venous pressure, pulmonary catheter wedge pressure, and careful monitoring of all fluid intake and losses.[2,30] UNa measurement is essential in order to determine the involvement of renal function in the onset of hyponatremia. Hypervolemic hyponatremia is a consequence of either loss of urine diluting capacity (due to failure) or chronic non-osmotic release of ADH/AVP together with the chronic activation of the RAA system. This is typical of edemigen chronic diseases (in which there is a continuous baroceptor activation due to low arterial volume). Euvolemic hyponatremia in the neurocritical setting is most often caused by brain disease or injury-induced SIADH and by glucocorticoid deficiency. Hypovolemic hyponatremia may result from extrarenal volume depletion. In this case UNa should be less than 30 mmol/l, but metabolic alkalosis may cause a misleading increased value so that urine chloride should be dosed as well. If hypovolemic hyponatremia is corrected with normal saline, it is) expected that UOsm could drop under 100 mmol/l because of the resolution of hypovolemia (a major stimulus for ADH/AVP incretion).[11] In the NCCU, hypotonic hyponatremia with renal loss of sodium is caused by CSWS, followed by inadequate hydration.[21] The importance in distinguishing between SIADH and CSW, the two main causes of hyponatremia in the NCCU, lays in the choice of proper treatment which can otherwise worsen the condition (see the section Management). A retrospective study on hyponatremic neurosurgical patients found an incidence of 62% and at least 5% for SIADH and CSWS, respectively, and at least 3% of patients co-existed with both.[21] Another study on patients with combined SIADH and CSWS after TBI found massive polyuria (more than 1 L/hour or 10 L/day) as the most typical clinical presentation.[31] Table 21.3 illustrates features and currently accepted diagnostic criteria for SIADH and CSWS. Pressure natriuresis caused by a large IV fluid administration, in order to maintain adequate blood pressure and brain perfusion in patients with ABI, may be clinically similar and further complicates accurate understanding and management.[30]

Management

To date, there are no evidence-based protocols for treating hyponatremia in any kind of ABI.[32] Generally, hyponatremia should be treated in case of severe disease (worsening vigilance impairment, seizures) and especially in fast onset acute disease. Hypotension or hypovolemia, when present, further require prompt treatment. In the NCCU, hyponatremia after ABI may be transient and self-limiting.[10,30] Careful monitoring of pNa and continuous fluid status assessment are the mainstay of management.[1] Rapidly developing hyponatremia may cause (or worsen) brain edema, putting the patient at risk for herniation. Irreversible neurological damage and death are reported in cases of overlooked acute hyponatremia. Correction within 48 hours is acceptable at a faster rate compared with chronic hyponatremia, yet if the onset time is unclear the patient should be treated as chronic.[11] From empirical observations, it is known that the brain cannot swell more than 5% of its volume.[1] Furthermore, it has been shown that an increase in pNa of 5 mmol/l, if other conditions are unchanged, decreases ICP by 50%.[11] An increase in pNa of 4 to 6 mmol/l in the first 6 hours is theoretically enough to prevent brain herniation and acute seizures. Severe acute hyponatremia can benefit from a 100 ml bolus (or 2 ml/kg if small patients) of 3% saline administered 3 times at intervals of 10 minutes. If symptoms are milder or after three boluses, 3% may be titrated to a 4 to 6 mmol/l increase in sodium levels in the first 6 hours, knowing that in the absence of urinary loss of water 1 ml/kg of 3% saline increases sodium concentration by 1 mmol/l.[1] In acutely symptomatic patients, faster corrections allowing a 1.5 to 2 mmol/l/h increase for the first 2 to 4 hours are tolerated.[10] To lower the incidence of osmotic demyelination syndrome, a pNa increase should be within 10 mmol/l/day. Reportedly, osmotic demyelination is followed in many cases by full recovery.[1] Management may get more complicated

Table 21.3 Differential diagnosis between SIADH and CSWS

	SIADH	CSWS
sNa (mmol/L)	<135	<135
uNa (mmol/L)	>25	>25
Total body sodium	Normal	Reduced
BUN	Reduced	Increased
Creatinine	Reduced	Increased
Uric acid	Reduced	Reduced
sK (mmol/L)	Decreased/no change	Increased/no change
Bicarbonate	Reduced	Increased
Hematocrit	Reduced/no change	Increased
Serum albumin concentration	Normal	Increased
Serum osmolality (mOSm/kg)	<285	<285
Urine osmolality (mOsm/kg)	>200	>200
Fluid balance	Positive	Negative
Jugular venous distension	Yes	No
ECF	Increased/no change	Reduced
CVP	>6	<6
PWP	>8	<8
Weight	Increased/higher	Reduced/lower

Source: Kirkman MA, Minerva Endocrinol. 2014;39(1):13-26.

when patients have unexpected water diuresis (for example in a spontaneous recovery from hyponatremia) and, thereby, may be at increased risk for overcorrection of hyponatremia.[1] An interesting strategy that may enhance the control of a pNa decrease slope is titrating an IV infusion of 3% saline with the concurrent administration of synthetic ADH/AVP agonist desmopressin at 1 to 2 µg q6 to 8h to antagonize unexpected and undesired water losses.[33] If SIADH is evident, indications for treatment are the same.[34] However, the first line of treatment, if the clinical conditions are mild enough to allow it, is free water restriction to 800 to 1000 mL/day, which usually leads to a slow rise of pNa by 1.5 mmol/l/day. Typically, acute patients with SAH/TBI cannot tolerate fluid restriction, since they are at risk of cerebral ischemia and cardiovascular instability. In these cases, infusing 1.8% or 3% saline is preferred. Once a sNa of 120 to 125 is reached, correction may be continued with enteral tablets.[35] In SAH-induced SIADH Ringer or normal saline solution should not be used to maintain cerebral perfusion because the infused sodium is secreted in hypertonic urine leading to net water retention and worsening of hyponatremia.[1] Pharmacological treatment of SIADH is indicated only when the diagnosis is clear and first line treatments have failed. It consists of inhibitors of ADH/AVP signaling acting at the renal duct, where they cause aquaresis. Demeclocycline, which impairs ADH/AVP-induced generation of intracellular cyclic adenosine monophosphate (cAMP) at the renal collecting duct, has been successfully used at doses of 150 to 300 mg q12h. Vaptans are ADH/AVP receptor antagonists which prevent the hormone from binding to V2 receptors in the renal collecting duct.[7] They have been administered in NCCU patients with hyponatremia and ABI. So far, experience is limited, yet promising. A single dose of conivaptan produces a valid response in patients with hyponatremia and ABI.[36] Furthermore, in normonatremic patients with TBI and raised ICP, conivaptan safely reduces intracranial hypertension with a controlled raise of pNa.[37] CSWS is a hypovolemic state so both fluid restriction and inhibition of aquaresis are inappropriate. Management requires volume repletion with 0.9% normal saline, or in severe cases, hypertonic solutions.[10] The mineralocorticoid properties of fludrocortisone have been successfully used to increase sodium

reabsorption from the renal tubule and thereby reduce water loss.[8] In a recent retrospective study, patients who coexist with SIADH and CSWS better responded to treatment when they received vasopressin and cortisone acetate together with appropriate saline infusion.[31]

OTHER ELECTROLYTE DISORDERS

Potassium

Potassium serum concentration (sK) derangements are common in NCCU patients, with SIADH being associated with hypokalemia (sK <3.5 mmol/l) and CSWS frequently causing hypokalemia in patients with ABI.[30] It has been known for more than 20 years that during severe ABI, potassium levels increase in the ECF and this is associated with higher ICPs and fatal outcomes. Unfortunately, this does not necessarily translate into hyperkalemia (sK >5 mmol/l).[38] Interestingly, a recent study indicates that patients with TBI and sK <3.5 mmol/L on admission have a better neurologic outcome when allocated to mild therapeutic hypothermia (MTH) compared with fever control, while on the contrary, patients with normal potassium levels on admission have better outcomes when treated just with fever control compared with MTH.[39] Hypokalemia and hyperkalemia are both associated with increased mortality in any critical care patient and must be promptly recognized and treated.[40] Clinical signs are mostly neurologic (paresthesia, motor paralysis, quadriplegia) and muscular (weakness including respiratory failure, constipation, fatigue, rhabdomyolysis), including cardiac (QT prolongation, ST depression, flat T waves, and U waves in hypokalemia; asystole, sine wave, loss of P waves, widening QRS and peaked T waves in hyperkalemia; ventricular arrhythmias can occur in both cases). Physical examination and electrocardiogram may also be unremarkable.[40–42] Table 21.4 looks at the causes of potassium disturbances.[42,43] Treating hypokalemia in the emergency setting consists of an IV infusion (rather than oral correction) under ECG monitoring, preferably using a central venous line and with a replacement that should not exceed 20 mmol/l/h to decrease the risk for unstable arrhythmias (unless one is already present).[44] Blood clotting creates a difference between plasma potassium concentration (pK) and sK, so pseudohyperkalemia (sK exceeding pK by more than 0.4 mmol/l)

Table 21.4 Causes of hypokalemia and hyperkalemia

Hypokalemia	Hyperkalemia
Increased excretion	**Impaired excretion**
Gastrointestinal loss	Renal failure
Diarrhea	CSWS
Enema	Adrenal insufficiency
Laxatives	Mineralocorticoid deficiencies
Renal loss	Drugs
Drugs	Angiotensin-converting enzyme inhibitors
Diuretics	Angiotensin receptor blockers
Glucocorticoids	Potassium-sparing diuretics
Aminoglycosides	Heparin and derivatives
Penicillin and derivates	Trimethoprim
Amphotericin B	**Shift to extracellular fluid**
Foscarnet	Drugs
Tenofovir	Succinylcholine
Cisplatin	Adrenergic blockers
CDI	Insulin deficiency or resistance
SIADH	Tissue damage
Metabolic alkalosis	Rhabdomyolysis
Osmotic diuresis	Burns
Renal tubular acidosis	Trauma
Bartter's syndrome	**Iatrogenic**
Mineralocorticoid excess	
Metabolic causes	
Liddle's syndrome	
Hypomagnesemia	
Shift to intracellular fluid	
Drugs	
Adrenergic agonists	
Methylxanthines	
Insulin	
Quetiapine	
Risperidone	
Delirium tremens	
Hyperthyroidism	
Familial hypokalemic periodic paralysis	
Barium poisoning	
Decreased intake	

Sources: Lee JW, *Electrolyte Blood Press.* 2010;8(2):72-81; Unwin RJ et al., *Nat Rev Nephrol.* 2011;7(2):75-84; Li M et al., *Injury.* 2013;44(9):1213-1218; Kirkman MA, *Minerva Endocrinol.* 2014;39(1):13-26.

should be excluded together with other falsely elevating conditions such as sample lysis or excessive cooling, thrombocytosis, leukocytosis, and delayed processing time. Emergency treatment is indicated when ECG abnormalities arise and/or sK reaches 6 mmol/l.[45] Treating hypokalemia has three main targets. Antagonization of potassium at the cell membrane is obtained with a slow infusion of 1 gram of calcium chloride or gluconate (onset within minutes), unless digoxin toxicity is suspected (possible enhancement of toxicity).[41] The shifting of potassium towards the intracellular space may be accomplished with 10 to 20 mg of nebulized albuterol over 30 minutes. This intervention has a synergistic effect with insulin infusion (10 units with 12.5 to 25 grams of glucose, onset within 30 minutes). Sodium bicarbonate should be administered only in situations with concurrent metabolic acidosis. Polystyrene sulfonate can be given as an enema (30–50 g) for a faster onset compared with oral administration. Loop diuretics (if hypovolemia and cerebral perfusion are not an issue and if renal function is preserved) and dialysis are effective, with a fast onset.[46,47]

Calcium

Hypocalcemia is very frequent (90% of incidence in the ICU) and is associated with increased mortality. The most common causes are a massive infusion of fluids, trauma, renal failure, sepsis, hypomagnesemia (and its causes) hypoparathyroidism, vitamin D deficiency, and the infusion of citrate, phosphate, albumin, and alkali. Gadolinium may affect total calcium concentration (sCa) but not ionized free calcium (Ca++). Clinical manifestations may include papilledema, seizures, tetany, and cardiac arrest. Urgent management is needed in cases of severe (sCa <7.5 mg/dL or Ca++ <0.9 mmol/l) or symptomatic hypocalcemia. An infusion of 1 g of calcium chloride or 3 g of calcium gluconate over 10 minutes should be immediately administered to control symptoms, followed by a continuous infusion of calcium gluconate (not chloride). The infusion should be titrated to 0.4–0.75 mmol/l to avoid cardiac arrhythmias. This can be obtained by diluting 1 to 2 g in 100 ml of 0.9% normal saline or 5% glucose and administering it within 30 to 60 minutes. If hypocalcemia cannot be corrected, hypomagnesemia should be sought and corrected first. Metabolic alkalosis should be treated after hypocalcemia because alkalization of blood further decreases hypocalcemia possibly leading to worsening of neurological symptoms or cardiac arrest.[42] Hypercalcemia (sCa >10.4 mg/dL) is a rarity in NCCU patients, mostly caused by hyperparathyroidism and malignancy, less commonly in sarcoidosis, after therapy with thiazide diuretics or prolonged immobility. Clinical symptoms are neurological (delirium, psychosis, confusion to coma), muscular (weakness, constipation, ileus), and cardiovascular (hypotension, hypovolemia, shortening of QT interval).[40] Basic treatment includes hydration and stimulation of diuresis, and pamidronate may be added.

Magnesium

Hypomagnesemia has a prevalence of 50% in ICU patients, and serum magnesium concentration (sMg) should be more than 1.5 mg/dL (1.7 mg/dL for patients with acute myocardial infarction) in order to prevent fatal arrhythmias like torsade de pointes. Neurologic symptoms may include seizures and coma. Hypomagnesemia frequently coexists with hypokalemia and hypocalcemia. Causes include trauma (and burns), surgery, infections (and sepsis), renal or gastrointestinal losses, starvation and malnutrition (including alcoholism), transfusion with citrated blood products, and treatment with drugs like diuretics, digoxin, aminoglycosides, amphotericin B, cyclosporine, and cisplatin.[40] CDI associated with ABI may present with hypomagnesemia together with hypernatremia.[15] Fractional excretion of magnesium is useful in establishing the cause. Treatment is empirical and aimed at keeping sMg between 1.5 and 2.4 mg/dL. In severe (<0.9 mg/dL) or symptomatic hypomagnesemia, IV administration is preferred considering rapid renal excretion (50% of infused dose if preserved function). Doses of 16 to 32 mg and up to 0.75 mg/kg are needed and infusions are titrated to last 8 to 12 hours. If more than 6 grams are needed (eg, for patients in CRRT), doses are infused over 24 hours. If renal impairment is present, dosages should be reduced to avoid hypermagnesemia, which is mainly a iatrogenic condition.[41]

Chloride

Plasma chloride concentration is regulated at the cellular level where it is fundamental for acid-base equilibrium. Disorders in plasma chloride are mostly iatrogenic and caused by saline infusions. The typical derangement in NCCU patients is hyperchloremia, which determines metabolic acidosis and its consequences.[48]

ENDOCRINOLOGIC CARE

NCCU patients may develop acute endocrine dysfunction at any level, especially after TBI, SAH, pituitary surgery (or apoplexy), and brain death. The most relevant disorders after ABI involve the HPA axis and are CDI (see section hypernatremia), secondary adrenal insufficiency (with glucocorticoid and/or mineralocorticoid dysfunction), and thyroid dysfunction.[49] Autoptic studies reveal evident hypothalamic and pituitary structural anomalies in over 40% of patients after fatal severe TBI.[50] CDI and adrenal insufficiency may complicate damage to these structures and are in fact life threatening conditions[51] characterizing 80% of brain dead organ donors, who often develop hypothyroidism as well.[52] The possibility of an ongoing endocrine failure must always be considered in these patients to provide appropriate management.[48] Patients who survive TBI and/or SAH are at risk of maintaining or developing a chronic endocrine dysfunction later after the acute phase with considerable effects on their quality of life. 27.5% and 40% to 47% of patients who have suffered from TBI and SAH, respectively, will develop a disturbance of at least one pituitary axis, according to two systematic reviews.[16,53] Range of incidence between single follow-up studies is wide and this is due to significant methodological differences: hormone stimulation tests are not always performed and scheduled visits vary remarkably.[16] This paragraph focuses mainly on the endocrinologic care of acute NCCU patients.

GENERAL ASPECTS IN PHYSIOPATHOLOGY

The anterior pituitary gland secretes hormones which are master regulators of vital functions acting peripherally on target hormones. Adrenocorticotropic hormone (ACTH, stimulating cortisol production in the adrenal cortex), thyroid stimulating hormone (TSH), growth hormone (GH), prolactin (PRL), follicle-stimulating hormone (FSH), and luteinizing hormone (LH) are secreted by specialized hormone-specific cells with a finely tuned regulation. This is allowed by a unique portal vascular system in which both hypothalamic (releasing hormones, like CRH which stimulates ACTH secretion, and inhibitory factors) and peripheral systemic hormones and substances concur. Any ABI can alter this delicate system, which may easily become vulnerable to watershed phenomenon, causing endocrine malfunctions. Among these, secondary adrenal insufficiency may be life-threatening.[49] Half of the damage can be either from direct TBI trauma and/or vascular when caused by high ICP-related brain stem ischemia in TBI or SAH and can lead to necrosis, fibrosis,

infarction and/or hemorrhage.[49] Half of all patients with ABI has a vascular insult compromising the hypothalamic-pituitary axis, yet 6% of patients with proven dysfunction have no sign of vascular damage.[54] Other mechanisms involved may be the spam of small vessels, which supply the hypothalamic-pituitary axis in SAH, the brain injury-induced release of substances that alter hormone release, the lower input from the cortex, and other brainstem structures.[55–57] Certain apolipoprotein E haplotypes associated with the development of Alzheimer's disease may influence the risk for developing hypopituitarism after TBI. Furthermore, circulating antibodies with anti-hypothalamic and anti-pituitary activity may be associated with developing endocrinologic failure after the acute phase. Their role, however, has to be further investigated.[58] Any axonal damage involving the posterior pituitary gland may cause CDI (see section Hypernatremia) and impair oxytocin release. High CSF levels of this hormone after SAH has been associated with poorer outcomes.[59] Eventual development of chronic oxytocin release deficiency after ABI is of marginal interest, given its widespread use as an exogenous drug in obstetrics.

GENERAL ASPECTS IN DIAGNOSIS

Early assessment in the acute phase and repeated assessment during follow-up have been recommended in all patients suffering from moderate-to-severe TBI. During the first two weeks following injury, major attention should be drawn to adrenal failure and CDI, while in the subsequent months, assessment should focus on the whole anterior and the posterior hormonal axes. Symptomatic patients with a history of mild brain injury are in fact at risk for hypopituitarism and should receive neuroendocrine testing.[58] Elements that may warrant a hormonal assessment in the acute neurocritical patient are prolonged unresponsiveness, which is not related to the severity of brain injury, evidence of cranial nerve deficits, skull fractures, vasopressor need, polyuria, hyponatremia, and hypoglycemia.[49] Imaging findings suggesting hormonal assessment are evidence of direct injury in the hypothalamic-pituitary region (such as edema, ischemia, or hemorrhage) and fractures involving the sella. No treatment should be started in the presence of radiologic findings.[60] The presence of subdural hemorrhage in patients with TBI attributes and odds ratio of 21 of having a pituitary hemorrhage and of 12 of having a pituitary stalk rupture.[50] Some authors suggest that the need for high dose vasopressors in an intubated patient is sufficient to start a neuroendocrine screening.[61] Evidence of diffuse axonal injury, basal skull fracture, and older age are important risk factors for the development of hypopituitarism following TBI.[57]

Adrenal failure

Around 10% of patients affected by TBI develop adrenal insufficiency within the first 7 days after trauma.[62] Inappropriately low plasma cortisol levels are found in up to 78% of patients with TBI after 10 days; this finding is predictive of mortality.[51] Total adrenal failure with hypotension is more often a complication of elective pituitary surgery rather than TBI and is a medical emergency needing treatment of consequent acute adrenal insufficient and cardiovascular support.[63] Anyway, adrenal failure following TBI is associated with more episodes of hypotension and increased vasopressor requirements in younger patients and in those with more severe injury.[61] More than 24% and more than 12% of patients who survived brain injury show failure to ACTH stimulation after 3 and 12 months, respectively.[64] Brain injury is more often associated with a failure of ACTH release by the anterior pituitary gland, defining a secondary adrenal failure. Primary failure of the adrenal gland though, may also complicate managing ABI and this is usually related to the co-presence of a systemic inflammatory response.[65] The clinical features of adrenal failure include hypotension, hypoxia, and severe anemia. The presence of CDI may suggest the possible coexistence of adrenal failure and vice versa.[58] Hypoglycemia and classic electrolyte derangements like hyponatremia and hypercalcemia may not be present at all.[66] Glucocorticoids are tonic inhibitors of ADH/AVP secretion and during adrenal insufficiency, ADH/AVP is inappropriately secreted. Furthermore, adrenal insufficiency causes decreased cardiac output so the non-osmotic release of ADH/AVP is also stimulated. The RAA system response is, instead, intact. The resulting euvolemic hyponatremia is very similar to that seen in SIADH, with low BUN and uric acid levels.[11] Hyperkalemia, a classic sign, is usually absent because mineralocorticoid secretion (aldosterone) is spared in TBI-induced adrenal failure. Skin hyperpigmentation is absent as well because ACTH and cortisol secretion are impaired. Diagnosis requires the dosing of morning serum cortisol. Levels of at least 18 μg/dL exclude disruption of the HPA axis, while levels of 3 μg/dL or less are diagnostic. In the acute phase, cortisol levels may be suppressed by medications like propofol, barbiturates, and etomidate. Corticosteroid binding globulin (CBG) levels should be measured also given that high CBG values (oral estrogen therapy, pregnancy) and low CBG values (acute illness, malnutrition) may lead to underestimation and overestimation, respectively, of cortisol levels. Patients with intermediate morning cortisol levels (3.1–17.9 μg/dL) may be treated if suggestive clinical findings are present in the acute phase and require a full endocrinologic evaluation in the chronic phase (3 months after TBI and later). This consists of ACTH dosage (to assess pituitary failure) and serum cortisol measurement after stimulation with exogenous ACTH and/or an insulin tolerance test (to assess glandular hypotrophy which is secondary to pituitary failure).[58] Managing acute patients with known or suspected adrenal failure consists of administration hydrocortisone 50–100 mg q6 to 8 h even without a biochemical diagnosis.[58,67] More stable patients can receive hydrocortisone 15–25 mg qd in divided doses or prednisone 2.5 to 5 mg qd. Mineralocorticoid replacement is not needed.[58]

OTHER ENDOCRINE DYSFUNCTIONS

Thyroid dysfunction

After TBI, 8% to 15% of patients will develop central hypothyroidism, characterized by inappropriately low TSH in the presence of low serum free tetraiodothyronine (T_4).[58,68] Acute patients often show the so-called "euthyroid sick syndrome" which may be difficult to distinguish from central hypothyroidism because TSH may be low as well. Current evidence suggests postponing an evaluation of the hypothalamic-pituitary-thyroid axis for at least 4 weeks after the onset of TBI in patients without suspected or documented preexisting hypothyroidism. Treatment in the acute setting is not usually indicated, and is also given the average half-life of T4 (7 days). A full replacement dose of 1.6 μg/kg qd (lower doses may be warranted in older patients and in those with cardiovascular comorbidities) should be administered carefully in patients with documented central hypothyroidism and after evidence of intact adrenal function or ongoing adequate glucocorticoid therapy, in order to avoid adrenal crisis.[58]

Growth hormone deficiency

Growth hormone (GH) deficiency can be found in 12% to 18% of patients after TBI.[58,69] An assessment of GH secretion should be performed several months after a TBI, although accumulating evidence suggests that early correction of GH deficiency improves the quality of life and cognition in the rehabilitation phase. Children should receive a continuous and complete neuroendocrine surveillance routine for at least 1 year.[58]

Hypogonadotropic hypogonadism

Hypogonadotropic hypogonadism is the single most prevalent endocrinopathy during follow up of TBI, with an incident rate that reaches 25%. Testosterone is prescribed in up to 8% of men who have suffered from moderate to severe TBI or SAH.[70]

Wake-sleep disorders

Recent works have focused on TBI-induced disturbed sleep and wakefulness. TBI can cause widespread damage to structures regulating circadian rhythms and accumulating evidence indicates that sleeping disorders are endowed with considerable morbidity and should be assessed and treated early in the management of these patients.[71]

GLYCEMIC CONTROL IN THE NCCU

Hyperglycemia typically complicates the clinical course of patients with ABI and its presence is associated with increased morbidity and mortality after TBI, SAH, and ischemic stroke.[72] Elevated blood glucose levels may be the consequence of preexisting diabetes mellitus (DM) and/or an epiphenomenon of stress response. Glucose is the main energy source of CNS, with 95% of adenosine triphosphate (ATP) being derived from its aerobic oxidation.[72] In anaerobic conditions like ischemia, all glucose is oxidized within 30 seconds and all ATP is hydrolyzed within 1 minute. Cell

death pathways and related inflammatory responses set up early, so that reperfusion fuels detrimental mechanisms (many of which are cell-mediated and based on glucose oxidation) thereby amplifying damage. If perfused blood is hyperglycemic, these mechanisms are more efficient and the resulting damage is increased, as shown by various animal models and retrospective clinical studies.[72] Blood glucose is normally tightly regulated between 3 and 5.5 mmol/l (55–100 mg/dL), although in pathological conditions (including critical care) levels between 2 and 10 mmol/l (36–180 mg/dL) may often be observed. Glucose enters the CNS through facilitated diffusion mechanisms at the BBB that couple (even more tightly) brain metabolism and glucose transport. Resulting CSF glucose concentrations vary between 0.5 and 2.5 mmol/l (10–45 mg/dL).[72] The most reliable tools to assess glucose availability in the CNS are microdialysis catheters that measure glucose concentration in the interstitial fluid. Their extended use has improved knowledge on the existing relationship between blood glucose and cerebral glucose in various clinical conditions. Furthermore, proper use can predict and detect ischemic areas. Hyperglycemia and hypoglycemia are not necessarily associated with high and low cerebral glucose levels in patients with SAH. Instead, the two compartments show a more linear correlation in patients affected by TBI, although this seems to be true only in the non-damaged tissue. Given the established role of hyperglycemia in the pathogenesis of brain tissue damage, several clinical trials have addressed the most appropriate glycemic target to optimize the outcome of these patients.[72] Insulin use is necessary to achieve a targeted blood glucose concentration and every administration endows a risk of hypoglycemia. A systemic meta-analysis of randomized clinical trials (RCTs) performed in NCCU patients showed that better outcomes are associated with a threshold for insulin administration higher than 11.1 mmol/l (200 mg/dL).[73] The milestone NICE-SUGAR RCT on TBI patients indicated that tight glycemic control between 4.5 and 6 mmol/l (80–105 mg/dL) was associated with more severe hypoglycemic episodes when compared with a conventional control within 10 mmol/l (180 mg/dL) without differing in any major clinical outcome.[74] For blood glucose monitoring, POC should be preferred over capillary glucometers, although frequent calibrations with central laboratory values are recommended.[75]

REFERENCES

1. Sterns RH. Disorders of plasma sodium—Causes, consequences, and correction. *N Engl J Med*. 2015;372(1):55-65.

2. Rahman M, Friedman WA. Hyponatremia in neurosurgical patients: Clinical guidelines development. *Neurosurgery*. 2009;65(5):925-35; discussion 935-936.

3. Bhave G, Neilson EG. Body fluid dynamics: Back to the future. *J Am Soc Nephrol*. 2011; 22(12):2166-2181.

4. Rose B, Post T. *Clinical Physiology of Acid-Base and Electrolyte Disorders.* New York, NY: McGraw-Hill Education; 2001.

5. Erstad BL. Osmolality and osmolarity: Narrowing the terminology gap. *Pharmacotherapy*. 2003;23(9):1085-1086.

6. Waldegger S, Jentsch TJ. From tonus to tonicity: Physiology of CLC chloride channels. *J Am Soc Nephrol*. 2000;11(7):1331-1339.

7. Wright WL. Sodium and fluid management in acute brain injury. *Curr Neurol Neurosci Rep*. 2012;12(4):466-473.

8. Bhardwaj A. Neurological impact of vasopressin dysregulation and hyponatremia. *Ann Neurol*. 2006;59(2):229-236.

9. Levin ER, Gardner DG, Samson WK. Natriuretic peptides. *N Engl Med*. 1998;339(5): 321-328.

10. Tisdall M, Crocker M, Watkiss J, Smith M. Disturbances of sodium in critically ill adult neurologic patients: A clinical review. *J Neurosurg Anesthesiol*. 2006;18(1):57-63.

11. Buffington MA, Abreo K. Hyponatremia: A review. *J Intensive Care Med*. 2016;31(4): 223-236.

12. Goldwasser P, Ayoub I, Barth RH. Pseudohypernatremia and pseudohyponatremia: A linear correction. *Nephrol Dial Transplant*. 2015;30(2):252-257.

13. Lindner G, Funk GC. Hypernatremia in critically ill patients. *J Crit Care*. 2013;28(2): 216.e11-220.

14. Bataille S, Baralla C, Torro D et al. Undercorrection of hypernatremia is frequent and associated with mortality. *BMC Nephrol*. 2014;15(1):37.

15. Li M, Hu YH, Chen G. Hypernatremia severity and the risk of death after traumatic brain injury. *Injury*. 2013;44(9):1213-1218.

16. Schneider HJ, Kreitschmann-Andermahr I, Ghigo E, Stalla GK, Agha A. Hypothalamopituitary dysfunction following traumatic brain injury and aneurysmal subarachnoid hemorrhage: A systematic review. *JAMA*. 2007;298(12):1429-1438.

17. Ryu JH, Walcott BP, Kahle KT et al. Induced and sustained hypernatremia for the prevention and treatment of cerebral edema following brain injury. *Neurocrit Care*. 2013; 19(2):222-231.

18. Tan SK, Kolmodin L, Sekhon MS et al. The effect of continuous hypertonic saline infusion and hypernatremia on mortality in patients with severe traumatic brain injury: A retrospective cohort study. *Can J Anaesth*. 2016;63(6):664-673.

19. Hays AN, Lazaridis C, Neyens R, Nicholas J, Gay S, Chalela JA. Osmotherapy: Use among neurointensivists. *Neurocrit Care*. 2011;14 (2):222-228.

20. Achinger SG, Arieff AI, Kalantar-Zadeh K, Ayus JC. Desmopressin acetate (DDAVP)-associated hyponatremia and brain damage: A case series. *Nephrol Dial Transplant*. 2014;29(12):2310-2315.

21. Sherlock, M, O'Sullivan E, Agha A et al. Incidence and pathophysiology of severe hyponatraemia in neurosurgical patients. *Postgrad Med J*. 2009;85(1002):171-175.

22. Corona G, Giuliani C, Parenti G et al. Moderate hyponatremia is associated with increased risk of mortality: Evidence from a meta-analysis. *PLoS One*. 2013;8(12): e80451.

23. Zheng B, Qiu Y, Jin H et al. A predictive value of hyponatremia for poor outcome and cerebral infarction in high-grade aneurysmal subarachnoid haemorrhage patients. *J Neurol Neurosurg Psychiatry*. 2011;82(2): 213-217.

24. Qureshi AI, Suri MF, Sung GY et al. Prognostic significance of hypernatremia and hyponatremia among patients with aneurysmal subarachnoid hemorrhage. *Neurosurgery*. 2002;50(4):749-755; discussion 755-6.

25. Mewasingh L, Aylett S, Kirkham F, Stanhope R. Hyponatraemia associated with lamotrigine in cranial diabetes insipidus. *Lancet.* 2000;356(9230):656.

26. Rabinstein AA, Wijdicks EF. Hyponatremia in critically ill neurological patients. *Neurologist.* 2003;9(6):290-300.

27. Manzanares W, Aramendi I, Langlois PL, Biestro A. Hyponatremia in the neurocritical care patient: An approach based on current evidence. *Med Intensiva.* 2015;39(4):234-243.

28. Nathan BR. Cerebral correlates of hyponatremia. *Neurocrit Care.* 2007;6(1):72-78.

29. Hannon MJ, Behan LA, O'Brien MM et al. Hyponatremia following mild/moderate subarachnoid hemorrhage is due to SIAD and glucocorticoid deficiency and not cerebral salt wasting. *J Clin Endocrinol Metab.* 2014;99(1):291-298.

30. Kirkman MA. Managing hyponatremia in neurosurgical patients. *Minerva Endocrinol.* 2014;39(1):13-26.

31. Wu X, Zhou X, Gao L et al. Diagnosis and management of combined central diabetes insipidus and cerebral salt wasting syndrome after traumatic brain injury. *World Neurosurg.* 2016;88:483-487.

32. Human T, Cook AM, Anger B et al. Treatment of hyponatremia in patients with acute neurological injury. *Neurocrit Care.* 2017;27(2):242-248.

33. Sood L, Sterns RH, Hix JK, Silver SM, Chen L. Hypertonic saline and desmopressin: A simple strategy for safe correction of severe hyponatremia. *Am J Kidney Dis.* 2013;61(4):571-578.

34. Ellison DH, Berl T. Clinical practice. The syndrome of inappropriate antidiuresis. *N Engl J Med.* 2007;356(20):2064-2072.

35. Diringer MN, Zazulia AR. Hyponatremia in neurologic patients: Consequences and approaches to treatment. *Neurologist.* 2006;12(3):117-126.

36. Human T, Onuoha A, Diringer M, Dhar R. Response to a bolus of conivaptan in patients with acute hyponatremia after brain injury. *J Crit Care.* 2012;27(6):745.e1-5.

37. Galton, C, Deem S, Yanez ND et al. Open-label randomized trial of the safety and efficacy of a single dose conivaptan to raise serum sodium in patients with traumatic brain injury. *Neurocrit Care.* 2011;14(3):354-360.

38. Reinert M, Khaldi A, Zauner A, Doppenberg E, Choi S, Bullock R. High level of extracellular potassium and its correlates after severe head injury: Relationship to high intracranial pressure. *J Neurosurg.* 2000;93(5):800-807.

39. Hifumi T, Kuroda Y, Kawakita K et al. Plasma potassium concentration on admission correlates with neurologic outcome in traumatic brain injury patients treated with targeted temperature management: A post hoc analysis of a multicenter randomized controlled trial. *World Neurosurg.* 2016;94:437-441.

40. McMahon GM, Mendu ML, Gibbons FK, Christopher KB. Association between hyperkalemia at critical care initiation and mortality. *Intensive Care Med.* 2012;38(11):1834-1842.

41. Cohen R, Ramos R, Garcia C et al. Electrocardiogram manifestations in hyperkalemia. *World J Cardiovasc Dis.* 2012;2(2):57-63.

42. Lee JW. Fluid and electrolyte disturbances in critically ill patients. *Electrolyte Blood Press.* 2010;8(2):72-81.

43. Unwin RJ, Luft FC, Shirley DG. Pathophysiology and management of hypokalemia: A clinical perspective. *Nat Rev Nephrol.* 2011;7(2):75-84.

44. Alfonzo AV, Isles C, Geddes C, Deighan C. Potassium disorders—Clinical spectrum and emergency management. *Resuscitation.* 2006;70(1):10-25.

45. Asirvatham JR, Moses V, Bjornson L. Errors in potassium measurement: A laboratory perspective for the clinician. *N Am J Med Sci.* 2013;5(4):255-259.

46. Elliott MJ, Ronksley PE, Clase CM, Ahmed SB, Hemmelgarn BR. Management of patients with acute hyperkalemia. *CMAJ.* 2010;182(15):1631-1635.

47. Mahoney BA, Smith WA, Lo DS, Tsoi K, Tonelli M, Clase CM. Emergency interventions for hyperkalaemia. *Cochrane Database Syst Rev.* 2005(2):CD003235.

48. McIntosh E, Andrews PJ. Is sodium chloride worth its salt? *Crit Care.* 2013;17(3):150.

49. Powner DJ, Boccalandro C, Alp MS, Vollmer DG. Endocrine failure after traumatic brain

injury in adults. *Neurocrit Care.* 2006;5(1): 61-70.

50. Idowu OE, Obafunwa JO, Soyemi SO. Pituitary gland trauma in fatal nonsurgical closed traumatic brain injury. *Brain Inj.* 2017;31(3): 359-362.

51. Hannon MJ, Crowley RK, Behan LA et al. Acute glucocorticoid deficiency and diabetes insipidus are common after acute traumatic brain injury and predict mortality. *J Clin Endocrinol Metab.* 2013;98(8):3229-3237.

52. Ranasinghe AM, Bonser RS. Endocrine changes in brain death and transplantation. *Best Pract Res Clin Endocrinol Metab.* 2011; 25(5):799-812.

53. Gasco V, Prodam F, Pagano L et al. Hypopituitarism following brain injury: When does it occur and how best to test? *Pituitary.* 2012; 15(1):20-24.

54. Benvenga S, Campenní A, Ruggeri RM, Trimarchi F. Clinical review 113: Hypopituitarism secondary to head trauma. *J Clin Endocrinol Metab.* 2000;85(4):1353-1361.

55. Vespa PM. Hormonal dysfunction in neurocritical patients. *Curr Opin Crit Care.* 2013;19 (2):107-112.

56. Hackl JM, Gottardis M, Wieser C et al. Endocrine abnormalities in severe traumatic brain injury—A cue to prognosis in severe craniocerebral trauma? *Intensive Care Med.* 1991;17(1):25-29.

57. Schneider M, Schneider HJ, Yassouridis A, Saller B, von Rosen F, Stalla GK. Predictors of anterior pituitary insufficiency after traumatic brain injury. *Clin Endocrinol (Oxf).* 2008;68 (2):206-212.

58. Tritos NA, Yuen KC, Kelly DF. American association of clinical endocrinologists and american college of endocrinology disease state clinical review: A neuroendocrine approach to patients with traumatic brain injury. *Endocr Pract.* 2015;21(7):823-831.

59. Martin J, Kagerbauer SM, Schuster T, Blobner M, Kochs EF, Landgraf R. Vasopressin and oxytocin in CSF and plasma of patients with aneurysmal subarachnoid haemorrhage. *Neuropeptides.* 2014;48(2): 91-96.

60. Schneider HJ, Stalla GK, Buchfelder M. Expert meeting: Hypopituitarism after traumatic brain injury and subarachnoid

haemorrhage. *Acta Neurochir (Wien).* 2006; 148(4):449-456.

61. Cohan P, Wang C, McArthur DL et al. Acute secondary adrenal insufficiency after traumatic brain injury: A prospective study. *Crit Care Med.* 2005;33(10):2358-2366.

62. Alavi SA, Tan CL, Menon DK, Simpson HL3, Hutchinson PJ. Incidence of pituitary dysfunction following traumatic brain injury: A prospective study from a regional neurosurgical centre. *Br J Neurosurg.* 2016;30(3): 302-306.

63. Pal A, Capatina C, Tenreiro AP et al. Pituitary apoplexy in non-functioning pituitary adenomas: Long term follow up is important because of significant numbers of tumour recurrences. *Clin Endocrinol (Oxf).* 2011;75 (4):501-504.

64. Schneider HJ, Schneider M, Saller B et al. Prevalence of anterior pituitary insufficiency 3 and 12 months after traumatic brain injury. *Eur J Endocrinol.* 2006;154(2): 259-265.

65. Dimopoulou I, Alevizopoulou P, Dafni U et al. Pituitary-adrenal responses to human corticotropin-releasing hormone in critically ill patients. *Intensive Care Med.* 2007;33(3): 454-459.

66. Kromah F, Tyroch A, McLean S, Hughes H, Flavin N, Lee S. Relative adrenal insufficiency in the critical care setting: Debunking the classic myth. *World J Surg.* 2011;35(8):1818-1823.

67. Schneider HJ, Aimaretti G, Kreitschmann-Andermahr I, Stalla GK, Ghigo E. Hypopituitarism. *Lancet.* 2007;369(9571):1461-1470.

68. Bondanelli M, De Marinis L, Ambrosio MR et al. Occurrence of pituitary dysfunction following traumatic brain injury. *J Neurotrauma.* 2004;21(6):685-696.

69. Agha A, Rogers B, Mylotte D et al. Neuroendocrine dysfunction in the acute phase of traumatic brain injury. *Clin Endocrinol (Oxf).* 2004;60(5):584-591.

70. Tölli A, Borg J, Bellander BM, Johansson F, Höybye C. Pituitary function within the first year after traumatic brain injury or subarachnoid haemorrhage. *J Endocrinol Invest.* 2017;40(2):193-205.

71. Singh K, Morse AM, Tkachenko N, Kothare SV. Sleep disorders associated with traumatic

brain injury—A review. *Pediatr Neurol.* 2016;60:30-36.

72. Rostami E. Glucose and the injured brain- monitored in the neurointensive care unit. *Front Neurol.* 2014;5:91.

73. Kramer AH, Roberts DJ, Zygun DA. Optimal glycemic control in neurocritical care patients: A systematic review and meta-analysis. *Crit Care.* 2012;16(5):R203.

74. Finfer S, Chittock D, Li Y, Foster D et al. Intensive versus conventional glucose con- trol in critically ill patients with traumatic brain injury: Long-term follow-up of a subgroup of patients from the NICE-SUGAR study. *Intensive Care Med.* 2015;41(6):1037-1047.

75. Badjatia N, Vespa P. Monitoring nutrition and glucose in acute brain injury. *Neurocrit Care.* 2014;21(Suppl 2):S159-S167.

22

Neuromuscular care

ANKUR KHANDELWAL AND HEMANSHU PRABHAKAR

INTRODUCTION

Neuromuscular blocking agents (NMBAs) play an important role in managing a large number of hospital patients. NMBAs paralyze skeletal muscles by blocking the transmission of nerve impulses at the myoneural junction. They do not possess sedative, amnestic, or analgesic properties. Initially marketed for muscle relaxation to ease endotracheal (ETT) intubation and provide optimal operating conditions, the application of NMBAs has been expanded to include critically ill patients in the intensive care unit (ICU) and emergency department (ED). Some indications for their use are listed in Table 22.1.

However, sick patients in ICU often have multiple organ failure and also receive concomitant medications. The pharmacokinetic and pharmacodynamics properties of NMBAs in this population are poorly understood. There have been repeated reports of prolonged neuromuscular (NM) block after long-term administration of NMBAs in the critically ill resulting from overdosage, prolonged excretion of the NMBA and its metabolite, or critical illness myopathy.[1] As such, it is inappropriate to extrapolate NMBA usage experience in the operating theater whether in healthy patients or in managing the critically ill.

CHARACTERISTICS OF THE IDEAL NMBA

There are no data to suggest that any one muscle relaxant (MR) is superior to another, and the choice of MR should be based on specific criteria including contraindications to the drug, its cardiovascular effects, duration of action, ease of administration, and cost.

An ideal NMBA for use in the ICU should have a rapid and predictable onset and offset of effect, stable cardiovascular profile, inactive metabolites, no propensity to accumulate, elimination independent of hepatic or renal function, no interaction with other drugs, suitable for continuous infusion, and low cost. No presently available agent meets all these requirements.

CLASSIFICATION

NMBAs are broadly classified as depolarizing or non-depolarizing MRs:

1. Depolarizing—Suxamethonium
2. Non-depolarizing
   a. Long acting—Pancuronium, pipecuronium, doxacurium, tubocurarine

Table 22.1 Indications

1. Facilitation of tracheal intubation
2. Improve patient-ventilator synchrony by preventing uncoordinated respiratory movements and reducing peak airway pressures
3. To aid oxygenation in refractory hypoxemia by decreasing oxygen consumption, improving chest wall compliance and allowing inverse ratio, high frequency or prone position ventilation
4. Control of increases in intracranial pressure by preventing bucking and coughing on the endotracheal tube and decreasing oxygen consumption and cerebral metabolism
5. To facilitate targeted temperature management by easing rapid attainment of target temperature and controlling shivering
6. Ablation of muscle spasms, eg, tetanus, neuroleptic malignant syndrome, status epilepticus
7. In selected patients with cardiovascular instability
8. In a patient who must remain immobile (ie, to protect a surgical repair or vascular device such as a membrane oxygenator or heart assist device)
9. Facilitation of procedures and tests, eg, inter-hospital and intra-hospital patient transport, bronchoscopy, tracheostomy, MRI, CT scanning

b. Intermediate acting—Atracurium, cisatracurium, vecuronium, rocuronium
c. Short acting—Mivacurium
d. Ultrashort acting—Gantacurium

On the basis of chemical structure, nondepolarizing MRs can be further divided into:

1. Benzylisoquinolinium compounds—Tubocurarine, doxacurium, atracurium, cisatracurium, mivacurium
2. Aminosteroid compounds—Pancuronium, Vecuronium, Rocuronium

MECHANISM OF ACTION

Depolarizing NMBAs act as agonists at postsynaptic nicotinic acetylcholine receptors. They hold open the ion-gated channels, leading to muscular fasciculation, until the ion potential is depleted, and then to paralysis. Non-depolarizing MRs produce NM blockade by competing with acetylcholine for the postsynaptic α subunits; this leads to inhibition of sodium channels and excitatory postsynaptic potential.

The muscle relaxants that are commonly used in ICU are atracurium, cisatracurium, pancuronium, vecuronium, and rocuronium.

Atracurium

Atracurium 0.5–0.6 mg/kg produces adequate conditions for tracheal intubation within 3 to 5 minutes. Clinical recovery occurs in about 25 to 35 minutes. Continuous infusion dosing ranges from 5 to 20 μg/kg/min. Atracurium is metabolized through two pathways: Hofmann elimination and nonspecific ester hydrolysis. Hofmann elimination is a purely chemical process characterized by spontaneous degradation of atracurium in the plasma at a physiological pH and at temperature into laudanosine and a monoquaternary acrylate. Ester hydrolysis also contributes to its disposition. Renal elimination accounts for 10% to 40% of the total drug elimination. Atracurium also causes dose-dependent histamine release. Atracurium's onset and duration of effect are predictable, however sick the patient. These properties make it useful for managing the critically ill patient.

Cisatracurium

Cisatracurium, the 1R cis–1′R cis isomer of atracurium, comprises approximately 15% of atracurium by weight, but more than 50% in terms of NM blocking activity. Cisatracurium 0.1 to 0.2 mg/kg produces adequate conditions for tracheal intubation within 2–3 minutes. Clinical recovery occurs in about 45 to 60 minutes. Continuous infusion dosing ranges from 1 to 3 μg/kg/min. Like atracurium, cisatracurium is metabolized by Hofmann elimination to laudanosine and a monoquaternary acrylate. In contrast, however, no ester hydrolysis of the parent molecule occurs. It is approximately four times as potent as atracurium and produces five times less laudanosine in contrast to atracurium. Moreover, it does not cause histamine release. Renal clearance is about 16% of total.

Pancuronium

Pancuronium is a long-acting NMBA. It produces adequate intubating conditions in 2.5 to 3.0 minutes after a dose of 0.1 to 0.15 mg/kg. Clinical recovery occurs within 90 to 100 minutes. Continuous infusion dosing ranges from 0.8 to 1.7 µg/kg/min. Pancuronium and its 3-OH metabolite, which has at least 50% of the NM blocking potency of the parent compound, are dependent upon renal (45%–70%) and hepatic clearance (10%–15%). The elimination half-life and duration of action of pancuronium are increased in patients with renal dysfunction. An increase in elimination half-life has also been demonstrated in patients with acute liver failure, cirrhosis, and total biliary obstruction. Pancuronium is no longer indicated for use in the critically ill. Its sympathomimetic effects are also disadvantageous in these patients.

Vecuronium

Vecuronium is the 2-desmethyl derivative of pancuronium. It provides good intubating conditions within 3 to 4 minutes after a dose of 0.08 to 0.1 mg/kg. Clinical recovery occurs in about 35 to 45 minutes. Continuous infusion dosing ranges from 0.8 to 1.7 µg/kg/min. Vecuronium is more lipid soluble and is metabolized two to three times more than pancuronium. It is taken up into the liver by a carrier-mediated transport system, and it is then deacetylated at the 3 position by liver microsomes. Approximately 12% of vecuronium is cleared by converting it to 3-desacetylvecuronium, and 30% to 40% of the drug is cleared in the bile as the parent compound. Although the liver is the principal organ of elimination for vecuronium, the drug also undergoes significant renal excretion (up to 25%). The principal metabolite of vecuronium, 3-desacetylvecuronium, is a potent (≈80% of vecuronium) NMBA in its own right. The metabolite, however, has a slower plasma clearance and a longer duration of action than vecuronium. In ICU patients with renal failure, 3-desacetylvecuronium can accumulate and produce prolonged NM blockade.

Rocuronium

Rocuronium is approximately six to 10 times less potent than pancuronium and vecuronium,

respectively. The usual intubating dose ranges from 0.6 to 1 mg/kg and the duration of action is similar to vecuronium. However, increasing the dosage of rocuronium from 0.6 mg/kg to 1.2 mg/kg shortens the onset time of complete NM block from 89 seconds to 55 seconds, but essentially doubles the clinical duration of recovery from 37 minutes to 73 minutes.[2] Continuous infusion dosing ranges from 8 to 12 µg/kg/min. Rocuronium is eliminated primarily by the liver (>70%), with a small percentage (≈10%) eliminated in the urine. The putative metabolite, 17-desacetylrocuronium has not been detected in significant quantities.

MUSCLE RELAXANTS AND CEREBRAL PHYSIOLOGY

Depolarizing muscle relaxant

Many studies have demonstrated that succinylcholine elevates intracranial pressure (ICP) in animals and in humans irrespective of the presence or absence of space-occupying intracranial lesions.[3,4] The rise in ICP with succinylcholine is accompanied by muscle fasciculation, an increase in muscle spindle afferent activity, electroencephalographic (EEG) arousal, and an elevation in cerebral blood flow (CBF). Fasciculation in the muscles of the neck, causing stasis in the jugular veins, might also contribute to increased ICP with succinylcholine. Succinylcholine-induced increase in serum potassium in a patient with subarachnoid hemorrhage is another concern. It seems independent of the presence of motor dysfunction. Nevertheless, succinylcholine use has been diminishing in clinical neuroanesthesia and neurointensive units, except for emergency situations, such as a patient with a full stomach where a rapid-sequence induction is recommended. In this situation, prior administration of small doses of non-depolarizing MR or lidocaine is recommended. Also, it has been demonstrated that a single dose of succinylcholine does not increase ICP either in patients sedated with propofol and opioid infusions or those previously hyperventilated.[5,6]

Non-depolarizing muscle relaxant

Benzylisoquinolinium MRs such as atracurium appear to have no significant effect on cerebral blood flow (CBF), cerebral metabolic rate of oxygen consumption ($CMRO_2$), or ICP. However, high doses of atracurium have the potential to release histamine, though the potential is considerably less than that of d-tubocurarine. Histamine can reduce cerebral perfusion pressure (CPP) because of increased ICP caused by cerebral vasodilation and the decrease in mean arterial pressure (MAP). Cisatracurium, one of the isomers of atracurium, produces and releases less histamine than atracurium and therefore less interference with CPP.

Steroidal compounds such as pancuronium, vecuronium, and rocuronium have little or minimal effect on CBF, $CMRO_2$, or ICP. Pancuronium raises blood pressure and heart rate, which could be detrimental for certain patients, including those with hypertension, especially if they have disturbed autoregulation. In these patients, a substantial elevation of ICP can occur. Vecuronium doesn't induce histamine release and doesn't change blood pressure or heart rate, and may be preferable. Rocuronium, because of its rapid onset of action when compared to other non-depolarizing MRs and its lack of adverse activity, such as histamine release, may be preferable to succinylcholine during rapid induction of anesthesia.

Two observational studies have investigated the ability of NM blockade to attenuate the rise in ICP and the fall in CPP that can accompany tracheal suctioning in brain injured patients with elevated ICP.[7,8] These studies are few in number, small in size, observational in design, and focused on physiologic changes, rather than on clinically important outcomes. Nevertheless, they provide evidence that pretreatment with an NMBA may mitigate procedure-related increases in ICP. It has been postulated that as an NMBA decreases intrathoracic pressure due to decreased muscular tone, improvement in cerebral venous return could result in a decrease in ICP.[9]

In contrast, two retrospective evaluations of prospective data have investigated NMBAs for managing intracranial hypertension, with a focus on clinically important outcomes.[10,11] One study of 514 patients with traumatic brain injury (TBI) and a Glasgow Coma Scale (GCS) score of less than 8 found that patients treated with early NM blockade for more than 12 hours had a higher risk of pneumonia and of having a prolonged ICU stay than patients treated with NMBAs for less than 6 hours; even after controlling for age, preresuscitation GCS and hypotension, CT findings, and single-versus multiple-system trauma. There was no difference in time with elevated ICP. The use of NMBAs was associated with a longer length of stay, more pneumonia, and a higher proportion of survivors who suffered from a persistent vegetative state or severe disability.[10] A similar retrospective evaluation (N = 326) found no difference in mortality or length of stay between patients with TBI who did, versus did not, receive an NMBA.[11] In summary, although these two studies provide important preliminary data regarding the role for NMBAs in managing intracranial hypertension, they do not provide support for evidence-based recommendations to guide clinical practice.

COMPLICATIONS

NMBAs are now routinely used in the ICU despite the relative paucity of literature regarding their use, safety, and efficacy in this setting. They are frequently used with sedatives and analgesics in ICUs. In the current era, the use of NMBAs in the ICU has decreased considerably because of the large number of both short and long term complications associated with their use. Of particular concern in the ICU setting is the risk that paralyzed patients receive inadequate analgesia and sedation.[12] Inadequate ventilation in the event of a ventilator failure, circuit disconnection or accidental extubation in the presence of muscle relaxation can be disastrous. Drug specific complications such as laudanosine (metabolite of atracurium)-associated seizures and vecuronium/atracurium/pancuronium-associated cerebral excitation and the consequent increased cerebral oxygen demand are undesirable in the ICU even though the reported evidences exist from animal studies.[13,14] Active metabolites of vecuronium and pancuronium accumulate in patients with renal dysfunction, producing prolonged residual paralysis, and rocuronium metabolism is decreased if there is hepatic dysfunction.[15] Investigators have also suggested that non-depolarizing NMBAs can gain access to nerves during systemic inflammatory response syndrome, resulting in direct neurotoxicity.[14]

Long term muscle weakness associated with the use of NMBAs and their subsequent complications is the main reason for their declining use in the ICU. It has been observed that prolonged recovery from NM blockade occurs more frequently when steroidal NMBAs are used.[16,17] Co-existing sepsis, the dysfunction of two or more organs, administration of steroids and hypercapnia exacerbates NMBAs induced myopathy. Drug–drug interactions that potentiate the depth of motor blockade may also prolong recovery (Table 22.2).[18,19] Hypothermia and electrolyte and metabolic derangements may also potentiate the NM blockade. Prolonged muscle weakness is the harbinger of immobility associated complications such as deep vein thrombosis, peripheral nerve injuries, and decubitus ulcers. Other complications long term use of NMBA include the inability to cough, which leads to the retention of secretions and consequent atelectasis or pneumonia as well as the infrequent or absent blinking of eyelids predisposing a patient to corneal drying, abrasion, and ulceration. NMBAs ablate abdominal rigidity, therefore, diagnosing

acute abdominal infection or perforation may be delayed in these patients. In neurocritically ill patients, the use of NMBAs obfuscates assessing the neurological status of patients. The use of NMBAs can also result in the subluxation of unstable spinal fractures.[20]

In contrast, the infusion of succinylcholine is not recommended due to its potential complications such as arrythmias, myalgia, elevated intracranial, intraocular and intragastric pressures, histamine release and the induction of malignant hyperthermia. It is usually contraindicated in patients with sepsis, massive trauma, burns, spinal cord transection, CNS injuries/infections, prolonged immobilization, disuse atrophy, Guillain-Barre´ syndrome, and peripheral nerve injury, because of the risk of an exaggerated and potentially fatal increase in serum potassium.[20]

These complications of NMBAs are associated with increased morbidity, prolonged ICU and hospital stay, and prolonged rehabilitation. No MR should be regarded as completely safe for long-term administration in the ICU.

Table 22.2 Drug–drug interactions of neuromuscular blocking agents (NMBAs)

Drugs that potentiate the action of non-depolarizing NMBAs	Drugs that antagonize the actions of non-depolarizing NMBAs
Antimicrobials (aminoglycosides, polymyxin B, clindamycin, tetracycline)	Phenytoin Carbamazepine Theophylline Ranitidine
Antiarrhythmics (quinidine, procainamide, bretylium)	
Local anesthetic agents	
Magnesium	
Calcium channel blockers	
β-Adrenergic blockers	
Immunosuppressive agents (cyclophosphamide, cyclosporine)	
Inhalation anesthetic gases	
Dantrolene	
Furosemide	
Lithium carbonate	

MONITORING

The best way to monitor an NMBA's effect in the ICU is not clear. There have been studies that have tried to ascertain the best method of monitoring the depth of NM blockade in critically ill patients. Although peripheral nerve stimulation using train of four (TOF) monitoring may result in using lower doses of NMBAs and faster recovery from NM blockade,[21,22] clinical evaluation may be equally effective.[23,24] The clinical practice guidelines for sustained NM blockade in adult patients suggests that TOF monitoring alone is not beneficial in those receiving a continuous infusion of NMBAs. It should be incorporated into a more inclusive assessment of the patient that includes clinical assessment.[25] When non-depolarizing NMBAs are used, certain recommendations described in various studies may minimize the incidence of complications. These have been listed in Table 22.3. Patients who are being treated for seizures and who also take NMBAs should have EEG monitoring to ensure that they are not actively seizing while paralyzed.

Table 22.3 Recommendations for the use of NMBAs in the ICU

1. Dosing of NMBAs should be done based on ideal body weight, particularly in obese patients
2. Avoid the use of NM blockers by:
   - Maximal use of analgesics and sedatives
   - Manipulation of ventilatory parameters and modes
3. Minimize the dose of NM blockers by:
   - Using a clinical and peripheral nerve stimulator with train-of-four monitoring
   - Do not administer for more than 2 days continuously
   - Administering by bolus rather than infusion
   - Administering only when required and in order to achieve a well-defined goal
   - Continually allow recovery from paralysis
4. Minimize complications by:
   - Correcting and optimizing acid-base disorders, electrolyte disturbances and other conditions known to exacerbate NMBAs induced by prolonged muscle weakness
   - Using an NMBA with minimal hepatic metabolism
   - Adapting structured physiotherapy regimen
   - Prophylaxis for deep vein thrombosis
   - Frequently changing position
   - Scheduling eyecare with lubricating eye drops or gel, eye covers or eyelid closure

CONCLUSION

Neuromuscular blockade is an essential modality for an intensivist and is intended to fulfill multiple indications. NMBA choice should be based on patient specific (eg, comorbidities) and drug-specific (eg, onset, offset, route of elimination) factors. However, based on recent evidences, NMBAs should be considered an intervention of last resort due to the multiple complications associated with their use. Careful administration and monitoring is warranted whenever NMBAs are used.

REFERENCES

1. Murphy GS, Vender JS. Neuromuscular-blocking drugs. Use and misuse in the intensive care unit. *Crit Care Clin.* 2001;17: 925-942.
2. Magorian T, Flannery KB, Miller RD. Comparison of rocuronium, succinylcholine, and vecuronium for rapid-sequence induction of anesthesia in adult patients. *Anesthesiology.* 1993;79:913-918.
3. Stirt JA, Grosslight KR, Bedford RF, Vollmer D. Defasciculation with metocurine prevents succinylcholine-induced increases in intracranial pressure. *Anesthesiology.* 1987;67: 50-53.
4. Minton MD, Grosslight K, Stirt JA, Bedford RF. Increases in intracranial pressure from succinylcholine: Prevention by prior non-depolarizing blockade. *Anesthesiology.* 1986;65:165-169.
5. Brown MM, Parr MJ, Manara AR. The effect of suxamethonium on intracranial pressure and cerebral perfusion pressure in patients with severe head injuries following blunt trauma. *Eur J Anaesthesiol.* 1996;13:474-477.
6. Kovarik WD, Mayberg TS, Lam AM, Mathisen TL, Winn HR. Succinylcholine does not change intracranial pressure, cerebral blood flow velocity, or the electroencephalogram in patients with neurologic injury. *Anesth Analg.* 1994;78:469-473.
7. Werba A, Klezl M, Schramm W et al. The level of neuromuscular block needed to suppress diaphragmatic movement during tracheal suction in patients with raised intracranial pressure: A study with vecuronium and atracurium. *Anaesthesia.* 1993;48:301-303.
8. Kerr ME, Sereika SM, Orndoff P et al. Effect of neuromuscular blockers and opiates on the cerebrovascular response to endotracheal suctioning in adults with severe head injuries. *Am J Crit Care.* 1998;7:205-217.
9. Greenberg SB, Vender J. The use of neuromuscular blocking agents in the ICU: Where are we now? *Crit Care Med.* 2013;41:1332-1344.

10. Hsiang JK, Chesnut RM, Crisp CB, Klauber MR, Blunt BA, Marshall LF. Early, routine paralysis for intracranial pressure control in severe head injury: Is it necessary? *Crit Care Med.* 1994;22:1471-1476.

11. Juul N, Morris GF, Marshall SB, Marshall LF. Neuromuscular blocking agents in neurointensive care. *Acta Neurochir Suppl.* 2000;76:467-470.

12. Loper KA, Butler S, Nessly M, Wild L. Paralyzed with pain: The need for education. *Pain.* 1989;37:315-316.

13. Gwinnutt CL, Eddleston JM, Edwards D, Pollard BJ. Concentrations of atracurium and laudanosine in cerebrospinal fluid and plasma in three intensive care patients. *Br J Anaesth.* 1990;65:829-832.

14. Szenohradszky J, Trevor AJ, Bickler P et al. Central nervous system effects of intrathecal muscle relaxants in rats. *Anesth Analg.* 1993;76:1304-1309.

15. Chamorro C, Borrallo JM, Romera MA, Silva JA, Balandín B. Anesthesia and analgesia protocol during therapeutic hypothermia after cardiac arrest: A systematic review. *Anesth Analg.* 2010;110:1328-1335.

16. Segredo V, Caldwell JE, Matthay MA, Sharma ML, Gruenke LD, Miller RD. Persistent paralysis in critically ill patients after long-term administration of vecuronium. *N Engl J Med.* 1992;327:524-528.

17. Op de Coul AA, Lambregts PC, Koeman J, van Puyenbroek MJ, TerLaak HJ, Gabreëls-Festen AA. Neuromuscular complications in patients given Pavulon (pancuronium bromide) during artificial ventilation. *Clin Neurol Neurosurg.* 1985;87:17-22.

18. Murray MJ, Cowen J, DeBlock H, Erstad B, Gray AW Jr, Tescher AN et al. Clinical practice guidelines for sustained neuromuscular blockade in the adult critically ill patient. *Crit Care Med.* 2002;30:142-156.

19. Warr J, Thiboutot Z, Rose L, Mehta S, Burry LD. Current therapeutic uses, pharmacology, and clinical considerations of neuromuscular blocking agents for critically ill adults. *Ann Pharmacother.* 2011;45:1116-1126.

20. Sharpe MD. The use of muscle relaxants in the intensive care unit. *Can J Anaesth.* 1992;39:949-962.

21. Frankel H, Jeng J, Tilly E, St Andre A, Champion H. The impact of implementation of neuromuscular blockade monitoring standards in a surgical intensive care unit. *Am Surg.* 1996;62:503-506.

22. Tavernier B, Rannou JJ, Vallet B. Peripheral nerve stimulation and clinical assessment for dosing of neuromuscular blocking agents in critically ill patients. *Crit Care Med.* 1998;26:804-805.

23. Strange C, Vaughan L, Franklin C, Johnson J. Comparison of train-of-four and best clinical assessment during continuous paralysis. *Am J Respir Crit Care Med.* 1997;156:1556-1561.

24. Baumann MH, McAlpin BW, Brown K et al. A prospective randomized comparison of train-of-four monitoring and clinical assessment during continuous ICU cisatracurium paralysis. *Chest.* 2004;126:1267-1273.

25. Murray MJ, DeBlock H, Erstad B et al. Clinical practice guidelines for sustained neuromuscular blockade in the adult critically ill patient. *Crit Care Med.* 2016;44:2079-2103.

23

Systemic care—Renal, hematologic, gastrointestinal

PANUMART MANATPON AND ANDREW W. KOFKE

RENAL SYSTEM

Acute kidney injury (AKI) terminology and scores

Acute kidney injury (AKI) is a common problem found in critically ill patients. It is described as an acute decline in kidney function (hours to days) and leads to a decreased ability to excrete nitrogenous waste products and urea and the dysregulation of fluid, electrolytes, and acid-base balance. AKI correlates with increased hospitalization, the risk of cardiovascular events, and the progression to chronic renal failure which may need renal replacement therapy and increases mortality.[1] However, the knowledge of AKI in the neurointensive care unit (NICU) setting regarding incidences, risk factors, mechanisms of injury, treatments, and outcomes is still limited. Patients admitted to NICU are complicated and usually require numerous investigations and treatments, thereby posing a high risk of acute kidney injury

(AKI). Thus, meticulous care must be taken in these patients to prevent AKI and further brain damage.

The term AKI has been suggested in order to emphasize smaller reductions in kidney function, whereas the term acute renal failure (ARF) generally means severe AKI wherein renal replacement therapy may be needed. This is important because a large variety of AKI definitions that are used in published studies make it difficult to compare studies, and contributes to difficulties in generalizing results and misconceptions in accurately understanding the epidemiology of AKI. Accordingly, the Acute Dialysis Quality Initiative (ADQI) group, comprising intensivists and nephrologists, proposed the so-called RIFLE criteria in 2004 to provide standardized definition and classification of the continuum of acute kidney injury.[2] The RIFLE criteria are divided into 5 classes and are based on two criteria: (1) a change in serum creatinine or a change in glomerular filtration rate (GFR) from baseline within 7 days and (2) urine output within a specific period of time (Table 23.1). However, RIFLE criteria

Table 23.1 The RIFLE, AKIN, and KDIGO criteria

RIFLE Criteria[2]

● Risk	Serum creatinine increase to 1.5 fold or a GFR decrease >25% from baseline	Urine output <0.5 mL/kg/h for 6 h
● Injury	Serum creatinine increase to 2.0 fold or a GFR decrease >50% from baseline	Urine output <0.5 mL/kg/h for 12 h
● Failure	Serum creatinine increase to 3.0 fold or a GFR decrease >75% or serum creatinine >4 mg/dL	Anuria for 12 h
● Loss	Persistent ARF = complete loss of kidney function >4 weeks	
● ESRF	End stage kidney disease >3 months	

AKIN Criteria[4]

● Stage 1	Serum creatinine increase ≥0.3 mg/dL to an increase of 1.5–2.0 fold from baseline	Urine output <0.5 mL/kg/h for 6 h
● Stage 2	Serum creatinine increase 2.0–3.0 fold from baseline	Urine output <0.5 mL/kg/h for 12 h
● Stage 3	Serum creatinine increase ≥ 3.0 fold from baseline or serum creatinine >4 mg/dL with an acute increase of at least 0.5 mg/dL	Urine output <0.3 mL/kg/h for 24 h or anuria for 12 h

KDIGO Criteria[6]

● Stage 1	Serum creatinine increase ≥0.3 mg/dL or an increase of 1.5–1.9 fold from baseline	Urine output <0.5 mL/kg/h for 6–12 h
● Stage 2	Serum creatinine increase 2.0–2.9 fold from baseline	Urine output <0.5 mL/kg/h for ≥12 h
● Stage 3	Serum creatinine increase ≥3.0 fold from baseline or serum creatinine >4 mg/dL or initiation of renal replacement therapy or in patients <18 years, decrease in eGFR to 35 mL/min/1.73 m^2	Urine output <0.3 mL/kg/h for ≥ 24 h or anuria for ≥12 h

may be invalid for defining AKI in the context of chronic renal dysfunction with chronically elevated serum creatinine, but without overriding AKI. Moreover, Pickering et al.[3] demonstrated no correlation between an increase in serum creatinine and a decrease in GFR in the same classification in RIFLE criteria. Therefore, in 2007, the RIFLE criteria were modified with the Acute Kidney Injury Network (AKIN) score where the GFR criteria are eliminated, the time frame is shortened (within 48 hours), and the absolute increase in serum creatinine concentration (≥0.3 mg/dL) is added.[4] The AKIN criteria categorizes AKI into stages 1, 2, and 3 which correspond to risk, injury, and failure as described in the RIFLE criteria, respectively. Loss and end stage renal failure (ESRF) are eliminated from the staging system. Nevertheless, the study showed that the AKIN criteria did not improve sensitivity or the ability to predict hospital mortality compared with the RIFLE criteria.[5] Following these scores, the KDIGO (Kidney Disease: Improving Global Outcomes) criteria, which is currently the most widely accepted criteria, was released in 2012,[6] classifying AKI into 3 stages based on serum creatinine and urine output. This is similar to the AKIN criteria except for stage 3 where the estimated GFR is taken into account in children younger than 18 years. The KDIGO criteria combines AKIN and RIFLE criteria together, considering an absolute increase in serum creatinine level of ≥0.3 mg/dL within 48 hours while using a 7-day timeframe for a ≥50% increase in serum creatinine. In fact, serum creatinine alone is not a very sensitive marker, only changing when significant kidney injury occurs. Notably, serum creatinine and urine output are affected by several other factors including medications, muscle wasting/injury, and nutritional status. All of these are commonly found in NICU patients, and may contribute to misinterpreting the indicators of kidney function. More recently, the new biomarkers, such as cystatin C, neutrophil gelatinase-associated lipocalin (NGAL), insulin-like growth factor binding protein 7 (IGFBP7), and tissue inhibitor metalloproteinase 2 (TIMP-2), have been introduced for early AKI detection and providing additional information regarding etiologies and stage of AKI.[7]

PATHOPHYSIOLOGY OF AKI IN TBI

To date, there has been limited information on the incidence of acute kidney injury (AKI) in traumatic brain injury (TBI) patients. Li et al.[8] reported that the incidence of AKI, as defined by AKIN criteria, was 23% in severe TBI patients; of those, 68%, 22%, and 10% were stage 1, stage 2, and stage 3, respectively. Ahmed et al.[9] performed a retrospective review of 95 severe TBI patients who were undergoing surgery for severe TBI and survived and were discharged from the hospital within a year. It revealed an AKI incidence of 11.6% and was divided into stage 1 (63.6%), stage 2 (27.3%), and stage 3 (9.1%). TBI patients with concomitant AKI are associated with higher mortality, poorer GCS at discharge, and an increased duration of mechanical ventilation, ICU length of stay, and hospital stay compared with those without AKI.[8-10]

Risk factors for AKI include age >75 years, hypotension, hypovolemia, sepsis, chronic kidney disease, vascular disease, congestive cardiac failure, diabetic mellitus, hypertension, proteinuria, jaundice, use of radiocontrast agents, and nephrotoxic medications such as NSAIDs, aminoglycosides, vancomycin, and hyperosmolar agents.[11,12] Chronic renal failure is a strong risk factor of AKI[12] in the NICU and it can increase the risk of several neurological complications, including intracranial hypertension, intracranial hypotension, subdural hematoma, hemorrhagic stroke, dementia, encephalopathy, cerebrovascular disease, osmotic myelinolysis, movement disorder, opportunistic infections, neoplasms, and neuropathy, caused by either uremic state or consequences of AKI treatments such as dialysis, kidney transplant, or immunosuppressive medications.[13]

In the NICU setting, there are a number of factors that can predispose critically ill patients to AKI. These factors include rhabdomyolysis, infection, and medication nephrotoxicity.

1. Rhabdomyolysis is associated with severe head injury related to trauma, a prolonged deteriorated mental status with protracted muscle compression/ischemia, convulsive seizure, and hyperosmolar states.[14] In such situations, rhabdomyolysis can contribute to AKI by renal vasoconstriction, intraluminal cast formation, and direct myoglobin toxicity. The incidence of AKI following rhabdomyolysis has been reported to be 33% to 50%.[15]

2. Infection. Cellular immune function can be suppressed after severe head injury,[16] which poses an increased risk of infection and systemic sepsis. Sepsis can contribute to AKI, which is thought to be associated with nitric oxide-mediated arterial vasodilation.[17] The mortality is far higher in patients with AKI in combination with sepsis (70%) compared with those with AKI alone (45%).[18]

3. Medication nephrotoxicity. Radiocontrast agents and potential nephrotoxic medications, including antibiotics, propofol, mannitol, and hypertonic saline, are commonly used in NICU patients. Propofol, a popular sedative agent in the ICU, can cause propofol infusion syndrome when high doses and/or prolonged duration are administered. The manifestations of propofol infusion syndrome include cardiac arrhythmia, metabolic acidosis, rhabdomyolysis, acute renal failure, hyperlipidemia, and enlarged or fatty liver. Mannitol is a hyperosmolar agent routinely employed to treat increased intracranial pressure (ICP) by drawing water from intracellular into extracellular compartments along osmotic gradients. One study showed that an accumulative dose of mannitol is an independent risk factor of AKI following cerebral trauma.[19] In patients with normal kidney function, a total mannitol dose of more than 1100 g may contribute to AKI, whereas only a lower dose of 300 g may promote AKI in patients with preexisting kidney disease. Risk factors associated with developing AKI in NICU patients receiving mannitol are congestive heart failure and a high APACHE II score.[20] The mechanism of mannitol-induced kidney injury is unclear. Renal vasoconstriction and tubular vacuolization are

believed to play a crucial role. Hypertonic saline is increasingly utilized to treat cerebral edema especially when mannitol is ineffective or contraindicated (eg, anuric renal failure). The problem of hypertonic saline is hyperchloremia potentially contributing to AKI. A study of SAH patients reported that the likelihood of developing AKI increases 5.4% for every 1 mEq/L increase in serum sodium.[21] Mechanisms of AKI are demonstrated in Table 23.2.

Table 23.2 Mechanisms of acute kidney injury[22]

Prerenal causes	Renal hypoperfusion due to:
	• Hypovolemia: Osmotic diuresis, diuretics, vomiting, diarrhea, blood loss
	• Intrarenal vasoconstriction: NSAIDs, angiotensin-converting enzyme inhibitors (ACEI), angiotensin receptor blockers (ARB)
	• Systemic vasodilation: Sepsis, neurogenic shock
Intrarenal causes	Glomerular: Post-infection, other glomerulonephritis
	Interstitial
	• Medications: NSAIDs, phenytoin, proton pump inhibitors, penicillin, cephalosporin, sulfonamide
	• Infection: Bacteria, virus, fungi
	• Systemic disease: Sarcoidosis, lupus
	Tubular
	• Ischemic due to prolong hypoperfusion
	• Nephrotoxic: Radiocontrast agents, aminoglycosides, amphotericin B, hemolysis, rhabdomyolysis
	Vascular: Renal vein thrombosis, malignant hypertension
Postrenal causes	Intra-renal or extra-renal obstruction

Source: Adapted from Rahman M et al. Am Fam Physician. 2012;86(7):631-639.

MANAGEMENT OF AKI IN NICU

The current standard of care for AKI includes identification of high-risk patients (discussed above), early AKI recognition, and developing strategies for prevention and management of AKI. Even with attention to these factors, renal failure may still arise in the correct adverse context in a NICU patient. The new biomarkers are a very promising tool for the early detection of AKI. They may enable its timely management and help to attenuate or completely reverse AKI in the early stages of AKI or to prevent progression to chronic renal failure. Nonetheless, there have been no studies validating the role of the new biomarkers in the context of TBI patients associated with AKI.

Strategies to prevent AKI are demonstrated in Table 23.3. Radiocontrast agents can contribute to the contrast-induced AKI (CI-AKI). Intravenous volume expansion with isotonic saline or sodium bicarbonate is the only intervention thought to help prevent the CI-AKI. The role of other pharmacologic interventions, such as N-Acetylcysteine (NAC), dopamine, fenoldopam, theophylline, nebivolol, prostaglandin, and atrial naturetic peptide (ANP), are still debated. Despite inconsistent outcome studies, oral NAC is recommended in combination with intravenous volume expansion (not with high chloride such as normal saline) in order to prevent CI-AKI in high-risk patients, since many studies support its benefits, which include low cost and low adverse effects.[23] The recommended dosage of NAC is 1200 mg orally twice daily both the day before and the day of the procedure.

Table 23.3 Strategies to prevent AKI

• Identify risk factors and alter modifiable risk factors
• Avoid nephrotoxic medications and replace by non-nephrotoxic equivalents whenever possible
• Use a low radiocontrast dose, avoid repeated radiocontrast agents, avoid using high-osmolar radiocontrast agents, and consider adequate hydration and oral N-Acetylcysteine (NAC)
• Maintain adequate hydration
• Optimize hemodynamic: Avoid hypotension, hypertension

Uncertain volume status is a common problem which can aggravate AKI. In a retrospective cohort study of 351 moderate to severe TBI patients admitted to the NICU, low (<637 mL) and high (>3673 mL) fluid balance were associated with poor short-term outcome. The higher incidence of refractory intracranial hypertension and AKI were identified in the high fluid balance group.[24] Adequate hydration is necessary and can be assessed by measuring intake and output, or more effectively by stroke volume variation (SVV) or pulse pressure variation (PPV). Mean arterial pressure should be optimized to ensure adequate perfusion to the kidneys and the brain. Hypotension, regardless of etiologies, can result in prerenal azotemia and cerebral ischemia, whereas hypertension is related to acute lung injury in TBI patients.[25]

There is no pharmacologic medication capable of reversing kidney injury process. Supportive treatments include optimization of volume status (avoid volume overload and hypovolemia), maintenance of adequate kidney perfusion, correction of electrolytes abnormalities (hyperkalemia, hyperphosphatemia, hypocalcemia) and acid-base imbalance (metabolic acidosis), adequate nutritional support, avoiding nephrotoxic agents whenever possible, and adjusting medication dosage based on kidney function.

In general, the indications for acute renal replacement therapy (RRT) are fluid overload refractory to diuretics, hyperkalemia unresponsive to medical therapy, metabolic acidosis wherein bicarbonate is not indicated or is ineffective, and uremia. During hemodialysis, plasma urea and osmolarity are rapidly reduced, thereby precipitating brain swelling. A decrease in arterial pressure can also occur during acute RRT, resulting in decreased cerebral perfusion pressure that triggers autoregulatory vasodilation of cerebral blood vessels, leading to increased CBV and further increased ICP. Thus, more gradual continuous renal replacement therapy (CRRT) is recommended for severe brain injury with cerebral edema since CRRT removes water and waste products slower and is more physiologic. This results in greater cerebrovascular stability and less osmotic exacerbation of cerebral swelling.

In those patients who are at risk of hemorrhage such as TBI or having an intraventricular catheter, anticoagulation free circuits or regional anticoagulation (ie, citrate or nafamostat) techniques are suggested. Acute intermittent hemodialysis (IHD) can be used successfully when CRRT is not available or patients are clinically stable without ICP issues. A modified prescription can be employed to reduce risk of further brain injury that can include no or regional anticoagulation, gradually increased blood flow, small surface area dialyzer, a start with 2-hour duration then increasing regarding stability, daily frequency, and dialysate: flow 500 mL/min, ≤10 mEq/L above serum sodium, bicarbonate 30 mEq/L, higher potassium and calcium, and 35°C temperature or isothermic dialysis.[26] Both mannitol and hypertonic saline, well known high osmolarity agents, may be utilized during RRT to stabilize plasma osmolarity to prevent cerebral edema.[26] Notably, although partially dialyzed, a use of mannitol in anuric ESRD[27] and repeated use during dialysis[28] in the TBI setting, where blood–brain barrier is impaired, is not recommended due to potential drug accumulation in the brain and possible greater osmotic gradients that are attributable to the partial dialysis of mannitol, which results in paradoxical cerebral edema and further elevated ICP.

Peritoneal dialysis (PD) is seldom used in the NICU. However, occasionally it is relevant for patients with chronic renal failure who use it during preadmission. The exchange volume exceeding 2 L in PD is associated with a reduction in cardiac output[29] which can be explained by increased intraabdominal pressure and can result in decreased right atrial pressure filling, both of which can contribute to a rise in ICP.

HEMATOLOGIC SYSTEM

Anemia

Anemia is very common in critically ill patients and can have detrimental effects on the brain. Oxygen delivery (DO_2) to the brain is directly proportional to cerebral blood flow (CBF) and arterial oxygen content (CaO_2) which depends on hemoglobin (Hb) and arterial oxygen saturation (SaO_2): $DO_2 = CBF \times (Hb \times SaO_2 \times 1.39)$. Thus, anemia results in a decrease in brain oxygenation that eventually stimulates compensatory mechanisms. These include increased cardiac output (CO) by sympathetic activation and decreased systemic vascular resistance, increased oxygen extraction, and cerebral vasodilation triggered by anemia-induced nitric oxide production in the brain.[30] In a rodent study with induced normovolemic anemia, a decline in the Hb level was proportional to an increase in CBF initially mainly due to a reduction in blood viscosity; however, it was observed that at Hb levels below 9 g/dL CBF substantially rose beyond the expected level that could be attributed only to a blood viscosity effect. This phenomenon can be explained by decreased blood viscosity followed by cerebral vasodilation (Figure 23.1).[31] In a normal brain with intact cerebrovascular reserve, maximal vasodilation is reached at a Hb level below 5 to 6 g/dL, beyond which no further vasodi-

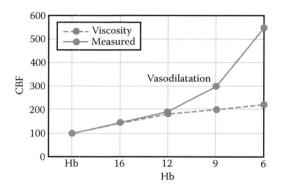

Figure 23.1 The dashed line demonstrates the effect of blood viscosity alone on CBF. At Hb levels below 9–10 g/dL, active cerebral vasodilation (solid line) occurs in order to increase CBF. (Reproduced from Kofke WA, Protection of the central nervous system in surgical patients. *Anesthesiology*, 2nd ed., McGraw-Hill, 2012.)

lation can be achieved and results in inadequate oxygen delivery to the brain and consequently an increase in brain oxygen extraction to maintain adequate brain oxygenation (Figure 23.2). Conversely, in an injured brain with impaired vascular reserve, an inability to develop compensatory vasodilation with anemia will lead to inadequate oxygen supply, reflecting the limited cerebrovascular reserve in TBI patients with edema or significant vascular injury (Figure 23.3).[32] These concepts are described in Figures 23.1 through 23.3 and physiologically have been reported in NICU patients via microdialysis[33] and PbO_2[34] monitoring. Moreover, in subarachnoid (SAH) patients who have impaired vascular reserve and are undergoing PET studies, Diringer et al. measured cerebral oxygen delivery (CBF × arterial O_2 content) [DO_2] in response to transfusion in anemic patients.[35–37] Following transfusion, CBF did not change but DO_2 rose and reduced the number of regions with low DO_2 by 47%.

Etiologies of anemia in brain injury patients are usually multifactorial. These include blood loss (eg, multiple trauma, gastrointestinal bleeding, surgery, and multiple phlebotomies), hemodilution caused by aggressive fluid resuscitation, decreased red blood cell (RBC) production, and increased RBC destruction.

The effects of anemia on the outcome of brain injury patients have been documented in several studies. Anemia, defined by a Hb level <9 g/dL, was

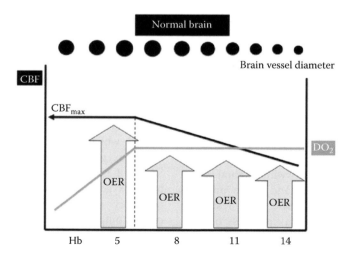

Figure 23.2 In the normal brain, at Hb levels below 6 g/dL, cerebral blood vessels cannot further vasodilate (ie, maximal CBF achieved) and the oxygen extraction ratio (OER) rises to compensate a fall of oxygen delivery to the brain. (Reproduced from Lelubre C et al. *Crit Care*. 2016;20(1):152. With permission.)

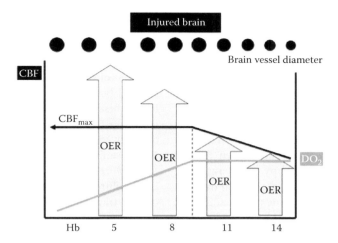

Figure 23.3 A lower CBF is demonstrated in the injured brain compared with the normal brain at corresponding Hb levels. Maximal vasodilation is obtained at a Hb level of 9 g/dL; Hb levels below this point contribute to a reduction in cerebral oxygen delivery and increased OER. (Reproduced from Lelubre C et al. *Crit Care.* 2016;20(1):152. With permission.)

associated with a poor outcome and increased mortality in TBI patients.[38,39] A retrospective study in severe TBI patients identified that a brain tissue oxygen tension (PbtO$_2$) of less than 20 mmHg, a critical value predicting cerebral ischemia, occurred when the Hb level fell below 9 g/dL (congruent with preclinical studies) with low PbtO$_2$, but not anemia alone, was a predictor of unfavorable neurological outcomes regardless of injury severity.[40]

The incidence of red blood cell transfusion (RBCT) in TBI patients is as high as 36%.[41] Several risks related to RBCT include infections, coagulopathy, hyperkalemia, hypocalcemia, hypothermia, 2,3-diphosphoglycerate deficiency, immunosuppression, and immune-mediated reactions such as hemolytic transfusion reaction and transfusion-related acute lung injury (TRALI). Predisposing factors to TRALI include female donor[42] especially with multiparity,[43] which is thought to be due to the greater amount of human leukocyte antigen (HLA) antibodies, critical illness,[43] and stored PRBC.[44]

To date, there has been no consensus of transfusion strategies in TBI patients and no sufficient data supporting the benefits of RBCT in these patients. Conversely, many studies have identified RBCT as an independent risk factor of poor long-term functional outcome[45] and increased hospital mortality.[38] A study in brain injury patients with anemia demonstrated that brain tissue oxygen tension (PbtO$_2$) was improved in 57% of the

patients after receiving RBCT, whereas 43% of those experienced unchanged or decreased PbtO$_2$; moreover, no association between RBCT and lactate pyruvate ratio (LPR) was found.[46] Due to the uncertainty of its benefits and a concern about its potential complications, RBCT in brain injury patients should be restricted and given only if necessary, as suggested by clinical condition, knowledge of impaired vascular reserve, or individualized information from neuromonitors (eg, PbO$_2$, microdialysis, oxygen extraction fraction).

The optimal Hb threshold triggering RBCT in unmonitored brain injury patients is still inconclusive. Given that maximal vasodilation occurs at a Hb level of 9 mg/dL in an injured brain, it may be reasonable to use this threshold to determine RBCT in TBI patients with cerebrovascular reserve impairment. Unfortunately, there is seldom good physiologic information in a given patient regarding cerebrovascular reserve status.

These issues were underscored in a subgroup analysis of the TRICC trial on 67 TBI patients comparing restrictive RBCT (RBCT if Hb <7 g/dL) to liberal RBCT (RBCT if Hb <10 g/dL). There was no difference in 30-day mortality, length of stay in the ICU and hospital, and the presence and change of multiple organ dysfunctions.[47] From this and knowledge regarding the human physiology of anemia and RBCT, we suggest that the use of restrictive RBCT (Hb levels <7 g/dL) may reasonably be accepted in patients admitted to the neuro-intensive care unit, who are awake and conscious. It is less clear in poor grade patients who likely have an (unknown) element of impaired cerebrovascular reserve. A reasonable approach in such patients would be to give consideration to systemic triggers [eg, mixed venous oxygen saturation (SvO$_2$), superior vena cava oxygen saturation (ScvO$_2$), or lactate level] or cerebral triggers [eg, venous saturation in jugular vein (SjvO$_2$), brain tissue oxygen tension (PbtO$_2$), microdialysis lactate/pyruvate ratio, or measures of oxygen extraction fraction] in order to determine the need of RBCT. The potential triggers of RBCT include ScvO$_2$ <60%, high lactate level, SjvO$_2$ <55%, and PbtO$_2$ <15 mmHg[32] or LPR >25; however, the published literature validating the use of these triggers for determining RBCT in TBI patients is limited.

Coagulopathy

TBI is associated with coagulation abnormalities including hypercoagulable and hypocoagulable states. The exact mechanisms of coagulopathy after brain injury are not well understood.[48–50] The widely accepted postulates of TBI-associated coagulopathy include the release of tissue factor, hyperfibrinolysis, decreased platelet count and/or function, and the activation of protein C pathway.[48] A meta-analysis study reported that 32.7% of TBI patients experienced coagulopathy that was associated with increased mortality and poor outcome.[49] Risk factors for developing TBI-associated coagulopathy include Abbreviated Injury Scale (AIS) head ≥5, GCS ≤8 at scene, systolic blood pressure (SBP) ≤90 mmHg at scene or ER, prehospital intravenous fluid ≥2000 mL, and age ≥75 years.[50]

Secondary brain injury can be attributable to both hypo and hypercoagulation abnormalities. The hypocoagulable state contributes to new hemorrhage or the progression of initial brain lesions, whereas the hypercoagulable state leads to microthrombi which can block small blood vessels and result in cerebral ischemia. In a subgroup analysis of blunt severe TBI patients, 80% of those who have at least one abnormal parameter (INR, PTT, platelet count) on admission experienced progression of intracranial hemorrhage (ICH) compared with 36% of patients with normal coagulation, and all patients with prolonged PTT had

ICH progression.[51] Oertel et al. performed a cohort study of 142 TBI patients and reported a rate of hemorrhagic progression of 42.3%. The risk factors associated with the progression of hemorrhage include older age, male sex, the shorter time interval between injury and the first CT scan, the longer first PTT, and SBP ≤90 mmHg.[52] However, coagulopathy in TBI patients may also be attributed to other etiologies that are frequently found in the NICU setting such as dilutional coagulopathy due to fluid resuscitation, anticoagulant medications, liver failure, and DIC caused by sepsis or extracranial trauma, all of which need to be differentiated from TBI-associated coagulopathy.

Conventional blood tests such as PT, PTT, and platelets are generally obtained to diagnose coagulopathy. Recently, thromboelastography (TEG) has been introduced in many clinical situations such as the perioperative periods and after trauma resuscitation. It provides a more comprehensive coagulation evaluation and help tailors specific therapies to individual patients. However, studies of TEG in TBI patients are scanty. A prospective observational study of 169 traumatic intracranial hemorrhage patients demonstrated that TEG values acquired after admission was not related to progression of traumatic intracranial hemorrhage, the need for surgery, and mortality rate.[53] Nonetheless, further studies are still needed to validate its use in this context.

There is no standard guideline of TBI-associated coagulopathy management. Generally, coagulopathy can be successfully treated by FFP and/or vitamin K, but their use may be hindered if acute reversal effect is needed or volume overload is a concern. Additionally, a prophylaxis role of FFP to prevent coagulopathy in head injury patients has not been established.[54] Recombinant factor VIIa (rFVIIa) has been widely demonstrated to be a safe adjunctive treatment modality to reverse severe coagulopathy in trauma and TBI coagulopathy,[55] with quick correction of coagulopathy, decreased time to intervention, and reduced progression of hemorrhagic lesions in high-risk patients[48]; however, the risk of thromboembolic events may increase after rFVIIa administration. Notably, a low dose of rFVIIa of 20 μg/kg was shown to effectively treat coagulopathy without an increased risk of thromboembolic events.[56] Prothrombin complex concentration (PCC) comprising vitamin-K clotting factors has also been demonstrated to successfully treat TBI-associated coagulopathy regardless of preinjury warfarin use. Joseph et al. compared PCC to rFVIIa in TBI patients with coagulopathy showing that patients treated with PCC had lower PRBC need, FFP need, mortality, and mean cost of treatment, but no difference in craniotomy rate and mean time to intervention.[57]

Conversely, the hypercoagulable state can lead to thromboembolic events (eg, cerebral venous thrombosis) resulting in cerebral ischemia and thereby exacerbating post-TBI secondary brain injury. Antiplatelet agents and/or anticoagulation agents such as heparin and vitamin K antagonists are the mainstay treatment of thromboembolic events. However, potential major bleeding, especially cerebral bleeding, the possibility of heparin-induced thrombocytopenia, and the lack of clinical human studies justifying their efficacy and safety in TBI patients impede their use. Recently, novel oral anticoagulants (NOACs), such as dabigatran, rivaroxaban, and apixaban, have emerged as alternatives for the prevention of venous thromboembolism with some advantages over traditional anticoagulants including easy administration due to fixed dose and less drug interaction. Mendonca et al. reported on 15 patients with cerebral vein thrombosis who were treated with dabigatran, an oral direct thrombin inhibitor. 87% had an excellent outcome and 80% had full or partial recanalization.[58] Notably, the risk of major bleeding may be lower with NOACs.[59,60] Bacchus et al. demonstrated the lower incidence of major bleeding or clinically relevant non-major bleeding with dabigatran compared with warfarin.[60] Although NOACs appear to be a promising treatment of thromboembolic diseases, there is little in the literature about their use.

GASTROINTESTINAL CARE

Stress ulcer-related GI bleeding

Critically ill patients are at risk of stress-related gastrointestinal ulcers and subsequent GI hemorrhage, which are associated with a prolonged ICU stay and increased mortality. Only 1% to 6% of patients with a GI ulcer who are admitted to the ICU develop bleeding.[61] The pathophysiology of a GI stress ulcer is multifactorial and it is not fully understood. A loss of the balance between protec-tive and destructive factors is thought to play an important role. A gastric ulcer related to brain injury is referred to as a Cushing ulcer which is initially identified with and attributable to elevated intracranial pressure. Risk factors for stress-ulcer GI bleeding include respiratory failure requiring mechanical ventilation for >48 h, coagulopathy (platelet count <50,000, INR >1.5, or PTT more than two times the control value), hepatic injury, acute kidney injury, maximum creatinine level, acute respiratory failure, sepsis, hypotension, severe head or spinal cord injury, anticoagulation, history of gastrointestinal bleeding, low intragastric pH, thermal injury involving more than 35% of the body surface area, major surgery longer than 4 hours, high dose steroid (>250 mg/day) use, age >50 years, and male sex.[61–64] In TBI patients, factors predisposing a patient to stress ulcer (ie, acid, pepsin, and cortisol) have been found to increase[63,64] and the incidence of GI bleeding in these patients strongly correlates with the severity of a head injury.[65]

Early enteral feeding is an effective non-pharmacological approach for ulcer prophylaxis. Pharmacological approaches include histamine-2 receptor antagonists (H_2A), proton pump inhibitors (PPIs), antacids, and sucralfate. PPIs suppress gastric production by irreversibly binding to H^+/K^+ ATPase on parietal cells in the stomach. They are considered to be safe and effective medications, and are available in oral and intravenous formulations. However, the potential adverse effects of PPIs include a disturbance in vitamin and mineral absorption (vitamin B12, calcium, magnesium, and iron) and an increased risk of infections (pneumonia, Clostridium difficile infection, bacterial gastroenteritis), both of which are the consequences of acid suppression. Moreover, drug interactions among PPIs, diazepam, phenytoin, warfarin, and clopidogrel have been reported.[66] The routine use of H_2A is not recommended in the NICU setting since H_2A may cause encephalopathy, drug interactions with many agents especially anticonvulsants, and an increased risk of pneumonia.[67] A meta-analysis of 1720 critically ill patients demonstrated that PPIs were more effective than H_2A in preventing upper GI bleeding with no differences in the risk of nosocomial pneumonia, ICU mortality, or ICU length of stay.[68] Antacids increase gastric pH with potential side effects including diarrhea, constipation, metabolic alkalosis, and electrolyte imbalances. Sucralfate binds to an ulcer and acts as a physical barrier to prevent acid penetration. It can reduce the bioavailability of many drugs such as phenytoin, digoxin, ciprofloxacin, norfloxacin, theophylline, tetracycline, and amitriptyline, and can lead to lower drug plasma concentration; however, this can be prevented by separating administration for at least 2 hours.[69] A large RCT of 1200 critically ill patients requiring mechanical ventilation demonstrated a lower rate of GI bleeding in patients receiving intravenous ranitidine compared with those receiving sucralfate.[70]

Altered gastric emptying

Altered gastric emptying is a common problem following head injury or spinal cord injury and can be presented as a delayed, rapid, or biphasic response. Delayed gastric emptying can contribute to increased gastric residual volume and feeding intolerance associated with increases in ICU length of stay, ICU mortality, and the risk of infections.[71] A study in severe TBI patients showed that during the first week after the injury a delay in gastric emptying was very common, while a biphasic response (fast gastric emptying in early stage then slow in later stage) was most frequently found during the second week. By the third week, the majority of the patients had improved gastric emptying.[72]

Managing delayed gastric emptying consists of dietary modification, nutritional and hydration support, and medications. A low-fat diet with small frequent meals is recommended. Prokinetic drugs help promote GI motility and are widely used to improve enteral feeding in critically ill patients. Cisapride stimulates gut motility by activating 5-HT$_4$ receptors, but it has been withdrawn from many countries because of cardiac toxicity. Metoclopramide is the only medication approved by the FDA and improves gut motility by inhibiting dopamine D2 receptor and presynaptic muscarinic receptors. The possible best dosage is 10 mg intravenously three times a day.[73] However, its use is hindered by the potential CNS-related adverse effects such as extrapyramidal side effects and increasing frequency and severity of seizures. Therefore, metoclopramide should be avoided in patients with seizure disorders. Erythromycin is a macrolide antibiotic that stimulates motilin receptors on enteric nerves and intestinal smooth muscle which leads to increased gastric emptying. The prolonged use of erythromycin causes tachyphylaxis which can be managed by discontinu-

ation for 2 weeks and then resuming. A retrospective study in TBI patients demonstrated that the efficacy of metoclopramide 10 mg, metoclopramide 20 mg, and metoclopramide 10 mg plus erythromycin 250 mg intravenously every 6 hours to treat gastric feeding intolerance were 55%, 62%, and 79%, respectively; thus, the authors suggested combination therapy (metoclopramide and erythromycin) as first line treatment of gastric feeding intolerance in head injury patients.[74] Antiemetic medications can be used if patients experience nausea and vomiting.

Diarrhea

Diarrhea is defined as ≥3 loose stools per day. The etiologies are categorized into infectious and noninfectious due to the different treatment approaches required. Infectious diarrhea related to the ICU is mainly caused by *Clostridium difficile*. Tripathy et al.[75] reported that the prevalence of *C. difficile* diarrhea in the NICU was 0.4% (9 of 2212 patients) and important risk factors include age >65 years and antibiotics, with cephalosporin being the most frequently prescribed. The manifestations of *C. difficile* diarrhea are various, ranging from mild diarrhea to more serious conditions such as pseudomembranous colitis and fatal intestinal perforation. The recommended therapies are shown in Table 23.4.

Antibiotic use, such as erythromycin, clarithromycin, clavulanic acid, and ceftriaxone, can cause antibiotic-associated diarrhea (AAD), a noninfectious diarrhea, by reducing the concentration of normal flora in the intestine, changing the osmolarity, or irritating the bowel. Enteral feeding-associated diar-

Table 23.4 Therapeutic approaches to *C. difficile* infection[76]

Enteric prevention and control
Start empiric *C. difficile* therapy in patients with strong pre-test suspicion
Discontinue any inciting antibiotics
Avoid anti-peristaltic agents
Mild-moderate infection: Metronidazole 500 mg orally three times a day x 10 days; or standard dose vancomycin if allergic/intolerant to metronidazole or for pregnant woman
Severe infection: Vancomycin 125 mg orally four times a day x 10 days

Source: Adapted from Surawicz CM et al. *Am J Gastroenterol.* 2013;108(4):478-498.

Table 23.5 Therapeutic approaches to non-infectious diarrhea

Discontinue drugs that can cause diarrhea (stool softeners, erythromycin, clarithromycin, amoxicillin/clavulanic acid, ceftriaxone)

Consider alternative antibiotics if coverage still required

Choose low osmolarity enteral formula

Consider a reduced infusion rate; do not stop enteral feeding

Add fiber in enteral formula[82]; highly water-soluble and low viscosity fiber are preferred

Avoid excessive use of opioid including loperamide

rhea is an important problem in ICU patients and is frequently found when high osmolarity formulas or high infusion rates are given, which can lead to excessive intraluminal volume and consequent diarrhea. Gramlich et al. conducted a systematic review in critically ill patients showing no increased risk of diarrhea in patients receiving enteral feeding compared with those receiving parenteral feeding.[77] Moreover, enteral feeding can reduce the incidence of diarrhea by preserving gastrointestinal mucosal structure and function.[78] Managing noninfectious diarrhea is depicted in Table 23.5. Recently, a meta-analysis demonstrated that probiotics reduced the incidence of *C. difficile*–associated diarrhea[79] and are considered as a safe and effective option to preventing *C. difficile*–associated diarrhea[80] in non-immunosuppressed patients. A pilot study of 46 severe TBI patients showed that patients receiving a probiotic had a lower incidence of nosocomial infections and shorter ICU stays compared with those without probiotic.[81] Despite the beneficial effects of probiotics identified in TBI patients, the data in these patients has been scarce and the effects of probiotics are primarily dependent on dose, strain and species-specific, and specific combination of probiotics.

Constipation

Constipation is defined as no bowel movement for 3 consecutive days and has an incidence in the ICU as high as 83%.[83] The risk factors for constipation in critically ill patients include immobility, the use of opioids or anticholinergic drugs, and a high severity of disease.[84] Constipation was associated with pro-

longed weaning from mechanical ventilator, delayed enteral feeding,[83] and delirium.[85] Most recently, a systemic review and meta-analysis of 534 ICU patients demonstrated that the use of a bowel protocol was associated with a trend toward a reduction in constipation, but no reduction in enteral feeding intolerance and duration of mechanical ventilation.[86] To date, there has been no widely accepted guideline or pharmacologic regimen for the treatment or prophylaxis of constipation in the ICU. Patanwala et al.[84] demonstrated the effectiveness of stimulants (senna and bisacodyl) or osmotic laxatives (lactulose) in producing a bowel movement in ICU patients. Stool softeners, bulk laxatives, and fiber-based laxatives may not be appropriate options for any patients experiencing fluid overload since these agents require adequate fluid intake.

SUMMARY

Traumatic brain injury is a major cause of disability and death in the United States. The goals of TBI management include maintaining intracranial homeostasis and preventing secondary brain insults. Systemic complications are common after TBI and are independent contributors to unfavorable outcomes; moreover, they potentially cause secondary brain injury, thereby escalating morbidity and mortality. Systemic care focusing on prevention, early detection, and appropriate treatment of systemic complications is an important element of TBI treatment in neurocritical care, which can improve TBI outcome and reduce mortality.

REFERENCES

1. Parr SK, Siew ED. Delayed consequences of acute kidney injury. *Adv Chronic Kidney Dis.* 2016;23(3):186-194.
2. Bellomo R, Ronco C, Kellum JA, Mehta RL, Palevsky P. Acute renal failure - definition, outcome measures, animal models, fluid therapy and information technology needs: The second international consensus conference of the acute dialysis quality initiative (ADQI) group. *Crit Care (London, England).* 2004;8(4):R204-R212.
3. Pickering JW, Endre ZH. GFR shot by RIFLE: Errors in staging acute kidney injury. *Lancet (London, England).* 2009;373(9672):1318-1319.

4. Mehta RL, Kellum JA, Shah SV et al. Acute kidney injury network: Report of an initiative to improve outcomes in acute kidney injury. *Crit Care (London, England)*. 2007;11(2):R31.

5. Bagshaw SM, George C, Bellomo R, ANZICS Database Management Committee. A comparison of the RIFLE and AKIN criteria for acute kidney injury in critically ill patients. *Nephrol Dial Transplant*. 2008;23(5):1569-1574.

6. Palevsky PM, Liu KD, Brophy PD et al. KDOQI US commentary on the 2012 KDIGO clinical practice guideline for acute kidney injury. *Am J Kidney Dis*. 2013;61(5):649-672.

7. Ostermann M, Joannidis M. Acute kidney injury 2016: Diagnosis and diagnostic workup. *Crit Care*. 2016;20:299.

8. Li N, Zhao WG, Zhang WF. Acute kidney injury in patients with severe traumatic brain injury: Implementation of the acute kidney injury network stage system. *Neurocritical Care*. 2011;14(3):377-381.

9. Ahmed M, Sriganesh K, Vinay B, Umamaheswara Rao GS. Acute kidney injury in survivors of surgery for severe traumatic brain injury: Incidence, risk factors, and outcome from a tertiary neuroscience center in India. *Br J Neurosurg*. 2015;29(4):544-548.

10. Corral L, Javierre CF, Ventura JL, Marcos P, Herrero JI, Manez R. Impact of non-neurological complications in severe traumatic brain injury outcome. *Crit Care (London, England)*. 2012;16(2):R44.

11. Finlay S, Bray B, Lewington AJ et al. Identification of risk factors associated with acute kidney injury in patients admitted to acute medical units. *Clin Med (London, England)*. 2013;13(3):233-238.

12. Hsu CY, Ordonez JD, Chertow GM, Fan D, McCulloch CE, Go AS. The risk of acute renal failure in patients with chronic kidney disease. *Kidney Int*. 2008;74(1):101-107.

13. Brouns R, De Deyn PP. Neurological complications in renal failure: A review. *Clin Neurol Neurosurg*. 2004;107(1):1-16.

14. Park YJ, Kim SW. Fatal rhabdomyolysis in a patient with head injury. *J Korean Neurosurg Soc*. 2013;53(5):303-304.

15. Lima RS, da Silva Junior GB, Liborio AB, Daher Ede F. Acute kidney injury due to rhabdomyolysis. *Saudi J Kidney Dis Transpl*. 2008;19(5):721-729.

16. Quattrocchi KB, Frank EH, Miller CH et al. Suppression of cellular immune activity following severe head injury. *J Neurotrauma*. 1990;7(2):77-87.

17. Landry DW, Oliver JA. The pathogenesis of vasodilatory shock. *N Engl J Med*. 2001;345(8):588-595.

18. Schrier RW, Wang W. Acute renal failure and sepsis. *N Engl J Med*. 2004;351(2):159-169.

19. Fang L, You H, Chen B et al. Mannitol is an independent risk factor of acute kidney injury after cerebral trauma: A case-control study. *Renal Fail*. 2010;32(6):673-679.

20. Gondim Fde A, Aiyagari V, Shackleford A, Diringer MN. Osmolality not predictive of mannitol-induced acute renal insufficiency. *J Neurosurg*. 2005;103(3):444-447.

21. Kumar AB, Shi Y, Shotwell MS, Richards J, Ehrenfeld JM. Hypernatremia is a significant risk factor for acute kidney injury after subarachnoid hemorrhage: A retrospective analysis. *Neurocrit Care*. 2015;22(2):184-191.

22. Rahman M, Shad F, Smith MC. Acute kidney injury: A guide to diagnosis and management. *Am Fam Physician*. 2012;86(7):631-639.

23. Pattharanitima P, Tasanarong A. Pharmacological strategies to prevent contrast-induced acute kidney injury. *Biomed Res Int*. 2014;2014:236930.

24. Zhao Z, Wang D, Jia Y et al. Analysis of the association of fluid balance and short-term outcome in traumatic brain injury. *J Neurol Sci*. 2016;364:12-18.

25. The Brain Trauma Foundation. The American Association of Neurological Surgeons. The joint section on neurotrauma and critical care. *J Neurotrauma*. 2007;24:S1-106.

26. Davenport A. Practical guidance for dialyzing a hemodialysis patient following acute brain injury. *Hemodial Int*. 2008;12(3):307-312.

27. Rifkin SI, Malek AR, Behrouz R. Use of hypertonic continuous venovenous hemodiafiltration to control intracranial hypertension in an end-stage renal disease patient. *Int J Nephrol*. 2010;2010:391656.

28. Swamy AP, Cestero RV. Mannitol and maintenance hemodialysis. *Artif Organs*. 1979;3(2):116-119.

29. Ivarsen P, Povlsen JV, Jensen JD. Increasing fill volume reduces cardiac performance in

peritoneal dialysis. *Nephrol Dial Transplant.* 2007;22(10):2999-3004.

30. McLaren AT, Mazer CD, Zhang H, Liu E, Mok L, Hare GM. A potential role for inducible nitric oxide synthase in the cerebral response to acute hemodilution. Canadian journal of anaesthesia. *J Cana D'anesthesie.* 2009;56(7):502-509.

31. Borgstrom L, Johannsson H, Siesjo BK. The influence of acute normovolemic anemia on cerebral blood flow and oxygen consumption of anesthetized rats. *Acta Physiol Scand.* 1975;93(4):505-514.

32. Lelubre C, Bouzat P, Crippa IA, Taccone FS. Anemia management after acute brain injury. *Crit Care (London, England).* 2016;20(1):152.

33. Chen HI, Stiefel MF, Oddo M et al. Detection of cerebral compromise with multimodality monitoring in patients with subarachnoid hemorrhage. *Neurosurgery.* 2011;69(1):53-63; discussion.

34. Smith MJ, Stiefel MF, Magge S et al. Packed red blood cell transfusion increases local cerebral oxygenation. *Crit Care Med.* 2005;33(5):1104-1108.

35. Dhar R, Scalfani MT, Zazulia AR, Videen TO, Derdeyn CP, Diringer MN. Comparison of induced hypertension, fluid bolus, and blood transfusion to augment cerebral oxygen delivery after subarachnoid hemorrhage. *J Neurosurg.* 2012;116(3):648-656.

36. Dhar R, Zazulia AR, Videen T, Diringer M. Red blood cell transfusion increases cerebral oxygen delivery after subarachnoid hemorrhage. *Neurology.* 2009;72(11):A64-A.

37. Dhar R, Zazulia AR, Videen TO, Zipfel GJ, Derdeyn CP, Diringer MN. Red blood cell transfusion increases cerebral oxygen delivery in anemic patients with subarachnoid hemorrhage. *Stroke.* 2009;40(9):3039-3044.

38. Salim A, Hadjizacharia P, DuBose J et al. Role of anemia in traumatic brain injury. *J Am Coll Surgeons.* 2008;207(3):398-406.

39. Van Beek JG, Mushkudiani NA, Steyerberg EW et al. Prognostic value of admission laboratory parameters in traumatic brain injury: Results from the IMPACT study. *J Neurotrauma.* 2007;24(2):315-328.

40. Oddo M, Levine JM, Kumar M et al. Anemia and brain oxygen after severe traumatic brain injury. *Intensive Care Med.* 2012;38(9):1497-1504.

41. Boutin A, Chasse M, Shemilt M et al. Red blood cell transfusion in patients with traumatic brain injury: A systematic review and meta-analysis. *Transfus Med Rev.* 2016;30(1):15-24.

42. Toy P, Gajic O, Bacchetti P et al. Transfusion-related acute lung injury: Incidence and risk factors. *Blood.* 2012;119(7):1757-1767.

43. Babaev A, Pozzi F, Hare G, Zhang H. Storage of red blood cells and transfusion-related acute lung injury. *J Anesth Crit Care.* 2014;1(1):00002.

44. Tung JP, Fraser JF, Nataatmadja M et al. Age of blood and recipient factors determine the severity of transfusion-related acute lung injury (TRALI). *Crit Care (London, England).* 2012;16(1):R19.

45. Warner MA, O'Keeffe T, Bhavsar P et al. Transfusions and long-term functional outcomes in traumatic brain injury. *J Neurosurg.* 2010;113(3):539-546.

46. Zygun DA, Nortje J, Hutchinson PJ, Timofeev I, Menon DK, Gupta AK. The effect of red blood cell transfusion on cerebral oxygenation and metabolism after severe traumatic brain injury. *Crit Care Med.* 2009;37(3):1074-1078.

47. McIntyre LA, Fergusson DA, Hutchison JS et al. Effect of a liberal versus restrictive transfusion strategy on mortality in patients with moderate to severe head injury. *Neurocrit Care.* 2006;5(1):4-9.

48. Laroche M, Kutcher ME, Huang MC, Cohen MJ, Manley GT. Coagulopathy after traumatic brain injury. *Neurosurgery.* 2012;70(6):1334-1345.

49. Harhangi BS, Kompanje EJ, Leebeek FW, Maas AI. Coagulation disorders after traumatic brain injury. *Acta Neurochir.* 2008;150(2):165-175; discussion 75.

50. Wafaisade A, Lefering R, Tjardes T et al. Acute coagulopathy in isolated blunt traumatic brain injury. *Neurocrit Care.* 2010;12(2):211-219.

51. Allard CB, Scarpelini S, Rhind SG et al. Abnormal coagulation tests are associated with progression of traumatic intracranial hemorrhage. *J Trauma.* 2009;67(5):959-967.

52. Oertel M, Kelly DF, McArthur D et al. Progressive hemorrhage after head trauma:

Predictors and consequences of the evolving injury. *J Neurosurg.* 2002;96(1):109-116.

53. Rao AJ, Laurie A, Hilliard C et al. The utility of thromboelastography for predicting the risk of progression of intracranial hemorrhage in traumatic brain injury patients. *Neurosurgery.* 2016;63(Suppl 1):173-174.

54. Winter JP, Plummer D, Bottini A, Rockswold GR, Ray D. Early fresh frozen plasma prophylaxis of abnormal coagulation parameters in the severely head-injured patient is not effective. *Ann Emerg Med.* 1989;18(5):553-555.

55. Dutton RP, McCunn M, Hyder M et al. Factor VIIa for correction of traumatic coagulopathy. *J Trauma.* 2004;57(4):709-718; discussion 18-9.

56. Yuan Q, Wu X, Du ZY et al. Low-dose recombinant factor VIIa for reversing coagulopathy in patients with isolated traumatic brain injury. *J Crit Care.* 2015;30(1):116-120.

57. Joseph B, Hadjizacharia P, Aziz H et al. Prothrombin complex concentrate: An effective therapy in reversing the coagulopathy of traumatic brain injury. *J Trauma Acute Care Surg.* 2013;74(1):248-253.

58. Mendonca MD, Barbosa R, Cruz-e-Silva V, Calado S, Viana-Baptista M. Oral direct thrombin inhibitor as an alternative in the management of cerebral venous thrombosis: A series of 15 patients. *Int J Stroke.* 2015;10 (7):1115-1118.

59. Finazzi G, Ageno W. Direct oral anticoagulants in rare venous thrombosis. *Intern Emerg Med.* 2016;11(2):167-170.

60. Bacchus F, Schulman S. Clinical experience with the new oral anticoagulants for treatment of venous thromboembolism. *Arterioscler Thromb Vasc Biol.* 2015;35(3):513-519.

61. Bardou M, Quenot JP, Barkun A. Stress-related mucosal disease in the critically ill patient. *Nat Rev Gastroenterol Hepatol.* 2015;12(2):98-107.

62. Quenot JP, Thiery N, Barbar S. When should stress ulcer prophylaxis be used in the ICU? *Curr Opin Crit Care.* 2009;15(2):139-143.

63. Idjadi F, Robbins R, Stahl WM, Essiet G. Prospective study of gastric secretion in stressed patients with intracranial injury. *J Trauma.* 1971;11(8):681-688.

64. Li ZM, Wang LX, Jiang LC, Zhu JX, Geng FY, Qiang F. Relationship between plasma cor-

tisol levels and stress ulcer following acute and severe head injury. *Med Princ Pract.* 2010;19(1):17-21.

65. Kamada T, Fusamoto H, Kawano S, Noguchi M, Hiramatsu K. Gastrointestinal bleeding following head injury: A clinical study of 433 cases. *J Trauma.* 1977;17(1):44-47.

66. Yang YX, Metz DC. Safety of proton pump inhibitor exposure. *Gastroenterology.* 2010; 139(4):1115-1127.

67. Schirmer CM, Kornbluth J, Heilman CB, Bhardwaj A. Gastrointestinal prophylaxis in neurocritical care. *Neurocrit Care.* 2012;16 (1):184-193.

68. Alhazzani W, Alenezi F, Jaeschke RZ, Moayyedi P, Cook DJ. Proton pump inhibitors versus histamine 2 receptor antagonists for stress ulcer prophylaxis in critically ill patients: A systematic review and meta-analysis. *Crit Care Med.* 2013;41(3):693-705.

69. McCarthy DM. Sucralfate. *N Engl J Med.* 1991;325(14):1017-1025.

70. Cook D, Guyatt G, Marshall J et al. A comparison of sucralfate and ranitidine for the prevention of upper gastrointestinal bleeding in patients requiring mechanical ventilation. Canadian critical care trials group. *N Engl J Med.* 1998;338(12):791-797.

71. Blaser AR, Starkopf J, KirsimÄGi Ü, Deane AM. Definition, prevalence, and outcome of feeding intolerance in intensive care: A systematic review and meta-analysis. *Acta Anaesthesiol Scand.* 2014;58(8):914-922.

72. Ott L, Young B, Phillips R et al. Altered gastric emptying in the head-injured patient: Relationship to feeding intolerance. *J Neurosurg.* 1991;74(5):738-742.

73. Doherty WL, Winter B. Prokinetic agents in critical care. *Crit Care (London, England).* 2003;7(3):206-208.

74. Dickerson RN, Mitchell JN, Morgan LM et al. Disparate response to metoclopramide therapy for gastric feeding intolerance in trauma patients with and without traumatic brain injury. *JPEN J Parenter Enteral Nutr.* 2009;33(6):646-655.

75. Tripathy S, Nair P, Rothburn M. *Clostridium difficile* associated disease in a neurointensive care unit. *Front Neurol.* 2013;4:82.

76. Surawicz CM, Brandt LJ, Binion DG et al. Guidelines for diagnosis, treatment, and

prevention of *Clostridium difficile* infections. 2013;108(4):478-498; quiz 99.

77. Gramlich L, Kichian K, Pinilla J, Rodych NJ, Dhaliwal R, Heyland DK. Does enteral nutrition compared to parenteral nutrition result in better outcomes in critically ill adult patients? A systematic review of the literature. *Nutrition (Burbank, Los Angeles County, CA)*. 2004;20(10):843-848.

78. Wiesen P, Van Gossum A, Preiser JC. Diarrhoea in the critically ill. *Curr Opin Crit Care*. 2006;12(2):149-154.

79. Johnston BC, Ma SS, Goldenberg JZ et al. Probiotics for the prevention of *Clostridium difficile*–associated diarrhea: A systematic review and meta-analysis. *Ann Intern Med*. 2012;157(12):878-888.

80. Goldenberg JZ, Ma SS, Saxton JD et al. Probiotics for the prevention of *Clostridium difficile*–associated diarrhea in adults and children. *Cochrane Database Syst Rev*. 2013 (5):Cd006095.

81. Tan M, Zhu JC, Du J, Zhang LM, Yin HH. Effects of probiotics on serum levels of Th1/Th2 cytokine and clinical outcomes in severe traumatic brain-injured patients: A prospective randomized pilot study. *Crit Care (London, England)*. 2011;15(6):R290.

82. Elia M, Engfer MB, Green CJ, Silk DB. Systematic review and meta-analysis: The clinical and physiological effects of fibre-containing enteral formulae. *Aliment Pharmacol Ther*. 2008;27(2):120-145.

83. Mostafa SM, Bhandari S, Ritchie G, Gratton N, Wenstone R. Constipation and its implications in the critically ill patient. *Br J Anaesth*. 2003;91(6):815-819.

84. Patanwala AE, Abarca J, Huckleberry Y, Erstad BL. Pharmacologic management of constipation in the critically ill patient. *Pharmacotherapy*. 2006;26(7):896-902.

85. Smonig R, Wallenhorst T, Bouju P et al. Constipation is independently associated with delirium in critically ill ventilated patients. *Intensive Care Med*. 2016;42 (1):126-127.

86. Oczkowski SJ, Duan EH, Groen A, Warren D, Cook DJ. The use of bowel protocols in critically ill adult patients: A systematic review and meta-analysis. *Crit Care Med*. 2017.

24

Post-traumatic cognitive dysfunction

ASHIMA NEHRA, MANJU MOHANTY, AND SHIVANI SHARMA

INTRODUCTION

While traumatic brain injury (TBI) can be caused by either open or closed head injuries, most result from the latter. Brain injuries occur because of acceleration-deceleration forces, blunt trauma, or both. TBIs occur on a broad continuum of severity, from very mild transient injuries to catastrophic injuries resulting in death or severe disability.[1]

TBI is often associated with cognitive impairments that may be transient, long lasting, or permanent. Based on the time of onset and resolution, they can be classified into four phases. The initial phase is the period of loss of consciousness or coma, which occurs soon after injury. The second phase is characterized by a mixture of both cognitive and behavioral abnormalities. Agitation, confusion, disorientation, alteration in psychomotor activity, inability to recall events, sequence time, and inability to learn new information are all common during this period. The third phase is known as the period of spontaneous recovery of cognitive functions which lasts from about 6–12 months and is followed by the plateauing of recovery over a 12–24 month period that is subsequent to the injury. The fourth phase is characterized by permanent cognitive sequela that includes impairment of attention, arousal, concentration, memory, language, and executive function.[2,3] Cognitive outcome depends on a number of factors, such as the degree of diffuse axonal injury, the duration of loss of consciousness (LOC) and post-traumatic amnesia (PTA), the clinical evidence of brain stem dysfunction at the time of injury, and the presence and size of focal hemispheric injury (Figure 24.1).[4]

Common cognitive impairments include:

- **Attention:** Attention and memory are relatively basic cognitive functions that provide a base for other complex cognitive functions. Even mild disruptions in these may cause or exacerbate additional deficits in executive functions, communication, or other higher mental functions. Frequently reported deficits include mental slowing, trouble following conversation, difficulty in focusing attention, sustaining attention for long periods of time, and attending simultaneously to more than one thing. According to Dockree et al. (2004), control of behavior is required to maintain a goal-directed focus without support from the environment. This control is modulated by the fronto-parietal lobe, and after a head injury, this ability to attend to things of the environment is compromised and leads to increased lapses of attention.[5–7]
- **Memory:** Memory deficits are the most prevalent complaint following TBI that may be either temporary or permanent. The degree of memory impairment is associated with the length of PTA. The circumscribed damage to structure in diencephalon or medial temporal lobe structure may cause selective impairment of memory. Both

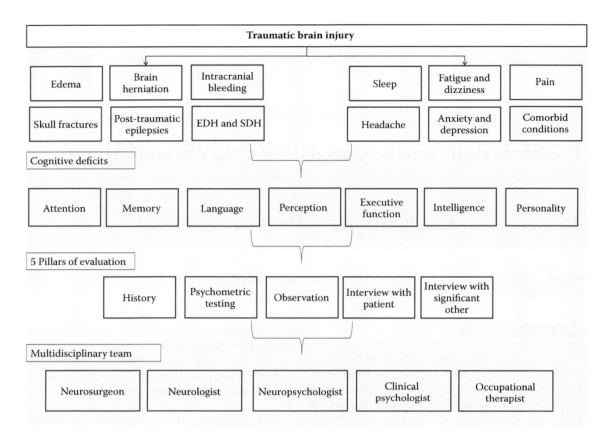

Figure 24.1 An overview of the diverse factors of TBI that can affect cognitive functioning and can be rehabilitated by a multidisciplinary team after evaluation.

recent and remote memory may be impaired but immediate memory may be spared. Most often, the newly acquired knowledge is forgotten.[8,9]

- **Language:** Difficulties in word findings and anomia are present after head injury. Expressive aphasias are more common compared with receptive aphasias. Recovery from aphasia and any related disorder is found to be greater than recovery from other cognitive deficits. According to a study conducted by Levin et al. (1990), patients were characterized by their impairment of memory and slowed information processing; in contrast, their language and visuospatial ability recovered to within the normal range.[10,11]

- **Perception:** Severe head injury as a part of general cognitive decline may be accompanied by visuo-perceptual disturbances such as figure ground perception and constructional abilities. Visual function affects about 50% of head injury

patients. Focal visuo-constructive disabilities are rare.[12,13]

- **Executive functioning:** TBI damages the frontal lobes in a higher percentage of patients that results in impaired executive functions. It involves self-regulatory functions that organize, direct, and manage other cognitive activities, emotional responses, and behavior. This regulatory function includes the ability to initiate behavior, inhibit competing actions or stimuli, select relevant task goals, plan and organize, solve complex problems, shift problem-solving strategies appropriately when necessary, regulate emotions, monitor and evaluate behavior, and hold information in mind in order to guide cognition and behavior. Executive functions are a critical determinant in functional outcome after TBI and among the most disabling aspects of cognitive impairment following TBI. Executive functioning like planning, organizing, sequencing, and set shifting are all impaired. These are further accompanied by impaired judgment and impulse control.[14–16]

- **Intelligence:** Acute and chronic phases of severe head injury lead to a reduction of both performance and verbal IQ, but this is not the case after mild head injury. Performance IQ may remain lower even after 3 years, but recovery of verbal IQ is faster. Approximately 10% of head injury patients with prolonged coma develop some degree of hydrocephalus, which may be present as progressive intellectual deterioration.[17,18]

- **Personality changes:** Changes in behavior and personality may be associated with TBI including a reduction in motivation and self-esteem, difficulty with empathy, emotional processing, loss of insight, psychosocial difficulties, post-traumatic stress disorder, depression, anxiety, and fatigue.[19–21]

A systematic review by Dikmen et al. (2009) revealed persistent cognitive impairment even six months postinjury.[22] However, individual differences and the severity of trauma determine the time and rate at which recovery proceeds. Stulemeijer et al. (2007) showed that 39% of mTBI patients reported cognitive complaints six months postinjury.[23] Schretlen and Shapiro (2003) believe that improvement postinjury in moderate to severe TBI cases occurs in 6 to 12 months; however, recovery slows down and plateaus by 2 years.[24]

Additionally, while some studies show no residual or significant cognitive impairment in patients three months postinjury, others reveal long-term neuropsychological deficits in attention and working memory even 8 years post mild head injury.[25,26]

Another interesting finding states that the risk of disability one year postinjury increases in patients with diagnosed cognitive impairment three months postinjury. Thus, early cognitive impairment has been found to be an important risk factor for future disability.[25]

The following factors contribute to complications in moderate and severe TBI and are associated with positive neuropsychological outcome.[27–29]

- **Edema:** A swelling of the brain that increases its intracranial pressure (ICP). In moderate to severe cases, uncontrollable ICP may even cause death.

- **Brain herniation:** A pathological process associated with increasing intracranial pressure, which may result in displacement and deformation of the brain.

- **Extradural and subdural hemorrhage:** While extradural hemorrhage is a condition in which blood appears between the dura mater and the skull, in subdural hemorrhage, blood gathers between the inner layer of the dura mater and the arachnoid mater.

- **Intracranial bleeding:** This refers to bleeding that occurs inside the skull/cranium. This is different from the above mentioned EDH and SDH since that includes bleeding around or in the brain itself.

- **Skull fractures:** Two types of skull fractures exist. The first is the benign linear fracture which results in a distinct straight line. The second is a more complicated depressed skull fracture in which the impact usually drives fragments of the skull into the underlying brain. Additionally, the presence of a skull fracture creates the possibility of infection, cerebrospinal fluid, and bleeding. The relation between skull fractures and neurospsychological functioning has been debated. While the skull by itself may absorb much of the kinetic energy, thereby protecting the brain from damage, brain damage may be more likely since the initial forces that fractured the skull may be high.

- **Post-traumatic epilepsies:** Seizures are a major complication after TBI. Research suggests that 10% of severe closed head wounds and 40% of penetrating TBIs lead to post-traumatic epilepsy.

Additionally, these following factors can cause cognitive dysfunction, but are not related to neural trauma:

- **Altered sleep cycle:** Sleep is a primitive behavior and an integral part of life, essential for restoring body and mind. It is required for good mental health, and insufficient sleep has been found to have negative effects on mood, cognitive performance, and motor function.[30] Sleep disturbance is common following TBI, and affects 30%–70% of individuals with insomnia, fatigue, and sleepiness.[31] Interestingly, these stated complaints are more common in mild TBIs than in severe

TBIs and patients with mTBIs are pressured to reintegrate back into their daily life.[32] A growing amount of literature points to decreased memory ability and reaction times of individuals suffering from insomnia.[33]

- **Fatigue and dizziness:** Fatigue can be defined as a condition of decreased physical and mental efficiency. Despite being commonly identified as a sign or a symptom of a disease or side effect of a treatment, fatigue has been considered a subjective experience.[34] Literature reveals mental fatigue induces a decline in executive function such as executive attention, sustained attention, goal-directed attention, alternating attention, divided attention, response inhibition, planning, and novelty processing.[35] A significant proportion of people with brain injury (32%–73%) reportedly experience fatigue. Whereas fatigue resolves within days or weeks for most people with mild injuries, it can persist over many years after moderate to severe injuries and impact participation in numerous activities, including work, study, leisure, and social pursuits.[36]

- **Pain:** Long lasting and persistent pain is a common consequence of TBI. Most studies indicate that about two-thirds of patients experience chronic pain after the injury.[37] Cognitive impairment in patients with chronic pain has been associated with mood changes and emotional distress and with symptoms and clinical features such as increased somatic preoccupation, depression, sleep disturbance, fatigue, and perceived interference with daily activities that are potential sources of chronic stress.[38]

- **Headache:** Headache is one of the most common symptoms after a TBI. One in three patients continue to experience headaches 12 months after an MTBI. An emerging term, "Cogniphobia," (avoidance of mental exertion due to a fear of developing or exacerbating a headache) may help explain why some patients with persistent headaches perform poorly on neuropsychological testing and in daily life long after an MTBI.[39]

- **Other comorbid conditions:** Depression has also been found to be a common consequence of head injury. Further, it has been found that treating depression leads to improvement in neuropsychological performance. This emotion-cognition interface in TBI is still relatively untouched by research.[40] The overall prevalence of significant depression for TBI has been found to be 20% to

50% with 6% to 39% specifically for mild TBI.[41] Further, a close connection between anxiety and TBI has been found with 11% to 70% of the cases reporting high levels of anxiety.[42] Other psychiatric conditions like psychosis (3%–8%), aggression (30%), apathy (10%), and insomnia (30%–70%) have been commonly reported.[43]

Additionally, TBI is also associated with other neurological conditions such as seizures and dementia six months or more postinjury.[44] An equal incidence of frontal and temporal lobe hypoperfusion indicates why patients with TBI have an increased risk of developing Alzheimer's disease.[45] Further, SPECT findings can also aid in the early detection of dementia,[46] validating the importance of extensive assessment and history taking in order to delineate the exact nature of complications and sequelae.

The five pillars of evaluation following are:[47]

- **History:** The importance of taking a complete history cannot be emphasized enough. Details can be solicited from various sources; eg, eyewitnesses are pivotal for details regarding the mechanism of injury, and the duration of loss of consciousness to name a few. Family members and close friends can provide additional details about any history of substance use, past medical and concussion history, and current medications. All these are pivotal from a neuropsychological testing point of view.

- **Psychometric testing:** Understanding the nature, severity, and modality of cognitive complaints can be accomplished through standardized neuropsychological tests that assess the functioning of various cognitive and emotional domains. The neuropsychological profiles that are yielded aid in diagnosis and rehabilitation planning. However, due to the wide ranging neurological, psychological, and psychosocial consequences of TBI, other factors and subtleties that may affect cognitive functioning should not be overlooked.

- **Observation during testing:** Interpreting body language and non-verbal cues can also reveal additional information for further questioning. An important factor to consider here is the possibility of *malingering*, which makes a clinician's job more challenging yet warrants further testing. Malingering is the intentional production of false or grossly exaggerated physical or psychological symptoms for secondary gains. However, it may coexist with genuine psychosocial problems too.[48]

- **Interview with patient** and **Interview with significant other**: Interviews help gather information about aspects that are either not covered in formal psychological testing or are just touched upon. Further, family members may provide a different picture than the one given by the patient, thus reiterating the importance of inputs from knowledgeable informants for diagnosis.

The survivors of TBI often have residual deficits in physical functioning that are visible and well accepted by the patients and family. But the cognitive and psychological deficits often remain unrecognized, hence, they significantly impact the quality of life and return to premorbid level of functioning. Therefore, it is essential to develop efficacious programs for prevention and intervention. In recent years neuropsychological rehabilitation has gained importance as a method that has proven to be efficacious.[49] It not only addresses the issue of cognitive deficits, but also focus on emotional and behavioral consequences. The role of neuronal plasticity is well recognized and allows the neurons in the brain to compensate for injury and adapt to their environment. Zangwill described three processes of rehabilitation; restoration, substitution, and compensation. Restoration refers to the process of restoring lost or impaired functions; substitution refers to replacing impaired functions by alternate functional strategies; while compensation requires using external sources that help to overcome limitations to a certain extent.[50]

Along with neuropsychological rehabilitation, an increasing number of studies have reiterated the importance of a multidisciplinary team (neurologist, neurosurgeon, clinical psychologist, occupational therapist, physiotherapist) to help survivors of TBI obtain functional autonomy.

CONCLUSION

Research suggests that TBI patients report post traumatic seqeulae ranging from headaches and behavioral problems to neuropsychological deficits. This type of postinjury disability is significantly associated with anxiety, depression, and low self-esteem. These impairments act as a hindrance to resuming activities carried out before injury.[51]

REFERENCES

1. Lee GP. The little black book of neuropsychology: A syndrome-based approach. *Arch Clin Neuropsychol.* 2011;26(7):698-699.
2. Levin HS, High WM, Goethe KE et al. The neurobehavioural rating scale: Assessment of the behavioural sequelae of head injury by the clinician. *J Neurol Neurosurg Psychiatry.* 1987;50(2):183-193.
3. Cripe LI. The neuropsychological assessment and management of closed head injury: General guidelines. *Cognitive Rehabilitation.* 1987 Jan:270.
4. Chaudhury S, Pande V, Saini R, Rathee SP. Neuropsychiatric sequelae of head injury. *Indian J Neurotrauma.* 2005;2:13-21.
5. Dockree PM, Kelly SP, Roche RA, Hogan MJ, Reilly RB, Robertson IH. Behavioural and physiological impairments of sustained attention after traumatic brain injury. *Cogn Brain Res.* 2004;20(3):403-414.
6. Chan RC, Hoosain R, Lee TM, Fan YW, Fong D. Are there sub-types of attentional deficits in patients with persisting post-concussive symptoms? A cluster analytical study. *Brain Inj.* 2003;17(2):131-148.
7. Fleminger S, Ponsford J. Long term outcome after traumatic brain injury: More attention needs to be paid to neuropsychiatric functioning. *BMJ: Br Med J.* 2005;331(7530):1419.
8. Menon P, Rao SL. Memory storage and encoding in patients with memory deficits after closed head injury. *NIMHANS J.* 1997;15(1):83-92.
9. Rabinowitz AR, Levin HS. Cognitive sequelae of traumatic brain injury. *Psychiatr Clin North Am.* 2014;37(1):1-11.
10. Levin HS, Gary HE Jr, Eisenberg HM et al. Neurobehavioral outcome 1 year after severe head injury: Experience of the traumatic coma data bank. *J Nneurosurg.* 1990;73(5):699-709.
11. Sharp DJ, Scott G, Leech R. Network dysfunction after traumatic brain injury. *Nat Rev Neurol.* 2014;10(3):156-166.
12. Jones RD, Anderson SW, Cole T, Hathaway-Nepple J. Neuropsychological sequelae of traumatic brain injury. In: Rizzo M, Tranel D, eds. *Head Injury and Postconcussive Syndrome.* New York: Churchill Livingstone; 1996:395-414.

13. Berger S, Kaldenberg J, Selmane R, Carlo S. Effectiveness of interventions to address visual and visual-perceptual impairments to improve occupational performance in adults with traumatic brain injury: A systematic review. *Am J Occup Ther.* 2016;70 (3):7003180010p1-7.

14. Hannay HJ, Howieson DB, Loring DW, Fischer JS, Lezak MD. Neuropathology for neuropsychologists. *Neuropsychol Assessment.* 2004;4(4):157-194.

15. Silver JM, McAllister TW, Yudofsky SC. *Textbook of Traumatic Brain Injury.* American Psychiatric Pub; 2011.

16. Goldberg E, Bougakov D. Neuropsychologic assessment of frontal lobe dysfunction. *Psychiatr Clin North Am.* 2005;28(3):567-580.

17. McCunney RJ, Russo PK. Brain injuries in boxers. *Phys Sportsmed.* 1984;12(5):52-67.

18. Königs M, Engenhorst PJ, Oosterlaan J. Intelligence after traumatic brain injury: Meta-analysis of outcomes and prognosis. *Eur J Neurol.* 2016;23(1):21-29.

19. Fleminger S. Long-term psychiatric disorders after traumatic brain injury. *Eur J Anaesthesiol.* 2008;25(S42):123-130.

20. Saunders JC, McDonald S, Richardson R. Loss of emotional experience after traumatic brain injury: Findings with the startle probe procedure. *Neuropsychology.* 2006;20(2):224.

21. Iverson GL. Misdiagnosis of the persistent postconcussion syndrome in patients with depression. *Arch Clin Neuropsychol.* 2006;21 (4):303-310.

22. Dikmen SS, Corrigan JD, Levin HS, Machamer J, Stiers W, Weisskopf MG. Cognitive outcome following traumatic brain injury. *J Head Trauma Rehabil.* 2009;24 (6):430-438.

23. Stulemeijer M, Vos PE, Bleijenberg G, Van der Werf SP. Cognitive complaints after mild traumatic brain injury: Things are not always what they seem. *J Psychosom Res.* 2007;63 (6):637-645.

24. Schretlen DJ, Shapiro AM. A quantitative review of the effects of traumatic brain injury on cognitive functioning. *Int Rev Psychiatry.* 2003;15(4):341-349.

25. Skandsen T, Finnanger TG, Andersson S, Lydersen S, Brunner JF, Vik A. Cognitive impairment 3 months after moderate and severe traumatic brain injury: A prospective follow-up study. *Arch Phys Med Rehabil.* 2010;91(12):1904-1913.

26. Vanderploeg RD, Curtiss G, Belanger HG. Long-term neuropsychological outcomes following mild traumatic brain injury. *J Int Neuropsychol Soc.* 2005;11(03):228-236.

27. Zillmer EA, Spiers MV, Culbertson W. *Principles of Neuropsychology.* Nelson Education; 2007.

28. Lee YK, Lee CW, Huang MY, Hsu CY, Su YC. Increased risk of ischemic stroke in patients with mild traumatic brain injury: A nationwide cohort study. *Scand J Trauma Resusc Emerg Med.* 2014;22(1):66.

29. Yellinek S, Cohen A, Merkin V, Shelef I, Benifla M. Clinical significance of skull base fracture in patients after traumatic brain injury. *J Clin Neurosci.* 2016;25:111-115.

30. Durmer JS, Dinges DF. Neurocognitive consequences of sleep deprivation. *Semin Neurol.* 2005;25(1):117-129.

31. Viola-Saltzman M, Watson NF. Traumatic brain injury and sleep disorders. *Neurol Clin.* 2012;30(4):1299-1312.

32. Mahmood O, Rapport LJ, Hanks RA, Fichtenberg NL. Neuropsychological performance and sleep disturbance following traumatic brain injury. *J Head Trauma Rehabil.* 2004;19(5):378-390.

33. Crenshaw MC, Edinger JD. Slow-wave sleep and waking cognitive performance among older adults with and without insomnia complaints. *Physiol Behav.* 1999;66(3):485-492.

34. Abd-Elfattah HM, Abdelazeim FH, Elshennawy S. Physical and cognitive consequences of fatigue: A review. *J Adv Res.* 2015;6(3):351-358.

35. Tanaka M, Ishii A, Watanabe Y. Neural effects of mental fatigue caused by continuous attention load: A magnetoencephalography study. *Brain Res.* 2014;1561:60-66.

36. Pensford J. *Fatigue following brain injury.* Available from http://www.internationalbrain.org/fatigue-following-brain-injury/.

37. Nampiaparampil DE. Prevalence of chronic pain after traumatic brain injury: A systematic review. *JAMA*. 2008;300(6):711-719.

38. Hart RP, Wade JB, Martelli MF. Cognitive impairment in patients with chronic pain: The significance of stress. *Curr Pain Headache Rep*. 2003;7(2):116-126.

39. Silverberg ND, Iverson GL, Panenka W. Cogniphobia in mild traumatic brain injury. *J Neurotrauma*. 2017;34(13):2141-2146.

40. Ruttan LA, Heinrichs RW. Depression and neurocognitive functioning in mild traumatic brain injury patients referred for assessment. *J Clin Exp Neuropsychol*. 2003;25(3):407-419.

41. Ardila A. Head trauma: Neurobehavioral aspects. *MedLink Neurol*. 2006.

42. Rao V, Lyketsos CG. Psychiatric aspects of traumatic brain injury. *Psychiatr Clin North Am*. 2002;25(1):43-69.

43. Lauterbach MD, Notarangelo PL, Nichols SJ, Lane KS, Koliatsos VE. Diagnostic and treatment challenges in traumatic brain injury patients with severe neuropsychiatric symptoms: Insights into psychiatric practice. *Neuropsychiatr Dis Treat*. 2015;11:1601-1607.

44. Bazarian JJ, Cernak I, Noble-Haeusslein L, Potolicchio S, Temkin N. Long-term neurologic outcomes after traumatic brain injury. *J Head Trauma Rehabil*. 2009;24(6):439-451.

45. Jordan BD. The clinical spectrum of sport-related traumatic brain injury. *Nat Rev Neurol*. 2013;9(4):222-230.

46. Habert MO, Horn JF, Sarazin M et al. Brain perfusion SPECT with an automated quantitative tool can identify prodromal Alzheimer's disease among patients with mild cognitive impairment. *Neurobiol Aging*. 2011;32(1):15-23.

47. Kaushansky M. Perspective of Long Term Management after Brain Injury. Invited talk presented at Neurosciences Centre, All India Institute of Medical Sciences, New Delhi, India, 2017.

48. Adetunji BA, Basil B, Mathews M, Williams A, Osinowo T, Oladinni O. Detection and management of malingering in a clinical setting. *Prim Psychiatry*. 2006;13(1):61.

49. Cicerone KD, Langenbahn DM, Braden C et al. Evidence-based cognitive rehabilitation: Updated review of the literature from 2003 through 2008. *Arch Phys Med Rehabil*. 2011;92(4):519-530.

50. Wilson BA, Evans J, Brentnall S, Bremner S, Keohane C, Williams H. The Oliver Zangwill Center for Neuropsychological Rehabilitation. In: *International Handbook of Neuropsychological Rehabilitation*. Springer US; 2000:231-246.

51. Ryan LM, Warden DL. Post concussion syndrome. *Int Rev Psychiatry*. 2003;15(4):310-316.

25

Psychological care

SARA LAXE AND NEUS FÀBREGAS

INTRODUCTION

Entering into an intensive care unit (ICU) may initiate a dramatic change in the lives of both the patients, and also their families or caregivers. These individuals can endure a substantial challenge and stress and they might need care, support, and follow up. The importance of this care is a well-recognized part of good quality practice.

The mortality rate in the ICU is high and previous research shows that 50% of those who survive a critical illness are discharged with some level of disability that will affect not only their functional outcome but also their quality of life[1] (see Table 25.1).

The number of people entering the ICU has followed an ascending curve in the last few decades due to an aging population but also because of the advances in technology and treatment developments, which increase the survival rate after intensive care.[2] Despite an increase in survival rates, there is also increased attention on the functional outcomes and quality of life after discharge.

If the cause of entering an ICU is due to a brain injury, the patient will suffer from a range of cognitive, behavioral, and emotional symptoms, in addition to physical changes. Even those with less-severe injuries suffer from memory, attention, concentration, behavioral, and emotional problems that can impact the ability to perform daily life activities. Moreover, these impairments have a direct impact on the family and on society as a whole.[3]

In recent years, researchers have detected long-term consequences of any critical illness in both the physical domains, such as fatigue or muscle weakness, and also in cognitive problems like mental fatigue, lack of concentration, difficulties in sleep, or emotional problems such as anxiety or depression. Studies have shown that a prolonged stay in ICU leads to adverse psychological problems in patients, and also with their families. These problems have a repercussion in functioning and well-being and can be present long after the recovery, even one year after the ICU discharge despite solving the medical condition that led to the admission.[4] All of these

Table 25.1 Changes in people's functioning after intensive care, according to the ICF (International Classification of Functioning Framework)

International Classification of Functioning Disability and Health (ICF)		
Body Functions	**Body Structures**	
• Cognitive changes: Memory and attention • Sleep changes • Sensory problems such as changes in vision, hearing or altered sensation • Swallowing problems • Nausea, vomiting • Constipation • Respiratory problems • Difficulty in speaking due to phonorespiratory coordination impairment • Pain • Urinary problems (due to long use of catheters, medication, infections of the urinary tract)	• Muscle atrophy • Bone mass loss • Contractions • Skin sores • Structures related to comorbidity (fractures, operations, catheters, prosthesis, etc.)	
Activities and Participation	**Environmental Factors**	
Difficulties	**Facilitators**	**Barriers**
• Unable to sit • Difficulty standing up • Difficulty in walking around the house • Difficulty in walking in the street • Unable to climb stairs • Maintaining a conversation • Making decisions • Need help to sit up, rolling in bed, going to the toilet • Complex daily routines, such as organizing the house bills, shopping	• Provision of information about management of basic daily life activities • Recommendation for returning to complex daily life activist • Information about driving and a return to work • Benefits from the Social Security and insurance • Provide guidance about support groups or continuing care from which the patient may benefit • Provide with leaflets for information that can reinforce verbal information • Provide with a diary	• Poor communication skills • Isolation in intensive care • Depersonalization of care in intensive care: catheters, machines, alarms, etc. • Financial problems that may arise • Lack of sleep of family members

Source: Laxe S et al., NeuroRehabilitation. 2011;29(1):99-110.

symptoms altogether are known as a postintensive care syndrome (PICS).[5]

There is also an increasing awareness of the "postintensive care syndrome–Family" and improving outcomes in family caregivers can also improve patient outcomes.[5] Despite this fact, most of the services do not have standardized procedures for early psychological support, but there is a growing interest to search for a better understanding of how these emotional factors can be monitored and counseled over time in order to improve health and wellness.

The objective of this chapter is to inform the health professional about the nonphysical changes or symptoms that can develop in patients and their families after being admitted to an ICU. It also provides information about validated checklists or questionnaires that can detect these symptoms and explain some possibilities for their treatment.

PSYCHOLOGICAL SYMPTOMS

Patients admitted into intensive care, especially those who do not have consciousness disorders, can understand the severity of their condition and the possibility of complications or even death and may suffer from anxiety and depression that can worsen their medical condition. In fact, depression and anxiety are predictors of moderate to severe disability in patients discharged from ICU.[6] Additionally, patients in the ICU normally complain about the coldness of the ICU, the isolation from their families, sensorial deprivation (if they need hearing aids or glasses), lack of intimacy, and stress from the alarms and machines that can have a negative impact in their perception of the experience. Other studies have reported what the patients recall from their ICU stay is and this variety is important. Some patients report no memories at all whereas others report pain, suctioning, lack of sleep, and/or hallucinations.[7,8]

Anxiety and depression can be present since ICU admission and they depend on different variables, such as the severity of the medical condition, gender, age, level of education, personality, or previous experiences as well as the level of disability or functional impairment after their discharge. In general, these symptoms tend to decrease over time, although there is usually an increase in symptoms when they are transferred to a normal ward. This is due to the perception that the care in the ICU is better than in a normal ward.[9,10]

Cognitive problems also seem to appear in up to 80% of cases after 1 year post-ICU discharge.[11]

More severe forms of psychiatric symptoms can also arise due to multifactorial causes, such as the lack of sleep and the use of drugs that have a psychotropic effect.[12,13] Studies suggest that between 40% to 80% of critically ill patients suffer from sleep disturbances that continue for 2 months after their discharge[14,15] and this increases to one out of two patients for those who had an acute respiratory syndrome, according to Dhooria.[16] A slow wave sleep reduction seems to play a role in the confusional syndrome and the recall of memories.[7]

POSTINTENSIVE CARE SYNDROME

Postintensive care syndrome is similar to post-traumatic stress disorder (PTSD) and this has been described at ICU discharge. Patients report feeling negative emotions when remembering things related to the disease that put them into intensive care. Examples could be hearing sirens or alarms on TV or in the street; stress that develops while driving near a hospital; as well as descriptions of fear, worrying, and panic attacks (see Table 25.2 for detailed diagnostic criterion). Spending more than 4 days in the ICU is a risk factor for suffering from PTSD[11,17,18] Its physiopathologic cause is still unknown, but those patients in the ICU who were admitted due to severe trauma or sepsis (together with acute respiratory distress syndrome), and those who have undergone mechanical ventilation have been found to have the worst outcomes in terms of quality of life.[1,19,20] Fluctuations in the level of sedation have increased the incidence of PTSD, anxiety, or depression, and, therefore, affect the patient's quality of life and prognosis of recovery.[13] Other independent factors that have been associated with psychological distress are age, sex, duration of mechanical ventilation, unemployment, personality traits, pain, and education status.

Delirium can be present in patients despite the absence of a non-preexisting condition, although premorbid depression has been associated independently with a higher incidence of delirium. Since there have been studies that have identified brain atrophy and white matter hyperintensity in people with delirium, there might also be a premorbid condition that had not been identified before admission.[12,13,21] Delirium itself has been shown to be an independent factor in increasing morbidity after ICU discharge.[12]

POST INTENSIVE CARE SYNDROME—FAMILY

Currently, it is often said that intensive care provides a patient with family-centered medicine, highlighting the important role that the family plays in the treatment process. Family is defined, by guidelines from the American College of Critical

Table 25.2 DSM-5 criterion for PTSD

DSM-5 Criterion for PTSD

Criterion A (one required)
- Direct exposure
- Witnessing trauma
- Learning that a relative or close friend was exposed to a trauma
- Indirect exposure to aversive details of the trauma (eg, a doctor)

Criterion B (one required)
- Intrusive thoughts
- Nightmares
- Flashbacks
- Emotional distress after exposure to traumatic reminders
- Physical reactivity after exposure to traumatic reminders

Criterion C (one required): Avoidance of trauma-related stimuli after the trauma, in the following way(s):
- Trauma-related thoughts or feelings
- Trauma-related reminders

Criterion D (two required): Negative thoughts or feelings that began or worsened after the trauma, in the following ways:
- Inability to recall key features of the trauma
- Overly negative thoughts and assumptions about oneself or the world
- Exaggerated blame of self or others for causing the trauma
- Negative affect
- Decreased interest in activities
- Feeling isolated
- Difficulty experiencing positive affect

Criterion E: Trauma-related arousal and reactivity that began or worsened after the trauma, in the following way(s):
- Irritability or aggression
- Risky or destructive behavior
- Hypervigilance
- Heightened startle reaction
- Difficulty concentrating
- Difficulty sleeping

Criterion F (required): Symptoms last for more than 1 month

(Continued)

Table 25.2 (Continued) DSM-5 criterion for PTSD

Criterion G (required): Symptoms create distress or functional impairment (eg, social, occupational)

Criterion H (required): Symptoms are not due to medication, substance use, or other illness

Source: Norris FH et al., *Am J Disaster Med.* 2008;3 (4):201-212.
Abbreviation: PTSD: Post-traumatic stress disorder.

Care Medicine (ACCM) and the Society of Critical Care Medicine (SCCM), as those individuals related or unrelated to the patient who provide support and with whom the patient has a significant relationship.[5]

Increased emotional distress appears in different degrees and at different times when the patient is in the ICU. The adjusting process begins within the first minutes and continues for a long time and even after discharge from the ICU. Depending on the aetiology of the cause of the admission as well as the relation to the person, the reactional impact may be different. As expected, traumatic brain injury (TBI) due to aggression leaves a family more unprepared and with greater feelings of anger than a family of an 80-year-old cardiovascular patient with a respiratory insufficiency.

There are some nonmodifiable factors, such as female gender, preexisting mental illness, spouse of an ICU patient, parent-child relationship, and sudden or violent incidents that can cause a critical illness, such as a traumatic brain injury (TBI).[22]

The emotional condition of relatives is very important, not only because of their direct effects on the patient, but also because medical professionals need to deal with the family members in order to make the appropriate decisions. The way family members cope with this stress also depends on many factors. The severity of the injury, the degree of relation to the patient, the chances of recovery, and previous experiences matter, but studies are controversial in finding linear associations with emotional stress reactions.[23] The personality of the relative seems to play an important role. In psychology, people's reactions to problems can be widely divided and either emotionally oriented or problem solving; they are also at a higher risk of suffering from either depression or anxiety.

One of the first studies to investigate the emotional burden of family members in the ICU was the one conducted among traumatic brain injury patients by Oddy et al. in 1978. He stated that the greatest level of stress appeared during the first month after the onset of the trauma with a progressive decrease at 6 months, and stabilized but without being back to normal during the first year.[24,25] Professionals should be trained in communication skills as well as psychological support in order to help families maintain a stable emotional status that will help during the clinical encounter but will also help in the future.

Health professionals are more familiar with relatives showing signs of depression and anxiety, but it is also important to highlight some cognitive bias that can influence decision making such as the optimistic bias. This term refers to the fact that the majority of the population, and more specifically, those who are not depressed, tend to have an unrealistic view of what their future can be.[26] And studies have shown how even objective information given by professionals does not always have the desired impact on people. As an example, this can have important repercussions in a young patient with an unresponsive wakefulness syndrome following cardiac arrest who is unlikely to recover consciousness in the next few months. Therefore, the family should make realistic decisions about the destination and transfer of the patient after the ICU and avoid futile treatments. Also, the optimistic bias has been shown to affect how people react to objective news, meaning that people have a tendency to ignore news that doesn't match their expectations.

HOW TO DETECT COGNITIVE PROBLEMS

It is important that professionals working in the ICU are aware of the emotional problems that may arise among patients and their families. Patients and families are unlikely to come to the doctor with complaints of depression or anxiety, therefore professionals should take into account some indirect signs or direct the medical interview during the anamnesis to detect emotional problems and transfer the individual to the right professional. There are several self-reported questionnaires that can help with the interview or that can be given to the patients or their families. These questionnaires

have been validated in the ICU populations and give a score that can be used as a guide to whether the symptoms are severe enough to need treatment.

Scores for the detection of post-traumatic stress disorder

- The UK-PTSS-14 is a screening tool used to identify patients at risk of suffering PTSD in the ICU; it has shown good concurrent validity, predictive validity, and internal reliability for screening acute PTSD, according to a NICE guideline review.[17,18]
- The post-traumatic stress diagnostic scale, the Traumatic Stress Diagnostic Scale (PDS), is a 49-item, self-report score that was developed for its use in clinical or research to measure the severity of PTSD. The PDS adds to the measurement of the severity of the symptoms, as well as the information about traumatic events, duration of symptoms, and disturbances on daily functioning.[27,28]
- Post-traumatic stress disorder TSS-10[29,30] is a 10-item questionnaire tool. This scale possesses a good accuracy test and internal reliability for screening chronic or delayed onset PTSD in critical care adults in Germany, according to the review conducted by the NICE organization.
- With the Post-traumatic Stress Disorder Checklist (PCLS), a score over 44 suggests that the person is at risk of having a PTSD. This questionnaire asks the patient to check if he or she has been bothered about stressing memories in the ICU, if he/she had bad dreams, if they have physical reactions such as trouble breathing or sweating when remembering a stressful situation, if they avoid thinking or talking about a stressful situation, if they have difficulty in concentrating, or whether they feel irritable or have anger outbursts.

Scores to detect depression and anxiety

The NICE guidelines recommend the use of the Hospital Anxiety and Depression Scale (HADS) and the State-Trait Anxiety Inventory (STAI-X1).

The HADS[31] is a scale with 14 items divided in two subscales with seven items that are used to determine depression symptoms, and seven items that measure anxiety symptoms. It is a self-reported scale in which the patients score from 0 to 3 each item and the total score is the sum of items ranging from 0–21. Scores of 8–10 are considered borderline and scores above 11 are considered a significant mood disorder.

The STAI-X1[32] has 20 items and is used to detect anxiety. The cutting points differ according to the studies but helps the professional to identify items that may not appear in a non-directed interview.

Both the HADS and the STAI-X1 have showed good test accuracy for screening depression and anxiety in adult critical care.

Scores for relatives

- Family Strain Questionnaire[33]: This is a questionnaire that assesses the burden of the family members of patients. It is a self-rating questionnaire in which the families describe if they need to help their relative more than before, if they have stopped being engaged in social activities due to the dependency, if they feel they have less privacy at home because of the care, or if they feel they don't have enough money to take care of the relative's expenses. It is a questionnaire that has been used by health professionals without any specific psychological training and is useful to measure the caregiver's strain.*
- The Family Interview Schedule (FIS)[34] is a measure intended to capture the impact of relatives with mental problems that ask questions about social problems, interpersonal strain among family members, work-related problems, and financial difficulties.

COMMUNICATION IN THE ICU

Communication, in general, is one of the "missing topics" of health professionals. The literature provides evidence that there is a lack of satisfaction among patients and families with the physicians' communication styles and techniques.[35–39] This fact can be more remarkable under circumstances such as the ICU setting, with dynamic and sometimes unexpected changes in the status of the patient.

Families are also separated physically from their loved ones, since traditionally the care in the ICU requires specific measures that make it difficult for the families to visit the patients.

Professionals in the ICU are among those with more stress and burn out[40,41] and the task of communicating bad news is often uncomfortable and can contribute to a detachment between patients and their doctors. Doctors tend to focus on technical and medical knowledge and avoid emotional contact. In a situation where the patient lives in the ICU, talking about outcome measures, such as survival rate or functional status, can be difficult; therefore, the answers to the family's main preoccupation are vague. Additionally, a family's stress and emotional reactions can affect their cognitive process of new, and normally undesirable, information.

Needless to say, a good communication is one of the most important aspects of the clinical encounter since it is not only important as a part of the medical anamnesis (as a way of establishing a therapeutic alliance), but it is also essential to making informed decisions and to making plans for the future. However, it can also help the patients and families to deal with their emotions more productively, and, therefore, can contribute in a positive way to a positive outcome.[42–46] One of the current highlights in the delivery of bad news is the communication style. In modern society medicine, practice has shifted from a paternalistic orientation to a patient-centered practice in which doctors are the providers of information and possibilities and the patients make decisions over their own bodies and their health based on their beliefs and personal situations. There is also a tendency for shared decision making that follows the principle of autonomy, and, in essence, represents the biopsychosocial perspective of understanding the person's experience of his or her health. Studies have shown that patients prefer when their doctors take time to explain to them the situation in a way that they can understand. They also want their doctors to empathize by letting them express their feelings, emotions, and fears. They also want to understand the repercussions of the disease as it relates to their previous life.[35,47,48]

Patient-centered medicine has been correlated with a higher feeling of well-being and satisfaction with the provided service according to several studies. At the same time, there have been found a fewer number of complaints in those situations in which the physician behaved more empathically compared with those with a more authoritarian approach.[48,49]

Table 25.3 Tips for good psychological care

1. Provide a good environment and effective communication to make the person as calm as possible. The hospitals should encourage policies that enhance environmental hygiene to reduce noise, alarms, lights, and give space for intimacy.
2. Through clinical assessment, identify those patients with risk factors for not only developing physical but also nonphysical morbidity.
3. When a patient or a relative has been identified as being at risk, due a comprehensive clinical assessment or the situation and transfer to the competent professional for treatment.
4. When a patient is going to be discharged from the ICU, beside all of the medical items, such as blood pressure, lack of infections, etc., a functional assessment should be done in order to detect muscle weakness, weight loss, fatigue, etc., that can impair walking or basic daily life activities. Additionally, the patient should be checked again for cognitive and emotional problems, such as lack of concentration, memory problems, problems with sleep, etc. Questions such as "Do you feel depressed?" are not of much help, since many people don´t want to recognize that they are depressed or they are possibly not aware of it. Therefore, the use of questionnaires is of great interest and help.
5. The work on a multidisciplinary team should be the ideal treatment of the patient and family. The implication of rehabilitation in the ICU can help prevent problems and help with treatment.
6. Short-term rehabilitation goal: Those goals that should be given to the patient before he or she is discharged from the hospital.
7. Medium-term rehabilitation goals: Goals to help the patient to return home and progressively be able to get back to his or her previous daily life activities.
8. Coordinating with other services to guarantee a continuum of treatment of the patients and their families as well as including the service of other professionals, such as social workers, but also provide spiritual support.

Sources: Fields SA, Johnson WM, *W V Med J.* 2012;108(2):32-35; Friedemann-Sánchez G et al., *Rehabil Nurs.* 2008;33 (5):206-213; Schmid Mast M et al., *Patient Educ Couns.* 2007;68(1):16-22.

Good communication and providing information to the patient and/or to their families is very important since it may reduce stress and can increase coping abilities. Research has found that there are significant associations between the doctor's support and low levels of stress in patients and/or their family members[50] (see Table 25.3).

RECOMMENDATIONS FOR GOOD COMMUNICATION

Prepare for the encounter

The delivery of news should be prepared in advance. Since time is precious in the ICU, whenever a patient is admitted to the ICU, a member of the team should provide information to the family about the rules of the ICU, including visiting hours, the names of professionals to contact, and advice about the possibility of sudden unwanted information.

It is advisable to ask the family to identify a family member who can be the contact person and can communicate information to the rest of the family. If the doctor realizes that the "contact" person is vulnerable, he/she should ask if that person wants a support contact to be present during the interview. This is very important in order to prevent an emotional shock and to make sure that the family member understands the news that the doctor anticipates and prepares them mentally. Daily encounters with the family should be desirable, even if there are no changes in the process but to reassure the information and detect possible emotional complications in the family members.

The doctors who are going to participate in the encounter should also be prepared. Besides checking all the clinical and related issues of the patients again, they should prepare themselves emotionally. Delivering bad news is also stressful for doctors and there are known circumstances that can aggravate the situation, including a long-call shift that leads to reduced attention; lack of empathy, concern, and sensitivity as well as increased irritability and a tendency to objectify patients.[40,41] All of these characteristics are not compatible with patient-oriented medicine and an open communication style and can rectify a misperception of the treatment.

The setting

The environment for delivering bad news is important. In a study by Lloyd-Williams et al.[51] one of the most important complaints was the location where the bad news was delivered. The ideal location should be a room with privacy where families can openly talk without fear that strangers are listening to them; but it should also be a place where they can sit. In western societies, people appreciate when doctors sit next to them and not on the other side of the table so that they can make physical contact with them, such as touching the forearm. Telephone conversations should be avoided since they do not provide the emotional support that the family may need. Needless to say, while delivering the news, doctors should indicate that it's the time for that specific patient or family member; therefore cell phones and pagers should be silenced.

The news provider

The senior medical professional with the most experience in the patient's case should be the one delivering the information. Residents or students in teaching hospitals can be present if the family was asked for permission. Some studies suggest that a nurse should be present during the encounter, since families feel quite close to the nurses and since they are the professionals who are closer to the patient.[52–54] Since the patients admitted into the ICU are followed by a multidisciplinary team involving doctors who would do the follow-up, it's reasonable to think that the delivery of news could be done within a team. However, the literature is controversial. On one hand, the team meeting could transmit the feeling of better care, but on the other hand, it can also give the impression of a less-intimate space and families may need to restrain their emotions in front of the team, while it would not be such a great thing in front of a team, this wouldn't present a problem in front of a doctor.

In a systematic literature review conducted with oncologic patients,[50] very few of the patients or families wanted other professionals to be present during the meeting; however, there are some cross-cultural differences. For instance, 78% of patients in Japan wanted to have families present while 81% of the patients in the United States did not wish anyone else to be present.[50] The doctor and nurse providing the news should not only be acquainted with the current clinical situation, but with any previous clinical history as well as with their social status. If the patient is conscious, he or she should be invited to participate in the discussion or asked if he or she prefers to delegate the responsibility of receiving the news to another family member. Needless to say, doctors should introduce themselves to the families and provide an opportunity to find them or ask for a meeting with them if needed in the future.

The delivery of bad news

In general, doctors and health professionals benefit from the awareness that different factors such as cultural differences, personality characteristics, age, and so on, can change the preferences of patients and they should tailor their communication style for each person.

There are studies that have identified associated factors, such as age, gender, and education, with the delivery of bad news.[50,55] Younger female patients with a higher education consistently want to know as many details as possible. Cultural aspects cannot be avoided when communicating the news. There are some studies that regard the discussion of end-of-life situations that show that 30% or fewer of Asian patients prefer to discuss it. This is in contrast to Western countries where 60% of the people do so.[51] Even within western societies, there is a difference in the disclosure of news between Europe and America, where, due to the legislation, doctors tend to be more aggressive regarding the release of information.[56,57]

Religion had also has an impact on information and prognosis. In a study by Ascaso,[58] many participants believed that their recovery was going to be influenced by their beliefs. If they had faith, they would benefit from that. Another interesting study by Berges, which was conducted in a population of

Mexican Americans, found that those who were connected to some organized religion improved significantly.[59,60]

There is a vast body of literature that indicates that patients preferred an empathic communication, meaning that besides being informed clearly, honestly, and without their doctors using jargon and words that they don't understand, they want their doctors to understand how the illness can affect their lives. They want them to know how they feel and how it is going to impact their abilities to perform their normal activities. They understand that there are situations with no clinical solution, but they want to have a window for hope.

Typically, patients or families ask for the prognosis relating to the disease, but this data is difficult to provide and when given, the professional should enhance the fact that population-based data from studies are difficult to apply in specific individual circumstances. Regarding a patient who is in a coma after a severe traumatic brain injury, an experienced doctor can say "I have never seen anyone recover their previous life after this status."

Rapport

After delivering the news, the doctors should check the patient's or family's level of understanding. It is well known that people under stressful circumstances can avoid integrating information that they dislike. A study by Diez-Ascaso prospectively analyzed how patients react to their medical news.[58] In general, they were satisfied with the information but it was contrasted with the lack of knowledge about their disease despite being told about it.[58] It is a good strategy to try to make sure that the recipient has understood the message regarding strategy, such as making him or her repeat it. They should also allow the individual to ask questions or offer the possibility of another talk, if needed.

INTERVENTIONS FOR PSYCHOLOGICAL CARE

Throughout this chapter we have seen how being in the ICU involves specific emotional problems as well as the different types of emotional problems that can arise in both patients and families. It is very important to notice any of these symptoms not only

improve or ameliorate them in the acute phase, but to avoid its later consequences.

Health professionals can use the different questionnaires mentioned previously in order to guide their clinical interviews and be able to detect whether further interventions need to be pursued. Good communication is the first step not only to detect possible syndromes, but it can also act as a treatment itself, making the patients or the families more confident.

Psychological care should start within the first 24 hours of admission, and if possible, a psychologist should also visit with the family, especially in those cases where the cause of admission was due to violent trauma such as a terrorist attack or gender violence.

Interventions can include:

- Counseling: Through family conferences to facilitate communication and the expression of feelings.
- Educational interventions: These can be leaflets with information about the ICU setting. The written information should be a continuation of the verbal ones, and constitute a mechanism of enhancing the verbal cues. The recommendation to start a diary has been shown to reduce anxiety. It can help with the enormous mental effort that families tend to have in processing the information that professionals give to them and help them to remember the clinical history as well as names of professionals, hours of visit, and contact numbers.
- Stress management: Can be done either in individual consults or in groups. Psychologists normally tend to work these areas and try to train families or patients in developing coping strategies to manage depression, feelings of destruction, fear, hopelessness, isolation, and desperation.
- Professional education: Education professionals in the delivery of bad news, in detecting the PCIS and in counselling techniques can help.
- Environmental changes: Hospital policies can be changed regarding physical space so that families can be closer to the patient. The majority of the patients and the families complain about the restrictions regarding visiting hours and there is dissatisfaction associated with the restriction of

visits. They feel their presence is important to safeguard the patient and to diminish their stress. Families sitting in the waiting room waiting for news can be very stressed. Some studies have shown that if families can be beside the patient, this can increase the outcome when coupled with an education program.[5] However, without an educational program, the presence of the patient's family can increase staff stress and increase their workload.

REFERENCES

1. Oeyen SG, Vandijck DM, Benoit DD, Annemans L, Decruyenaere JM. Quality of life after intensive care: A systematic review of the literature. *Crit Care Med.* 2010;38 (12):2386-2400.

2. Hashem MD, Nallagangula A, Nalamalapu S et al. Patient outcomes after critical illness: A systematic review of qualitative studies following hospital discharge. *Crit Care [Internet].* October 26, 2017;20(1):345.

3. Laxe S, Zasler N, Tschiesner U, López-Blazquez R, Tormos JM, Bernabeu M. ICF use to identify common problems on a TBI neurorehabilitation unit in Spain. *NeuroRehabilitation.* 2011;29(1):99-110.

4. Sharma BG, Evs M, Ms K, BG. Psychological evaluation of patients in critical care/intensive care unit and patients admitted in wards. *J Clin Diagn Res.* 2014;8(12):WC01-WC03.

5. Davidson JE, Aslakson RA, Long AC et al. Guidelines for family-centered care in the neonatal, pediatric, and adult ICU. *Crit Care Med.* 2017;45(1):103-128.

6. Hodgson CL, Udy AA, Bailey M et al. The impact of disability in survivors of critical illness. *Intensive Care Med.* 2017;43(7):992-1001.

7. Jones C, Griffiths RD, Humphris G, Skirrow PM. Memory, delusions, and the development of acute posttraumatic stress disorder-related symptoms after intensive care. *Crit Care Med.* 2001;29(3):573-580.

8. Iedema R, Allen S, Britton K et al. Patients' and family members' views on how clinicians enact and how they should enact incident disclosure: The "100 patient stories" qualitative study. *BMJ.* 2011;343:d4423.

9. Momennasab M, Ghahramani T, Yektatalab S, Zand F. Physical and mental health of patients immediately after discharge from intensive care unit and 24 hours later. *Trauma Mon [Internet].* 2017;21(1):e29231.

10. McCairn AJ, Jones C. Does time of transfer from critical care to the general wards affect anxiety? A pragmatic prospective cohort study. *Intensive Crit Care Nurs.* 2014;30 (4):219-225.

11. Chung CR, Yoo HJ, Park J, Ryu S. Cognitive impairment and psychological distress at discharge from intensive care unit. *Psychiatry Investig.* 2017;14(3):376-379.

12. Pandharipande PP, Ely EW, Arora RC et al. The intensive care delirium research agenda: A multinational, interprofessional perspective. *Intensive Care Med.* 2017;43(9):1329-1339.

13. Svenningsen H. Associations between sedation, delirium and post-traumatic stress disorder and their impact on quality of life and memories following discharge from an intensive care unit. *Dan Med J.* 2013;60(4):B4630.

14. Huang W, Bliwise DL, Johnson TM, Long Q, Kutner N, Stringer AY. Correlates of persistent sleep complaints after traumatic brain injury. *NeuroRehabilitation.* 2013;23(5):698-714.

15. Da Costa D, Dritsa M, Verreault N, Balaa C, Kudzman J, Khalifé S. Sleep problems and depressed mood negatively impact health-related quality of life during pregnancy. *Arch Womens Ment Health.* 2010;13(3):249-257.

16. Dhooria S, Sehgal IS, Agrawal AK, Agarwal R, Aggarwal AN, Behera D. Sleep after critical illness: Study of survivors of acute respiratory distress syndrome and systematic review of literature. *Indian J Crit Care Med.* 2016;20 (6):323-331.

17. Twigg E, Humphris G, Jones C, Bramwell R, Griffiths RD. Use of a screening questionnaire for post-traumatic stress disorder (PTSD) on a sample of UK ICU patients. *Acta Anaesthesiol Scand.* 2008;52(2):202-208.

18. Jackson JC, Pandharipande PP, Girard TD et al. Depression, post-traumatic stress disorder, and functional disability in survivors of critical illness in the BRAIN-ICU study: A longitudinal cohort study. *Lancet Respir Med.* 2014;2(5):369-379.

19. Arango-Lasprilla JC, Krch D, Drew A, De Los Reyes Aragon CJ, Stevens LF. Health-related quality of life of individuals with traumatic brain injury in Barranquilla, Colombia. *Brain Inj.* 2012;26(6):825-833.

20. Chahraoui K, Laurent A, Bioy A, Quenot JP. Psychological experience of patients 3 months after a stay in the intensive care unit: A descriptive and qualitative study. *J Crit Care.* 2015;30(3):599-605.

21. Nitchingham A, Kumar V, Shenkin S, Ferguson KJ, Caplan GA. A systematic review of neuroimaging in delirium: Predictors, correlates and consequences. *Int J Geriatr Psychiatry.* 2017 Jun 2. [Epub ahead of print].

22. Warrillow S, Farley KJ, Jones D. How to improve communication quality with patients and relatives in the ICU. *Minerva Anestesiol.* 2016;82(7):797-803.

23. Norup A, Siert L, Lykke Mortensen E. Emotional distress and quality of life in relatives of patients with severe brain injury: The first month after injury. *Brain Inj.* 2010;24(2):81-88.

24. Oddy M, Humphrey M, Uttley D. Subjective impairment and social recovery after closed head injury. *J Neurol Neurosurg Psychiatry.* 1978;41(7):611-616.

25. Oddy M, Humphrey M, Uttley D. Stresses upon the relatives of head-injured patients. *Br J Psychiatry J Ment Sci.* 1978;133:507-513.

26. Harris AJL, Hahn U. Unrealistic optimism about future life events: A cautionary note. *Psychol Rev.* 2011;118(1):135-154.

27. Norris FH, Hamblen JL, Brown LM, Schinka JA. Validation of the short posttraumatic stress disorder rating interview (expanded version, Sprint-E) as a measure of postdisaster distress and treatment need. *Am J Disaster Med.* 2008;3(4):201-212.

28. Dragan M, Lis-Turlejska M, Popiel A, Szumiał S, Dragan WŁ. The validation of the Polish version of the posttraumatic diagnostic scale and its factor structure. *Eur J Psychotraumatol.* 2012;3. doi:10.3402/ejpt.v3i0.18479. Epub 2012 Aug 9.

29. Baranyi A, Krauseneck T, Rothenhäusler HB. Posttraumatic stress symptoms after solid-organ transplantation: Preoperative risk factors and the impact on health-related quality of life and life satisfaction. *Health Qual Life Outcomes.* 2013;11:111.

30. Stoll C, Kapfhammer HP, Rothenhäusler HB et al. Sensitivity and specificity of a screening test to document traumatic experiences and to diagnose post-traumatic stress disorder in ARDS patients after intensive care treatment. *Intensive Care Med.* 1999;25(7):697-704.

31. Zigmond AS, Snaith RP. The hospital anxiety and depression scale. *Acta Psychiatr Scand.* 1983;67(6):361-370.

32. Vedana L, Baiardi P, Sommaruga M et al. Clinical validation of an anxiety and depression screening test for intensive in-hospital rehabilitation. *Monaldi Arch Chest Dis Arch Monaldi Mal Torace.* 2002;58(2):101-106.

33. Vidotto G, Ferrario SR, Bond TG, Zotti AM. Family strain questionnaire—Short form for nurses and general practitioners. *J Clin Nurs.* 2010;19(1-2):275-283.

34. Sartorius N, Janca A. Psychiatric assessment instruments developed by the World Health Organization. *Soc Psychiatry Psychiatr Epidemiol.* 1996;31(2):55-69.

35. Butalid L, Verhaak PFM, Boeije HR, Bensing JM. Patients' views on changes in doctor-patient communication between 1982 and 2001: A mixed-methods study. *BMC Fam Pract.* 2012;13:80.

36. García Díaz F. Breaking bad news in medicine: Strategies that turn necessity into a virtue. *Med Intensiva.* 2006;30(9):452-459.

37. Grainger KP, Masterson S, Jennings M. Things aren't the same, are they?: The management of bad news delivery in the discourse of stroke care. *Commun Med.* 2005;2(1):35-44.

38. Merckaert I, Liénard A, Libert Y et al. Is it possible to improve the breaking bad news skills of residents when a relative is present? A randomised study. *Br J Cancer.* 2013;109(10):2507-2514.

39. Lefebvre H, Levert MJ. The needs experienced by individuals and their loved ones following a traumatic brain injury. *J Trauma Nurs.* 2012;19(4):197-207.

40. Chuang CH, Tseng PC, Lin CY, Lin KH, Chen YY. Burnout in the intensive care unit professionals: A systematic review. *Medicine (Baltimore).* 2016;95(50):e5629.

41. Passalacqua SA, Segrin C. The effect of resident physician stress, burnout, and empathy

on patient-centered communication during the long-call shift. *Health Commun.* 2012;27 (5):449-456.

42. Boyd EA, Lo B, Evans LR et al. "It's not just what the doctor tells me:": Factors that influence surrogate decision-makers' perceptions of prognosis. *Crit Care Med.* 2010;38(5):1270-1275.

43. Dosser I, Kennedy C. Family carers' experiences of support at the end of life: Carers' and health professionals' views. *Int J Palliat Nurs.* 2012;18(10):491-497.

44. Falk AC, von Wendt L, Söderkvist BK. Families' perceptions of given information in relation to their child's head injury. *Scand J Caring Sci.* 2009;23(1):125-129.

45. Fields SA, Johnson WM. Physician-patient communication: Breaking bad news. *W V Med J.* 2012;108(2):32-35.

46. Friedemann-Sánchez G, Griffin JM, Rettmann NA, Rittman M, Partin MR. Communicating information to families of polytrauma patients: A narrative literature review. *Rehabil Nurs.* 2008;33(5):206-213.

47. Schmid Mast M, Hall JA, Roter DL. Disentangling physician sex and physician communication style: Their effects on patient satisfaction in a virtual medical visit. *Patient Educ Couns.* 2007;68(1):16-22.

48. Epstein RM, Franks P, Fiscella K et al. Measuring patient-centered communication in patient-physician consultations: theoretical and practical issues. *Soc Sci Med.* 2005;61 (7):1516-1528.

49. Storstein A. Communication and neurology—Bad news and how to break them. *Acta Neurol Scand Suppl.* 2011;(191):5-11.

50. Fujimori M, Akechi T, Uchitomi Y. Factors associated with patient preferences for communication of bad news. *Palliat Support Care.* 2017;15(3):328-335.

51. Lloyd-Williams M, Morton J, Peters S. The end-of-life care experiences of relatives of brain dead intensive care patients. *J Pain Symptom Manage.* 2009;37(4):659-664.

52. Graugaard PK, Rogg L, Eide H, Uhlig T, Loge JH. Ways of providing the patient with a prognosis: A terminology of employed strategies based on qualitative data. *Patient Educ Couns.* 2011;83(1):80-86.

53. Hollyday SL, Buonocore D. Breaking bad news and discussing goals of care in the intensive care unit. *AACN Adv Crit Care.* 2015;26(2):131-141.

54. Michelson KN, Patel R, Haber-Barker N, Emanuel L, Frader J. End-of-life care decisions in the PICU: Roles professionals play. *Pediatr Crit Care Med.* 2013;14(1):e34-e44. doi:10.1097/PCC.0b013e31826e7408.

55. Fujimori M, Parker PA, Akechi T, Sakano Y, Baile WF, Uchitomi Y. Japanese cancer patients' communication style preferences when receiving bad news. *Psychooncology.* 2007;16(7):617-625.

56. Chittem M, Butow P. Responding to family requests for nondisclosure: The impact of oncologists' cultural background. *J Cancer Res Ther.* 2015;11(1):174-180.

57. Bousquet G, Orri M, Winterman S, Brugière C, Verneuil L, Revah-Levy A. Breaking bad news in oncology: A metasynthesis. *J Clin Oncol.* 2015;33(22):2437-2443.

58. Díez-Ascaso O, Martinez-Sánchez P, Fuentes B, Díez-Tejedor E. Sociocultural study on the self-perception of stroke and an analysis of doctor-patient communication. *Neurol Barc Spain.* 2011;26(2):81-91.

59. Reyes-Ortiz CA, Berges IM, Raji MA, Koenig HG, Kuo YF, Markides KS. Church attendance mediates the association between depressive symptoms and cognitive functioning among older Mexican Americans. *J Gerontol A Biol Sci Med Sci.* 2008;63(5):480-486.

60. Berges IM, Kuo YF, Markides KS, Ottenbacher K. Attendance at religious services and physical functioning after stroke among older Mexican Americans. *Exp Aging Res.* 2007;33(1):1-11.

PART IX

Special considerations

26

Pediatric neurotrauma

ANKUR KHANDELWAL AND HEMANSHU PRABHAKAR

INTRODUCTION

Neurotrauma broadly encompasses traumatic brain injury (TBI) and spinal cord injury (SCI). Among all traumatic injuries, neurotrauma is now the leading cause of morbidity and mortality in children although, over the last decade, substantial improvement in understanding the pathophysiology of neurotrauma has improved prehospital and in-hospital management including rehabilitation.[1,2] This is due to tremendous heterogeneity in mechanism, pathology, type, and severity of injury including wide discrepancies in management protocols in different neurotrauma centers of the world. Apart from physical, cognitive, and emotional burden, neurotrauma also accentuates socioeconomic loss. The mechanism by which neurotrauma disrupts developing, widespread neural networks in pediatric patients is poorly understood, and is a subject of intense research and is undoubtedly consequential.

EPIDEMIOLOGY

Traumatic brain injury

According to the Centers for Disease Control and Prevention (CDC), almost half a million (473,947) emergency department visits for TBI are made annually by children aged 0 to 14 years; of these up to 90% return home with mild injuries (Glasgow Coma Scale ≥13), 37,000 are hospitalized, and 2685 die because of their injuries. The death rate is higher for children younger than 4 years than for those 5 to 14 years of age. Head trauma affects male children more than their female counterparts (M: F3:2). Moreover, boys have a four times higher risk of fatal TBI compared with girls.[3] The observed types of TBI and mechanisms of injury differ with child age and development. According to the CDC, falls are the most common mechanism for TBI in the age group of 1–4 years. In older children and adolescents, common mechanisms of head injury include falls, unintentional blunt trauma (eg, being hit by an object), motor vehicle accidents (MVAs) including bicycle-related crashes, assault, and sports-related injuries. Abusive head trauma (AHT) is particularly common in children aged less than 2 years; approximately 30 of every 100,000 infants less than 1 year were hospitalized for AHT.[4] Apart from gender and age, race also appears to have an impact on the risk of suffering from TBI. Recently, Haider and colleagues studied 7778 pediatric patients between 2 and 16 years from the National Pediatric Trauma Registry and concluded that African-American children have a less favorable clinical and functional outcome after TBI.[5] Racial disparities in outcomes may be explained because of the differences in healthcare and/or health status. The mortality rate was however identical for all studied races.

SPINAL CORD INJURY

Pediatric SCI is relatively rare because of the greater flexibility of their tissues compared with adults. In a large retrospective study of the National Pediatric Trauma Registry over a 10-year period, the overall incidence of cervical spine injuries (CSI) was 1.5%.[6] Approximately 72% of spinal injuries in children under 8 years old occur in the cervical spine.[7] In one study, 88 pediatric patients were identified based on the analysis of a database of 1770 traumatic SCI patients. In this study, the level of injury differed based on the child's age category, with C2 lesions occurring in the pre-teen groups, C4 lesions occurring in the teen group, and C4–C5 lesions occurring in the adult group.[8] This is related to the fulcrum of cervical motion which is C1–C3 in younger children (<8 years) and C5–C6 in older children and adolescents. Regarding the mechanism of injury, MVA usually affects younger children whereas adolescents are commonly injured during sporting activities.[9] Similar to TBI, males are more commonly affected than females.[8-11] SCI without radiological anomaly, (SCIWORA) accounts approximately for 43% of injuries[9] whereas CSI

without radiological abnormality occurs in 17% of patients.[6] Although the exact association of CSI and TBI is not known in children, as many as 50% to 60% of the CSI in children may be associated with head injury.[12-14]

SUSCEPTIBILITY TO NEUROTRAUMA: ANATOMIC AND PHYSIOLOGIC BASIS

Traumatic brain injury

Children are more susceptible to TBI because they have a larger head to body size ratio and thinner cranial bones that provide less protection to the intracranial contents. These characteristics may result in profound consequences from acceleration-deceleration injuries. Additionally, since children and adolescents often have little extra subarachnoid space compared with older adults, even relatively small volumes of swollen tissue can lead to dangerous tissue shifts and elevations of intracranial pressure (ICP). Moreover, less myelinated neural tissue and inflammatory mediators in the developing brain further increases its vulnerability to damage. The scalp is highly vascularized and a potential cause of lethal blood loss.[15,16]

The cerebral metabolic rate of oxygen consumption ($CMRO_2$) at rest is higher in children (5.2 mL/100 gm/min of brain tissue) compared with adults (3–3.5 mL/100 gm/min of brain tissue) which makes them less tolerant to hypoxia. This is also evident from low oxygen extraction fraction (OEF) commonly observed after pediatric TBI.[17] Moreover, the autoregulatory curve in neonates is maintained within a narrow range of mean arterial pressure (MAP) of 20–60 mmHg.[18] Beyond these limits, CBF becomes pressure passive resulting in a linear correlation between CBF and systemic blood pressure (Figure 26.1).[19] Neonates are especially vulnerable to cerebral ischemia and intraventricular hemorrhage due to this narrow autoregulatory range.

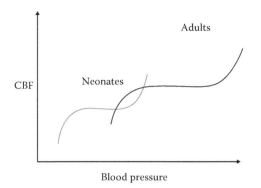

Figure 26.1 Autoregulation of cerebral blood flow (CBF) in neonates and adults. The slope of the autoregulatory curve drops and rises significantly at the lower and upper limits of the curve, respectively, and is shifted to the left in neonates and infants (left curve) when compared with adults (right curve). (Reprinted from *Cottrell and Patel's Neuroanesthesia*, In: Cottrell JE, Patel P, eds. 6th ed., Soriano SG III, McManus ML, Pediatric neuroanesthesia and critical care, 337-350, Copyright 2016, with permission from Elsevier.)

SPINAL CORD INJURY

In children, cranio-cervical stability is more dependent on the ligaments and soft tissues than on the vertebrae. The immature spine is hypermobile because of ligamentous laxity, shallow and angled facet joints, underdeveloped spinous processes, and physiologic anterior wedging of vertebral bodies, all of which contribute to high torque and shear forces acting on the C1-C2 region. Incomplete ossification of the odontoid process, a relatively large head, and weak neck muscles are other factors that predispose a child to instability of the pediatric cervical spine. These features predispose younger children (<8 years) to upper CSI, SCIWORA, or severe ligamentous injuries and conversely, more fracture-subluxations in the older children.[20,21] Younger children are also much more likely to sustain complete (ASIA Grade A) and severe (ASIA Grade B

and C) cord injuries than older children.[22,23] This trend reflects the inadequacy of the immature vertebral column to protect the spinal cord. Again, complete lesions of the cord are associated more frequently with lower C-spine injuries.[9]

PATHOPHYSIOLOGY

Regardless of the mechanism/etiology of neurotrauma, consequences depend on both primary and secondary injuries. Primary injury (mechanical) occurs at the time of initial impact and results from the displacement of the structures of the brain or spinal cord or both. The primary injury serves as the nidus from which secondary mechanisms of injury evolves in minutes or hours or days and involves a cascade of vascular, cellular, and biochemical events.[24–26] Mild injury elicits fewer inflammatory and secondary sequels than the moderate or severe types.[27,28] These secondary injuries lead to alterations in cell function and propagation of injury through processes such as depolarization, excitotoxicity, disruption of calcium homeostasis, free-radical generation, mitochondrial dysfunction, and membrane damage, which in turn aggravates inflammation, edema, ischemia, and necrosis (Figure 26.2).[29] If timely and expert interventions are delayed, life-threatening intracranial hypertension and herniation (brain) and accentuation of sensory-motor deficit (brain/spinal cord) can soon ensue. The best hope for improving outcome in neurotrauma patients is a better understanding of these processes and the development of therapies that can limit secondary brain injury.

Classification

Primary head injuries can be:

1. Extraaxial (eg, epidural hematoma [EDH], subdural hematoma [SDH], subarachnoid hemorrhage [SAH], and intraventricular hemorrhage [IVH])

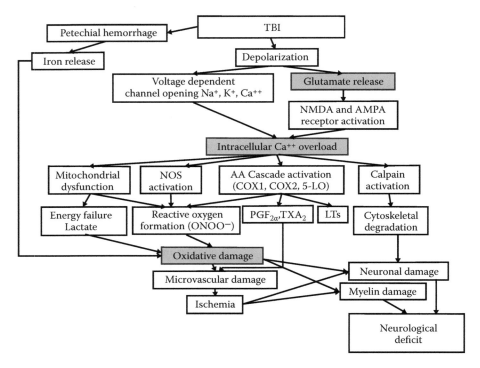

Figure 26.2 Schematic of post-traumatic secondary injury showing the cascade of pathophysiological and pathochemical players and their inter-relationships. Note: AA = Arachidonic acid; AMPA = α-amino-3-hydroxy-5-methyl-4-isoxazolepropionic acid; COX1 = cyclooxygenase 1; COX2 = cyclooxygenase 2; LTs = leukotrienes; NMDA = N-methyl-D-aspartic acid; NOS = nitric oxide synthase; ONOO– = peroxynitrite; PGF2α = prostaglandin 2α; TBI = traumatic brain injury; TXA2 = thromboxane A2; 5-LO = 5-lipoxygenase. (Reprinted from *Comprehensive Medicinal Chemistry II*, In: Taylor JB, Triggle DJ, eds, 2nd ed., Hall ED, Stroke/traumatic brain and spinal cord injuries, 253-277, Copyright 2007, with permission from Elsevier.)

2. Intra-axial (eg, diffuse axonal injury [DAI], cortical contusion, and intracerebral hematoma)
3. Vascular (eg, vascular dissection, carotid cavernous fistula, arteriovenous dural fistula, and pseudo aneurysm)

Secondary injuries include both:

1. Acute injuries (eg, diffuse cerebral swelling, brain herniation, infarction, or infection)
2. Chronic injuries (eg, hydrocephalus, encephalomalacia, cerebrospinal fluid [CSF] leak, and leptomeningeal cyst)

CSI is broadly classified as:

1. Based on their stability (stable versus unstable)
2. Level (axial versus subaxial)
3. Mechanism of injury (hyperflexion, hyperextension, rotation, vertical compression, distraction, and shear forces)

Various patterns of CSI can be:

1. Fracture
2. Fracture without subluxation
3. Subluxation without fracture
4. SCI with radiological abnormality
5. SCIWORA

Imaging evaluation

Computed tomography (CT) of the brain is the mainstay of radiological investigation in the setting of acute TBI. A CT scan of the brain is often combined with a cervical spine CT to rule out CSI, especially when the history of trauma is unclear. CT findings found to be suggestive of nonaccidental injury include combinations of chronic and acute injury, for example, atrophy, ex vacuo dilatation of ventricles, subdural hygromas, subdural hematoma, and multiple acute and chronic extra-axial hematomas. In contrast, skull fractures, intra-parenchymal hematomas, and epidural hematomas have been found to be more common in accidental TBI.[30,31] The limitation of a CT scan includes its low sensitivity in diagnosing diffuse axonal injury (DAI). Patients with DAI may initially have a normal CT scan despite significant neurological findings and increased ICP; a repeat CT scan often shows secondary injury due to cerebral edema.[32] Moreover, the use of ionizing radiation involved in CT scanning limits its practicality for use in the longitudinal studies of children. In contrast, advanced magnetic resonance imaging (MRI) techniques that study microstructural injuries, including diffusion-weighted imaging (DWI), diffusion tensor imaging (DTI), and susceptibility weighted imaging (SWI) have demonstrated an increased sensitivity and specificity to DAI. In addition, MRI findings correlate with neuropsychological and psychiatric outcomes in children.[33]

In suspected CSI, lateral, anteroposterior (AP), and open-mouth odontoid views of the cervical spine should be obtained initially. However, open-mouth odontoid images are difficult to acquire in young children who have a short neck and are often in a collar and unable to open their mouth on command.[34] Of the AP and lateral images routinely acquired, the lateral image has the highest sensitivity to CSI and additional images (odontoid and oblique views) do not increase sensitivity or specificity.[35] Flexion-extension radiography (FER) is not indicated in the setting of an acutely traumatized young child since it places the patient at risk for SCI in the setting of an unstable spine. Moreover, FER offers no additional information when AP and lateral radiographs are normal.[36,37] However, FER is useful in the follow-up evaluation of the child previously found to have ligamentous injury associated with instability.[37] If the patient is medically unstable, cross-table lateral radiography may be performed until the patient's condition permits complete evaluation of the cervical spine.

CT is superior to radiography in detecting cervical spine fractures. Multidetector CT shows exquisite bone detail and allows fast acquisition of thin-section images. Coronal and sagittal reconstructed imaging should be performed routinely. Given the proclivity for ligamentous injury in infants and the insensitivity of CT to ligamentous injury, it is debatable whether CT should be performed at all for suspected CSI in children under

5 years old. MR imaging is especially helpful in evaluating trauma-related SCI. MR imaging facilitates evaluation of the extradural spaces and of the integrity of the spinal ligaments. Increased intraspinous distance, divergence of the articular processes, and widening of the posterior aspect of the disk space are indicative of pediatric cervical spine instability.[38]

Clinical management

INITIAL ASSESSMENT

An aggressive multisystem and multidisciplinary team approach forms the initial pillar of effective management of a trauma victim. Initial assessment in a trauma patient should begin with primary survey (A—Airway maintenance with cervical spine protection, B—Breathing and ventilation, C—Circulation with hemorrhage control, D—Disability, E—Exposure and environmental control) followed by secondary survey (head to toe examination) as emphasized in Advanced Trauma Life Support (ATLS) protocol.[39] Around the time of the secondary survey, clarification of the history is important to ensure that no injuries or relevant comorbidities are missed. And finally, the tertiary survey is a repetition of the secondary survey that again aims to pick up "missed" injuries. This may occur on multiple occasions. The Glasgow Coma Scale (GCS) is the most widely used tool for assessing consciousness. A modified version of the GCS score for assessing consciousness in infants and children is outlined in Table 26.1.[40] In TBI, a GCS score of 13 to 15 signifies mild TBI, 9–12 is moderate TBI, and 3–8 is severe TBI. GCS score ≤ 8 suggests the need for urgent endotracheal (ET) intubation and ventilation, both for airway protection and the management of increased ICP. Predictors of outcome after pediatric TBI are listed in Table 26.2.[41–46]

In suspected CSI, the immobilization of the neck should be ensured until excluded by clinical examination and/or radiological investigation in order to avoid spinal cord compression and aggravation of neurological injury. Several techniques have been used in children to restrict cervical spine movement. These include the application of a spine board with a tape across the forehead, blankets or towels around the forehead, sandbags or rigid cervical collars, depending on the child's age and

Table 26.1 Modified Glasgow Coma Scale (GCS) for infants and children

Area assessed	Infants	Children	Score
Eye opening (E)	Open spontaneously	Open spontaneously	4
	Open in response to verbal stimuli	Open in response to verbal stimuli	3
	Open in response to pain only	Open in response to pain only	2
	No response	No response	1
Verbal response (V)	Coos and babbles	Oriented, appropriate	5
	Irritable cries	Confused	4
	Cries in response to pain	Inappropriate words	3
	Moans in response to pain	Incomprehensible words or non-specific sounds	2
	No response	No response	1
Motor response (M)	Moves spontaneously and purposefully	Obeys commands	6
	Withdraws to touch	Localizes painful stimulus	5
	Withdraws in response to pain	Withdraws in response to pain	4
	Responds to pain with decorticate posturing (abnormal flexion)	Responds to pain with decorticate posturing (abnormal flexion)	3
	Responds to pain with decerebrate posturing (abnormal extension)	Responds to pain with decerebrate posturing (abnormal extension)	2
	No response	No response	1

Source: Adapted from Morray JP et al., Crit Care Med. 1984;12:1018-1020.

Table 26.2 Predictors of poor outcome after pediatric TBI and CSI

TBI	CSI
Younger age	Younger age
High Injury Severity Score (ISS)	Motor vehicle–related mechanism
GCS ≤7	Atlanto-occipital dislocation
Hypoxia (PaO$_2$ <60 mmHg)	Upper cervical injury
Hypotension (SBP <5th percentile for age)	High Injury Severity Score (ISS)
Hyperventilation (PaCO$_2$ <35 mmHg)	Associated closed head injury
Hyperglycemia (glucose >250 mg/dL)	
Hyperthermia (temperature >38°C)	
Immediate blood transfusion (≥20 mL/kg)	
Intracranial hypertension (ICP >20 mmHg)	
Cerebral perfusion pressure <40 mmHg	

physical maturity. In children more than 6 months of age, neck immobilization using a small rigid cervical collar is the most commonly used technique. However, no single technique ensures complete immobilization; indeed a combination of techniques is an effective approach. Since younger children have a prominent occiput, a pad placed under the thoracic spine provides neutral alignment of the spine and avoids excessive flexion that may occur in the supine position.[47] Alternatively, the head can be placed in an occipital recess to achieve a more neutral position for immobilization of the cervical spine. Treloar and Nypaver found that semi-rigid cervical collars placed on children less than 8 years of age did not prevent this positional forced flexion when placed supine on standard, rigid spinal boards.[48] Rapid assessment of the sensory

Table 26.3 Modified American Spinal Injury Association Impairment (ASIA) scale

Grade A	Complete: No motor or sensory function is preserved in the sacral segments S4–S5
Grade B	Sensory incomplete: Sensory but not motor function is preserved below the neurological level (includes sacral segments S4–S5)
Grade C	Motor incomplete: >50% of key muscles below the single neurological level of injury have a muscle strength grade <3
Grade D	Motor incomplete: >50% of key muscles below the single neurological level of injury have a muscle strength grade ≥3
Grade E	Normal: Sensory and motor function normal

Source: Adapted from Kirshblum SC et al., *J Spinal Cord Med.* 2011;34:535-546.

and motor functions helps to determine the level of SCI. The extent of spinal injury is most commonly done using the modified American Spinal Injury Association (ASIA) Impairment Scale (Table 26.3).[49] Predictors of outcome after pediatric CSI have been listed in Table 26.2.[9]

The management of severe neurotrauma in children must be based on a precise strategy including step-by-step increments in both sophisticated neuromonitoring and therapeutic interventions.

AIRWAY MANAGEMENT

The management of a pediatric airway presents a special challenge due to anatomical and physiological differences compared with an adult airway (Table 26.4). Additionally, uncertainties in the diagnosis of CSI, blood, and vomitus in the mouth, laryngopharyngeal injury, and intracranial hypertension following trauma can cause complications during airway management. Inadequate assessment of respiratory status, leading to inadequate resuscitation, can lead to precipitous deterioration and subsequent hypoxia. All TBI patients requiring ET intubation should be presumed to have a full stomach and thus should undergo rapid sequence induction (RSI). However, recently controversies pertaining to RSI have questioned the benefit of this technique.[50] All TBI patients should be presumed to have CSI unless excluded. Extreme caution should be exercised in order to prevent neck movement during laryngoscopy and intubation. Established techniques such as manual in line

Table 26.4 Unique features of the pediatric airway

Anatomical	Physiological
Narrower and highly compliant airways	Obligate nasal breathers (up to 6 months of age)
Larger tongue	Negative intrathoracic pressure is poorly maintained (highly compliant chest wall)
Longer, narrower, and floppy epiglottis	2–3 times higher oxygen consumption—hypoxia is poorly tolerated
Cephalad and anterior larynx	Closing volume greater than functional residual capacity (up to 6–8 years of age)
Acute angulation between epiglottis and larynx	Weak intercostal muscles
Angulated vocal cords	High vagal tone
Funnel-shaped larynx	
Subglottic region—narrowest portion (at the level of cricoid cartilage)	
Shorter trachea	
Smaller and lesser alveoli	
Larger occiput	

stabilization alone or in combination with video laryngoscopes should be used. Flexible fiber-optic laryngoscopy does not seem feasible during emergency situations. Moreover, smooth and gentle intubation should be attempted so as to prevent undue hemodynamic responses and increase of ICP. Nasotracheal intubation should be avoided in basilar skull fractures.[51]

Oxygenation and ventilation

Hypoxemia (PaO_2 < 60 mmHg) linearly increases cerebral blood flow (CBF), cerebral blood volume (CBV), and ICP and thus should be avoided. It is an independent predictor of mortality. In pediatric patients, optimal positive end expiratory pressure (PEEP) that can improve oxygenation without increasing ICP is not exactly defined. In adults, high PEEP therapy has been shown to increase ICP and compromise CPP.[52,53] Hyperventilation reduces ICP at the expense of cerebral blood flow (CBF) and cerebral perfusion pressure (CPP). The effects on CBF are compounded in the multisystem trauma patient with TBI whose injuries place them at greater risk for superimposed hypotension. The beneficial effects of hyperventilation are at best short-lived and predicated on delaying herniation to allow more definitive interventions. The 2012 pediatric TBI guidelines recommended avoidance of prophylactic severe hyperventilation to a $PaCO_2$ < 30 mmHg within the first 48 hours of TBI. If hyperventilation is to be used, advanced neuromonitoring for evaluating cerebral ischemia may be considered (Level III evidence).[54]

Circulatory support

Hypotension frequently accompanies TBI in children. The causes are multifactorial. These include acute blood loss from polytrauma (50%),[55] scalp laceration,[15,16] extensive intracranial hemorrhage, and neurogenic hypotension resulting from the exhaustion of endogenous catecholamines.[56] Hypotension is independently associated with an increased mortality rate in children with TBI.[44,57] The degree and duration of relative hypotension that can safely be tolerated by children remains unclear. While systolic blood pressure (SBP)<5th percentile defines hypotension, in the absence of ICP monitoring and suspected increased ICP, supranormal systemic BP may be needed in order

to maintain cerebral perfusion pressure (CPP).[58] Isotonic crystalloid solutions (0.9% normal saline, plasmalyte-A) are commonly used for cerebral resuscitation. Hypotonic crystalloids should be avoided and the role of colloids is controversial. Hypertonic saline (HS) solutions have the advantages of efficiently increasing arterial pressure with a small volume resuscitation and decreasing intracranial hypertension.[59] When vascular loading is insufficient to maintain arterial pressure, vasopressors must be added rapidly. Both noradrenaline and phenylephrine have been shown to produce a consistent and predictable effect in increasing MAP and augmenting CPP.[60,61]

Coagulopathy and transfusion trigger

Anemia is common in patients with severe TBI and can result in decreased cerebral oxygen delivery and secondary brain injury.[62] Acute traumatic coagulopathy (ATC) is an acquired coagulation disorder that has been described in the context of isolated TBI. Blood loss and hemodilution secondary to fluid resuscitation is not the most likely mechanism for coagulopathy associated with head injury.[63] Direct injury with the activation of coagulation by tissue factor, insufficient control of fibrinogenesis and fibrinolysis, platelet function abnormalities, abnormalities of protein C, elevated thrombomodulin, activation of inflammatory mediators, and reduction of factor V levels may all play a role in the causation of ATC. Risk factors for ATC in children include GCS ≤8, increasing age, a higher severity of illness score, and brain contusions/lacerations.[64] Coagulation function may be further compromised by hypoperfusion, hypothermia, acidosis, and hypocalcemia. Therefore, early monitoring of the coagulation profile and correction are warranted. In a recent systematic review and meta-analysis, Epstein et al. reported that ATC was uniformly associated with high transfusion rates of 41% and high mortality (17% to 86%).[65] Little is known regarding optimal RBC transfusion practices in pediatric patients with TBI. A recent retrospective study reviewed outcomes in 1607 pediatric patients with TBI, of which 178 received RBC transfusion.[66] The authors demonstrated that RBC transfusions in these patients were associated with poor outcomes and increased mortality. They, therefore, suggested that a transfusion trigger of 8.0 g/dl be considered in children with TBI.

Future studies will need to consider additional triggers (eg, PbtO$_2$), timing, and dose of packed RBC, while minimizing confounding.

Glycemic control

Hyperglycemia worsens outcome after pediatric TBI.[45,67,68] Causes of hyperglycemia after TBI include an increase in gluconeogenesis and glycogenolysis from catecholamine response, cortisol release, and glucose intolerance.[69-71] As such, dextrose containing fluids should ideally be avoided except in cases of established hypoglycaemia. However, aggressive treatment of hyperglycemia should also be performed cautiously due to the potential for an increased risk of hypoglycemia and its potentially devastating neurologic consequences if unrecognized and untreated.[72] Given the potential impact of both hyperglycemia and hypoglycemia, intermittent monitoring of blood glucose concentrations during intraoperative care is suggested.

Temperature management

Earlier studies showed an improvement in neurological outcome following initiation of moderate hypothermia (32–33°C) in children with severe TBI.[73-75] However, recent studies have shown no benefit of moderate hypothermia versus normothermia in pediatric TBI.[76-78] The 2012 pediatric TBI guidelines emphasized that moderate hypothermia beginning within 8 hours after severe TBI for up to 48 hours duration (Level II evidence) can be used as a neuro-protective measure and for refractory intracranial hypertension. Rewarming at a rate more than 0.5°C should be avoided.[54] Moreover, the therapeutic effects of hypothermia is offset by complications like hypotension, bradycardia, arrhythmias, hyperglycemia, sepsis, coagulopathy, and rebound increase in ICP during and after rewarming.[79,80]

Hyperthermia, on the other hand, invariably worsens prognosis after TBI. The pathophysiologic mechanism includes fever induced increased metabolic demand, lipid peroxidation, inflammation and excitotoxicity, and reduction of seizure threshold.[46,81]

Nutritional support

Nutritional support is an important component of the care of the neurotrauma patient. Caloric expenditure in such patients can be almost twice that of the expected resting energy expenditure (REE) and may be influenced by temperature, muscle tone, GCS, and time of measurement in relation to injury.[82] There is a significantly greater mortality rate as a consequence of undernutrition for a 2-week period after injury, when compared with receiving full nutrition by 7 days.[83] Fewer infectious and overall complications have been demonstrated by starting feedings that meet the estimated energy and nitrogen requirements on day one following injury.[84] As such, nutritional support should begin by 72 hours with full replacement by the 7th day. The 2012 pediatric TBI guidelines does not support the use of an immune-modulating diet to improve outcome.[54]

Intracranial hypertension

The normal ICP in children and term infants ranges from 3–7 mmHg and 1.5–6 mmHg, respectively.[85] The etiology of an increase in ICP after TBI is multifactorial. It can be due to a traumatic mass lesion, vascular engorgement, and/or cerebral edema.[86] The optimal ICP threshold for pediatric TBI is not yet defined. The 2012 pediatric TBI guidelines recommended that immediate intervention should be undertaken at ICP ≥20 mmHg (Level III evidence) with the aim of maintaining CPP >40 mmHg (Level III evidence).[54] Specifically, in the age groups 2–6, 7–10, and 11–16 years, CPP values of 43, 54, and 58 mmHg, respectively, have been shown to be associated with good outcomes.[87] Various initial measures to reduce ICP includes head up position (up to 30°), sedation and analgesia, intubation and controlled mechanical ventilation, CSF drainage, diuretics/osmotherapy (mannitol, HS), and controlled hyperventilation. In refractory cases barbiturate coma, moderate hypothermia, and surgical decompression may be helpful.

STEROIDS

A number of studies in adults including the large multicenter CRASH study have shown no benefit of steroid use in TBI.[88-90] Complications like adrenal suppression, hyperglycemia, increased risk of infection, and gastrointestinal bleeding attributed to steroid administration have been shown to worsen outcome. The 2012 pediatric TBI guidelines also stated that there is no role for steroids to improve outcome or lower ICP in TBI patients (Level II evidence).[54]

Antiseizure prophylaxis

Post-traumatic seizure (PTS) rates as high as 19% have been reported in children with severe TBI.[91] PTS most commonly occurs within the first 24 hours after injury.[92] PTS affect patients through multiple mechanisms: increasing or prolonging cerebral hypoxia, increasing the release of excitotoxic neurotransmitters, increasing $CMRO_2$ and ICP, and causing fluctuations in systemic BP.[93,94] Younger age (<2 years), mechanism of injury (non-accidental trauma), GCS ≤8, skull fracture, and the presence of a subdural hematoma have all been shown to be associated with higher rates of early (within 7 days of injury) PTS following severe TBI.[95–97]

Prophylactic administration of phenytoin has been shown to reduce the incidence of early PTS, but not late PTS (after 7 days of injury).[98,99] The 2012 pediatric TBI guidelines also recommended the prophylactic use of phenytoin to reduce the incidence of early PTS (Level III evidence).[54]

Antibiotic prophylaxis

The risk of infection is much higher in pediatric TBI (particularly penetrating brain injury) and is associated with higher morbidity and mortality.[100] Local wound infection, meningitis, ventriculitis, or cerebral abscess formation may be caused by a contaminated foreign object and the presence of skin, hair, bone fragments, or other materials inside the brain. The incidence is even higher if there is a CSF leak, air sinus injury, transventricular injury, or injuries crossing the midline. Broad spectrum antibiotic prophylaxis is universally recommended to be started as early as possible in all TBI cases and continued for at least 6 weeks.[101]

NEUROMONITORING

The goal of neuromonitoring is to supplement the continuous evaluation of the head-injured patient beyond what serial neurologic exams and serial imaging can provide. ICP monitoring may be considered for children who have an abnormal initial head CT scan and an initial GCS score <8.[102]

Typically, the choice of monitor is between an intraparenchymal device and an intraventricular device connected by a catheter to an external drain gauge. However, it is still unclear whether ICP monitoring improves the outcome of severe TBI in children. In a recent U.S. National Trauma Database review of pediatric patients with severe TBI from 2001 to 2006, only 7.7% of patients meeting the criteria underwent ICP monitoring. Notably, ICP monitoring in this study was associated with decreased mortality only when the GCS was 3, but was associated with a longer ICU stay, longer hospitalization, and more days on the ventilator, potentially reflecting the population most likely to be chosen to undergo monitoring.[103]

Other monitoring modalities such as brain tissue oxygen tension, transcranial Doppler, jugular venous oximetry, cerebral microdialysis, and near-infrared reflective spectroscopy have shown variable results regarding favorable outcome in pediatric TBI. As such, the role of multimodal monitoring is now evolving to obtain real-time information and aiming for faster responses in management.

BIOMARKERS

Investigations into various biomarkers have been utilized as an adjunct to predicting neurological outcomes in the pediatric TBI. Ubiquitin c-terminal hydrolase (UCH-L1), alpha II spectrin breakdown product 145 kDa (SPDP 145), glial fibrillary acidic protein (GFAP), neuron-specific enolase (NSE), S100B, and myelin basic protein (MBP) have specifically been investigated. Increases in UCH-L1 and alpha II spectrin and SPDP 145 have specifically been seen in pediatric subjects with moderate and severe TBI. UCH-L1 and SPDP 145 have also been found to have a stronger correlation with the Glasgow Outcome Scale than NSE, S100B, and MBP.[104] GFAP is not found outside the central nervous system and is thus a more specific biomarker.[105] Correlation between various biomarkers to different subtypes of brain injuries can be tested to provide a stronger and more specific prognostic value to particular markers.

SURGICAL INDICATIONS

The perioperative period is an extension of ongoing resuscitation with the goals of restricting further

Table 26.5 Indications for surgery in neurotrauma

Indications for operative management in TBI	Indications for operative management in CSI
1. Open, compound, depressed compound fracture that causes a mass effect	1. Irreducible fracture subluxation
2. Clinical deterioration	2. Unstable fractures requiring stabilization
3. More than 1 cm thick extracerebral clot, more than 25 ml intracerebral hematoma	3. Pure ligamentous instability
4. Midline shift >5 mm	4. Progressive deformity
5. Enlargement of contralateral ventricle	5. Compression of neural structures
6. Raised or increasing intracranial pressure (ICP)	

injury and preventing secondary insults. The majority of surgeries following TBI deal with the removal of mass lesions mainly to relieve dangerous tissue shifts and decrease globally increased ICP and thus prevent life threatening herniation. On the contrary, the vast majority of pediatric CSI can be effectively treated nonoperatively. The most effective immobilization appears to be accomplished with either halo devices or Minerva jackets. The specific treatment varies with the injury types. SCIWORA is, by definition, not associated with overt instability and therefore only requires external immobilization.[106] The outcome of spinal injuries in children is more favorable than in adults, especially in patients with incomplete injuries. This is attributed to plasticity and capacity for greater functional recovery of the immature spinal cord. However, the prognosis for children with complete SCI is still gloomy. Common indications for operative management in TBI and CSI are listed in Table 26.5.

REHABILITATION

Apart from the therapeutic strategies described above, a multidisciplinary rehabilitation approach should be employed to promote early recovery and facilitate a smooth transition to positive long term outcomes.[107,108] Attention must be given to maintain adequate oxygenation and stability of blood pressure. Appropriate analgesia (multimodal approach) and sedation should be ensured to prevent deleterious complications of pain. Early tracheostomy is recommended to reduce mechanical ventilation days when the overall benefit is felt to outweigh the complications associated with such a procedure. However, there is no evidence that early tracheostomy reduces mortality or the rate of nosocomial pneumonia. Optimizing glucose levels, temperature, electrolytes and acid-base status, correcting coagulation abnormalities, and ensuring optimal nutritional support should be the utmost concerns. In addition, early mobilization, vocational and speech rehabilitation, occupational therapy, and peer acquaintance should be instituted simultaneously for early improved outcomes.

SUMMARY

Neurotrauma continues to increase as a cause of fatality worldwide. As access to motorized transportation expands, more children are subjected to risk as passengers, pedestrians, and cyclists in contexts in which traffic and vehicle safety developments may not have kept pace with the increase in volume. Children have unique injury patterns and responses to injury. The next evolution in neurotrauma care may be towards adding more sophisticated management algorithms into the care of patients, based on an individual patient's unique pathophysiology of injury. This care might be guided by using advanced imaging and monitoring techniques that might allow targeted treatment and individualized treatment thresholds. Effective neuroprotection or neurorescue therapy is desperately needed for both TBI and SCI. Attention should be paid to employ effective rehabilitation to ultimately restore quality of life and dignity after trauma.

REFERENCES

1. Heron M, Sutton PD, Xu J, Ventura SJ, Strobino DM, Guyer B. Annual summary of vital statistics: 2007. *Pediatrics*. 2010;125:4-15.

2. Faul M, Coronado V. Epidemiology of traumatic brain injury. *Handb Clin Neurol.* 2015;127:3-13.

3. Faul M, Xu L, Wald MM, Coronado VG. Traumatic Brain Injury in the United States: Emergency Department Visits, Hospitalizations and Deaths 2002–2006. Atlanta (GA): Centers for Disease Control and Prevention, National Center for Injury Prevention and Control; 2010.

4. Keenan HT, Runyan DK, Marshall SW, Nocera MA, Merten DF, Sinal SH. A population-based study of inflicted traumatic brain injury in young children. *JAMA.* 2003;290:621-626.

5. Haider AH, Efron DT, Haut ER, DiRusso SM, Sullivan T, Cornwell EE 3rd. Black children experience worse clinical and functional outcomes after traumatic brain injury: An analysis of the national pediatric trauma registry. *J Trauma.* 2007;62:1259–1262.

6. Patel JC, Tepas JJ 3rd, Mollitt DL, Pieper P. Pediatric cervical spine injuries: Defining the disease. *J Pediatr Surg.* 2001;36: 373-376.

7. Hall DE, Boydston W. Pediatric neck injuries. *Pediatr Rev.* 1999;20:13-9.

8. Apple DF Jr, Anson CA, Hunter JD, Bell RB. Spinal cord injury in youth. *Clin Pediatr.* 1995;34:90-95.

9. Brown RL, Brunn MA, Garcia VF. Cervical spine injuries in children: A review of 103 patients treated consecutively at a level 1 pediatric trauma center. *J Pediatr Surg.* 2001;36:1107-1114.

10. Carreon LY, Glassman SD, Campbell MJ. Pediatric spine fractures: A review of 137 hospital admissions. *J Spinal Disord Tech.* 2004;17(6):477-482.

11. Wang MY, Hoh DJ, Leary SP, Griffith P, McComb JG. High rates of neurological improvement following severe traumatic pediatric spinal cord injury. *Spine (Phila Pa 1976).* 2004;29:1493-1497.

12. Michael DB, Guyot DR, Darmody WR. Coincidence of head and cervical spine injury. *J Neurotrauma.* 1989;6:177-189.

13. Givens TG, Polley KA, Smith GF, Hardin WD Jr. Pediatric cervical spine injury: A three-year experience. *J Trauma.* 1996;41:310-314.

14. Birney TJ, Hanley EN Jr. Traumatic cervical spine injuries in childhood and adolescence. *Spine.* 1989;14:1277-1282.

15. Araki T, Yokota H, Morita A. Pediatric traumatic brain injury: Characteristic features, diagnosis, and management. *Neurol Med Chir (Tokyo).* 2017;57:82-93.

16. Bhalla T, Dewhirst E, Sawardekar A, Dairo O, Tobias JD. Perioperative management of the pediatric patient with traumatic brain injury. *Paediatr Anaesth.* 2012;22:627-640.

17. Ragan DK, McKinstry R, Benzinger T, Leonard J, Pineda JA. Depression of whole–brain oxygen extraction fraction is associated with poor outcome in pediatric traumatic brain injury. *Pediatr Res.* 2012;71:199-204.

18. Pryds O. Control of cerebral circulation in the high-risk neonate. *Ann Neurol.* 1991;30:321-329.

19. Soriano SG III, McManus ML. Pediatric neuroanesthesia and critical care. In: Cottrell JE, Patel P, eds. *Cottrell and Patel's NEUROANESTHESIA.* 6th ed. Philadelphia: Elsevier; 2016:337-350.

20. Dickman CA, Zabramski JM, Hadley MN, Rekate HL, Sonntag VK. Pediatric spinal cord injury without radiographic abnormalities: Report of 26 cases and review of the literature. *J Spinal Disord.* 1991;4:296-305.

21. Apple JS, Kirks DR, Merten DF, Martinez S. Cervical spine fractures and dislocations in children. *Pediatr Radiol.* 1987;17:45-49.

22. Hadley MN, Zabramski JM, Browner CM, Rekate H, Sonntag VK. Pediatric spinal trauma. Review of 122 cases of spinal cord and vertebral column injuries. *J Neurosurg.* 1988;68:18-24.

23. Hamilton MG, Myles ST. Pediatric spinal injury: Review of 174 hospital admissions. *J Neurosurg.* 1992;77:700-704.

24. Prins M, Greco T, Alexander D, Giza CC. The pathophysiology of traumatic brain injury at a glance. *Dis Model Mech.* 2013;6:1307-1315.

25. Anderson AJ. Mechanisms and pathways of inflammatory responses in CNS trauma: Spinal cord injury. *J Spinal Cord Med.* 2002;25:70-79.

26. Greve MW, Zink BJ. Pathophysiology of traumatic brain injury. *Mt Sinai J Med.* 2009;76:97-104.

27. Kloos AD, Fisher LC, Detloff MR, Hassenzahl DL, Basso DM. Stepwise motor and all-or-none sensory recovery is associated with nonlinear sparing after incremental spinal cord injury in rats. *Exp Neurol.* 2005;191:251-265.

28. Siegenthaler MM, Tu MK, Keirstead HS. The extent of myelin pathology differs following contusion and transection spinal cord injury. *J Neurotrauma.* 2007;24:1631-1646.

29. Hall ED. Stroke/traumatic brain and spinal cord injuries. In: Taylor JB, Triggle DJ, eds. *Comprehensive Medicinal Chemistry II.* 2nd ed. New York: Elsevier; 2007:253-277.

30. Ewing-Cobbs L, Prasad M, Kramer L et al. Acute neuroradiologic findings in young children with inflicted or noninflicted traumatic brain injury. *Childs Nerv Syst.* 2000;16:25-33.

31. Keenan HT, Runyan DK, Marshall SW, Nocera MA, Merten DF. A population-based comparison of clinical and outcome characteristics of young children with serious inflicted and noninflicted traumatic brain injury. *Pediatrics.* 2004;114:633-639.

32. Hollingworth W, Vavilala MS, Jarvik JG et al. The use of repeated head computed tomography in pediatric blunt head trauma: Factors predicting new and worsening brain injury. *Pediatr Crit Care Med.* 2007;8:348-356.

33. Smitherman E, Hernandez A, Stavinoha PL et al. Predicting outcome after pediatric traumatic brain injury by early magnetic resonance imaging lesion location and volume. *J Neurotrauma.* 2016;33:35-48.

34. Buhs C, Cullen M, Klein M, Farmer D. The pediatric trauma C-spine: Is the 'odontoid' view necessary? *J Pediatr Surg.* 2000; 35:994-997.

35. Silva CT, Doria AS, Traubici J, Moineddin R, Davila J, Shroff M. Do additional views improve the diagnostic performance of cervical spine radiography in pediatric trauma? *Am J Roentgenol.* 2010;194:500-508.

36. Dwek JR, Chung CB. Radiography of cervical spine injury in children: Are flexion-extension radiographs useful for acute trauma? *Am J Roentgenol.* 2000;174:1617-1619.

37. Ralston ME, Chung K, Barnes PD, Emans JB, Schutzman SA. Role of flexion-extension radiographs in blunt pediatric cervical spine injury. *Acad Emerg Med.* 2001;8:237-245.

38. Lustrin ES, Karakas SP, Ortiz AO et al. Pediatric cervical spine: Normal anatomy, variants, and trauma. *Radiographics.* 2003;23:539-560.

39. ATLS Subcommittee; American College of Surgeons' Committee on Trauma; International ATLS working group et al. Advanced trauma life support (ATLS®): The ninth edition. *J Trauma Acute Care Surg.* 2013;74:1363-1366.

40. Morray JP, Tyler DC, Jones TK, Stuntz JT, Lemire RJ. Coma scale for use in brain-injured children. *Crit Care Med.* 1984; 12:1018-1020.

41. Chiaretti A, Piastra M, Pulitanò S et al. Prognostic factors and outcome of children with severe head injury: An 8-year experience. *Childs Nerv Syst.* 2002;18:129-136.

42. Marshall LF, Becker DP, Bowers SA et al. The national traumatic coma data bank. Part 1: Design, purpose, goals, and results. *J Neurosurg.* 1983;59:276-284.

43. Tepas JJ 3rd, DiScala C, Ramenofsky ML, Barlow B. Mortality and head injury: The pediatric perspective. *J Pediatr Surg.* 1990;25:92-95.

44. Luerssen TG, Klauber MR, Marshall LF. Outcome from head injury related to patient's age. A longitudinal prospective study of adult and pediatric head injury. *J Neurosurg.* 1988;68:409-416.

45. Elkon B, Cambrin JR, Hirshberg E, Bratton SL. Hyperglycemia: An independent risk factor for poor outcome in children with traumatic brain injury. *Pediatr Crit Care Med.* 2014;15:623-623.

46. Natale JE, Joseph JG, Helfaer MA, Shaffner DH. Early hyperthermia after traumatic brain injury in children: Risk factors, influence on length of stay, and effect on short-term

neurologic status. *Crit Care Med.* 2000; 28:2608-2615.

47. Kannan N, Ramaiah R, Vavilala MS. Pediatric neurotrauma. *Int J Crit Illn Inj Sci.* 2014; 4:131-137.

48. Treloar DJ, Nypaver M. Angulation of the pediatric cervical spine with and without cervical collar. *Pediatr Emerg Care.* 1997; 13:5-8.

49. Kirshblum SC, Burns SP, Biering-Sorensen F et al. International standards for neurological classification of spinal cord injury (revised 2011). *J Spinal Cord Med.* 2011; 34:535-546.

50. El-Orbany M, Connolly LA. Rapid sequence induction and intubation: Current controversy. *Anesth Analg.* 2010;110:1318-1325.

51. Tobias JD. Airway management for pediatric emergencies. *Pediatr Ann.* 1996;25:317-320, 323-328.

52. Shapiro HM, Marshall LF. Intracranial pressure responses to PEEP in head-injured patients. *J Trauma.* 1978;18:254-256.

53. Videtta W, Villarejo F, Cohen M et al. Effects of positive end-expiratory pressure on intracranial pressure and cerebral perfusion pressure. *Acta Neurochir Suppl.* 2002; 81:93-97.

54. Kochanek PM, Carney N, Adelson PD et al. Guidelines for the acute medical management of severe traumatic brain injury in infants, children, and adolescents—Second edition. *Pediatr Crit Care Med.* 2012;13 (Suppl 1):S1-82.

55. Orliaguet GA, Meyer PG, Blanot S et al. Predictive factors of outcome in severely traumatized children. *Anesth Analg.* 1998; 87:537-542.

56. Chesnut RM, Gautille T, Blunt BA, Klauber MR, Marshall LF. Neurogenic hypotension in patients with severe head injuries. *J Trauma.* 1998;44:958-963.

57. Pigula FA, Wald SL, Shackford SR, Vane DW. The effect of hypotension and hypoxia on children with severe head injuries. *J Pediatr Surg.* 1993;28:310-314.

58. Williams M, Lee JK. Intraoperative blood pressure and cerebral perfusion: Strategies to clarify hemodynamic goals. *Paediatr Anaesth.* 2014; 24:657-667.

59. Simma B, Burger R, Falk M, Sacher P, Fanconi S. A prospective, randomized, and controlled study of fluid management in children with severe head injury: Lactated Ringer's solution versus hypertonic saline. *Crit Care Med.* 1998;26:1265-1270.

60. Kroppenstedt SN, Sakowitz OW, Thomale UW, Unterberg AW, Stover JF. Norepinephrine is superior to dopamine in increasing cortical perfusion following controlled cortical impact injury in rats. *Acta Neurochir Suppl.* 2002;81:225-227.

61. Sookplung P, Siriussawakul A, Malakouti A et al. Vasopressor use and effect on blood pressure after severe adult traumatic brain injury. *Neurocrit Care.* 2011;15:46-54.

62. LeRoux P. Haemoglobin management in acute brain injury. *Curr Opin Crit Care.* 2013;19:83-91.

63. Zhang J, Jiang R, Liu L, Watkins T, Zhang F, Dong JF. Traumatic brain injury-associated coagulopathy. *J Neurotrauma.* 2012;29: 2597-2605.

64. Talving P, Lustenberger T, Lam L et al. Coagulopathy after isolated severe traumatic brain injury in children. *J Trauma.* 2011;71:1205-1210.

65. Epstein DS, Mitra B, O'Reilly G, Rosenfeld JV, Cameron PA. Acute traumatic coagulopathy in the setting of isolated traumatic brain injury: A systematic review and meta-analysis. *Injury.* 2014;45:819-824.

66. Acker SN, Partrick DA, Ross JT, Nadlonek NA, Bronsert M, Bensard DD. Blood component transfusion increases the risk of death in children with traumatic brain injury. *J Trauma Acute Care Surg.* 2014;76: 1082-1087.

67. Smith RL, Lin JC, Adelson PD et al. Relationship between hyperglycemia and outcome in children with severe traumatic brain injury. *Pediatr Crit Care Med.* 2012; 13:85-91.

68. Cochran A, Scaife ER, Hansen KW, Downey EC. Hyperglycemia and outcomes from pediatric traumatic brain injury. *J Trauma.* 2003;55:1035-1038.

69. Sharma D, Jelacic J, Chennuri R, Chaiwat O, Chandler W, Vavilala MS. Incidence and risk factors for perioperative hyperglycemia in

children with traumatic brain injury. *Anesth Analg.* 2009;108:81-89.

70. Young B, Ott L, Dempsey R, Haack D, Tibbs P. Relationship between admission hyperglycemia and neurologic outcome of severely brain-injured patients. *Ann Surg.* 1989;210:466-472.

71. Lipshutz AK, Gropper MA. Perioperative glycemic control: An evidence-based review. *Anesthesiology.* 2009;110:408-421.

72. Bilotta F, Caramia R, Cernak I et al. Intensive insulin therapy after severe traumatic brain injury: A randomized clinical trial. *Neurocrit Care.* 2008;9:159-166.

73. Hendrick EB. The use of hypothermia in severe head injuries in childhood. *Arch Surg.* 1959;79:362-364.

74. Biswas AK, Bruce DA, Sklar FH, Bokovoy JL, Sommerauer JF. Treatment of acute traumatic brain injury in children with moderate hypothermia improves intracranial hypertension. *Crit Care Med.* 2002;30:2742-2751.

75. Adelson PD, Ragheb J, Kanev P et al. Phase II clinical trial of moderate hypothermia after severe traumatic brain injury in children. *Neurosurgery.* 2005;56:740-754.

76. Hutchison JS, Ward RE, Lacroix J et al. Hypothermia therapy after traumatic brain injury in children. *N Engl J Med.* 2008; 358:2447-2456.

77. Beca J, McSharry B, Erickson S et al. Hypothermia for traumatic brain injury in children—A phase II randomized controlled trial. *Crit Care Med.* 2015;43:1458-1466.

78. Tasker RC. Hypothermia did not improve mortality or disability in severe traumatic brain injury. *Arch Dis Child Educ Pract Ed.* 2014;99:119.

79. Bourdages M, Bigras JL, Farrell CA, Hutchison JS, Lacroix J; Canadian Critical Care Trials Group. Cardiac arrhythmias associated with severe traumatic brain injury and hypothermia therapy. *Pediatr Crit Care Med.* 2010;11:408-414.

80. Sandestig A, Romner B, Grände PO. Therapeutic hypothermia in children and adults with severe traumatic brain injury. *Ther Hypothermia Temp Manag.* 2014; 4:10-20.

81. Bao L, Chen D, Ding L, Ling W, Xu F. Fever burden is an independent predictor for prognosis of traumatic brain injury. *PLoS One.* 2014;9:e90956.

82. Clifton GL, Robertson CS, Grossman RG, Hodge S, Foltz R, Garza C. The metabolic response to severe head injury. *J Neurosurg.* 1984; 60: 687-96.

83. Rapp RP, Young B, Twyman D et al. The favorable effect of early parenteral feeding on survival in head-injured patients. *J Neurosurg.* 1983;58:906-912.

84. Taylor SJ, Fettes SB, Jewkes C, Nelson RJ. Prospective, randomized, controlled trial to determine the effect of early enhanced enteral nutrition on clinical outcome in mechanically ventilated patients suffering head injury. *Crit Care Med.* 1999;27:2525-2531.

85. Dunn LT. Raised intracranial pressure. *J Neurol Neurosurg Psychiatry.* 2002;73 (Suppl 1):i23-i27.

86. Kukreti V, Mohseni-Bod H, Drake J. Management of raised intracranial pressure in children with traumatic brain injury. *J Pediatr Neurosci.* 2014;9:207-215.

87. Chambers IR, Stobbart L, Jones PA et al. Age-related differences in intracranial pressure and cerebral perfusion pressure in the first 6 hours of monitoring after children's head injury: Association with outcome. *Childs Nerv Syst.* 2005;21:195-199.

88. Gudeman SK, Miller JD, Becker DP. Failure of high-dose steroid therapy to influence intracranial pressure in patients with severe head injury. *J Neurosurg.* 1979;51:301-306.

89. Saul TG, Ducker TB, Salcman M, Carro E. Steroids in severe head injury: A prospective randomized clinical trial. *J Neurosurg.* 1981;54:596-600.

90. Edwards P, Arango M, Balica L et al. Final results of MRC CRASH, a randomised placebo-controlled trial of intravenous corticosteroid in adults with head injury-outcomes at 6 months. *Lancet.* 2005;365: 1957-1959.

91. Arango JI, Deibert CP, Brown D et al. Posttraumatic seizures in children with severe traumatic brain injury. *Childs Nerv Syst.* 2012;28:1925-1929.

92. Mazzola CA, Adelson PD. Critical care management of head trauma in children. *Crit Care Med*. 2002;30:S393-S401.

93. Engel J Jr, Kuhl DE, Phelps ME, Rausch R, Nuwer M. Local cerebral metabolism during partial seizures. *Neurology*. 1983;33:400-413.

94. Hunt RF, Boychuk JA, Smith BN. Neural circuit mechanisms of post-traumatic epilepsy. *Front Cell Neurosci*. 2013;7:89.

95. Liesemer K, Bratton SL, Zebrack CM, Brockmeyer D, Statler KD. Early posttraumatic seizures in moderate to severe pediatric traumatic brain injury: Rates, risk factors, and clinical features. *J Neurotrauma*. 2011;28:755-762.

96. Chung MG, O'Brien NF. Prevalence of early posttraumatic seizures in children with moderate to severe traumatic brain injury despite levetiracetam prophylaxis. *Pediatr Crit Care Med*. 2016;17:150-156.

97. O'Neill BR, Handler MH, Tong S, Chapman KE. Incidence of seizures on continuous EEG monitoring following traumatic brain injury in children. *J Neurosurg Pediatr*. 2015;16:167-176.

98. Lewis RJ, Yee L, Inkelis SH, Gilmore D. Clinical predictors of post-traumatic seizures in children with head trauma. *Ann Emerg Med*. 1993;22:1114-1118.

99. Khan AA, Banerjee A. The role of prophylactic anticonvulsants in moderate to severe head injury. *Int J Emerg Med*. 2010;3:187-191.

100. Koestler J, Keshavarz R. Penetrating head injury in children: A case report and review of the literature. *J Emerg Med*. 2001;21:145-150.

101. Pruitt BA. Guidelines for the management of penetrating brain injuries. *J Trauma*. 2001;51:S1-S86.

102. Hu CF, Fan HC, Chang CF, Chen SJ. Current approaches to the treatment of head injury in children. *Pediatr Neonatol*. 2013;54:73-81.

103. Alkhoury F, Kyriakides TC. Intracranial pressure monitoring in children with severe traumatic brain injury: National trauma data bank-based review of outcomes. *JAMA Surg*. 2014;149:544-548.

104. Berger RP, Beers SR, Richichi R, Wiesman D, Adelson PD. Serum biomarker concentrations and outcome after pediatric traumatic brain injury. *J Neurotrauma*. 2007;24:1793-1801.

105. Fraser DD, Close TE, Rose KL et al. Severe traumatic brain injury in children elevates glial fibrillary acidic protein in cerebrospinal fluid and serum. *Pediatr Crit Care Med*. 2011;12:319-324.

106. Pang D, Pollack IF. Spinal cord injury without radiographic abnormality in children—The SCIWORA syndrome. *J Trauma*. 1989;29:654-664.

107. Popernack ML, Gray N, Reuter-Rice K. Moderate-to-severe traumatic brain injury in children: Complications and rehabilitation strategies. *J Pediatr Health Care*. 2015;29:e1-e7.

108. Forsyth R, Basu A. The promotion of recovery through rehabilitation after acquired brain injury in children. *Dev Med Child Neurol*. 2015;57:16-22.

27

Geriatric neurotrauma

HOSSAM EL BEHEIRY

INTRODUCTION

Elderly neurotrauma patients have distinct characteristics requiring special considerations pertaining to their perioperative management. These elderly neurotrauma patients may undergo neurosurgical and non-neurosurgical procedures during their hospital stay for urgent, semi-urgent or elective surgery. Anesthesia can be challenging. A careful understanding of the mechanisms of neurologic injury and its effects on neurologic function as well as the physiologic and pharmacologic changes of aging is essential in order to deliver safe anesthesia for this subpopulation of unfortunate patients.

EPIDEMIOLOGY, MECHANISMS, AND PATHOPHYSIOLOGY OF INJURY

The epidemiologic patterns in traumatic brain injury (TBI) show an overall decrease, but in elderly patients, this incidence is increasing. Studies from North America and Europe have reported increased rates of neurotrauma in the elderly ranging from 7%–34%. In this elderly subpopulation, falls are the leading cause of TBI followed by motor vehicle accidents and struck pedestrian injuries.[1] Similarly, spinal cord injuries (SCI) are increasing among the elderly. For example, the SCI rate went from 84 cases/million to 131 cases/million in men aged 65 to 74 years. Much of this increase was due to falls.[2]

The pathophysiologic effects of TBI in the elderly, as in the general population, include primary and secondary effects.[3] Primary effects are the result of the traumatic impact and cause skull fractures, intracranial hemorrhages, brain contusion, or diffuse axonal injury. Traumatic subdural hemorrhages are more common in the elderly because of shrunken brain size, increased use of anticoagulants, and a higher likelihood of uncontrolled hypertensive heart disease. Primary effects of injury initiate a cascade of secondary effects in the form of brain ischemia and inflammation leading to cerebral edema, increased ICP, and apoptosis. Secondary effects can be enhanced by hypoxia, hypotension, hypercarbia, and hyperglycemia, which are more likely to occur in the elderly patient. In contrast, SCI effects are generally due to the initial primary physical injury and disruption of the spinal cord. Geriatric patients are much more predisposed to traumatic SCI because of degenerative changes in the spinal column, that is, disc space collapse, ligamentum flavum buckling, and osteophyte development. Such degenerative changes can result in spinal stenosis, cord compression, and clinical myelopathy. Additionally, these degenerative changes result in the creation of a rigid spinal column, so that an application of an external traumatic force on the spine is not dissipated and becomes focused on a limited area, resulting in a fracture and SCI. Usually, SCIs in the elderly tend to be incomplete (American Spinal Injury Association Grades C and D), with preservation of neurological function below the lesion or area of injury.[4] Secondary injury of the spinal cord results from ischemia, excitoxicity, and initiation of inflammatory processes.

PHYSIOLOGIC IMPLICATIONS OF NORMAL AGING FOR THE PATHOPHYSIOLOGY OF NEUROTRAUMA

Organ function declines gradually as a person ages. The onset, extent, and course of progression of these changes occur with considerable variability between elderly individuals. Therefore, the effects of the physiologic changes during aging on the pathology and outcome of neurotrauma are complex and multifactorial.

Central nervous system

The elderly central nervous system (CNS) shows several changes that will enhance the effects of CNS trauma. Such changes are mainly in the form of cerebral arteriosclerosis increasing the risk of injury, depressed free radical clearance enhancing oxidative damage after injury and cerebral atrophy, and adherent dura increasing the intracranial hemorrhage and brain contusion induced by the physical impact. The resting CBF is lower in the elderly but cerebral autoregulation during normal aging seems to be intact. In agreement with the literature, recent reports showed that static cerebral autoregulation efficiency was similar in young adults and older adults.[5] Also, previous investigations showed that aging up to 86 years is associated with an overall preservation of dynamic cerebral autoregulation. This leads to a sufficiency of cerebral cortical oxygenation during daily life activities, despite the decrease in absolute cerebral bloodflow velocity and increase in cerebrovascular resistance with advancing age.[6]

After several hours of head injury, there is an initial decrease in CBF. It results from increased intracranial pressure (ICP), and vasospasm leading to further brain damage in the elderly compared with younger individuals. This is expected because cerebral blood flow (CBF), and vascular reactivity to $PaCO_2$ and metabolic changes and tolerance to ischemia are excessively impaired in the elderly.[7] Hence, ICP or cerebral perfusion pressure (CPP) targeted therapy is particularly recommended in the aging patient. Similar changes occur in the injured spinal cord.

Subsequent to several hours of cerebral hypoperfusion, hyperemia or reperfusion occur and may lead to secondary CNS injury. This phenomenon is believed to be the major cause of "delayed deterioration" in the elderly. Delayed deterioration in an aged patient is associated with poor outcome and increased mortality.[8] Delayed deterioration is defined as a patient who present with a relatively good neurological condition during the initial period after a head injury, and then deteriorates into a severe morbid neurological state (eg, GCS score of <8) within 48 hours of injury. It is more common in the elderly than young adults, and occurs in 20%–30% of elderly patients with TBI. Delayed deterioration is often induced by delayed hyperemia or hyperperfusion, delayed traumatic intracerebral hematoma, delayed expansion of subdural hematoma, or delayed increase in cerebral edema due to brain contusion. This delayed deterioration is common in the elderly because they possess an enlarged subdural space, which initially buffers ICP elevation. Once delayed deterioration occurs, it is a rapidly progressive phenomenon because the intracranial tissue compliance is diminished in the elderly.

Cardiovascular system

Normal cardiovascular changes in old age include vascular and myocardial stiffening as well as autonomic dysfunction, including impaired beta receptor responsiveness. This leads to systolic hypertension, increased left ventricular after load, and diastolic dysfunction.[9] Consequently, there is a potential for a decrease in coronary blood flow and greater dependence of cardiac output on normal sinus rhythm, vascular tone, and preload. In TBI there is neurocardiac interaction that can enhance the normal cardiovascular changes of aging. For example, TBI is associated with increased endogenous catecholamines resulting in subendocardial ischemia, and myocardial dysfunction as well as dysautonomia and conduction abnormalities. The combined effects of the cardiovascular changes in aging and the TBI cardiac complications can limit the ability of the elderly to respond to the stresses of neurotrauma, mainly in the form of low cardiac output states. In spinal cord injury, neurogenic shock (hypotension, bradycardia, and hypothermia) that occurs in high cord transection above T6 can be exaggerated in the elderly because of decreased cardiovascular reserves and autonomic dysfunction. Similarly, hypotension that may accompany spinal shock post injury can be magnified.[10]

Respiratory system

Normal aging of the respiratory system decreases pulmonary reserve. This results from decreased chest wall compliance, diminished elasticity of lung parenchyma, and increased closing volume due to collapsible small airways. These changes lead to increased ventilation/perfusion mismatch and a reduction in baseline PaO_2 (PaO_2 in the elderly = $100 - 0.3 \times Age$).[9] The pulmonary complications of brain injury are synergistic to the aging induced changes in pulmonary function.[9] Severe head injury can cause respiratory depression/apnea, hypoxic ischemic encephalopathy, neurogenic pulmonary edema, aspiration pneumonitis, and lung infection with acute respiratory distress syndrome. These TBI respiratory complications together with normal respiratory aging can lead to early respiratory failure with the need for artificial ventilation in order to maintain adequate gas exchange.

Additionally, limited respiratory reserves can stall the efforts to restore targeted CPP. The latter is achieved by fluid loading, adequate oxygenation and maintenance of acceptable $PaCO_2$ levels, and the use of vasopressors. In SCI, lesions, above C3, C3–C5, and C6–T8 are accompanied with a decrease in vital capacity by >90%, 70%, and 20%, respectively. Elderly patients will not be able to tolerate such effects on pulmonary reserve given the aging consequences on the respiratory system. Therefore, ventilatory support is common in the elderly population with SCI.[11]

Endocrine system

The common endocrine changes in normal aging are decreased secretion of thyroxin and insulin, resulting in hypothyroidism and glucose intolerance. These are not usually affected directly by TBI. Acute posterior pituitary dysfunction with abnormal antidiuretic hormone secretion has not been described in normal aging. However, it is a common clinical disorder in TBI, including cerebral diabetes insipidus, a syndrome of inappropriate antidiuretic hormone secretion, and cerebral salt wasting.

Hematologic system

With advancing age, healthy individuals may have laboratory signs of heightened coagulation enzyme activity accompanied by increased plasma concentrations of fibrinogen, factor VIII, and Von Willebrand factor. These changes may explain the higher incidence of arterial and venous thrombosis in the elderly compared with young people.[9] In TBI, coagulopathy (early hypocoagulopathy followed by delayed hypercoagulable state) is common and correlates with injury severity and increased mortality.[12] It is not known how aging and TBI coagulopathy interact.

EFFECTS OF PHARMACOKINETIC AND PHARMACODYNAMIC CHANGES

Pharmacokinetic changes

Reduced total body water content and increased fat percentage result in a higher serum drug concentration and longer half-lives after bolus injection of lipid-soluble drugs. Declining cardiovascular function and increased arm-tongue circulation time can slow drug delivery to sites of action, resulting in a slower onset of drug peak effects. Decreased serum albumin results in a higher volume of distribution of acidic drugs. The opposite is seen for alkaline drugs. As the human body ages, gradual deterioration of all body systems results in reduced hepatic and renal metabolism and excretion, impaired cardiovascular distribution, and disrupted fluid homeostasis. Although the liver and kidneys display minimal structural changes with aging, it has been found that P450-dependent oxidation decreases, meaning that hepatically cleared drugs have a longer half-life. In the elderly patient, these pharmacokinetic changes may not have direct interaction with neurotrauma to further cause changes in drug distribution and metabolism.

Pharmacodynamic changes

The most important changes of normal aging that can interact with CNS trauma to modify drug actions are cardiac decline (diastolic dysfunction and dependence on sympathetic drive) and depressed CNS function.[13,14] Propofol cardiovascular and hypnotic actions are expected to be excessively potentiated in the elderly neurotrauma patient. Postinduction hypotension induced by propofol is enhanced due to lack of increased sympathetic outflow. Additionally, geriatric patients also exhibit a higher sensitivity to opioids and benzodiazepines as well as a decreased minimum alveolar concentration of inhaled anesthetics. Hence,

it is important for the anesthesiologist to carefully titrate anesthetic administration in elderly neurotrauma patients (Table 27.1).[14]

ANESTHETIC MANAGEMENT OF THE ELDERLY NEUROTRAUMA PATIENT UNDERGOING NEUROSURGICAL PROCEDURES

There is a paucity of information about CNS trauma in the elderly. This led to the implementation of guidelines derived from previous investigations primarily done in the young adult population. Thus, anesthetic management follows the same basic principles of geriatric anesthesia and anesthesia for patients with CNS trauma. Obviously, anesthetic management should take into account what we currently know about the interaction between the pathophysiology of aging and the effects of neurotrauma.

The decision to undergo surgery

The indications, timing, and techniques of neurosurgical interventions are equivalent to those for younger adults (Table 27.2). However, there are certain considerations for the elderly patient[15,16]: (1) less invasive procedures should be performed if possible to minimize surgical and anesthetic complications, (2) the chosen procedure should have a higher likelihood for improving quality of life, (3) competent patients should clearly understand the alternatives, risks, and benefits of the surgical intervention, and (4) incapacitated patients should

Table 27.1 Dose adjustments for anesthetic agents in the elderly

Drug	Dose modification
Barbiturates	Slight reduction of bolus and infusion rates
Etomidate	Decrease bolus by ~50%
Propofol	Reduction of ~40% in bolus and infusion rates
Volatile agents	Reduction in MAC by 4%–6% per decade
Midazolam	Reduction of 50% in bolus and infusion rates
Short-acting opioids	Reduction of 30%–50% in bolus dose and infusion rates
Non-depolarizing neuromuscular block	Reduction of infusion rates by 20%–40%
Local anesthetic in spinal block	Small reduction in dose to achieve same segmental block
Local anesthetic in epidural block	Small reduction in loading dose and infusion rates and top-ups

Table 27.2 Common neurosurgical interventions in head injury and spinal cord injury

Injury	Intervention	Timing
Closed depressed skull fracture	Bone elevation or repositioning by craniotomy	Early or delayed
Open depressed skull fracture	Debridement, dural closure, or duroplasty with or without cranioplasty	Within 24 hours to prevent infection
Penetrating injuries	Wound exploration with craniotomy and dural opening	As promptly as possible
Acute epidural hematoma	Craniotomy with hematoma evacuation	As promptly as possible
Acute subdural hematoma	Craniotomy, burr holes, or mini craniotomy with hematoma evacuation	As promptly as possible
Intracerebral hematoma and brain contusion	Craniotomy and hematoma evacuation ±brain resection and/or decompressive craniotomy	Early surgery is desirable depending on clinical picture
Traumatic CSF leakage	Duroplasty with craniotomy or transnasal endoscopic repair	Surgery is performed if conservative treatment fails
Fracture of the optic canal	Optic canal decompression	Surgery within few days or within 1–2 weeks of injury
Blow-out craniofascial fracture	Orbitoplasty	Emergency or elective depending on the injury
Zygomatic, mandibular or maxillary fracture	Open reduction and internal fixation according to type of fracture	Early after injury
Spinal cord injury	Decompression and fusion	Early surgery within 72 hours
Central cord injury	Decompression and fusion	No consensus

have their living wills respected and the final decision should be a collective decision between the immediate family and the multidisciplinary team managing the patient.

Preoperative assessment

The anesthesiologist evaluates the patient either in the ICU or in the operating room (OR) depending on the urgency of the surgical intervention. In any event, the patient would have been evaluated and stabilized in the emergency department and have had an initial CT scan.

In immediate or urgent cases, the anesthesiologist's first encounter with the patient is usually in the OR. Once the patient arrives in the OR, the anesthesia team performs rapid assessment that should begin with the airway, breathing, and circulation. This basic assessment is followed by a brief neurologic evaluation to identify and document the preoperative neurologic deficits whether focal or non-focal. Also, the mechanism of injury and possible extracranial injuries should be identified. During assessment, resuscitation is continued to maintain normal blood pressure and adequate oxygenation as well as controlling ICP.

In expedited or elective cases there is time for more thorough preoperative assessment to maximize good anesthetic outcomes. The anesthesiologist evaluates the vital signs, airway, breathing, and circulation. Extracranial injuries including concealed trauma, that is, small pneumothorax, should be identified by reviewing the history of injury, imaging studies and laboratory investigations, and performing a full physical examination. The preoperative neurologic status should be documented with the most recent GCS as well as the pupillary condition and motor function. Identifying cervical spine injuries and intracranial hypertension are essential components in the preoperative assessment. Additionally, the preoperative review should detect aggravating conditions for CNS injury such as medical conditions that existed before the trauma, intoxication, and previous treatments. An initial report showed that 73% of elderly patients with TBI have medical conditions consisting of arthritis, hypertension, coronary artery disease, diabetes, cerebrovascular disease, and warfarin anticoagulation.[17]

Monitoring

Most neuroanesthesiologists will agree on the indications for various monitors that should be applied in the elderly neurotrauma patients.[18] Arterial line insertion is specially recommended in elderly patients suffering moderate and severe TBI or in SCI for beat-to-beat blood pressure monitoring, and blood gas and blood sugar analysis. Core temperature should be measured continuously because elderly patients can easily become hypothermic. Central venous catheter insertion is needed for volume replacement and central pressure monitoring in cases of expected excessive surgical bleeding and in intubated patients or in patients who will be left intubated to facilitate total parenteral nutrition. Wedge pressure and cardiac output monitoring with a pulmonary artery catheter are seldom needed unless active congestive failure or neurogenic pulmonary edema is present. ICP monitoring should be considered in all patients with severe TBI (GCS <9) and a grossly abnormal CT scan (intracranial hemorrhage, severe edema, contusion, and herniation). In patients with immediate or urgent indication for surgery, invasive monitor placement should not delay surgery and can be inserted as the surgical team begins.

Anesthesia induction

Intubation in the elderly is potentially difficult in a neurotrauma situation because of the combination of the high possibility of C-spine injury, the possibility of a full stomach, and the anatomic upper airway changes of aging (peg or loose teeth, temporomandibular stiffness, edentulous jaws, cervical spondylosis, and arthritis of atlanto-occipital joint).[19] Therefore, the anesthetist should be prepared to use videolaryngoscopy or bronchoscopy for safe intubation in anticipated or unexpected difficult cases. Patients should be preoxygenated, and short acting hypnotics, narcotics, and muscle relaxants titrated judiciously to prevent post-induction hypotension. Bag and mask ventilation should be performed to prevent hypercarbia and increased ICP. Manual in-line neck stabilization should be maintained until the endotracheal tube is secured and a neck collar is applied if indicated. If awake intubation is necessary, good topicalization without excessive sedation and avoidance of coughing, straining, and blood pressure elevations will ensure stable ICP and CPP.

Maintenance of anesthesia

The aim during anesthetic delivery in patients with neurotrauma, particularly in the elderly, is the minimization of secondary injury.[20,21] Accordingly, the anesthetic goals are maintenance of optimal CPP, treatment of increased ICP, and maintenance of normothermia, euglycemia, and euvolemia. Moreover, coagulopathy should be corrected (Table 27.3).

There is no evidence for a superior anesthetic technique in neurotrauma. A balanced technique carefully titrated to maintain adequate hemodynamics of the patient is most frequently applied. The intravenous anesthetics propofol, etomidate, and thiopental are cerebral vasoconstrictors. They maintain the coupling ratio between CBF and cerebral metabolic demand for O_2 thus preventing hyperperfusion and increased ICP. In contrast, volatile anesthetics (isoflurane, sevoflurane, and desflurane) are cerebral vasodilators and de-couple CBF and cerebral metabolism in concentrations more than 1 MAC. In higher concentrations (>1.5 MAC), they can abolish cerebral autoregulation. Short acting opioids (fentanyl, alfentanil, sufentanil, and remifentanil) have virtually no effect on cerebral dynamics and ICP. Non-depolarizing muscle relaxants prevent bucking and straining, and therefore prevent increases in ICP. Depolarizing muscle relaxants, (ie, succinylcholine) can cause transient but insignificant increases in ICP, and it is not contraindicated in TBI patients. However, succinylcholine can cause dangerous hyperkalemia in patients with crush injuries, recent paraplegia, and certain pre-injury myopathies.

Osmotherapy may be initiated or continued during surgery. Mannitol is typically used in doses between 0.25 and 1 g/kg. Its brain dehydrating effect requires an intact blood–brain barrier. It causes initial hypervolemia and subsequent diuresis. The latter should be replaced by normal saline

Table 27.3 Goals of anesthetic management in neurotrauma particularly in the elderly

Clinical feature	Action
Oxygenation	Avoid hypoxemia
	Keep $PaO_2 > 60$ mmHg or $SaO_2 > 90\%$
Ventilation	Avoid routine and prophylactic hyperventilation ($PaCO_2 \leq 30$ mmHg)
	Initiate hyperventilation as an urgent measure to control ICP
Arterial blood pressure	Preferably invasive monitoring with an arterial line
	Avoid mean arterial pressure >80 mmHg
Cerebral perfusion pressure	Monitored in severe TBI
	Maintain between 50–70 mmHg
Jugular O_2 saturation	Not an essential monitor during anesthesia
	If already present, maintain between 55%–75%
Intracranial pressure	Monitored in severe TBI
	Initiate therapy and/or procedural management if >20 mmHg
Osmotherapy	Used as part of ICP control measures
	Avoid hypotension with mannitol
Fluid management	Maintain euvolemia
	Non-glucose-containing isotonic crystalloid preferred
Temperature	Maintain normothermia (36–37°C)
	Hypothermia not recommended as measure for neuroprotection
Blood sugar control	Avoid tight blood sugar control
	Maintain blood sugar <10 mmol/L (<180 mg/dL)
Hematology	Maintain hemoglobin ≥10 gm/dL
	Maintain platelet count >100,000
Coagulation profile	Maintain INR <1.3
	Maintain fibrinogen >200 mg/dL
Steroids	High-dose steroids not recommended in TBI
	High-dose steroids in SCI controversial

Abbreviations: ICP: intracranial pressure; SCI: spinal cord injury; TBI: Traumatic brain injury.

to maintain euvolemia. Serum osmolality may be monitored during mannitol administration. If serum osmolality becomes greater than 320 mOsm/L, mannitol should be discontinued unless the osmolar gap is less than 15. Hypertonic saline (2%, 3%, or 23.4%) can be used to reduce brain edema and ICP. Saline concentrations more than 3% should be infused through a central venous catheter. Hypertonic saline has been reported to be superior to mannitol for reducing ICP, and maintaining intravascular osmolarity.

Postoperative management

Contraindications for extubating elderly neurotrauma patients include: (1) preoperative intubation and mechanical ventilation, (2) elevated ICP, (3) severe cerebral edema, and (4) life-threatening extracranial injury. Extubation criteria are the return of consciousness, adequate respiratory drive and gas exchange, and reversal of muscle relaxation. During extubation, surges in blood pressure are obtunded by antihypertensive agents, preferably labetalol, because of its rapid onset of action and lack of cerebral vasodilation. The patient is transported to the ICU or NICU by the anesthesiologist. Great care is taken to prevent damage to monitoring devices as external ventricular drains.

REFERENCES

1. Dams-O'Connor K, Cuthbert JP,Whyte J, Corrigan JD, Faul M, Harrison-Felix C. Traumatic brain injury among older adults at level

I and II trauma centers. *J Neurotrauma.* 2013;30:2001-2013.

2. Pascal J, Fehlings M, Vaccaro AR, Harrop JS. Traumatic spine injuries in the geriatric population. *Neurosurg Focus.* 2008;25(5):E16.

3. Werner C, Engelhard K. Pathophysiology of traumatic brain injury. *Br J Anaesth.* 2007;99 (1):4-9.

4. DeVivo MJ, Kartus PL, Rutt RD, Stover SL, Fine PR. The influence of age at time of spinal cord injury on rehabilitation outcome. *Arch Neurol.* 1990;47:687-691.

5. Robertson AD, Edgell H, Hughson RL. Assessing cerebrovascular autoregulation from critical closing pressure and resistance area product during upright posture in aging and hypertension. *Am J Physiol Heart Circ Physiol.* 2014;307: H124-H133.

6. Oudegeest-Sander MH, van Beek AH, Abbink K, Olde Rikkert MG, Hopman MT, Claassen JA. Assessment of dynamic cerebral autoregulation and cerebrovascular CO_2 reactivity in ageing by measurements of cerebral blood flow and cortical oxygenation. *Exp Physiol.* 2014;99(3):586-598.

7. Thompson HJ, McCormick WC, Kagan SH. Traumatic brain injury in older adults: Epidemiology, outcomes, and future implications. *J Am Geriatr Soc.* 2006;54(10):1590-1595.

8. Karibe H, Hayashi T, Narisawa A, Kameyama M, Nakagawa A, Tominaga T. Clinical characteristics and outcome in elderly patients with traumatic brain injury: For establishment of management strategy. *Neurol Med Chir.* 2017;57(8):418-425.

9. Alvis BD, Hughes CG. Physiology considerations in the geriatric patient. *Anesthesiol Clin.* 2015;33:447-456.

10. Lo V, Esquenazi Y, Han MK, Lee K. Critical care management of patients with acute spinal cord injury. *J Neurosurg Sci.* 2013; 57:281-292.

11. Grossman RG, Frankowski RF, Burau KD. Incidence and severity of acute complications after spinal cord injury. *J Neurosurg Spine.* 2012;17:119-128.

12. Wijayatilake DS, Sherren PB, Jigajinni SV. Systemic complications of traumatic brain

injury. *Curr Opin Anaesthesiol.* 2015;28:525-531.

13. Rana MV, Bonasera LK, Bordelon GJ. Pharmacologic considerations of anesthetic agents in geriatric patients. *Anesthesiol Clin.* 2017;35:259-271.

14. Lele A, Algarra NN. Traumatic brain injury, Anesthesia for. In: Papadakos P, Gestring M, eds. *Encyclopedia of Trauma Care.* 1st ed. Berlin Heidelberg: Springer-Verlag; 2015: 1676-1684. https://link.springer.com/reference work/10.1007/978-3-642-36200-2.

15. Murthy S, Hepner DL, Cooper Z, Bader AM, Neuman MD. Controversies in anaesthesia for noncardiac surgery in older adults. *Br J Anaesth.* 2015;115(Suppl 2):ii15-ii25.

16. Shigemori M, and members of the Guidelines Committee on the Management of Severe Head Injury, the Japan Society of Neurotraumatology. Guidelines for the management of severe head injury, 2nd edition. *Neurologia Medico-Chirurgica.* 2012; 52:1-30.

17. Mosenthal AC, Livingston DH, Lavery RF et al. The effect of age on functional outcome in mild traumatic brain injury: 6-month report of a prospective multicenter trial. *J Trauma.* 2004;56:1042-1048.

18. Mantilla JHM, Arboleda LFG. Anesthesia for patients with traumatic brain injury. *Colombian J Anesthesiol.* 2015;43(Suppl 1):3-8.

19. Johnson KN, Botros DB, Groban L, Bryan YF. Anatomic and physiopathologic changes affecting the airway of the elderly patient: Implications for geriatric-focused airway management. *Clin Interv Aging.* 2015;10: 1925-1934.

20. Mitchell D, Hoefnagel A. Neurotrauma, anesthesia management. In: Papadakos P, Gestring M, eds. *Encyclopedia of Trauma Care.* 1st ed. Berlin Heidelberg: Springer-Verlag; 2015:1012-1016.

21. Brain Trauma Foundation. 2016. Guidelines for the management of severe traumatic brain injury. *Evidence synthesis and recommendations, Part III:* thresholds. https:// braintrauma.org/guidelines/guidelines-for -the-management-of-severe-tbi-4th-ed#/.

28

Pregnancy and neurotrauma

ALEXANDRA KISILEVSKY AND ALANA M. FLEXMAN

INTRODUCTION

Epidemiology

Trauma occurs in approximately 7% of all pregnancies and is the leading cause of non-obstetrical maternal death (>20%).[1] The majority of trauma in pregnancy is blunt trauma from motor vehicle accidents, domestic violence, and falls, but other reported mechanisms include penetrating trauma, toxic exposures, burns, and self-inflicted injuries. Traumatic brain injury (TBI) and hemorrhagic shock are responsible for most maternal fatalities and even minor trauma can be associated with poor fetal outcomes. Indeed, trauma is associated with multiple increased risks to the fetus, including spontaneous abortion, uterine rupture, placental abruption, cesarean, and pre-term delivery.[2] In the trauma setting, only 11% of fetal mortality is attributable to maternal mortality and early assessment of fetal well-being is paramount.[3]

PRESENTATION

The presentation of neurotrauma in the pregnant patient is similar to the non-pregnant patient and frequently includes signs and symptoms of central nervous system (CNS) hemorrhage, brainstem herniation (eg, fixed and dilated pupil), and a decreased level of consciousness.[4–6] This presentation can differ from that of brain tumors and cerebrovascular (CVS) lesions in pregnancy; focal neurological deficits, seizure, and hydrocephalus commonly arise in the setting of tumors while severe headache, photophobia, and neck pain are common with intracranial CVS lesions, particularly in the postpartum period.[7,8] The presentation of eclampsia can mimic head injury and should be suspected in late pregnancy if hypertension, seizures, and end organ dysfunction are present. A high-energy mechanism and the presence of skull injury should increase the index of suspicion for significant neurotrauma. In the setting of trauma, the gestational age of pregnancy does not appear to affect the severity of maternal neurological injury.[9]

Radiological evaluation

Parturients with overt signs and symptoms of TBI (ie, GCS <13) should be evaluated expeditiously by a noncontrast computed tomography (CT) scan (the gold standard). If indicated, a radiological evaluation should not be delayed or avoided over concerns regarding fetal radiation exposure. The fetal radiation dose during a maternal CT head is estimated at close to zero.[10] Appropriate fetal shielding should be used as necessary.

For adult patients with minor traumatic head injury (GCS ≥13) in whom intracranial injury may be less obvious, the decision to proceed with CT imaging is often based on clinical prediction rules such as the Canadian CT Head Rule.[11] Importantly, however, this study specifically excluded pregnant patients. The New Orleans criteria is another clinical prediction rule used to guide CT imaging in patients ≥3 years of age with minor head injury and a GCS score of 15.[12] This study, which did not exclude parturients, identified the following factors as high risk for neurosurgical intervention: headache, vomiting, age >60 years, drug or alcohol intoxication, short-term memory deficit, visible trauma above the clavicle, and seizure.

Management

Management of the pregnant trauma patient should follow standard Advanced Trauma Life Support (ATLS) guidelines for non-pregnant patients including a primary and detailed secondary survey.[13] All female trauma patients of childbearing age should be suspected of pregnancy until proven otherwise; once maternal resuscitation has been initiated, evaluation for pregnancy via laboratory investigation or ultrasonography should be part of the routine workup. In the setting of the pregnant trauma patient, the American College of Obstetricians and Gynecologists (ACOG) recommends simultaneous (as opposed to sequential) assessment by both trauma and obstetrical services. Overall goals of management include aggressive maternal resuscitation and early assessment of fetal well-being via a continuous fetal heart rate (FHR) monitoring while recognizing that the best hope for fetal survival is maternal survival. When resuscitative measures have been instituted but the gravid uterus continues to interfere with maternal hemodynamics, perimortem cesarean delivery should be performed.[14] Regardless of gestational age, maternal supremacy is upheld with the caveat that, in the setting of fetal viability (≥23 weeks) and an unsalvageable mother, an emergency perimortem cesarean section may be warranted in order to save the fetus.

If head trauma is suspected or confirmed, the goal of initial management is to prevent secondary brain injury by maintaining adequate cerebral perfusion pressure (CPP) and oxygenation. To improve outcomes, the Brain Trauma Foundation TBI Guidelines recommend maintaining a systolic blood pressure ≥110 mmHg in patients aged 15 to 49 years and a target CPP of 60 to 70 mmHg.[15] Although these guidelines may be relevant to women of possible childbearing age, they make no specific recommendations regarding pregnancy. It is important to remember that uteroplacental perfusion is not autoregulated but is linearly related to maternal blood pressure; an abnormal fetal heart rate tracing may indicate impending maternal hemodynamic instability since blood is preferentially shunted to vital organs and away from the placenta. Therefore, a reassuring FHR is a targeted endpoint during resuscitation of the pregnant trauma patient with the maintenance of maternal systolic pressure within a narrow range of baseline (ie, 20%).

Specific treatment should be tailored to the individual pregnant patient and should involve multidisciplinary services including obstetrics, neonatology, neuroradiology, neurosurgery, and neuroanesthesia. Factors that must be taken into account during the formulation of a neurosurgical and neuroanesthetic plan that considers the timing of neurosurgery versus delivery of the fetus include current maternal neurological status, anticipated natural history of the underlying neuropathology, gestational age, and fetal well-being.

Timing of neurosurgery versus delivery of the fetus

In the setting of life-threatening or progressive maternal neurological injury, emergency neurosurgical intervention is indicated regardless of pregnancy or gestational age of the fetus. Delayed surgical intervention risks potential maternal neurological deterioration and death.[16] If surgical intervention is deemed non-urgent, the ACOG recommends surgery in the second trimester when the risk of preterm labor and spontaneous abortion are lowest.[17] In the setting of significant neurotrauma; however, this recommendation may rarely apply.

Once the need for maternal neurosurgical intervention has been determined, decisions must be made regarding possible fetal delivery and timing relative to neurosurgery (Figure 28.1). These decisions may be challenging and should involve

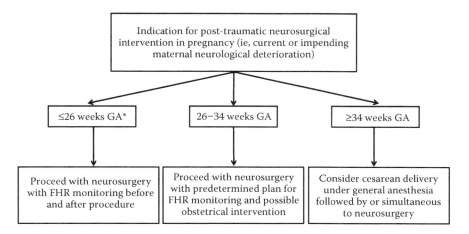

Figure 28.1 Suggested decision-making strategy for the timing of fetal delivery relative to maternal neurosurgical intervention in the setting of significant neurotrauma. *The lower limit of fetal viability is defined as ≤26 weeks gestational age (GA) but may differ based on institutional guidelines. Note that emergency perimortem cesarean delivery should be considered at any gestational age if the gravid uterus interferes with maternal hemodynamics.

multidisciplinary services while considering maternal neurological and hemodynamic status as well as gestational age and fetal well-being. In the setting of acute maternal neurological deterioration in the third trimester, cesarean delivery under general anesthesia, followed by neurosurgical decompression, is frequently recommended. The benefits of delivery before neurosurgical decompression include improved maternal hemodynamic control and eliminating possible adverse fetal effects secondary to the management of elevated maternal intracranial pressure (ICP). Simultaneous cesarean section and neurosurgical intervention have also been reported.[4] If the decision is made to proceed with neurosurgery before delivery due to concerns of fetal viability, a plan for fetal heart rate monitoring and potential emergent obstetrical intervention should be determined a priori. Regardless, the time from initial neurological insult to definitive surgical management should be minimized in order to optimize maternal neurological outcome. For concerns regarding a viable fetus and a stable mother, emergency cesarean section is indicated for fetal distress unresponsive to maternal resuscitative measures.

Intraoperative management

An appreciation for the normal anatomical and physiological changes of pregnancy is necessary for providing optimal anesthetic management to the head-injured parturient and for avoiding complications to the fetus (Table 28.1). In particular, management strategies for an elevated ICP, patient positioning with avoidance of aorto-caval compression, difficult airway management (including possible cervical spinal instability), the use of FHR monitoring, and the potential teratogenicity of medications must be taken into consideration.

HYPERVENTILATION

Normal pregnancy is associated with a 45% increase in minute ventilation mainly due to increased tidal volume resulting in a respiratory alkalosis. A typical arterial blood gas measurement during pregnancy can indicate respiratory alkalosis, with a reduction in $PaCO_2$ to approximately 30 mmHg. $PaCO_2$ values below those of normal pregnancy (ie, 28–32 mmHg) may result in uterine artery vasoconstriction, left shift of the maternal hemoglobin-oxygen dissociation curve, and fetal hypoxia.

Hyperventilation results in cerebral vasoconstriction and is recommended as a temporizing measure for reducing elevated ICP such as in the setting of acute brain herniation. In the absence of pregnancy, a $PaCO_2$ of 30–35 mmHg is often initially targeted. Hyperventilation to a $PaCO_2$ <25 mmHg is associated with adverse outcomes and is not advised.[15] Strong evidence for a specific

Table 28.1 Anesthetic considerations important to the management of the pregnant patient undergoing neurosurgical intervention

System	Considerations
Airway	Increased risk of difficult airway
	Increased risk of aspiration
	Potential cervical spinal injury
Respiratory	Increased risk of hypoxemia due to rapid desaturation with apnea
	Baseline respiratory alkalosis resulting in altered hyperventilation target (ie, 25–30 mmHg)
Cardiovascular	Avoidance of aorto-caval compression after 18–20 weeks gestation
	Increased cardiac output
Pharmacological	Altered pharmacokinetics
	Adjustment of AED dosing
	Effect of mannitol on the fetus
Fetus	Maintaining utero-placental perfusion
	Consideration for FHR monitoring
	Early mobilization of resources for possible fetal delivery
	Consideration for steroids for fetal lung maturation
	Teratogenicity of medication and ionizing radiation

Abbreviations: AED: Antiepileptic drugs; FHR: fetal heart rate.

ventilation target in the parturient is lacking.[18] Given the normal respiratory alkalosis of pregnancy and the established deleterious effects of a $PaCO_2$ <25 mmHg, titration of hyperventilation in pregnancy as necessary within the range of 25 to 30 mmHg is likely appropriate with the recognition that prolonged prophylactic hyperventilation should be avoided in order to ensure adequate cerebral blood flow. The Brain Trauma Foundation specifically recommends avoiding hyperventilation in the first 24 hours after injury when cerebral blood flow may be critically reduced.[15]

DIURETICS—MANNITOL

Diuretic agents such as mannitol and hypertonic saline are used to manage elevated ICP as they reduce intracranial volume by creating an osmotic gradient that enhances the flow of water out of brain tissue/cerebrospinal fluid and into the intravascular space. Mannitol crosses the placenta and is assigned a category C status in pregnancy by the U.S. Food and Drug Administration (FDA), indicating that risk cannot be ruled out as no controlled studies in pregnancy are available. The potential consequences of mannitol include maternal dehydration with resultant fetal hypoperfusion, reduced fetal urinary blood flow, and a reduction in amniotic fluid volume.[19] Case reports and case series on the management of neuropathology in pregnancy suggest mannitol is safe at clinically-relevant doses. The safe administration of mannitol at 0.5 to 1.5 mg/kg to manage ICP in parturients with intracranial tumors has been described.[5] In another case report, mannitol (0.25 mg/kg) administered for brain relaxation during awake craniotomy for tumor resection reduced amniotic fluid volume by 30% immediately postoperatively, but recovered to within 13% of baseline by 48 hours.[20] Finally, although historic data on chronic diuretic use suggested their association with fetal complications, a more recent meta-analysis concluded that chronic diuretics were not associated with an increased risk of adverse events.[21]

Loop diuretics (ie, furosemide) are an alternative to, or may be used in conjunction with, hyperosmotic agents in order to control elevated ICP. Similar to mannitol, furosemide crosses the placenta and is categorized by the FDA as a class C drug in pregnancy. The use of furosemide, in the setting of elevated ICP and pregnancy, is also limited to case reports and case series, which suggest safety with short-term and low-dose usage (ie, 20 or 40 mg IV).[5]

Given their ability to cross the placenta and produce changes in maternal and fetal volume status, as well as metabolic derangements, the use of diuretics in pregnancy should be reserved for the acute emergent treatment of elevated ICP when perceived benefit outweighs risk. Concurrent monitoring for and aggressive treatment of maternal hypotension is warranted.

DEXAMETHASONE

Corticosteroids such as dexamethasone are frequently administered when neuropathology, especially brain tumors, is present in order to reduce edema and control elevated ICP. High dose and chronic administration of prenatal dexamethasone has been implicated in potential adverse fetal affects including abnormal skeletal growth, cleft palate, and adrenal hypoplasia.[22] However, single dose antenatal steroid administration in premature infants has been shown to result in improved neuro-developmental outcomes and a single dose of antenatal corticosteroids is recommended by the ACOG for fetal lung maturation in the setting of prematurity.[23] Overall, the administration of single dose dexamethasone to the pregnant patient undergoing neurosurgical intervention is likely to be safe and is advocated by multiple groups.[18,24] Similar to diuretics, corticosteroids should be administered when the benefits outweigh the risks, and at the lowest possible therapeutic dose.

AIRWAY MANAGEMENT

Pregnancy increases airway edema and tissue friability, and results in a cephalad displacement of the stomach and reduced lower esophageal sphincter tone, which can lead to rapid desaturation with apnea as a consequence of reduced functional residual capacity and increased O_2 consumption. Together, the anatomic and physiologic changes of pregnancy place the parturient at high risk of aspiration and possible failed airway. As early as 12 to 18 weeks gestation, aspiration prophylaxis with a non-particulate antacid (ie, 0.3 M sodium citrate), an H_2 receptor antagonist, a proton pump inhibitor, and/or a pro-motility agent should be administered. Optimal patient positioning to align the pharyngeal and laryngeal axes (ie, the "sniffing" position) with maintenance of left uterine displacement should be adopted. A rapid sequence induction with adequate pre-oxygenation using 100% FiO_2 and the application of cricoid pressure is typically advocated.

In the setting of trauma, airway management may be further complicated by airway injury, hypovolemia, hypoxia and an uncooperative patient, and an unstable cervical spine with the potential for spinal cord injury during airway manipulation and patient positioning. An awake fiber-optic intubation or immobilization of the cervical spine via manual in-line stabilization can mitigate the risk of the latter.[25] The potential conflict between maintaining hemodynamic control on induction in order to ensure adequate cerebral perfusion pressure and the need for a rapid sequence induction to rapidly secure the airway in order to avoid aspiration and hypoxemia should be considered when formulating the anesthetic plan.

PATIENT POSITIONING

From 18 to 20 weeks gestation onwards, the parturient is at risk of aorto-caval compression in the supine position. Compressing major vessels by the gravid uterus can result in a reduction in cardiac output with resultant hypotension and uteroplacental insufficiency. The risk of aorto-caval compression when supine can be minimized by ensuring the maintenance of left uterine displacement. This is typically accomplished by wedging the parturient's right hip. If traumatic thoracolumbar spine injury is suspected, wedging should be avoided and a whole-body left lateral tilt adopted. The supine position allows for relative ease of access of the fundus for continuous fetal heart rate monitoring and potential obstetrical intervention.

Prone positioning presents the potential risk of compressing the gravid uterus. The technical challenge of adopting the prone position in pregnancy may be overcome by utilizing specific operating tables that ensure a free-hanging abdomen. Late gestational age should not be considered a contraindication to the prone position.[26] When adopted correctly, prone positioning provides complete relief of aorto-caval compression thus optimizing placental perfusion.[27] In the author's institution, the Jackson table has been used successfully on multiple occasions for safe prone positioning in the third trimester. Using both the Wilson and Relton-Hall laminectomy frame for prone positioning during spine surgery in the second and third trimesters has been reported successfully.[28,29] However, using the prone position renders continuous fetal heart rate monitoring and access for emergency operative delivery more challenging.

The use of the sitting position facilitates access for neurosurgical procedures involving the posterior fossa and cervical spine. This position has been successfully used for craniotomy and removing a cerebellopontine angle meningioma in a pregnant patient at 25 weeks gestation.[30] Venous air embolism is a potential catastrophic complication of the sitting position and requires continuous intraoperative monitoring with Doppler ultrasonography and capnography. Similar to the supine position, the sitting position allows for relative ease of access for FHR monitoring.

FHR monitoring

Gestational age with a distinction between pre-viability and viability should be used to guide fetal heart rate monitoring during non-obstetric surgery of the parturient.[17] In the setting of a pre-viable fetus, it is usually sufficient to assess fetal heart rate by Doppler before and after surgery. Regarding fetal viability, the ACOG recommends continuous intraoperative FHR when all of the following criteria are met: continuous FHR is physically possible, a qualified individual is available to interpret the FHR, obstetrical expertise is available and willing to intervene during the procedure, informed consent for operative delivery has been obtained if possible, and interrupting or modifying the surgical procedure is possible to allow for operative delivery. At a minimum, when the fetus is viable, FHR and contraction monitoring should be ascertained before and after the surgical procedure.

It is important to recognize that the provision of general anesthesia itself can result in reduced fetal heart rate variability. Thus, in the absence of alternative explanations for impaired uterine perfusion and oxygenation (ie, maternal hypotension or hypoxia), the presence of reduced variability concerning a normal fetal heart rate may be interpreted as normal. Fetal bradycardia, tachycardia, and late or variable decelerations, however, may signify fetal distress and warrant immediate and aggressive maternal resuscitation and preparation for possible delivery. Initial resuscitative measures should include administration of 100% FiO_2, assurance of left uterine displacement and normovolemia, and augmenting maternal mean arterial blood pressure up to 20% above baseline. Phenylepherine (as opposed to ephedrine) is the initial vasopressor of choice in pregnancy for maintaining uteroplacental perfusion secondary to improved fetal acid-base status.[31]

ANTIEPILEPTIC THERAPY

Although the majority of infants born to women on chronic antiepileptic therapy are healthy, fetal exposure to antiepileptic agents (AEDs) is associated with teratogenic consequences including intra-uterine growth restriction, major congenital malformations, long-term cognitive dysfunction, and increased risk of infant mortality.[32] These risks appear to be highest in the setting of sodium valproate monotherapy as well as AED polytherapy. Several of the newer anticonvulsants (ie, levetiracetam) have been shown to confer a lower risk of major congenital malformations, particularly when used as a monotherapy regimen.[33] The risk of antiepileptic therapy must be balanced against the potential risks of maternal seizure activity as generalized convulsions may result in both maternal and fetal hypoxia and acidosis. Whenever possible, AEDs should be used as monotherapy and serum drug concentrations monitored to ensure therapeutic levels regarding the altered pharmacokinetics of pregnancy.

UTEROTONIC AGENTS AND ICP

Medications which stimulate uterine smooth muscle contraction such as oxytocin are frequently administered post vaginal and operative delivery in order to reduce the risk of maternal postpartum hemorrhage. High quality data on the effects of uterotonic agents on ICP and cerebral blood flow in humans is lacking. Oxytocin, a vasodilator, may result in maternal hypotension and decreased cardiac output with indirect effects on cerebral perfusion pressure. In high bolus doses, it may further increase elevated ICP.[34] These effects should be minimized by using the lowest possible therapeutic dose.

Other uterotonic agents commonly used to manage postpartum bleeding include the ergot alkaloid ergonovine and the prostaglandin F_2 alpha analog carboprost. Both of these agents may result in systemic hypertension, which may increase cerebral blood flow, particularly in the setting of disrupted autoregulation following TBI. Ultimately, the anesthesiologist must balance the risks of potential maternal morbidity from significant postpartum hemorrhage with those of elevated ICP in the setting of reduced maternal intracranial compliance.

MATERNAL AND FETAL OUTCOMES FOLLOWING HEAD TRAUMA IN PREGNANCY

The incidence of neurosurgical intervention during pregnancy and trauma is scarce and difficult to precisely quantify. Descriptions of the anesthetic

Table 28.2 Case reports and case series of emergency neurosurgical intervention in pregnancy following trauma

Study	Mechanism of injury	Gestational age	LOC on presentation	Diagnosis	Neurosurgical intervention	Operative fetal delivery	Outcome Maternal	Outcome Fetal
Case series								
Cohen-Gadol et al. J Neurosurg. 2009	MVA	20	GCS 3	EDH/SDH	Craniotomy, evacuation hematoma	NO	Death	Stillborn HD #1
	MVA	4	GCS 4	SAH	ICP monitor insertion	NO	GOS2	D&C POD#15
	MVA	30	GCS 4	IPH	Delayed craniotomy, evacuation hematoma	NO Forceps 31w GA	GOS2	Low apgar at delivery, long-term outcome unknown
Nossek et al. Acta Neurochir. 2011	MVA	30	HA	EDH	Craniotomy, evacuation hematoma	YES Postoperatively 42w GA	No deficits reported	No OB complications reported
	MVA	12	GCS 5, fixed pupil	SDH	Craniotomy, evacuation hematoma	NO Vaginal 38w GA	No deficits reported	No OB complications reported
Kazemi et al. JNA. 2014	MVA	30	GCS 5	TBI	Burr hole, EVD insertion	YES Emergency 32w GA	GOS3	?
	MVA	16	GCS 2	TBI	Burr hole, EVD insertion	NO Therapeutic abortion POD#4	GOS4	Death

(Continued)

Table 28.2 (Continued) Case reports and case series of emergency neurosurgical intervention in pregnancy following trauma

Study	Mechanism of injury	Gestational age	LOC on presentation	Diagnosis	Neurosurgical intervention	Operative fetal delivery	Outcome Maternal	Outcome Fetal
Case report								
Goldschlager et al. *J Trauma.* 2009	MVA	34	GCS 9, fixed pupil	SDH	Craniotomy, evacuation hematoma	YES Simultaneous	Good	Good
Neville et al. *BMJ Case Rep.* 2012	MVA	13	GCS 6	Extensive contusion	Decompressive craniectomy	YES Postoperatively 35w GA	GOS3	Good
Whitney et al. *J Neurosurg.* 2012	MVA	21	GCS 3, fixed pupils	Extensive contusion	Bilateral decompressive craniectomies	YES Emergency postoperatively 26w GA	Death	Good
Dawar et al. *Neurol Ind.* 2013	MVA	36	GCS 11, fixed pupil	SDH	Craniotomy, evacuation hematoma	YES Simultaneous	Good	Good
Satapathy et al. *Ind J Neurotrauma.* 2014	MVA	24	GCS 11	SDH	Craniotomy, evacuation hematoma	NO	Good	?
Tawfik et al. *Saudi J Anesthesia.* 2015	Blunt trauma	37	GCS 11, fixed pupil	EDH	Craniotomy, evacuation hematoma	YES Preceding	Good	?Good

Abbreviations: D&C: Dilatation and curettage; EDH: epidural hematoma; EVD: external ventricular drain; GA: gestational age; GCS: Glasgow Coma Scale; GOS: Glasgow Outcome Scale; ICP: intracranial pressure; IPH: intraparenchymal hemorrhage; MVA: motor vehicle accident; OB: obstetrical; POD: postoperative day; SDH: subdural hematoma; TBI: traumatic brain injury; ?: unknown outcome.

management and outcome following head trauma during pregnancy are limited to case reports and case series and likely suffer from selection bias, as only potentially salvageable patients will undergo neurosurgical intervention and only those with favorable outcomes may be reported (Table 28.2).

A large, retrospective review of treating parturients with concomitant intracranial pathology from 1969 to 2005 in the United States identified 34 women of whom four (11.7%) were suffering from traumatic injury.[35] Three of these patients ultimately underwent neurosurgical intervention all with poor maternal outcome. Fetal outcomes were also generally negative. Another more recent retrospective review of parturients undergoing neurosurgical intervention at a single Canadian center identified nine patients of whom two (22%) were suffering from traumatic brain injury.[5] Both patients underwent emergency burr hole and extra-ventricular drain insertion with poor maternal neurologic outcome and one fetal demise. A third retrospective review of parturients with intracranial pathology from 2003 to 2010 in Israel describes managing 16 patients of whom two (12.5%) were suffering from TBI.[6] Both patients underwent craniotomy for hematoma evacuation (at 12 and 30 weeks gestation) and subsequently delivered full-term infants. Contrary to previous reports, no adverse short or long term maternal or fetal outcomes were reported.

Several case reports document emergency craniotomy for evacuating hematoma in the setting of altered level of consciousness in pregnancy with good short and long-term maternal and fetal outcomes. Neurosurgical decompression may immediately precede or occur simultaneously with emergency cesarean section in the third trimester as seen in one case report.[4] In two instances, emergency cesarean section of a full or near full-term fetus (36 and 37 weeks) was carried out immediately before neurosurgical decompression.[36,37] Another patient was discharged home postoperatively with a viable fetus in utero at 25 weeks gestation.[38] Finally, two case reports of decompressive craniectomy for elevated ICP following failure of medical management in pregnancy have been published.[39,40] Maternal outcomes were poor (one death, one severe, long-term neurologic impairment) but good fetal outcomes were reported at 6 months to 1 year. Ultimately, maternal and fetal outcomes likely depend on the degree of preexisting maternal and fetal injury as opposed to the anesthetic or neurosurgical management per se.

TRAUMATIC SPINAL CORD INJURY IN PREGNANCY

Many of the aforementioned special considerations for intracranial neurotrauma in pregnancy also apply to traumatic spinal cord injury in the parturient (ie, prone positioning). Overall goals in management include maintaining adequate maternal spinal cord perfusion pressure in order to avoid secondary spinal cord injury, protecting the spinal cord during left uterine displacement, as well as maintaining adequate uteroplacental perfusion. As with head trauma, progressive or threatened neurological deficit may constitute a maternal neurosurgical emergency and spinal surgery should be performed regardless of the gestational age of the fetus. After 34 weeks gestation, delivery of the fetus before surgery should be considered.

In the setting of spinal pathology, magnetic resonance imaging (MRI), which avoids maternal and fetal ionizing radiation, may be the initial imaging modality of choice and is considered safe in pregnancy. Fetal teratogenicity following exposure to the use of intraoperative fluoroscopy should be considered, along with the total dose and stage of pregnancy when considering the risks of exposure during pregnancy.

Although spinal surgery in the parturient in the lateral decubitus position is possible,[41] the prone position may be preferred for optimal surgical access. As discussed previously, this position can be safely adopted in pregnancy by using a four-post frame (see Positioning section above). An additional consideration is the theoretical risk of increased bleeding during spine surgery due to engorgement of the epidural venous plexus during pregnancy. Despite this risk, successful spine surgery has been performed without significant blood loss.[28,41]

CONCLUSIONS

The provision of anesthesia for the parturient concerning neurotrauma illustrates the many conflicts that can arise between ideal maternal and fetal care. Prime examples include the consequences of maternal elevated ICP management on the fetus, the timing of fetal delivery versus maternal neurosurgical intervention, and the potential teratogenicity of medications administered to the mother. Given the rare nature of this presentation, the literature provides limited guidance on optimal management. Early involvement of multidisciplinary services and an understanding of the normal anatomical and physiological changes of pregnancy are imperative in order to provide high-quality care to both patients. While maternal supremacy takes precedence, the consequences of maternal intervention on the fetus must also be considered and, whenever possible, tailored to ensure optimal maternal and fetal outcome.

REFERENCES

1. Mendez-Figueroa H, Dahlke JD, Vrees RA, Rouse DJ. Trauma in pregnancy: An updated systematic review. *Am J Obstet Gynecol.* 2013;209(1):1-10.

2. El-Kady D, Gilbert WM, Anderson J, Danielsen B, Towner D, Smith LH. Trauma during pregnancy: An analysis of maternal and fetal outcomes in a large population. *Am J Obstet Gynecol.* 2004;190(6):1661-1668.

3. Hill CC, Pickinpaugh J. Trauma and surgical emergencies in the obstetric patient. *Surg Clin North Am.* 2008;88(2):421-40, viii.

4. Goldschlager T, Steyn M, Loh V, Selvanathan S, Vonau M, Campbell S. Simultaneous craniotomy and caesarean section for trauma. *J Trauma.* 2009;66(4):E50-E51.

5. Kazemi P, Villar G, Flexman AM. Anesthetic management of neurosurgical procedures during pregnancy: A case series. *J Neurosurg Anesthesiol.* 2014;26(3):234-240.

6. Nossek E, Ekstein M, Rimon E, Kupferminc MJ, Ram Z. Neurosurgery and pregnancy. *Acta Neurochir (Wien).* 2011;153(9):1727-1735.

7. Bateman BT, Olbrecht VA, Berman MF, Minehart RD, Schwamm LH, Leffert LR. Peripartum subarachnoid hemorrhage: Nationwide data and institutional experience. *Anesthesiology.* 2012;116(2):324-333.

8. Terry AR, Barker FG 2nd, Leffert L, Bateman BT, Souter I, Plotkin SR. Outcomes of hospitalization in pregnant women with CNS neoplasms: A population-based study. *Neuro Oncol.* 2012;14(6):768-776.

9. Goldman SM, Wagner LK. Radiologic ABCs of maternal and fetal survival after trauma: When minutes may count. *Radiographics.* 1999;19(5):1349-1357.

10. Jain V, Chari R, Maslovitz S et al. Guidelines for the management of a pregnant trauma patient. *J Obstet Gynaecol Can.* 2015;37(6):553-574.

11. Stiell IG, Wells GA, Vandemheen K et al. The Canadian CT head rule for patients with minor head injury. *Lancet.* 2001;357(9266):1391-1396.

12. Haydel MJ, Preston CA, Mills TJ, Luber S, Blaudeau E, DeBlieux PM. Indications for computed tomography in patients with minor head injury. *N Engl J Med.* 2000;343(2):100-105.

13. ATLS Subcommittee, American College of Surgeons' Committee on Trauma, International ATLS working group. Advanced trauma life support (ATLS®): the ninth edition. *J Trauma Acute Care Surg.* 2013;74(5):1363-1366.

14. Jeejeebhoy FM, Zelop CM, Lipman S et al. Cardiac arrest in pregnancy: A scientific statement from the American Heart Association. *Circulation.* 2015;132(18):1747-1773.

15. Carney N, Totten AM, O'Reilly C et al. Guidelines for the management of severe traumatic brain injury, fourth edition. *Neurosurgery.* 2017;80(1):6-15.

16. Isla A, Alvarez F, Gonzalez A, Garcia-Grande A, Perez-Alvarez M, Garcia-Blazquez M. Brain tumor and pregnancy. *Obstet Gynecol.* 1997;89(1):19-23.

17. Practice ACoO. ACOG committee opinion no. 474: Nonobstetric surgery during pregnancy. *Obstet Gynecol.* 2011;117(2 Pt 1):420-421.

18. Wang LP, Paech MJ. Neuroanesthesia for the pregnant woman. *Anesth Analg.* 2008;107(1):193-200.

19. Lumbers ER, Stevens AD. Changes in fetal renal function in response to infusions of a hyperosmotic solution of mannitol to the ewe. *J Physiol.* 1983;343:439-446.

20. Handlogten KS, Sharpe EE, Brost BC, Parney IF, Pasternak JJ. Dexmedetomidine and mannitol for awake craniotomy in a pregnant patient. *Anesth Analg.* 2015;120(5):1099-1103.

21. Collins R, Yusuf S, Peto R. Overview of randomised trials of diuretics in pregnancy. *Br Med J (Clin Res Ed)*. 1985;290(6461):17-23.

22. Cheng X, Wang G, Lee KK, Yang X. Dexamethasone use during pregnancy: Potential adverse effects on embryonic skeletogenesis. *Curr Pharm Des*. 2014;20(34):5430-5437.

23. American College of Obstetricians and Gynecologists' Committee on Obstetric Practice; Society for Maternal–Fetal Medicine. Committee opinion No. 677: Antenatal corticosteroid therapy for fetal maturation. *Obstet Gynecol*. 2016;128(4):e187-e194.

24. Ng J, Kitchen N. Neurosurgery and pregnancy. *J Neurol Neurosurg Psychiatry*. 2008;79(7):745-752.

25. Kuczkowski KM, Fouhy SA, Greenberg M, Benumof JL. Trauma in pregnancy: Anaesthetic management of the pregnant trauma victim with unstable cervical spine. *Anaesthesia*. 2003;58(8):822.

26. Brookfield KF, Brown MD. How should pregnant women with spinal disease be managed? *Nat Clin Pract Neurol*. 2008;4 (12):652-653.

27. Nakai Y, Mine M, Nishio J, Maeda T, Imanaka M, Ogita S. Effects of maternal prone position on the umbilical arterial flow. *Acta Obstet Gynecol Scand*. 1998;77(10):967-969.

28. Brown MD, Levi AD. Surgery for lumbar disc herniation during pregnancy. *Spine (Phila Pa 1976)*. 2001;26(4):440-443.

29. Jea A, Moza K, Levi AD, Vanni S. Spontaneous spinal epidural hematoma during pregnancy: Case report and literature review. *Neurosurgery*. 2005;56(5):E1156.

30. Giannini A, Bricchi M. Posterior fossa surgery in the sitting position in a pregnant patient with cerebellopontine angle meningioma. *Br J Anaesth*. 1999;82(6):941-944.

31. Loubert C. Fluid and vasopressor management for Cesarean delivery under spinal anesthesia: Continuing professional development. *Can J Anaesth*. 2012;59(6):604-619.

32. Pennell PB. Antiepileptic drugs during pregnancy: What is known and which AEDs seem to be safest? *Epilepsia*. 2008;49(suppl 9):43-55.

33. Koubeissi M. Levetiracetam: More evidence of safety in pregnancy. *Epilepsy Curr/Am Epilepsy Soc*. 2013;13(6):279-281.

34. Thomas JS, Koh SH, Cooper GM. Haemodynamic effects of oxytocin given as i.v. bolus or infusion on women undergoing Caesarean section. *Br J Anaesth*. 2007;98 (1):116-119.

35. Cohen-Gadol AA, Friedman JA, Friedman JD, Tubbs RS, Munis JR, Meyer FB. Neurosurgical management of intracranial lesions in the pregnant patient: A 36-year institutional experience and review of the literature. *J Neurosurg*. 2009;111(6):1150-1157.

36. Tawfik MM, Badran BA, Eisa AA, Barakat RI. Simultaneous cesarean delivery and craniotomy in a term pregnant patient with traumatic brain injury. *Saudi J Anaesth*. 2015;9 (2):207-210.

37. Satapathy MC, Mishra SS, Das S, Dhir MK. Emergency management strategy for pregnant head trauma victims—Case reports and review of literatures. *Indian J Neurotrauma*. 2014;11:45-48.

38. Dawar P, Kalra A, Agrawal D, Sharma BS. Decompressive craniectomy in term pregnancy with combined cesarean section for traumatic brain injury. *Neurol India*. 2013;61 (4):423-425.

39. Neville G, Kaliaperumal C, Kaar G. 'Miracle baby': An outcome of multidisciplinary approach to neurotrauma in pregnancy. *BMJ Case Rep*. 2012.

40. Whitney N, Raslan AM, Ragel BT. Decompressive craniectomy in a neurologically devastated pregnant woman to maintain fetal viability. *J Neurosurg*. 2012;116(3):487-490.

41. Han IH, Kuh SU, Kim JH et al. Clinical approach and surgical strategy for spinal diseases in pregnant women: A report of ten cases. *Spine (Phila Pa 1976)*. 2008;33(17): E614-E619.

29

Polytrauma

MOHAMED SAMY ABDEL RAHEEM

INTRODUCTION

Polytrauma is a high-energy impact injury that involves more than one body system. It is one of the leading causes of death and disability worldwide.

Anesthetic management of polytrauma patients is highly challenging. The unique difficulties associated with polytrauma, in terms of the initial anatomical injury and the accompanying physiological deterioration, pose a huge burden on the trauma team.

The anesthesiologist's involvement in trauma management starts with, but is not limited to, the initial resuscitation. Therefore, for a successful outcome, it is paramount that the trauma anesthesiologist acquires adequate knowledge about the pathophysiology of polytrauma along with all recent management strategies. Additionally, the ability to work in a multidisciplinary team with technical as well as non technical skills are essential for managing the complex nature of polytrauma.

EPIDEMIOLOGY

In general, trauma is regarded as a global pandemic. It remains a leading cause of death and morbidity in children and young adults in the developed countries.[1] According to the WHO Global Status Report on Road Safety in 2013, 1.2 million people die annually on the roads and about 20 to 50 million sustain injury. This problem is more evident in low- and middle-income countries.[2] It was estimated that 8.4 million deaths per year are expected in 2020.[3]

Trauma not only presents risks to patients' lives, it also has a negative social and economic impact and presents a major burden on the healthcare system. In 2000, the U.S. Centers for Disease Control and Prevention estimated that US$117 billion was spent on injury-attributable medical care, amounting to approximately 10% of total U.S. medical expenditures.[4]

ETIOLOGY

The etiology of trauma varies depending on several factors including the lifestyle and the socioeconomic standards.[5] In addition to road traffic accidents, other causes include violence (16%), self-inflicted injuries (6%), falls (6%), and burns (5%). Wars, terrorism, and occupational injuries are among the known etiologies of polytrauma.

DEFINITION OF POLYTRAUMA

In 1975, Border and his colleagues first used the term polytrauma in Germany to describe patients with two or more significant injuries.[6] Thereafter, it was used across Europe. The terms "multiple trauma" and "major trauma" were used in the Angelo-American literature.

A consensus definition of polytrauma was lacking.[7] However, according to an international consensus opinion, the definition of polytrauma should include both anatomic and physiologic parameters. Hence, the abbreviated injury score (AIS)-based anatomic definition is the most practical. Therefore, a definition of polytrauma as an involvement of two (out of the six) body regions with AIS > 2 emerged as a better definition than the Injury Severity Score (ISS) cutoffs. The latter is the preferred definition for mono-trauma.[8]

The six body regions are:

1. Head, neck, and cervical spine
2. Face
3. Chest and thoracic spine
4. Abdomen and lumbar spine
5. Limbs and bony pelvis
6. Skin

Based on this definition, multiple extremity fractures or a bony pelvic and extremity fracture are not regarded as a polytrauma.

MORTALITY FOLLOWING POLYTRAUMA

The Trauma Audit Research Network (TARN) database includes patients who sustained trauma between 1989 to 2007 in England and Wales as well as some European hospitals. This database revealed that polytrauma represents 16% of all trauma cases, yet, it accounted for 43% of the deaths and 75% of this mortality was in children and young adults in the working age. Moreover, while large international databases only include trauma patients admitted to hospitals, a significant percentage (50%–60%) of trauma victims die before arriving at a hospital.[9]

According to the Major Trauma Outcome Study (MTOS), trauma registry[10] polytrauma (using AIS criteria) is mainly caused by road traffic collisions. It occurs in only 10% of cases, however, it causes nearly half of the overall deaths in children and adult patients younger than 65 years who reach the hospital alive. The mortality risk is highest following thoracic and abdominal trauma in the young age group. Though polytrauma is rare in those over 65 years, it has double the mortality rate compared with young adults, reflecting the vulnerability of this age group.

Traumatic brain injury (TBI) is the leading cause of death in polytrauma[11] followed by severe hemorrhage or exsanguination due to abdominal or thoracic injury.[12] The combination of both was regarded as highly lethal.[13]

In 1983, Donald Trunkey[14] proposed the "trimodal death distribution" with 3 peaks of mortality following trauma. *The first peak* is immediate at the scene and caused by non-survivable injuries. The only factor to deal with this peak is prevention. Baker et al.[15] and Trunkey[14] estimated the mortality during this peak as 64% and 53%, respectively. *The second peak* occurs within hours of experiencing the trauma. It accounts for 20% of deaths and is caused by severe cranial injury or exsanguination because of cardiovascular, abdominal, or pelvic injuries. The concept of *"golden hour"* was developed to reduce mortality during this peak. *The third peak* occurs within days to weeks of hospital admission and accounts for 80% of deaths. Mortality during the third peak is related to multiple organ dysfunction and sepsis. Improved critical care management and resuscitation can reduce mortality during this peak.[14]

Though the "Trimodal death distribution" is still used in trauma teaching, research, and literature, a recent systematic review revealed that the temporal death distribution after trauma is unimodal or bimodal.[16] While the immediate peak did not show a considerable change, the early peak showed a leftward shift (reduced) due to early hospital transport and aggressive treatment and the late peak was markedly diminished reflecting the ongoing improvement in resuscitation and critical care management.[17] Moreover, patients who sustain penetrating injuries often die immediately whereas those with blunt trauma rarely die immediately or within the first hour.[18]

The *"golden hour"* was a term used by R. Adams Cowley in 1975.[19] He stated that "the first hour after injury will largely determine a critically injured person's chances for survival." A recent controversy regarding the validity of the "golden hour" is emerging. However, there is not enough evidence to dispute the concept of "golden hour."[20] Based on some evidence from the battlefield,[21] the analogous concept of "Platinum 10 minutes" was introduced; limiting the allowable time for pre-hospital care before transport to a definitive trauma care center. Interestingly, several observational studies showed no beneficial impact of shorter rescue times on survival.[22,23]

PATHOPHYSIOLOGY

Following trauma, immediate death can result from severe TBI or exsanguinating hemorrhagic shock. In victims who survive the initial insult, several pathologic processes develop and contribute to the later deaths.[24,25] Managing a polytrauma victim should be directed towards targeting the following pathophysiologic changes in response to trauma.

Pathophysiologic processes

The pathophysiologic processes that take place after trauma (Figure 29.1) are induced by the first traumatic insult (first hit) followed by the second hit according to the "two-hit" theory. Soon, other processes ensue including a pro-inflammatory response (systemic inflammatory response syndrome—SIRS), an anti-inflammatory response (counter anti-inflammatory response syndrome—CARS), activation of plasmatic cascade (complement, kallikrein-kinin system, and coagulation) systems, synthesis of acute phase reactant, accumulation and activation of

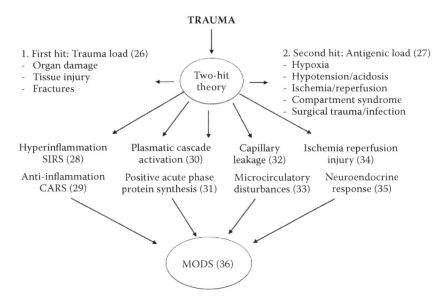

Figure 29.1 Pathophysiology of polytrauma.

leucocytes, capillary leak, microcirculatory disturbances, ischemia/reperfusion injury, and neuroendocrine changes. This sequence, if untreated in a timely manner, leads to multiple organ dysfunction (MODS) and failure.[26–36]

Organ crosstalk in polytrauma

The adverse effects of one organ's injury on other organ(s) further complicate the pathophysiology of polytrauma. The term "crosstalk" was used to describe this complex interaction. The "two-hit theory" is one of several pathophysiologic pathways proposed to describe this interaction.[37]

- Brain-lung crosstalk: TBI can lead to acute lung injury (ALI). Severe TBI is associated with a 5–10-fold increase in the risk of ALI[38] as well as an increased risk of neurogenic pulmonary edema.[39] Moreover, inflammatory mediators, originating from the microglia and astrocytes, may cross a "permeable" blood–brain barrier to the systemic circulation leading to extracerebral organ dysfunction.[40] On the other hand, lung trauma-induced respiratory failure and mechanical ventilation both appeared to be risk factors for increased mortality and neurologic morbidity in patients with TBI.[41]
- Brain-heart crosstalk: Neurogenic stunned myocardium (also called neurogenic stress cardiomyopathy) can result from TBI[42,43] and manifest as electrocardiographic changes, myocardial cell injury, and possible cardiac failure. Reciprocally, neurogenic stress cardiomyopathy is considered a secondary insult that can adversely affect the injured brain.[44]
- Spinal cord injury: Sympathetic nervous system dysfunction results in loss of peripheral vascular tone and hypotension with profound changes in heart rate and rhythm (neurogenic shock) that aggravates organ hypoperfusion.[45]
- Thoracic trauma: Major vascular injury, cardiac contusion, and tension pneumothorax/hemothorax result in a profound hypotension that impairs the perfusion of other organ systems. Likewise, pulmonary contusion and hemothorax/pneumothorax results in systemic hypoxia imposing a secondary organ injury.[46]
- Abdominal injury: In the context of abdominal organ injuries, other organs could be affected by the resulting massive hemorrhage, the release of

inflammatory mediators, and the development of intra-abdominal hypertension (IAH). The latter impairs abdominal organ perfusion, increases intrathoracic, central venous, and intracranial pressures.[47]
- Skeletal and pelvic fractures: Some extremity and pelvic fractures lead to a significant blood loss and mandate emergency care. A Fat embolism can influence the course and outcome in polytrauma patients with extremity and pelvic fractures.[48]

The lethal triad

Another recognizable detrimental factor in the pathophysiology of polytrauma is the *"lethal triad"* of acidosis, hypothermia, and coagulopathy. Since it is initiated by bleeding and ends by more bleeding, Kashuk and his colleagues[49] described this triad as the *"bloody vicious cycle."* Left untreated, the components of the triad worsen each other progressing to irreversible death.

1. *Metabolic acidosis:* In the setting of polytrauma, acidosis results from low cardiac output and impaired tissue perfusion secondary to blood loss and peripheral vasoconstriction. The resulting oxygen delivery/demand imbalance triggers anaerobic metabolism with the accumulation of lactate as a by-product which brings the body PH down below 7.35. During resuscitation, acidosis can be further aggravated by using large volumes of sodium chloride (normal saline) resulting in a state of hyperchloremic metabolic acidosis.[50,51]

2. *Hypothermia:* Hypothermia (core body temperature <35°C) is a common finding in trauma victims with an incidence of about 50% in those arriving to the emergency department.[52] Several factors contribute to the development of hypothermia in trauma including hemorrhagic shock, TBI, alcohol intoxication, prolonged environmental exposure, and severe burns.[53] During resuscitation, patient exposure to room temperature as well as the infusion of fluids further reduces core body temperature. Hypothermia is associated with a higher mortality. In one study,[54] core temperature <32°C was associated with 100% mortality irrespective of the severity of shock, the Injury Severity Score, or the

volume of resuscitation fluid used. Among many adverse effects of hypothermia in trauma, coagulopathy is considered the most devastating consequence.[54]

3. *Coagulopathy:* At the time of admission to the emergency department, coagulopathy is present in up to 25% to 35% of trauma patients and is associated with a fourfold increase in mortality.[55] Direct and indirect factors (Figure 29.2) contribute to the development of trauma-induced coagulopathy (TIC). Acute traumatic coagulopathy (ATC) has been identified in one out of four patients. Trauma and traumatic shock triggers the endogenous ATC.[56] Moreover, indirect factors including acidosis, hypothermia, and dilutional coagulopathy further exacerbate the ATC and lead to the TIC.[57]

Understanding the pathophysiology of ATC and TIC is the basis of the damage control resuscitation (DCR) concept.[58]

SCORING SYSTEMS AND RISK STRATIFICATION

In 1977, Baker and his colleagues[59] stated that "If you have never felt the need for any type of severity scoring system, then you probably have never had to explain how it is that the survival rate of 85% in your trauma center is actually better than the survival rate of 97% in some other hospital where the patients are much less seriously injured." This statement highlights the merit for using scoring systems in trauma. Assessing the severity of injury and trauma load serves several purposes including decision making, triaging, evaluating outcome and efficiency of trauma systems, auditing, epidemiologic and clinical research, setting up trauma systems, and cost estimation.[60] While easy-to-use scoring systems can serve the first two purposes, more sophisticated scores are needed for research and outcome evaluation purposes. The common goal of all scores is to make it easy for clinicians to speak a common language[61] and to allow comparing certain cohorts of patients by formulating the complex clinical data into an easy one-dimensional value.[62] However, it is unrealistic that one scoring system can reliably reflect the degree of critical illness in trauma patients. Therefore, many scoring systems were designed and categorized in different ways to: (1) address the impact of the trauma load using anatomic, physiologic, or combined criteria, (2) guide triaging, (3) describe the injury severity of the whole body or body regions, and (4) help predict outcome. Based on the first category, Table 29.1 illustrates the commonly used scoring systems in the trauma setting.

TRIAGE IN POLYTRAUMA

Trauma triage is the process of rapidly assessing the patient in order to prioritize treatment or transport

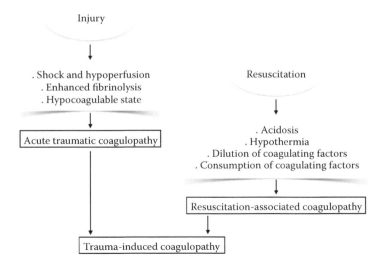

Figure 29.2 Trauma-induced coagulopathy.

Table 29.1 Commonly used scoring systems in trauma

Scoring System	Description
1. Anatomic	
Abbreviated Injury Scale (AIS)	Introduced in 1971, Scale: 1 to 6 (scores 5–6 indicate non-survivable). No comprehensive measure of severity. Not a linear scale, does not predict mortality.[63]
Injury Severity Score (ISS)	Introduced in 1977, incorporates AIS, Score form 1 to 75, Describes 6 body regions, The highest AIS in each region is used, The AIS score of the 3 most severely injured body region is squared. Different injury patterns can have the same ISS score. Unable to account for multiple injuries in the same body region. Not useful as a triage tool.[64]
New Injury Severity Score (NISS)	
Anatomic Profile (AP)	
Organ Injury Scales	Introduced in 1997, a modified version of ISS, Sums the squares of the top three AIS injuries regardless of the body region.[65]
	Includes serious injuries in any body region, head, and torso injuries are the most heavily weighted body regions, summarizes serious injuries (AIS > 3) into four categories from A to D. [66]
	Introduced in 1987, classify injury severity for individual organs, uses a scale from 1–5.[67]
2. Physiologic	
Revised Trauma Score (RTS)	Introduced in the 1980s. One of the most commonly used as a triage tool, uses 3 physiologic parameters (GCS, SPB, and RR). Each parameter has a score from 0–4 depending on the physiologic derangement. GCS inclusion makes it inaccurate for intubated and ventilated and intoxicated patients.[68]
Glasgow Coma Scale (GCS) and Pediatric GCS	Commonly used score to assess the level of consciousness especially in the context of TBI. Uses three parameters (1) Best eye response (2) Best verbal response and (3) Best motor response. The worst score is 3 and the best is 15.
APACHE I, II, and III	APACHE I introduced in 1981, II in 1985, and III in 1991. Widely used in ICU. It has two components: chronic health evaluation (comorbid conditions) and acute physiology score (uses the most abnormal physiologic variables in the first 24 hours).[69–70]
3. Combined	
Trauma Score–Injury Severity Score (TRISS)	Combines anatomic (ISS), physiologic (RTS) parameters and patient age. Determines the probability of survival. It is the standard method for outcome assessment. However, it carries the limitations of both ISS and RTS.[72]
A Severity Characterization of Trauma (ASCOT)	Introduced in 1990. Combine anatomic (AP) and physiologic scores (RTS) with age (in deciles) added in the final calculation. Compared with TRISS, it has almost the same predictive power, but higher complexity of calculation.[73]

according to their severity of injury. The triaging process is a dynamic one. It should be repeated before transport to the appropriate facility and at the emergency department of the trauma center/unit.

Field triage is a rather complex process that depends on the changing medical condition of the patient, the number of casualties, the nature of the incident, as well as the available resources. Resource availability includes transport, how far the appropriate trauma center/unit is from the scene, and its ability to deal with the trauma victim(s). Therefore,

it involves assessing the anatomy and physiology of trauma, its mechanism, and special patient considerations such as: extremes of age, pregnancy, burn injury, and preexisting comorbidities.[74] In situations where healthcare resources are limited or overwhelmed, such as in mass casualty incidents, the concept of field triage is modified, giving priority to those whose injuries are salvageable in order to save the maximum number of lives.[75] While several systems exist for field triage, they differ in the number of triage levels and the way patients are triaged to each level.[76] However, they have many features in common such as using the "walking filter" to identify those who can walk (to be labeled as minor injuries) and the use of color codes and tags to categorize patients according to the severity of injury.[77] Simple triage and rapid transport (START) is an example of the first civilian triage systems (Figure 29.3) that is widely used in many countries.[78] However, it was found to be neither sensitive enough nor specific.[79]

In-hospital triage aims at rapidly categorizing trauma victims according to the severity of their injury in order to receive treatment according to

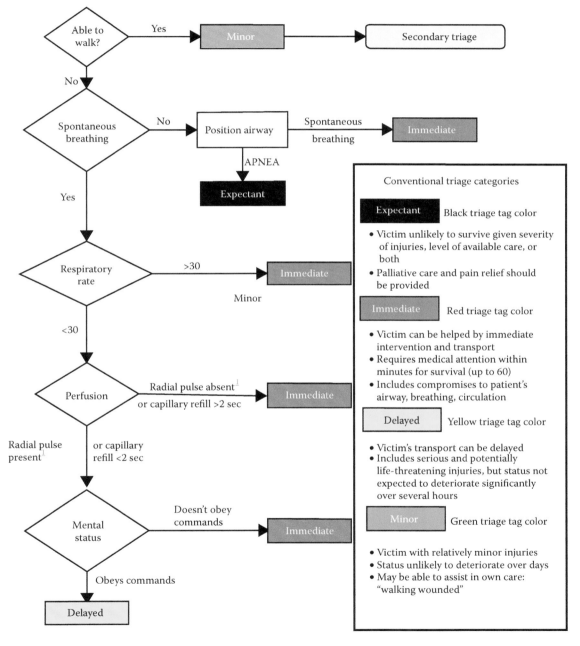

Figure 29.3 START algorithm. (Adapted from START Adult Triage Algorithm with permission. Developed by Hoag Hospital, Newport Beach and Newport Beach Fire Department, CA. 1983. Accessed June 7, 2017. http://www.start-triage.com.)

their clinical urgency. There are four well-known in-hospital triage systems: the Australian Triage Scale (ATS), the Canadian Triage and Acuity Scale (CTAS), the Manchester Triage System (MTS), and the American Emergency Severity Index (ESI). All of them use a five level triage algorithm.[80] They classify patients into immediate (red), very urgent (orange), urgent (yellow), standard (green), and non-urgent (blue).

MANAGEMENT OF POLYTRAUMA

Organization and preparedness

Rapid identification and appropriate response to polytrauma entails the need for good organization and teamwork. Organization starts at the pre-hospital setting, through the notification process, ambulance services, and ends by the major trauma centers and trauma units. A chain of arrangements and preparedness is required in order to provide the optimal medical care for trauma victims.

The main goal of any efficient trauma system is to save more lives. This goal can be achieved by ensuring that the injured patient gains the fastest access to the appropriate level of care with timely diagnosis and management by trained healthcare professionals.

Following polytrauma, time is of the essence. The presence of a predetermined multidisciplinary trauma team is pivotal. Factors needed for team efficiency include effective leadership, understanding roles and responsibilities by team members, good communication, proper documentation, technical and non technical skill training, and regular drills.[81]

Structured approach

The American College of Surgeons developed the Advanced Trauma Life Support (ATLS). The ATLS is the standard of care used in trauma patients providing a consistent structured approach to patient assessment and early management. The main merit of the ATLS is to rapidly assess and manage injuries according to their life-threatening potential.[82] The structured approach includes primary survey and resuscitation with its adjuncts, the secondary survey with its adjuncts, followed by postresuscitation and definitive care. A tertiary survey performed later was recommended to identify injuries not diagnosed during the first and secondary surveys.[83]

Primary survey and resuscitation (Figure 29.4)

In primary survey, life-threatening injuries should be assessed and managed. The concept is to treat first what kills the patient first. Therefore, managing the airway with cervical spine protection (Ac) takes priority followed by breathing (B), circulation and hemorrhage control (C), then disability (D) to assess the neurologic status, and finally exposure and environmental control (E). This stepwise longitudinal approach highlights the priority in management, however, with proper task allocation to the trauma team members, management can be done simultaneously.

AIRWAY AND CERVICAL SPINE (AC)

Airway loss is rapidly lethal. In trauma situations, maintaining airway patency is of utmost necessity to avoid asphyxia. In all trauma patients, cervical spine instability should be considered until proven otherwise. A high index of suspicion is needed to diagnose cervical spine injury, especially in those who sustained multisystem injuries, blunt trauma above the level of the clavicle, or in unconscious patients.

During airway management, high flow oxygen should be administered and manual-in-line stabilization (MILS) of the cervical spine should be maintained until the airway is secure. Airway opening can be achieved by:

1. Maneuvers (only jaw thrust should be used in trauma patients)
2. Airway adjuncts (oropharyngeal or nasal airway)
3. Supraglottic devices
4. Intubation using direct laryngoscopy, video-laryngoscopy, or a fiber-optic technique.

BREATHING (B)

Breathing includes assessing the adequacy of ventilation and oxygenation and managing life-threatening situations such as airway obstruction, tension or open pneumothorax, massive hemothorax, cardiac tamponade, or vascular injury and flail chest. Managing any of the above mentioned life-threatening breathing conditions might be as simple as inserting a chest drain or performing an emergency thoracotomy in order to control a massive hemothorax.

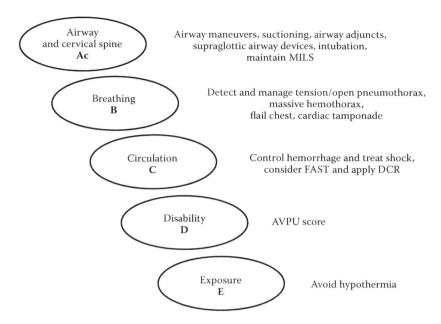

Figure 29.4 Primary survey and resuscitation. Abbreviations: MILS, Manual In-Line Stabilization; FAST, Focused Assessment with Sonography in Trauma; DCR, Damage Control Resuscitation; AVPU, Alert, Responds to verbal command, Responds to pain, Unresponsive.

CIRCULATION AND HEMORRHAGE CONTROL (C)

Exsanguinating hemorrhage is one of the two main causes of death following polytrauma. Assessing bleeding relies on the vital signs, estimating overt blood loss, and searching for an occult source of bleeding due to thoracic/abdominal injury or pelvic fracture. Focused assessment sonography for trauma (FAST) is a very useful diagnostic tool to diagnose internal bleeding.

Two wide bore peripheral venous access or intraosseous access allows rapid infusion of warmed balanced salt solution or blood to restore the circulating volume. In cases of massive hemorrhage, damage control resuscitation (vide infra) is a management strategy that includes permissive hypotension, hemostatic resuscitation by initiation of massive transfusion protocol (MTP) for blood, and component transfusion and damage control surgery.

DISABILITY (D)

Assessing the consciousness level helps identify traumatic brain injury, defining the resuscitation endpoints and setting management priorities.

In view of the time constraints, AVPU is the simple mnemonic used to describe the level of consciousness

of the patients as alert (A), responds to verbal stimuli (V), responds to pain (P), or unresponsive (U). GCS is used in the secondary survey for detailed assessment of the conscious level.

EXPOSURE AND ENVIRONMENT (E)

Exposure allows rapid initial survey for injury identification. During exposure, hypothermia should be avoided by using warm blankets and external warming devices.

DAMAGE CONTROL RESUSCITATION (DCR)

In severely injured polytrauma patients, prioritizing the physiology of the patient over the anatomic repair of injuries in order to avoid catastrophic deterioration led to the development of the DCR concept.

Damage control was first used in the Navy to describe the limited repair of damaged warships in a way that kept them operational rather than fully repairing them.[84] Schwab and his colleagues used this terminology in trauma in 1993.[85]

Surgical intervention for anatomic repair of serious abdominal, thoracic, or orthopedic injuries is one form of the "second hit." The stress response of surgery activates the immune-inflammatory response driving the body into the state of "systemic inflammatory response syndrome." In addition, other surgery-related factors including contamination, excessive blood loss, increased transfusion requirements, and heat loss aggravate the lethal triad of acidosis, hypothermia, and coagulopathy. Therefore, the main goal of DCR is to avoid tipping the physiologic balance towards the uncontrolled physiologic disequilibrium that can lead to organ dysfunction and failure. This goal is achieved by arresting hemorrhage in the shortest possible time, avoiding contamination, restoring the blood volume, correcting acidosis and coagulopathy followed by stabilization of the patient's physiologic status, and finally the anatomic surgical repair. The components of DCR are:

1. *Permissive hypotension*

   Applying permissive hypotension serves a dual role by maintaining organ perfusion while avoiding exacerbating hemorrhage due to clot disruption and the excessive need for crystalloids and blood. According to the most recent European guidelines on managing major bleeding and coagulopathy following trauma,[86] a target systolic blood pressure of 80 to 90 mmHg was recommended in the initial phase following trauma without TBI until bleeding is stopped (Grade 1C). However, in patients with severe TBI (GCS ≤8), the guideline recommends that a mean arterial pressure ≥80 mmHg be maintained (Grade 1C).

2. *Hemostatic resuscitation*

   Hemostatic resuscitation is a management strategy based on the better understanding of "Acute Traumatic Coagulopathy." The delayed administration of fluids in trauma was associated with reduced morbidity and mortality.[87] Restricted use of fluids (Grade 2C) and early administration of blood and blood products leads to restoring circulating blood volume while avoiding dilutional coagulopathy.[86] The immediate initiation of massive transfusion protocols (MTP) for red blood cell and component transfusion not only avoids dilutional coagulopathy but also reduces the overall blood products used.[88]

   The ratio of red blood cells (RBC): fresh frozen plasma (FFP)—Platelets of 1:1:1 was proposed as a "balanced transfusion" to avoid dilutional coagulopathy and exaggeration of the already initiated consumptive loss of platelets and other coagulation factors.[89] This ratio, however, has been the subject of controversy in view of the possible risks of infections, TRALI, and ALI mediated by the high FFP: RBC ratio.[90] Though a FFP: RBC ratio of 1: 2[86] was recently recommended (Grade 1B), nevertheless, the exact ratio is yet to be determined.

   Prevention of fibrinolysis by administrating tranexamic acid significantly reduced all-cause mortality and mortality due to bleeding.[90] Early administration of tranexamic acid was recommended (Grade 1A), preferably within the first 3 hours (Grade 1B) after injury.[86]

   Monitoring coagulation status together with initiating the measures to treat coagulopathy should start immediately after hospital admission (Grade 1B) using standard laboratory or viscoleastic tests (Grade 1C). The use of point of care (POC) testing to assess the coagulation derangement also determines the need for fibrinogen concentrate or cryoprecipitate.[86] Other measures include: avoiding hypothermia, monitoring and correcting ionized calcium levels, and the reversal of anticoagulant or antiplatelet agents.

3. *Damage control surgery*

   Stone and his colleagues were the first to describe the "truncated laparotomy" in 1983.[91] Later on, Rotondo and his coauthors[85] used the term "damage control laparotomy." The damage control surgery is currently applied, as part of damage control resuscitation, in abdominal, thoracic, vascular, cranial, and orthopedic surgery.

   The rationale of DCS is to prioritize physiologic optimization over anatomic repair of injuries by limiting the goals of initial surgical intervention to controlling hemorrhage and contamination, decompressing cavities, and deriding and splinting fractures. Johnson et al.[92] modified the three-stage DCS proposed earlier into a four-stage one to highlight the initial phase of resuscitation in the ED. These phases are[93]:

   - Phase DC0 (in emergency department): Damage control resuscitation
   - Phase DCI (in operating room): Performing the appropriate damage control procedure

(laparotomy, thoracotomy, craniotomy, orthopedic, or vascular procedure) involving surgical exploration, control of bleeding and contamination, and possible packing and temporary wound closure

- Phase DCII (in intensive care unit): During this phase, physiologic and biochemical stabilization of the patient is continued with thorough search for unidentified injuries via the tertiary survey
- Phase DCIII (in operating room): Following the stabilization phase, the patient is taken back to the operating room for definitive anatomic repair of injuries

Adjuncts to primary survey

It is challenging to detect multiple injuries and start a life or limb saving treatment within a short period of time. Adjuncts to a primary survey including conventional x-ray of cervical spine, chest, and pelvis as well as FAST are useful adjuncts in early management. The use of a multi-sliced computer tomography scan (MSCT) for injury diagnosis during the primary survey is emerging. It helps the rapid diagnosis of body injuries while resuscitation is underway. However, its use is limited by the cost and the need for adequate resources.[94] Although it seems to be a promising adjunct to a primary survey in polytrauma patients, a systematic review concluded that it was not associated with a reduction in mortality.[95]

SECONDARY SURVEY

A secondary survey only starts when the primary survey is completed and all the life-threatening injuries are managed, wounds are covered, and fractures are splinted. Moreover, it is important that a quick primary survey is repeated to rule out any physiologic deterioration during the secondary survey. The secondary survey includes a brief history, a thorough body examination from head to toe and front to back, a documentation of injuries, and performing the indicated investigations and imaging.

HISTORY

The acronym AMPLE is used to gather the important information that can influence patient management including allergies, medications, past medical illness, last meal, and events related to the accident.

EXAMINATION

The detailed examination of the patient includes the head and face, neck, chest, abdomen and pelvis, extremities and genitalia. Thereafter, careful logrolling of the patient with in-line manual stabilization of the cervical spine is performed in order to examine the back from top to bottom, including the spine and perineum with digital rectal examination to rule out injury or loss of tone if a spine injury is suspected.

INVESTIGATIONS

Further investigations and imaging procedures are performed as indicated to aid diagnosis, plan further management, and identify *"missed injuries."*

ADJUNCTS TO SECONDARY SURVEY

The adjuncts to a secondary survey include basic monitoring (electrocardiography, blood pressure, pulse oximetry, capnography, temperature, and urine output). In certain situations, invasive monitoring tools may be indicated such as direct arterial blood pressure, central venous pressure, intra-abdominal pressure, and cardiac output monitoring. Blood tests as well as x-ray, ultrasound (FAST), and CT imaging of the spine, thorax, and abdomen and pelvis are performed.

MISSED INJURIES IN POLYTRAUMA

There is no consensus on the definition of missed injury in different studies. The most commonly used definition is the failure to identify injuries during the primary and secondary survey.[96] In a systematic review,[97] three definitions were used. *Type I definition* refers to injuries missed during the primary and secondary survey but identified by the tertiary survey. *Type II* missed injuries were those not identified by the tertiary survey, while *Type III* were those missed during the entire hospital stay. Missed injuries in polytrauma patients are not uncommon. The incidence varied in different studies between 0.6%–39% depending on the definition used, the study population, and the methodology. The mean incidence using *Type I* definition was estimated as 4.3% with a range between 1.26% to 65% whereas *Type II* incidence was reported to be 1.5%.[98]

Head and neck, thoracic, and extremity injuries are the most commonly missed injuries.[99] Factors contributing to missing injuries are either related to the injury itself or to the healthcare professionals.[100] Injury-related factors include: multiple injuries, high ISS, and low GCS due to head injury or intoxication.[101] In addition, healthcare professionals may contribute to missed injuries in cases of overwhelming injuries or multiple casualties, an inadequate clinical survey, and insufficient or misinterpreted imaging.[101] Missed injuries are associated with a longer length of stay in the ICU and hospital and may also increase morbidity and mortality.[100]

Tertiary survey

The tertiary survey was introduced in the 1990s in order to reduce the incidence of missed injuries.[99] The tertiary survey is typically carried out within the first 24 hours of injury and is associated with a reduced incidence of missed injuries.[98]

DEFINITIVE MANAGEMENT: THE "WINDOW OF OPPORTUNITY"

A window of opportunity in polytrauma management refers to the time period when definitive surgical repair achieves the desired outcome with the least impact on the patient's physiological status. Following DCS, further surgical interventions are often needed for definitive anatomical repair during the stabilization period in the ICU. The impact of surgery on the patient's physiologic reserve depends on its type and timing. For orthopedic procedures, the window was set between the fifth and tenth days. Earlier interventions between the second to the fourth days after an injury has been reported to be unsuitable for performing definitive osteosynthesis.[102] The balance between the early surgical intervention with its impact on the patient's ongoing immune disturbance (as a second hit) vs. the delayed one with the risk of contamination or function loss is the rationale behind this concept.

ANESTHETIC CONSIDERATIONS IN POLYTRAUMA MANAGEMENT

The anesthesiologist's involvement in polytrauma management is not limited to airway and breathing management during the initial phase of resuscitation. It extends to circulation management during DCR, providing anesthesia for damage control surgery, intensive care management during the stabilization phase, and the delayed anesthetic management during subsequent definitive surgical repair procedures.

Anesthetic management of polytrauma patients is uniquely challenging. It requires a clear understanding of the pathophysiology of trauma, unique technical skills, and a great deal of anesthesia non-technical skills such as communication, situation awareness, and decision making.

Airway and breathing management

The following factors are among the main challenges in trauma airway management:

- Assessing airway and breathing in the noisy, high volume trauma unit can be rather difficult.
- Potential cervical spine instability requiring stabilization is crucial.
- There is clear evidence that emergency airway management in trauma is difficult with a high incidence of failed intubation, possible need for surgical airway, and serious complications.[103]
- Airway trauma with anatomic disruption, blood edema, and debris adds to the intubation difficulty.
- Competing priorities do exist in cases when induction is required for endotracheal intubation in a hemodynamically unstable patient or protective lung ventilation is indicated in a patient with TBI.
- Early establishment of a definitive airway is indicated in certain situations such as impending airway loss (facial burn or smoke inhalation) and TBI as per the National Institute for Health and Care Excellence (NICE) guideline.[104]

For airway and breathing management in polytrauma, the anesthetist normally assumes a non-leadership role. However, decisions related to such management should be shared with the team. Considering the anticipated difficulties and preparing for difficult airway management, senior anesthetic involvement, and skilled assistance are all crucial.

Cervical spine stabilization should be applied by MILS throughout airway management by a skilled assistant. Rapid sequence induction is a commonly used technique to avoid aspiration of gastric contents. In conjunction with MILS, lifting the anterior part of a hard cervical collar allows the application of cricoid pressure, however; techniques aiming at avoiding/minimizing cervical spine movement such as using a bougie should be considered.

Induction agents such as thiopentone and propofol can result in profound hypotension in a hemodynamically unstable or volume depleted patient. Etomidate, on the other hand, inhibits catecholamine release and adrenocortical suppression. Though Ketamine has a myocardial depressant effect; it is a popular induction agent in trauma patients. Its safe use in patients with TBI was reported in a systematic review.[105] Ketamine use in TBI patients was associated with a significant decrease in intracranial cranial pressure (ICP) and an increase in cerebral perfusion pressure (CPP).

The appealing pharmacologic profile of succinylcholine, including its rapid onset, short duration, and excellent intubating conditions rendered it the muscle relaxant of choice for RSI in patients with aspiration risk.[106] Nevertheless, the risk of serious hyperkalemia in burn and crush injuries as well as the transient rise in intraocular pressure and ICP should always be considered. In a recent Cochrane review, rocuronium was reported to be less superior to succinylcholine in terms of intubating conditions.[107] However, its rapid onset of action makes it a suitable alternative to succinylcholine for RSI whenever the latter use seems to be deleterious. The concern regarding the long duration of rocuronium in case of failed intubation no longer exists after the introduction of sugammadex.[108]

Alternative plans for failed intubation and the "cannot intubate, cannot ventilate" scenario should be considered. The UK Fourth National Audit Project (NAP4) addressed the difficulties in airway management after trauma. NAP4 recommended the concept of "right person, right place, right equipment and right preparation."[103]

Protective lung strategy with low tidal volume was associated with a proven mortality benefit.[109] However, its application with the possibility of induced hypercarbia is a clinical dilemma in patients with TBI. On the contrary, the use of PEEP (up to 15 cm H2O) was not associated with a reduced CPP or increased ICP.[110]

Circulation and DCR

The central role of the anesthesiologist during the delivery of DCR involves the immediate initiation of MTP coupled with establishing invasive monitoring in order to avoid overzealous fluid transfusion, provide timely blood transfusion, and apply permissive hypotension within the appropriate limits, depending on the guideline targets set for different situations.

Goal-directed hemostatic resuscitation is best achieved by using point of care testing (POC). In the setting of massive hemorrhage, the standard laboratory test (SLT)-guided hemostatic correction has considerable shortcomings.[111] SLTs are time consuming with a long "turnaround time" that may exceed 60 minutes. Additionally, they have limited diagnostic value being unable to detect platelet dysfunction, fibrinolysis, or clot instability. Therefore, POC-guided algorithmic correction of TIC not only corrects the derangement reliably, but it also reduces blood loss, transfusion requirements, and risks associated with blood transfusion.[112]

Fibrinogen is the most abundant coagulation factor. Its level rapidly falls to critically low levels during the early phase of trauma.[113] Upon arrival at the ED, low plasma fibrinogen levels were reported to be independent predictors of massive transfusion requirements and death in severe trauma.[114] Fibrinogen replacement can be achieved by using cryoprecipitate or fibrinogen concentrate. There is evidence that fibrinogen supplementation reverses coagulopathy, reduces bleeding, and increases survival in traumatic hemorrhage.[115]

Anesthesia for DCS and definitive surgical repair

During or after the stabilization phase, staged DCS or surgical procedures for definitive anatomical repair are often required. The anesthesia challenges include:

- The decision to perform DCS or definitive repair is not always easy. A joint decision should be made involving senior surgeons and critical care physicians based on the physiologic and anatomic status of the patient while considering the hemostatic and metabolic derangement.
- The anesthetic technique should be tailored individually to avoid physiologic deterioration.
- The continual monitoring of the hemodynamic, hemostatic, and metabolic status of the patient throughout the surgical procedure. The stabilization process has to continue throughout the perioperative phases.

- Transferring the patient between areas of care (ICU, imaging suites, and operating room) requires good preparation, skilled personnel, appropriate equipment, and great care.
- Anesthesia nontechnical skills including properly documentation of the patient's physiologic, neurologic, and anatomical condition as well as good communication, team work, situation awareness, and vigilance are extremely important for successful trauma management.

CONCLUSION

Polytrauma, being regarded as a global pandemic, is still one of the main causes of mortality, especially in the rather young and productive age group. Moreover, it represents a clear financial burden on the economy and healthcare. The management of polytrauma patients is a real challenge that mandates cooperation between several disciplines and organizations, and requires preparedness and expertise. New concepts in trauma management are emerging that aim at providing better care and reducing the overall morbidity and mortality. The anesthesiologist role in managing polytrauma is broad and pivotal. Dealing with such cases, anesthesia technical and nontechnical skills are both required.

REFERENCES

1. Krug EG, Sharma GK, Lozano R. The global burden of injuries. *Am J Public Health*. 2000;90(4):523-526.
2. World Health Organization. *Global Status Report on Road Safety 2013: Supporting a Decade of Action*. Geneva: World Health Organization; 2013.
3. Murray CL, Lopez AD. Alternative projections of mortality and disability by cause 1990–2020. *Lancet*. 1997;349(9064):1498-1504.
4. Centers for Disease Control and Prevention. Medical expenditures attributable to injuries—United States, 2000. *MMWR*. 2004;53:1-4.
5. Peden M, McGee K, Sharma G. *The Injury Chart Book: A Graphical Overview of the Global Burden of Injuries*. Geneva: World Health Organization; 2002.
6. Border JR, LaDuca J, Seibel R. Priorities in the management of the patient with polytrauma. *Prog Surg*. 1975;14:84-120.
7. Pape H. Classification of patients with multiple injuries—Is the polytrauma patient defined adequately in 2012? *Injury*. 2012;43 (2):127-128.
8. Butcher N, Balogh Z. Update on the definition of polytrauma. *Eur J Trauma Emerg Surg*. 2014;40(2):107-111.
9. Pfeifer R, Tarkin I, Rocos B, Pape H. Patterns of mortality and causes of death in polytrauma patients—Has anything changed? *Injury*. 2009;40(9):907-911.
10. Champion HC, Copes WS, Sacco WJ, Lawnick MM, Keast SC, Frey CF. The major trauma outcome study: Establishing national norms for trauma care. *J Trauma*. 1990;30:1356-1365.
11. Goris RJ, Draaisma J. Causes of death after blunt trauma. *J Trauma*. 1982;22(2):141-146.
12. Chiara O, Scott J, Cimbanassi S et al. Trauma deaths in an Italian urban area: An audit of pre-hospital and in-hospital trauma care. *Injury*. 2002;33(7):553-562.
13. Jin G, deMoya M, Duggan M et al. Traumatic brain injury and hemorrhagic shock: Evaluation of different resuscitation strategies in a large animal model of combined insults. *Shock*. 2012;38(1):49-56.
14. Trunkey DD. Trauma. Accidental and intentional injuries account for more years of life lost in the U.S. than cancer and heart disease. Among the prescribed remedies are improved preventive efforts, speedier surgery and further research. *Sci Am*. 1983;249(2):28-35.
15. Baker CC, Oppenheimer L, Stephens B, Lewis F, Trunkey DD. Epidemiology of trauma deaths. *Am J Surg*. 1980;140(1):144-150.
16. Pfeifer R, Teuben M, Andruszkow H, Barkatali B, Pape H. Mortality patterns in patients with multiple trauma: A systematic review of autopsy studies. *PlosOne*. 2016;11 (2):e0148844.
17. Gunst M, Ghaemmaghami V, Gruszecki A, Urban J, Frankel H, Shafi S. Changing

epidemiology of trauma deaths leads to a bimodal distribution. *Proc (Bayl Univ Med Cent).* 2010;23(4):349-354.

18. Demetriades D, Murray J, Charalambides K et al. Trauma fatalities: Time and location of hospital deaths. *J Am Coll Surg.* 2004;198 (1):20-29.

19. Cowley RA. A total emergency medical system for the state of Maryland. *Md State Med J.* 1975;24(7):37-45.

20. Rogers F, Rittenhouse K, Gross B. The golden hour in trauma: Dogma or medical folklore? *Injury.* 2015;46(4):525-527.

21. Battlefield Advanced Trauma Life Support (BATLS). *J R Army Med Corps.* 2000;146:110-114.

22. Lerner EB, Billittier AJ, Dorn JM, Wu YW. Is total out-of-hospital time a significant predictor of trauma patient mortality? *Acad Emerg Med.* 2003;10(9):949-954.

23. Di Bartolomeo S, Valent F, Rosolen V et al. Are pre-hospital time and emergency department disposition time useful process indicators for trauma care in Italy? *Injury.* 2007;38(3):305-311.

24. Keel M, Trentz O. Pathophysiology of polytrauma. *Injury.* 2005;36(6):691-709.

25. Tosounidis T, Giannoudis P. Pathophysiology of polytrauma. In: Pape H, Sanders R, Borrelli J, eds. *The Poly-Traumatized Patient with Fractures: a Multi-Disciplinary Approach.* Berlin Heidelberg: Springer; 2011:33-41.

26. Rotstein OD. Modeling the two-hit hypothesis for evaluating strategies to prevent organ injury after shock/resuscitation. *J Trauma.* 2003;54(5):203-206.

27. Waydhas C, Nast-Kolb D, Trupka A et al. Posttraumatic inflammatory response, secondary operations, and late multiple organ failure. *J Trauma.* 1996;40(4):624-631.

28. van Griensen M, Krettek C, Pape H. Immune reactions after trauma. *Eur J Trauma.* 2003;29(4):181-192.

29. Bone R. Sir Isaac Newton, sepsis, SIRS, and CARS. *Crit Care Med.* 1996;24(7):1125-1128.

30. Fosse E, Pillgram-Larsen J, Svennevig JL et al. Complement activation in injured patients occurs immediately and is dependent on the severity of the trauma. *Injury.* 1998;29(7):509-514.

31. Whicher JT, Evans SW. Acute phase proteins. *Hosp Update.* 1990;16:899-905.

32. Laroux FS, Pavlick KP, Hines IN et al. Role of nitric oxide in inflammation. *Acta Physiol Scand.* 2001;173(1):113-118.

33. Bateman RM, Sharpe MD, Ellis CG. Bench-to-bedside review: Microvascular dysfunction in sepsis—Hemodynamics, oxygen transport, and nitric oxide. *Crit Care.* 2003;7(1):359-373.

34. Dorweiler B, Pruefer D, Andrasi TB et al. Ischemia-reperfusion injury. *Eur J Trauma Emerg Surg.* 2007;33(6):600-612.

35. Woolf PD. Hormonal responses to trauma. *Crit Care Med.* 1992;20(2):216-226.

36. Ciesla DJ, Moore EE, Johnson JL et al. Multiple organ dysfunction during resuscitation is not postinjury multiple organ failure. *Arch Surg.* 2004;139(6):590-594.

37. Mascia L. Acute lung injury in patients with severe brain injury: A double hit model. *Neurocrit Care.* 2009;11(3):417-426.

38. Bratton SL, Davis RL. Acute lung injury in isolated traumatic brain injury. *Neurosurgery.* 1997;40(4):707-712.

39. Ledingham IM, Watt I. Influence of sedation on mortality in critically ill multiple trauma patients. *Lancet.* 1983;1(8336):1270.

40. Habgood MD, Bye N, Dziegielewska KM et al. Changes in blood–brain barrier permeability to large and small molecules following traumatic brain injury in mice. *Eur J Neurosci.* 2007;25(1):231-238.

41. Zygun DA, Kortbeek JB, Fick GH, Laupland KB, Doig CJ. Non-neurologic organ dysfunction in severe traumatic brain injury. *Crit Care Med.* 2005;33(3):654-660.

42. Riera M, Llompart-Pou JA, Carrillo A, Blanco C. Head injury and inverted Takotsubo cardiomyopathy. *J Trauma.* 2010;68(1):E13-E15.

43. Hasanin A, Kamal A, Amin S et al. Incidence and outcome of cardiac injury in patients with severe head trauma. *Scand J Trauma Resusc Emerg Med.* 2016;24:58.

44. Mazzeo AT, Micalizzi A, Mascia L, Scicolone A, Siracusano L. Brain-heart crosstalk: The

many faces of stress-related cardiomyopathy syndromes in anaesthesia and intensive care. *Br J Anaesth.* 2014;112(5):803-815.

45. Bilello JF, Davis JW, Cunningham MA, Groom TF, Lemaster D, Sue LP. Cervical spinal cord injury and the need for cardiovascular intervention. *Arch Surg.* 2003;138 (10):1127-1129.

46. Stawicki SP. Trends in nonoperative management of traumatic injuries: A synopsis. *OPUS 12 Scientist.* 2007;1(1):19-35.

47. Marinis A, Argyra E, Lykoudis P et al. Ischemia as a possible effect of increased intra-abdominal pressure on central nervous system cytokines, lactate and perfusion pressures. *Crit Care.* 2010;14(2):R31.

48. Nau T, Aldrian S, Koenig F, Vecsei V. Fixation of femoral fractures in multiple-injury patients with combined chest and head injuries. *ANZ J Surg.* 2003;73(12):1018-1021.

49. Kashuk JL, Moore EE, Millikan JS, Moore JB. Major abdominal vascular trauma—A unified approach. *J Trauma.* 1982;22(8):672-679.

50. Ho AM, Karmakar MK, Contardi LH, Ng SS, Hewson JR. Excessive use of normal saline in managing traumatized patients in shock: A preventable contributor to acidosis. *J Trauma.* 2001;51(1):173-177.

51. De Backer D, Cortes DO. Characteristics of fluids used for intravascular volume replacement. *Best Pract Res Clin Anaesthesiol.* 2012;26(4):441-451.

52. Helm M, Lampl L, Hauke J, Bock KH. Accidental hypothermia in trauma patients. *Is it relevant to preclinical emergency treatment?. Anaesthesist.* 1995;44(2):101-107.

53. Søreide E, Smith CE. Hypothermia in trauma victims—Friend or foe?. *Indian J Crit Care Med.* 2004;8(2):116-119.

54. Tsuei BJ, Kearney PA. Hypothermia in the trauma patient. *Injury.* 2004;35(1):7-15.

55. Maegele M, Lefering R, Yucel N et al. Early coagulopathy in multiple injury: An analysis from the German trauma registry on 8724 patients. *Injury.* 2007;38(3):298-304.

56. Brohi K, Singh J, Heron M, Coats T. Acute traumatic coagulopathy. *J Trauma.* 2003;54 (6):1127-1130.

57. Gando S, Otomo Y. Local hemostasis, immunothrombosis, and systemic disseminated intravascular coagulation in trauma and traumatic shock. *Crit Care.* 2015;19(1):72.

58. Kushimoto S, Kudo D, Kawazoe Y. Acute traumatic coagulopathy and trauma- induced coagulopathy: An overview. *J Intensive Care.* 2017;5(1):6.

59. Baker SP, O'Neill B, Haddon W Jr, Long WB. The Injury Severity Score: A method for describing patients with multiple injuries and evaluating emergency care. *J Trauma.* 1974;14(3):187-196.

60. Lefering R. Trauma score systems for quality assessment. *Eur J Trauma.* 2002;28(2):52-63.

61. McLellan BA. Trauma severity scoring: The language of trauma. In: McMurtry RY, McLellan BA, eds. *Management of Blunt Trauma.* Baltimore: Williams & Wilkins; 1990:11-19.

62. Wutzler S, Maegele M, Wafaisade, A et al. Risk stratification in trauma and haemorrhagic shock: Scoring systems derived from the trauma register DGU®. *Injury.* 2014;45(Suppl 3):S29-S34.

63. Committee on Medical Aspects of Automotive Safety: Rating the severity of tissue damage. 1. The abbreviated scale. *JAMA.* 1971;215(2):277-280.

64. Baker SP, O'Neill B, Haddon Jr W, Long WB. The Injury Severity Score: A method for describing patients with multiple injuries and evaluating emergency care. *J Trauma.* 1974;14(3):187-196.

65. Osler T, Baker SP, Long W. A modification of the Injury Severity Score that both improves accuracy and simplifies scoring. *J Trauma.* 1997;43(6):922-925.

66. Champion HR, Sacco WJ, Lepper RL, Atzinger EM, Copes WS, Prall RH. An anatomic index of injury severity. *J Trauma.* 1980;20(3):197-202.

67. Moore EE, Cogbill TH, Malangoni MA et al. Organ injury scaling, II: Pancreas, duodenum, small bowel, colon and rectum. *J Trauma.* 1990;30(11):1427-1429.

68. Champion HR, Sacco WJ, Copes WS, Gann DS, Gennarelli TA, Flanagan ME. A revision

of the trauma score. *J Trauma*. 1989;29 (5):623-629.

69. Knaus WA, Zimmerman JE, Wagner DP, Draper EA, Lawrence DE. APACHE-acute physiology and chronic health evaluation: A physiologically based classification system. *Crit Care Med*. 1981;9(8):591-597.

70. Knaus WA, Draper EA, Wagner DP, Zimmerman JE. APACHE II: A severity of disease classification system. *Crit Care Med*. 1985;13(10):818-829.

71. Knaus WA, Wagner DP, Draper EA et al. The APACHE III prognostic system. Risk prediction of hospital mortality for critically ill hospitalized adults. *Chest*. 1991;100 (6):1619-1636.

72. Boyd CR, Tolson MA, Copes WS. Evaluating trauma care: The TRISS method. Trauma score and the Injury Severity Score. *J Trauma*. 1987;27(4):370-378.

73. Markle J, Cayten CG, Byrne DW, Moy F, Murphy JG. Comparison between TRISS and ASCOT methods in controlling for injury severity. *J Trauma*. 1992;33(2):326-332.

74. Sasser SM, Hunt RC, Faul M et al. Guidelines for field triage of injured patients: Recommendations of the national expert panel on field triage, 2011. *MMWR*. 2012;61(RR-1):1-20.

75. Frykberg ER. Triage: Principles and practice. *Scand J Surg*. 2005;94(4):272-278.

76. Ryan JM. Triage: Principles and pressures. *Eur J Trauma Emerg Surg*. 2008;34:427-432.

77. Koenig KL. Schultz C, eds. *Disaster Medicine: Comprehensive Principles and Practise*. Cambridge, UK: Cambridge University Press; 2010.

78. START Adult Triage Algorithm. Developed by Hoag Hospital, Newport Beach and Newport Beach Fire Department, CA. 1983. Accessed June 7, 2017. http://www.start-triage.com.

79. Bhalla MC, Frey J, Rider C, Nord M, Hegerhorst M. Simple triage algorithm and rapid treatment and sort, assess, lifesaving, interventions, treatment, and transportation mass casualty triage methods for sensitivity, specificity, and predictive values. *Am J Emerg Med*. 2015;33(11):1687-1691.

80. Farrohknia N, Castrén M, Ehrenberg A et al. Emergency department triage scales and their components: A systematic review of the scientific evidence. *Scand J Trauma Resusc Emerg Med*. 2011;19:42.

81. McCullough AL, Haycock JC, Forward DP, Moran CG. Early management of the severely injured major trauma patient. *Br J Anaesth*. 2014;113(2):234-241.

82. ATLS Subcommittee, American College of Surgeons' Committee on Trauma, International ATLS working group. Advanced trauma life support (ATLS): The ninth edition. *J Trauma Acute Care Surg*. 2013;74 (5):1363-1366.

83. Ferree S, Houwert RM, van Laarhoven JJ, Smeeing DP, Leenen LP, Hietbrink F. Tertiary survey in polytrauma patients should be an ongoing process. *Injury*. 2016;47(4):792-796.

84. Ball CG. Damage control resuscitation: History, theory and technique. *Can J Surg*. 2014;57(1):55-60.

85. Rotondo MF, Schwab CW, McGonigal MD et al. 'Damage control': An approach for improved survival in exsanguinating penetrating abdominal injury. *J Trauma*. 1993;35 (3):375-382.

86. Rossaint R, Bouillon B, Cerny V et al. The European guideline on management of major bleeding and coagulopathy following trauma: Fourth edition. *Crit Care*. 2016; 20:100.

87. Bickell WH, Wall MJ Jr, Pepe PE et al. Immediate versus delayed fluid resuscitation for hypotensive patients with penetrating torso injuries. *N Engl J Med*. 1994;331(17):1105-1109.

88. Geeraedts LM Jr, Kaasjager HA, van Vugt AB, Frolke JP. Exsanguination in trauma: A review of diagnostics and treatment options. *Injury*. 2009;40(1):11-20.

89. Hirshberg A, Dugas M, Banez EI, Scott BG, Wall MJ Jr, Mattox KL. Minimizing dilutional coagulopathy in exsanguinating hemorrhage: A computer simulation. *J Trauma*. 2003;54(3):454-463.

90. Sperry JL, Ochoa JB, Gunn SR et al. An FFP:PRBC transfusion ratio >/=1:1.5 is

associated with a lower risk of mortality after massive transfusion. *J Trauma.* 2008;65(5):986-993.

91. Stone HH, Strom PR, Mullins RJ. Management of the major coagulopathy with onset during laparotomy. *Ann Surg.* 1983;197 (5):532-535.

92. Johnson JW, Gracias VH, Schwab CW et al. Evolution in damage control for exsanguinating penetrating abdominal injury. *J Trauma.* 2001;51(2):261-269.

93. Lamb CM, MacGoey P, Navarro AP, Brooks AJ. Damage control surgery in the era of damage control resuscitation. *Br J Anaesth.* 2014;113(2):242-249.

94. Banerjee P, Rudra S, Ghosh M, Panose P. CT scans in primary survey for polytrauma patients. *Adv Computed Tomography.* 2013;2(2):46-51.

95. Sierink JC, Saltzherr TP, Reitsma JB, Van Delden OM, Luitse JS, Goslings JC. Systematic review and meta-analysis of immediate total-body computed tomography compared with selective radiological imaging of injured patients. *Br J Surg.* 2012;99(Supp 1):52-58.

96. Giannakopoulos GF, Saltzherr TP, Beenen LFM et al. Missed injuries during the initial assessment in a cohort of 1124 level-1 trauma patients. *Injury.* 2012;43(9):1517-1521.

97. Keijzers GB, Giannakopoulos GF, Del Mar C, Bakker FC, Geeraedts LMG Jr. The effect of tertiary surveys on missed injuries in trauma: A systematic review. *Scand J Trauma Resusc Emerg Med.* 2012;20:77.

98. Tammelin E, Handolin L, Söderlund T. Missed injuries in polytrauma patients after trauma tertiary survey in trauma intensive care unit. *Scand J Surg.* 2016;105(4).

99. Enderson BL, Reath DB, Meadors J, Dallas W, DeBoo JM, Maull KI. The tertiary trauma survey: A prospective study of missed injury. *J Trauma.* 1990;30(6):666-669.

100. Buduhan G, McRitchie DI. Missed injuries in patients with multiple trauma. *J Trauma.* 2000;49(4):600-605.

101. Kremli MK. Missed musculoskeletal injuries in a university hospital in riyadh: Types of missed injuries and responsible factors. *Injury.* 1996;27(7):503-506.

102. Stahel PF, Heyde CE, Wyrwich W, Ertel W. Current concepts of polytrauma management: From ATLS to 'damage control.' *Orthopade.* 2005;34(9):823-836.

103. Cook TM, Woodall N, Frerk C, Fourth National Audit Project. Major complications of airway management in the UK: Results of the fourth national audit project of the royal college of anaesthetists and the difficult airway society. Part 1: Anaesthesia. *Br J Anaesth.* 2011;106(5):617-631.

104. National Institute for Health and Clinical Excellence. Head Injury: Triage, assessment, investigation and early management of head injury in infants, children and adults. 2014. www.nice.org.uk.

105. Zeiler FA, Teitelbaum J, West M, Gillman LM. The ketamine effect on ICP in traumatic brain injury. *Neurocrit Care.* 2014;21(1):163-173.

106. Scott RPF. Onset times and intubating conditions. *Br J Anaesth.* 1998;80:417-419.

107. Tran DT, Newton EK, Mount VA, Lee JS, Wells GA, Perry JJ. Rocuronium versus succinylcholine for rapid sequence induction intubation. *Cochrane Database Syst Rev.* 2015;(10):CD002788.

108. Sorensen MK, Bretlau C, Gatke MR, Sorensen AM, Rasmussen LS. Rapid sequence induction and intubation with rocuronium-sugammadex compared with succinylcholine: A randomized trial. *Br J Anaesth.* 2012;108(4):682-689.

109. Serpa Neto A, Cardoso SO, Manetta JA et al. Association between use of lung-protective ventilation with lower tidal volumes and clinical outcomes among patients without acute respiratory distress syndrome: A meta-analysis. *JAMA.* 2012;308(16):1651-1659.

110. Nemer SN, Santos R, Caldeira J et al. Positive end-expiratory pressure can increase brain tissue oxygen pressure in hypoxemic severe traumatic brain injury patients. *Crit Care.* 2011;15(Supp 2):41.

111. Haas T, Fries D, Tanaka KA, Asmis L, Curry NS, Schöchl H. Usefulness of standard plasma coagulation tests in the management of perioperative coagulopathic bleeding: Is there any evidence?. *Br J Anaesth.* 2015;114(2):217-224.

112. Meybohm P, Zacharowski K, Weber CF. Point-of-care coagulation management in intensive care medicine. *Crit Care*. 2013;17(2):218.

113. Hayakawa M, Gando S, Ono Y, Wada T, Yanagida Y, Sawamura A. Fibrinogen level deteriorates before other routine coagulation parameters and massive transfusion in the early phase of severe trauma: A retrospective observational study. *Semin Thromb Hemost*. 2015;41(1):35-42.

114. Hayakawa M, Maekawa K, Kushimoto S et al. High D-dimer levels predict a poor outcome in patients with severe trauma, even with high fibrinogen levels on arrival: A multicenter retrospective study. *Shock*. 2016;45(3):308-314.

115. Wafaisade A, Lefering R, Maegele M et al. Administration of fibrinogen concentrate in exsanguinating trauma patients is associated with improved survival at 6 hours but not at discharge. *J Trauma Acute Care Surg*. 2013;74(2):387-395.

PART X

Fluids

30

Fluid management

SHUMAILA HASAN AND MATTHEW A. KIRKMAN

INTRODUCTION

Fluid management in patients with neurotrauma can present specific challenges to the anesthesiologist. These patients can experience rapid fluctuations in intravascular volume, which may be the result of the use of osmotic diuretics, such as mannitol, the development of diabetes insipidus or significant intraoperative hemorrhage, for example. Particularly challenging is the balance between ensuring adequate fluid administration to maintain tissue perfusion while preventing fluid overload and significant increases in cerebral water content, which may result in or exacerbate secondary injury and intracranial hypertension.

The aim of this chapter is to briefly review the physiology of sodium and water homeostasis and the implications for fluid management in neurotrauma patients. The main methods of monitoring and managing fluid status are also discussed. Conditions associated with electrolyte disturbance, including the syndrome of inappropriate antidiuretic hormone secretion, cerebral salt wasting, and diabetes insipidus are covered elsewhere in this textbook, as is the transfusion of blood products.

PHYSIOLOGY OF FLUID BALANCE

Osmolality, osmolarity, and tonicity

Osmolality is a quantification of the number of osmotically active particles in a solvent, commonly expressed in milliosmoles per kilogram of solvent (mmol/kg or mOsm/kg). Normal plasma osmolality is 275 to 295 mOsm/kg, and this is regulated through osmoreceptors in the anterior hypothalamus (see below). Importantly, the size or molecular weight of the solute is of no importance in determining osmolality, solely the number of particles in the solution is the determining factor. As a result, equimolar concentrations of any substance (such as glucose or mannitol, for example) have the same osmolality.

Osmolarity is the total concentration of osmotically active particles per liter of solvent, expressed as mmol/L. For diluted solutions, which include most physiologic conditions, osmolality and osmolarity are considered interchangeable terms. The osmolarity of some commonly used intravenous (IV) fluids is shown in Table 30.1.

Tonicity is a measure of the effective osmotic pressure gradient and only reflects the concentration

Table 30.1 Osmolarity of a selection of commonly used intravenous fluids

Fluid name	Osmolarity (mOsm/L)	Oncotic pressure (mmHg)	Sodium (mEq/L)
0.9% Saline	308	0	154
0.45% Saline	154	0	77
Ringer's lactate solution	273	0	130
5% Albumin	290	19	130–160
Dextrose 0.45% saline	406	0	77

of solutes that penetrate a semipermeable membrane, in contrast to osmolarity, which reflects both penetrating and nonpenetrating solutes. Differences in tonicity between the cells and extracellular space is critical in determining the movement of fluid between the two. For example, if the extracellular solution is hypotonic relative to the cells, fluid will move into the cell to redress the discrepancy, which results in cell swelling, and vice versa. The regulation of sodium ions is a major determinant of intravascular fluid status, affecting tonicity and thus, fluid movement.

Blood–brain barrier

The brain is unique because it is isolated from the intravascular compartment by the blood–brain barrier (BBB), which is composed of endothelial cells connected via tight junctions. The normal BBB is impermeable to plasma proteins, water-soluble compounds, sodium, potassium and chloride ions, but permeable to gases and lipophilic substances. Because of the physical structure of the BBB, the primary determinant of fluid movement in and out of the central nervous system (CNS) is the osmolar gradient, that is, the relative concentrations of all osmotically active particles (including most electrolytes) between the plasma and extracellular fluid. This is in contrast to peripheral tissues where tight junctions are not found, and fluid movement is governed principally by the plasma concentration of large macromolecules—the so-called oncotic gradient.

Traumatic brain injury (TBI) can result in impairment of the BBB, leakage from capillaries, and vasogenic edema. In this setting, as is discussed later, the correct choice of fluids is critical to minimize neurologic injury. For example, hypotonic solutions are deleterious in patients with an impaired BBB, as it will increase cerebral swelling and thus intracranial pressure. Importantly, different from peripheral tissues, the plasma oncotic pressure has little influence on the formation of edema within the brain tissue. Attempts to prevent cerebral edema by fluid restriction may instead lead to hemodynamic instability and less-favorable outcomes, which is why they are not advocated.

Hormone influences on fluid homeostasis

In the healthy, awake human, thirst is stimulated by the activation of osmoreceptors in the anterior hypothalamus, which occurs at approximately ≥295 mOsm/kg. There are several hormones that influence sodium and fluid balance in physiologic conditions (Table 30.2).

Antidiuretic hormone (ADH) is produced in the supraoptic nuclei of the hypothalamus and secreted from the posterior pituitary gland. It works by binding to distal renal collecting tubules to stimulate the reabsorption of water and concentrates urine secondary not only to high osmolality but also to certain medications, hypovolemia, hypoglycemia, and stress. ADH also acts to stimulate the sensation of thirst.

Table 30.2 Hormones that influence fluid balance

Hormone	Effect
Antidiuretic hormone/ arginine vasopressin	• Increased water reabsorption
Natriuretic peptides	• Renal loss of sodium and water
Aldosterone	• Increased sodium reabsorption

Natriuretic peptides are produced in the hypothalamus and are located in the midbrain, median eminence, choroid plexus, and spinal cord. There are several types, including atrial natriuretic peptide (ANP), brain natriuretic peptide (BNP), and C-type natriuretic peptide (CNP). BNP fibers can be identified alongside the carotid, middle cerebral, posterior communicating, and anterior cerebral arteries. Natriuretic peptides work by causing renal sodium and fluid loss. Interestingly, recent evidence suggests that CNP appears to modulate permeability of the BBB.[1]

Aldosterone is a hormone that is secreted as a result of the detection of decreased intravascular volume/blood pressure by baroreceptors, which are located in several large arteries but particularly in the carotid sinus. The physiologic effect of aldosterone is the reabsorption of water and sodium retention.

ASSESSMENT OF FLUID BALANCE

There are several clinical, laboratory, and invasive methods available to assess fluid balance in patients with neurotrauma, and these are shown below in Table 30.3.

The specific methods used for assessing fluid balance is influenced by several variables, including the clinical condition of the patient, access to specific invasive monitoring techniques and expertise, and the setting (prehospital setting, emergency department, ward, operating room, or intensive care unit, for example). The use of advanced monitoring techniques has become increasingly common, possibly because they facilitate an accurate and continuous evaluation of fluid status and permit the monitoring of response to treatment. More details about the main invasive monitoring devices used are shown in Table 30.4.

Table 30.3 Assessment of fluid balance status[a]

Modality	Monitored variables	Indication of dehydration	Indication of fluid overload
Clinical assessment	Heart rate (bpm)	>110	–
	Systolic blood pressure (mmHg)	<90	–
	Respiratory examination	–	Crackles on auscultation
	Skin	Decreased skin swelling	Skin edema
	Urine color	Dark or amber	Clear
	Urine output (mL/kg/h)	<0.5	–
	Daily weight change	Lose >1 kg in 24 h	Gain >1 kg in 24 h
	Input/output balance chart	+1000 mL in 24 h	–1000 mL in 24 h
	Other clinical markers	Orthostatic hypotension	–
		Dry mucous membranes	
		Confusion/agitation	
		Weak/thready pulse	
		Slow capillary refill time	
Biochemical testing	Urine-specific gravity	>1.030	<1.010
	Serum osmolality (mOsm/kg)	>300	<280
	Hemoglobin (g/dL)	>15	<10
	Hematocrit (%)	>50	<30
	Blood urea nitrogen (mg/dL)	>18	<10
	Creatinine (mg/dL)	>1.3	<0.7
	pH on blood gas	Metabolic acidosis (negative base excess)	–
Invasive monitoring	CVP (mmHg)	<4	>9
	PADP (mmHg)	<6	>16
	PCWP (mmHg)	<6	>14

Abbreviations: bpm: Beats per minute; CVP: central venous pressure; PADP: pulmonary artery diastolic pressure; PCWP: pulmonary capillary wedge pressure.
[a] Reference ranges for some values may vary between laboratories.

Table 30.4 Overview of commoner invasive pressure and cardiac output monitors used to guide fluid management

Device		Comments
Invasive pressure monitors	CVP	• Right atrial pressure • Allows administration of potent vasoactive therapies • Can be used as a surrogate marker of pulmonary artery occlusion pressure (whose measurement would require a PAC) • Static CVP does not accurately indicate volume status or fluid responsiveness[29]
	Invasive ABP	• Allows frequent blood-gas monitoring and rapid recognition of hemodynamic instability • Facilitates the use of pulse pressure/PiCCO monitoring (see below)
Cardiac output monitors	PAC	• Traditionally considered the "gold standard" monitor, but measurements are not completely reliable • CO typically derived using temperature (cold) dilution curve analysis • Use declined in recent years owing to studies showing increased mortality in use of PAC, particularly in lower-risk patients[30,31]
	PiCCO (*Philips Healthcare, Guildford, UK*)	• Based on the principle that pulse pressure (difference between systolic and diastolic pressures) is proportional to SV • Requires a central line and arterial line (with the latter ideally sited in a large vessel, eg, femoral artery) • Hemodynamic measurements are acquired using thermodilution methods. A fixed volume of cold saline is injected through the central line to allow assessment of the temperature gradient and dissipation curve • Provides a continuous reading of CO (or SV) • Can also measure SVV in the fully ventilated patient with TV >8 mL/kg and no arrhythmias. SVV quantifies the cyclic change in SV with respiration to predict fluid responsiveness. SVV >12% predicts fluid responsiveness and <9% makes it unlikely
	LiDCO (*LiDCO Ltd, Cambridge, UK*)	• Similar to PiCCO, relies on arterial waveform analysis to estimate CO • Different from PiCCO in that calibration is performed using lithium dilution via peripheral cannula and thus does not require a central line (only an arterial line)
	ODM	• Increasingly used based on evidence of reduced complications,[2] LOS,[2] morbidity,[3] and mortality,[3] particularly in high-risk surgical patients • Involves placement of a Doppler probe into the esophagus at the level of T5/6 to measure aortic red cell velocity and flow time, which is converted into estimates of blood flow and thus SV using assumptions of the cross-sectional diameter of the descending aorta • Peak velocity as identified on the ODM waveform as a surrogate marker for left ventricular contractility

(*Continued*)

Table 30.4 (Continued) Overview of commoner invasive pressure and cardiac output monitors used to guide fluid management

Device	Comments
	• Corrected flow time (FTc), that is, time spent in systole "corrected" for heart rate, can identify changes in preload and afterload, with values <330 ms indicating hypovolemia or high SVR, and values >360 ms, indicating the opposite
	• Can average SV over a longer time period to reduce the influence of AF on measurements, for example
	• Like PiCCO, can also quantify SVV
	• Not practical to use in the extubated patient—nasal probes are available but uncomfortable in the awake patient
NiCOM (Cheetah Medical, Vancouver, WA)	• Quantifies thoracic bioimpedance
	• Need to differentiate changes resulting from CV and those from ventilation, through frequency and phase modulation of an applied voltage
	• Provides a reading of SV

Abbreviations: ABP: Arterial blood pressure; AF: atrial fibrillation; CVP: central venous pressure; EDM: esophageal Doppler monitor; LiDCO: lithium dilution technique for the measurement of cardiac output; LOS: length of stay; NiCOM: noninvasive cardiac output monitoring; PiCCO: pulse contour cardiac output; SV: stroke volume; SVR: systemic vascular resistance; SVV: stroke volume variation; TV: tidal volume.

MANAGEMENT

The main decisions that need to be made regarding fluid management pertain to the choice of fluids to use, the timing of administration, and the volume to use. Although not specific to patients with neurotrauma, there is a large amount of evidence from trials of early goal-directed therapy in surgical patients that prove that even relatively small differences in the volume and timing of fluid administered can significantly influence outcomes.[2,3]

Fluid choice

The type of fluid(s) used is critical when considering patients who have sustained TBI, as it may influence outcomes. There has been much debate over the superiority of crystalloids and colloids over each other. Blood product transfusions are discussed in a separate chapter.

CRYSTALLOIDS

Crystalloid fluids can be broadly classified into hypotonic, isotonic, and hypertonic. They are often used as maintenance fluids, the commonest examples include 0.9% saline and Ringer's lactate, both of which

have a similar osmolarity (are isotonic) to normal plasma. The use of 0.9% saline is associated with hyperchloremic metabolic acidosis,[4] so some medical professionals recommend the alternation of 0.9% saline with Ringer's lactate as maintenance fluids.

There is evidence that the administration of large amounts of crystalloids is deleterious. In resuscitation settings, overuse can influence the development of acute respiratory distress syndrome (ARDS), multiorgan failure, and compartment syndromes.[5] Use of more than 1.5 L of crystalloid in the emergency department was shown to independently predict mortality, especially in older patients.[6] It is recommended that no more than 2 L of crystalloids be administered to a patient in 1 day unless there are obvious sources of extracellular fluid losses.[7]

Crystalloids remain in the intravascular space for less time than colloids (often <60 minutes), and allow water to distribute equally over time to intravascular and interstitial spaces; administration of large volumes, therefore, leads to whole-body interstitial edema. For these reasons, crystalloids have not historically been preferred as resuscitation fluids. If crystalloids are to be used, Plasmalyte A is a better-balanced solution than others, producing less acid-base balance disturbance and improved renal cortical tissue perfusion than 0.9% saline, according to data from a randomized trial.[8]

Dextrose is another crystalloid that is available in a range of formulations, but it is hypotonic and its use in patients with neurotrauma is generally not advocated, particularly in the first 48 hours following injury. It is rapidly lost from the intravascular compartment, can lower serum osmolality and sodium, and it can increase cerebral brain content and ICP. Furthermore, hyperglycemia exacerbates secondary neuronal injury and is associated with worsened outcomes after severe TBI.[9] The only instance in which dextrose-containing solutions should be used is if the patient is hypoglycemic in the absence of nutritional support.

There has been significant interest in the routine use of hypertonic crystalloids, such as 3% saline in patients with TBI, although there is no evidence of superiority over isotonic crystalloids. Hypertonic saline has the advantage of raising sodium in patients with hyponatremia and can reduce intracranial pressure (ICP), although without judicious use and monitoring, hypernatremia could rapidly result in the risk of seizures and reduced level of consciousness. Thus, the use of hypertonic saline necessitates regular checks of serum sodium levels (every 4–6 hours). In addition, administration through a peripheral cannula can lead to phlebitis, and use of a central venous catheter may be preferred. Hypertonic saline can be administered in bolus form or as a continuous infusion, with dosing titrated according to serum sodium levels and/or osmolality.

Lactate was historically believed to solely be a by-product of anaerobic metabolism; however, there is emerging evidence that it can act as a preferential fuel in the injured brain. Preliminary clinical data suggest that hypertonic lactate solutions spare cerebral glucose, improve cerebral energy metabolism, and can effectively reduce elevated ICP.[10] However, additional data are required before its routine use in the brain-injured patient can be recommended.

COLLOIDS

Colloids are solutions containing large insoluble macromolecules that largely remain in the intravascular compartment, as they do not readily cross the BBB capillary wall. A variety of colloid solutions exist, including dextran, hydroxyethyl starch (HES), gelatin, and albumin preparations. Relative to crystalloids, colloids achieve a more rapid resuscitation, and smaller infusion volumes are required; however, they are generally more expensive.

HES is an enzymatically hydrolyzed amylopectin whose use has fallen out of favor due to concerns raised about its connection with renal impairment[11,12] and mortality,[12,13] particularly in surgical patients at risk of sepsis or renal failure. Dextran is a glucose polymer that can inhibit platelet aggregation and improve microcirculatory flow. However, like HES, dextrans have fallen out of favor because they impact normal blood coagulation and are associated with allergic as well as pseudoallergic reactions. Additionally, dextrans may have an impact on blood grouping and cross-matching. Gelatins are proteins that are formed by the hydrolysis of collagen and are available in three different forms: succinylated or modified fluid gelatins (eg, Gelofusine), oxypolygelatins (eg, Gelifundol), and urea-crosslinked gelatins (eg, Haemaccel). They have a negative charge that enhances intravascular retention and do not interfere with blood cross-matching; however, they are associated with a higher risk of allergic reactions than other colloids.[14] Gelatins are the most widely used colloids, and their main use is as a volume expander in resuscitation settings.

Human albumin solution (HAS) is another colloid, which is available in concentrations ranging from 5% to 25%. Although it is a blood product, HAS does not contain clotting factors or isoagglutinins, the latter meaning that no knowledge of the patient's blood type is required prior to administration. It has a plasma half-life of 16 hours in nonedematous patients. The most important study relating to the use of HASs was the SAFE multicenter, randomized, controlled trial.[15] In this study, almost 7000 patients with critical illnesses of varying etiologies were randomized to receive either 4% albumin or 0.9% saline as a resuscitation fluid for 28 days. There was no difference in mortality at 28 days following randomization. However, in a post-hoc follow-up study of the SAFE trial, which focused on 460 patients with TBI, the use of albumin was associated with a significantly higher mortality 2 years following randomization (33.2% [albumin] vs. 20.4% [saline], relative risk = 1.63, 95% confidence interval = 1.17–2.26, $P < 0.003$).[16] This difference appeared to be driven by patients with severe TBI (Glasgow Coma Scale [GCS] score 3–8; 41.8% [albumin] vs. 22.2% [saline], relative risk = 1.88, 95% confidence interval = 1.31–2.70, $P < 0.001$), and no significant difference in outcomes between the two treatment arms was seen in those with GCS scores between 9 and 12 (16.0% [albumin] vs. 21.6% [saline], relative risk = 0.74, 95% confidence interval = 0.31–1.79, $P = 0.50$).[16] This may have been due to a higher incidence of intracranial hypertension in patients with severe TBI within the first week following injury and also increased use of additional treatments to control intracranial hypertension in this group.[17]

Determining fluid volume required

The average adult patient who is afebrile will lose approximately 2400 mL per day from a range of sources (Table 30.5). However, in the neurotrauma patient, there may be additional losses from various sources, such as bleeding, vomiting, nasogastric suction, and diarrhea. Pyrexia is common in patients with TBI,[18] and increases respiratory as well as involuntary losses. Therefore, the meticulous documentation of fluid balance charts in combination with a thorough clinical assessment, laboratory markers, and/or invasive monitoring results, are crucial to ensuring adequate fluid administration.

Fluid resuscitation protocol

It is possible to broadly divide fluid resuscitation approaches into fixed (or recipe) and individualized. The fixed/recipe protocols are determined on a mL-per-kg-of-body-weight-per-hour basis and can be further divided into wet and dry protocols,

Table 30.5 Average estimated daily fluid loss in an adult

Type	Estimated volume (mL) per day
Sweat	100
Urine	1400
Feces	200
Involuntary losses—Skin	350
Involuntary losses—Lungs	350
Total	**2400**

depending on the volume of fluid prescribed. The main issue with these fixed approaches is that they fail to account for interindividual and situation-specific variance in fluid requirements. Studies evaluating different fluid resuscitation approaches have typically been performed in patients undergoing elective surgery, and thus, their applicability to the patient with neurotrauma is, at best, limited.

More individualized approaches to fluid resuscitation are based on optimizing physiologic targets, including global oxygen delivery (DO_2), which is the product of cardiac output (CO) and oxygen content of arterial blood (CaO_2), as follows:

$$DO_2 = CO \times CaO_2$$

Targeting DO_2 often involves the use of inotropic medications and blood transfusions. Patients under general anesthesia experience peripheral vasodilation and, in these instances, vasopressors are often required. Inotropic medications are useful in improving physiologic markers of CO and perfusion. However, they are associated with complications, including arrhythmias, myocyte death, and reduced renal perfusion. There is no reliable evidence that one vasopressor is superior to another,[19] but norepinephrine has a predictable and consistent effect on systemic blood pressure and cerebral hemodynamics and is widely used.

The management of hypovolemia can be particularly challenging, and it should be avoided because it can result in reduced CO and cerebral perfusion. Hypovolemic/hypotensive patients should be treated initially with intravenous fluid resuscitation, but a vasoactive agent may be required if adequate blood pressure cannot be achieved with fluid resuscitation alone. It is widely accepted that overly aggressive fluid resuscitation is detrimental, and euvolemia is the primary cardiovascular goal.[20]

Monitoring response to fluid treatment

There is increasing literature from patients with a range of pathologies (including nontraumatic) that states that when evaluating volume status, response to fluid administration, and titrating fluid administration, more dynamic hemodynamic parameters, such as changes in stroke volume and arterial pulse pressure, are superior to more static parameters, such as right atrial pressure, pulmonary artery occlusion pressure, and right ventricular end-diastolic volume.[21,22]

Clinical signs and biochemical parameters play a role in monitoring response to treatment. For example, a commonly used urine output target is 0.5 to 1.0 mL/kg/h. The use of venous saturations, lactate, and base excess can be used but there is no robust evidence that supports that targeting these improves outcomes.vh

SPECIFIC MANAGEMENT CHALLENGES

Prehospital fluid management

The use of prehospital fluid resuscitation has been controversial, in part due to conflicting evidence about the association between prehospital cannula insertion and mortality.[23] Permissive hypotension and limited fluid resuscitation have been recommended for the prehospital care of general trauma patients,[7] however, in patients with suspected traumatic brain injury (TBI), this must be balanced with the potential consequences of cerebral hypoperfusion.[24] The same applies to the patient with spinal cord injury (SCI). A single episode of hypotension (systolic BP <90 mmHg) is strongly associated with poorer outcomes in patients with TBI,[25] and thus prevention or rapid reversal of hypotension is essential in these patients. In the absence of active bleeding, more aggressive resuscitation approaches may be warranted. Patients with suspected TBI should receive prehospital fluid administration titrated to ensure a systolic blood pressure of >90 mmHg. The optimal prehospital fluid management of neurotrauma patients with polytrauma remains unclear.

There is little evidence to guide the choice and amount of fluid used in the prehospital setting. A sensible protocol is the use of 250 mL boluses of crystalloids up to a maximum of 1 L, given the risks associated with excessive crystalloid used in resuscitation settings.[7] Although the use of either 0.9% saline or Ringer's lactate is generally recommended, recent evidence from a post-hoc analysis of 791 patients in the PROMMTT (PRospective Observational Multicenter Major Trauma Transfusion) trial suggests that the prehospital use of Ringer's lactate is associated with increased mortality in TBI when compared with 0.9% saline.[26] However, this requires validation through further study.

Treating intracranial hypertension

There has been much debate about the optimal osmotic agent to use in the setting of intracranial hypertension. Mannitol (0.25–1.0 g/kg) is widely considered a standard of care for the acute treatment of elevated ICP, according to the Brain Trauma Foundation guidelines for the management of severe TBI,[27] but it has never been subject to a randomized comparison with placebo. It acts within minutes of administration and improves viscosity and cerebral blood flow. However, it also opens the BBB and, with multiple doses, can cross the interstitial space and cause hypotonicity. Side effects include initial fluid overload, subsequent hypotension, metabolic acidosis, and electrolyte imbalance, all of which can adversely affect the injured brain. Furthermore, repeated administration of mannitol may result in unacceptably high serum osmolality (>320 mOsm/L), neurologic complications, and acute kidney injury.

Hypertonic saline, which is available in concentrations ranging from 1.8% to 23.4%, may have a more profound and long-lasting effect on ICP compared with mannitol, but outcome benefits over mannitol have not been demonstrated.[28] There is extensive heterogeneity in clinical outcome studies in terms of dose, concentration, frequency, and mode (bolus or continuous infusion) of administration. Furthermore, the optimal osmolar load to lower elevated ICP is undefined. Hypertonic saline has several theoretical beneficial effects on the injured brain in addition to its osmotic action, including neurochemical, vasoregulatory, and immunologic actions. It also expands intravascular volume, potentially augmenting cerebral perfusion pressure, which is itself a therapeutic target in patients with TBI.

Spinal cord injury

Relative to TBI, there are sparse clinical data to guide the fluid management of patients with SCI. SCI is associated with decreased sympathetic tone, which results in vasodilation, hypotension, bradycardia, and impaired organ perfusion. It is important to ensure that patients with SCI do not receive excessive fluids as this can exacerbate spinal cord edema with potentially devastating consequences; however, similarly inadequate fluid resuscitation may lead to spinal cord ischemia with equally deleterious effects. Further research is required to better understand optimal treatment paradigms for patients with SCI.

CONCLUSIONS

There has been much debate and controversy about the optimal choice, amount, and timing of fluids to be administered to neurotrauma patients. In part, owing to the lack of a robust evidence base to guide decision making in several areas, and many unanswered questions, there is significant variation in the fluid management of patients between centers. Based on what is known to date, there are several key points that can be made about fluid management in neurotrauma.

First, the main determinant of fluid movement across the BBB is the presence of an osmotic gradient, and, where possible, routine use of fluids that exacerbate edema should be avoided, including those with dextrose, low sodium, and low tonicity. Second, although debate about the relative superiority of crystalloids and colloids continues, there is evidence from different population groups that the routine and frequent use of several colloids may be harmful. Third, although prehospital resuscitation of general trauma patients typically focuses on permissive hypotension and limited fluid resuscitation, in patients with neurotrauma, more aggressive fluid resuscitation may be warranted to prevent the harmful effects of cerebral and spinal cord hypoperfusion. The optimal fluid management of polytrauma patients with neurotrauma remains unclear. Finally, although the debate about the optimal agent to treat intracranial hypertension continues, hypertonic saline may be preferred over mannitol, particularly in the hypotensive patient, although, to date, no robust outcome benefits have been proven.

Additional research is required to further clarify the optimal monitoring and management paradigms for fluid management in neurotrauma patients, including for patients with SCI where relatively little research has been done to date. Ultimately, the choice and volume of fluids used should be determined on an individual, case-by-case basis, accounting for standard maintenance requirements as well as additional losses that are dependent on the clinical situation. This individualized care can be facilitated by the use of advanced monitoring techniques where appropriate, including in the intraoperative and critical care settings. A reasonable approach in these settings may involve use of a central venous line, arterial line, and CO monitor, with the use of fluid boluses to influence SV.

REFERENCES

1. Bohara M, Kambe Y, Nagayama T, Tokimura H, Arita K, Miyata A. C-type natriuretic peptide modulates permeability of the blood–brain barrier. *J Cereb Blood Flow Metab*. London, England: SAGE Publications Sage UK; 2014;34(4):589-596.

2. Phan TD, Ismail H, Heriot AG, Ho KM. Improving perioperative outcomes: Fluid optimization with the esophageal Doppler monitor, a metaanalysis and review. *J Am Coll Surg*. 2008;207(6):935-941.

3. Hamilton MA, Cecconi M, Rhodes A. A systematic review and meta-analysis on the use of preemptive hemodynamic intervention to improve postoperative outcomes in moderate and high-risk surgical patients. *Anesth Analg*. 2011;112(6):1392-1402.

4. Myles PS, Andrews S, Nicholson J, Lobo DN, Mythen M. Contemporary Approaches to Perioperative IV Fluid Therapy. *World J Surg*. Switzerland: Springer International Publishing; 2017;20(2):125-127.

5. Kasotakis G, Sideris A, Yang Y, de Moya M, Alam H, King DR et al. Aggressive early crystalloid resuscitation adversely affects outcomes in adult blunt trauma patients. *J Trauma Acute Care Surg*. 2013;74(5):1215-1222.

6. Ley EJ, Clond MA, Srour MK, Barnajian M, Mirocha J, Margulies DR et al. Emergency department crystalloid resuscitation of 1.5 L or more is associated with increased mortality in elderly and nonelderly trauma patients. *J Trauma: Injury, Infection, Crit Care*. 2011;70(2):398-400.

7. James MFM. Volume therapy in trauma and neurotrauma. *Best Pract Res Clin Anaesthesiol*. 2014;28(3):285-296.

8. Chowdhury AH, Cox EF, Francis ST, Lobo DN. A randomized, controlled, double-blind crossover study on the effects of 2-L infusions of 0.9% saline and plasma-lyte® 148 on renal blood flow velocity and renal cortical tissue perfusion in healthy volunteers. *Ann Surg*. 2012;256(1):18-24.

9. Salim A, Hadjizacharia P, Dubose J, Brown C, Inaba K, Chan LS et al. Persistent hyperglycemia in severe traumatic brain injury: An independent predictor of outcome. *Am Surg*. 2009;75(1):25-29.

10. Bouzat P, Oddo M. Lactate and the injured brain: Friend or foe? *Curr Opin Crit Care.* 2014;20(2):133-140.

11. Perner A, Haase N, Guttormsen AB, Tenhunen J, Klemenzson G, Åneman A et al. Hydroxyethyl starch 130/0.42 versus Ringer's acetate in severe sepsis. *N Engl J Med.* 2012;367(2):124-134.

12. Zarychanski R, Abou-Setta AM, Turgeon AF, Houston BL, McIntyre L, Marshall JC et al. Association of hydroxyethyl starch administration with mortality and acute kidney injury in critically ill patients requiring volume resuscitation: A systematic review and meta-analysis. *JAMA.* 2013;309(7):678-688.

13. Perel P, Roberts I, Ker K. Colloids versus crystalloids for fluid resuscitation in critically ill patients. In: Perel P, ed. *Cochrane Database Syst Rev.* Chichester, UK: John Wiley & Sons, Ltd; 2013;13(2):CD000567.

14. Laxenaire MC, Charpentier C, Feldman L. [Anaphylactoid reactions to colloid plasma substitutes: Incidence, risk factors, mechanisms. A French multicenter prospective study]. *Ann Fr Anesth Reanim [Internet].* 1994;13(3):301-310. Available from: http://eutils.ncbi.nlm.nih.gov/entrez/eutils/elink.fcgi?dbfrom=pubmed&id=7992937&retmode=ref&cmd=prlinks.

15. Finfer S, Bellomo R, Boyce N, French J, Myburgh J, Norton R et al. A comparison of albumin and saline for fluid resuscitation in the intensive care unit. *N Engl J Med.* 2004;350(22):2247-2256.

16. SAFE Study Investigators, Australian and New Zealand Intensive Care Society Clinical Trials Group, Australian Red Cross Blood Service, George Institute for International Health et al. Saline or albumin for fluid resuscitation in patients with traumatic brain injury. *N Engl J Med.* 2007;357(9):874-884.

17. Cooper DJ, Myburgh J, Heritier S, Finfer S, Bellomo R, Billot L et al. Albumin resuscitation for traumatic brain injury: Is intracranial hypertension the cause of increased mortality? *J Neurotrauma [Internet].* 2013;30(7):512-518.

18. Bohman L-E, Levine JM. Fever and therapeutic normothermia in severe brain injury: An update. *Curr Opin Crit Care.* 2014;20(2):182-188.

19. Sookplung P, Siriussawakul A, Malakouti A, Sharma D, Wang J, Souter MJ et al. Vasopressor use and effect on blood pressure after severe adult traumatic brain injury. *Neurocrit Care.* Totowa, NJ: Humana Press Inc; 2011;15(1):46-54.

20. Gantner D, Moore EM, Cooper DJ. Intravenous fluids in traumatic brain injury: What's the solution? *Curr Opin Crit Care.* 2014;20(4):385-389.

21. Michard F, Teboul J-L. Predicting fluid responsiveness in ICU patients. *Chest.* New York: Elsevier; 2002;121(6):2000-2008.

22. Berkenstadt H, Margalit N, Hadani M, Friedman Z, Segal E, Villa Y et al. Stroke volume variation as a predictor of fluid responsiveness in patients undergoing brain surgery. *Anesth Analg.* 2001;92(4):984-989.

23. Haut ER, Kalish BT, Cotton BA, Efron DT, Haider AH, Stevens KA et al. Prehospital intravenous fluid administration is associated with higher mortality in trauma patients: A National Trauma Data Bank analysis. *Ann Surg.* 2011;253(2):371-377.

24. Boer C, Franschman G, Loer SA. Prehospital management of severe traumatic brain injury: Concepts and ongoing controversies. *Curr Opin Anaesthesiol.* 2012;25(5):556-562.

25. McHugh GS, Engel DC, Butcher I, Steyerberg EW, Lu J, Mushkudiani N et al. Prognostic value of secondary insults in traumatic brain injury: Results from the IMPACT study. *J Neurotrauma.* 2007;24(2):287-293.

26. Rowell SE, Fair KA, Barbosa RR, Watters JM, Bulger EM, Holcomb JB et al. The impact of pre-hospital administration of lactated Ringer's solution versus normal saline in patients with traumatic brain injury. *J Neurotrauma.* 2016;33(11):1054-1059.

27. Carney N, Totten AM, O'Reilly C, Ullman JS, Hawryluk GWJ, Bell MJ et al. *Guidelines for the Management of Severe Traumatic Brain Injury.* 4th ed. *Neurosurgery.* 2017;80(1):6-15.

28. Diringer MN. New trends in hyperosmolar therapy? *Curr Opin Crit Care*. 2013;19(2): 77-82.

29. Osman D, Ridel C, Ray P, Monnet X, Anguel N, Richard C et al. Cardiac filling pressures are not appropriate to predict hemodynamic response to volume challenge. *Crit Care Med*. 2007;35(1):64-68.

30. Marik PE. Obituary: Pulmonary artery catheter 1970 to 2013. *Ann Intensive Care*. Paris, France: Springer; 2013;3(1):38.

31. Connors AF, Speroff T, Dawson NV, Thomas C, Harrell FE, Wagner D et al. The effectiveness of right heart catheterization in the initial care of critically ill patients. SUPPORT Investigators. *JAMA*. 1996;276(11):889-897.

31

Coagulopathy and blood transfusions

LAMIA NAYEB AND MATTHEW A. KIRKMAN

INTRODUCTION

Coagulopathy is common in patients with traumatic brain injury (TBI)[1] and is associated with the progression of hemorrhagic and ischemic lesions,[2,3] longer intensive care unit (ICU) stay,[4,5] single and multiple organ failure,[5] and overall morbidity and mortality.[4–6] Causes of coagulopathy in patients with trauma include acute traumatic coagulopathy (ATC) and delayed coagulopathy secondary to hemodilution. Its underlying pathophysiology is complex and not fully elucidated; although, at a high level the process appears to be dynamic, with an initial hypercoagulable state followed by bleeding diathesis.[7] Anemia is also common in patients with TBI, and may contribute to secondary injury and worsened outcomes.[8] The presence of coagulopathy and/or anemia have several important implications in the management of patients with TBI, including decisions regarding surgical intervention and its timing. Despite this, and the relative frequency with which coagulopathy and anemia are encountered in patients with TBI, the evidence base to guide decision making is suboptimal, and the management of neither coagulopathy nor anemia is discussed in the most recent (4th edition) guidelines on the

management of severe TBI from the Brain Trauma Foundation.[9]

The aims of this chapter are to: (i) review the epidemiology, risk factors, pathophysiology, investigation, and management of coagulopathy in patients with TBI; (ii) discuss the management of anemia in TBI, with a particular focus on blood transfusions; and (iii) briefly discuss particular management challenges, including the management of patients on anticoagulation and/or antiplatelet therapy, and decisions regarding venous thromboembolism (VTE) prophylaxis.

COAGULOPATHY

Epidemiology and risk factors

The exact prevalence of coagulopathy in patients with TBI is unknown, in part due to the lack of a universally accepted definition of what constitutes coagulopathy in a population group. A meta-analysis of 22 studies found the prevalence of ATC in patients with isolated TBI varied between 7% and 86.1% (pooled proportion: 35.2%).[1] Reasons for this wide variation in reported prevalence include differences in study design and the definitions of coagulopathy used. Timing of blood testing is also likely to influence the detection of coagulopathy. In one retrospective study of 278 patients with isolated severe TBI, a prolonged course of coagulopathy lasting more than 72 hours was observed in less than one-third of the patients.[10]

Several risk factors have been associated with the development of coagulopathy in TBI (Table 31.1).

Overview of coagulation cascade

The process of coagulation is complex and a detailed description of the molecular and cellular aspects is beyond the scope of this chapter. Instead, a summary is provided here.

Primary hemostasis occurs when vascular injury exposes the endothelium to circulating platelets that are captured to form a basic plug. Secondary hemostasis involves a coagulation cascade through an extrinsic (tissue factor) and an intrinsic (contact) pathway (Figure 31.1). In both cases, serial reactions between inactive enzyme protease precursors and

Table 31.1 Risk factors for the development of coagulopathy in patients with TBI

- GCS score ≤8 at scene[5]
- AIS-Head severity grade[5]
- Hypotension at the scene and/or in the emergency room[5]
- Prehospital IV fluids ≥2000 mL[5]
- Age ≥75[5]
- ISS ≥16[4]
- Cerebral edema[4]
- SAH[4]
- Midline shift on CT[4]

Abbreviations: AIS: Abbreviated injury scale; CT: computed tomography; GCS: Glasgow Coma Scale; ISS: Injury Severity Score; SAH: subarachnoid hemorrhage.

their respective glycoprotein cofactors result in the activation of factor X that catalyzes conversion of prothrombin to thrombin, thrombin in turn

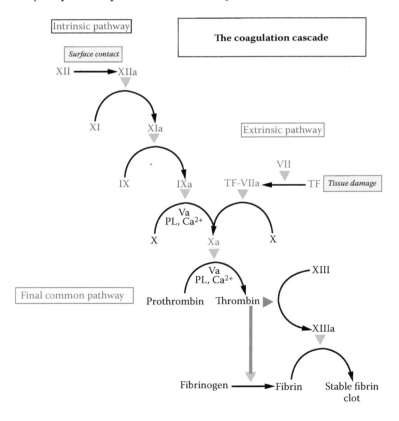

Figure 31.1 Overview of the coagulation cascade.
Abbreviations: PL: Platelet membrane phospholipid; TF: tissue factor.

catalyzes conversion of fibrinogen to fibrin. The final product of coagulation is a stabilized fibrin mesh formed by fibrin polymerization that stabilizes the platelet plug. Fibrin is in turn broken down by plasmin. Tissue factor (TF) [thromboplastin], a transmembrane receptor separated from its ligand factor VII by the endothelium, is highly expressed in brain tissue, possibly reflecting additional hemostatic protection.[11]

The fibrinolytic system acts to ensure basal hemostasis, providing negative feedback to prevent excessive thrombogenesis and to maintain vascular patency. Inactive circulating plasminogen, which is assimilated into clots as they form, is cleaved to plasmin by tissue plasminogen activator (tPA) released from injured vascular endothelial cells, and urokinase plasminogen activator (uPA). Production of tPA and urokinase further amplify plasmin generation and are both in turn inhibited by plasminogen activator inhibitor-1 and -2. Plasmin is inactivated by α-2-plasmin inhibitor and α-2-macroglobulin, and thrombin-activatable fibrinolysis inhibitor (TAFI).

Pathophysiology

Several theories to explain coagulopathy after TBI have been proposed, and the major ones are discussed in the following subsections.

TISSUE FACTOR

Central nervous system tissue is particularly rich in tissue factor (TF; factor III or thromboplastin),[12] a transmembrane lipoprotein expressed in fibroblasts, vascular smooth muscle cells, pericytes, and astrocytes, and not normally exposed to circulating blood. Release of TF from injured brain tissue into the blood circulation has been hypothesized to activate the extrinsic pathway and eventually result in disseminated intravascular coagulation (DIC) through ongoing amplification. There is evidence to suggest that extravascular blood-borne TF binds its ligand factor VIIa in the absence of injury,[13] potentially rapidly amplifying an injury-triggered coagulopathy.

TF has also been associated with the presence of circulating endothelial- and platelet-derived procoagulant microparticles (PMPs), released by apoptotic cells both in cerebrospinal fluid (CSF) and peripheral circulation following TBI. PMPs may contribute to ongoing activation of the coagulation cascade and worsen outcomes. In a small study of 16 patients with severe TBI, persistently high levels of PMPs in CSF at 10 days post-TBI was associated with poor clinical outcome, while high peripheral blood levels were associated with eventual DIC.[14] PMPs may directly aggravate coagulopathy through delivery of more TF to platelets and could even recruit other target cells not normally able to trigger coagulation, such as neurons through endocytosis of PMPs by target cells, for example, brain endothelial cells,[15] enabling them to potentiate the coagulation cascade.

PLATELETS

Multiple studies have found an association between TBI and decreased platelet count and/or function, independent of antiplatelet therapy.[16] Thrombocytopenia can result in progression of traumatic intracranial hemorrhage and independently predicts mortality in severe TBI.[3,17] Concomitant increased platelet activation with reduced platelet function has been observed in TBI[18] and the presence of post-TBI thrombocytopenia in the absence of significant hemorrhage[19–21] and the high incidence of intravascular microthrombosis following TBI[22] have both been used to suggest that platelets may be "hyperactive" following TBI.

The exact cause or causes of platelet dysfunction in TBI remain to be elucidated, but it may involve a neurohumoral factor triggered by brain injury,[23] platelet-activating factor (PAF)—an endogenous pro-inflammatory phospholipid that binds platelet receptors as well as receptors on leukocytes and endothelial cells,[12] the cyclooxygenase pathway, or an undiscovered platelet inhibitor.[21]

HYPERFIBRINOLYSIS

Hyperfibrinolysis may cause coagulopathy in TBI by TF-driven over activation of the extrinsic pathway, raised levels of tissue plasminogen activator (tPA) or activated protein C, or depletion of α-2-plasmin inhibitor resulting in increased plasmin.[24–26]

Assessment

CLINICAL AND RADIOLOGIC INDICATORS

Clinical signs, such as bleeding from wound(s) or sites of line insertion, may indicate the presence of an underlying coagulopathy. Imaging may also have a role in predicting the duration of coagulopathy

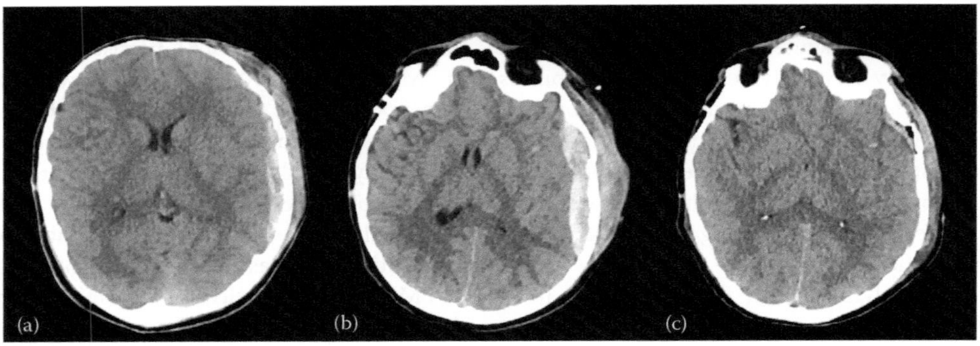

Figure 31.2 Noncontrast axial computed tomography (CT) imaging of a young male who fell off a skateboard at high velocity and hit a stationary car. He was intubated at the scene and taken to the nearest trauma center. (a) Initial CT scan demonstrating an acute extradural hematoma overlying the left frontal, anterior left parietal, and left temporal lobes. Small foci of acute contusional injury in the left frontal and temporal lobes were also present on the scan. There was associated mass effect and sulcal effacement in the left cerebral hemisphere. In addition, there were mildly displaced acute fractures of the left frontal, left parietal, and left squamous temporal bones, and also of the left zygomatic arch. (b) Repeat CT imaging performed 24 hours later demonstrates enlargement of the extradural hematoma. The patient was coagulopathic on blood testing, which was corrected in liaison with local hematologists. (c) CT imaging performed following craniotomy for evacuation of the extradural hematoma demonstrates a reduction in the volume and mass effect of the left-sided extradural hematoma.

(Figure 31.2); one prospective study ($n = 218$) found higher rates of intracranial hemorrhage and signs of raised intracranial pressure on the initial CT scan among patients with delayed/sustained coagulopathy relative to those with early coagulopathy only, with the former group also having worse outcomes in 6 months.[6] Despite this, blood testing is ultimately required to confirm the presence of coagulopathy and guide further treatment.

LABORATORY TESTING

As highlighted earlier in this chapter, there is no universally accepted definition of coagulopathy in TBI. Typically, a derangement of one or more of the commonly available laboratory parameters of coagulation (including platelet count, prothrombin time [PT]/international normalized ratio [INR], and/or partial prothrombin time [PTT]) are used (Table 31.2). Less specific but easily measured are D-dimer

Table 31.2 Laboratory tests used in the evaluation of coagulopathy

	Platelets	Enzymatic coagulation	Fibrinolysis
More commonly tested	• Platelet count • Platelet function testing (eg, PFA-100)	• Prothrombin time (PT), international normalized ratio (INR) • Partial prothrombin time (PTT) • Fibrinogen	• D-dimer
Less commonly tested/ research use	• Bleeding time • Thromboelastography • Whole blood impedance aggregometry • Rapid platelet function assay	• Thromboelastography • Thrombin time • Thrombin-antithrombin III complex • Prothrombin cleavage fragments 1 and 2	• Fibrinogen degradation products (FDP) • Thromboelastography • Plasminogen activator inhibitor-1

and fibrinogen levels. A variety of other markers, such as fibrinogen degradation products (FDP), plasmin–antiplasmin complex, and thrombin–antithrombin III complex, are available but they are largely restricted to research. While the use of these tests may indicate a hypocoagulable state, there is no specific routine laboratory test to confirm a hypercoagulable state.

THROMBOELASTOGRAPHY

Thromboelastography (TEG) uses a hemostatic assay to provide a global picture of coagulation status, including hypo-/hypercoagulability and fibrinolysis. A small whole blood sample is exposed to gentle rotation in order to activate the coagulation cascade, and the strength and viscoelastic properties of the clot formed are analyzed. The application of TEG has thus far been limited to resuscitation and perioperative settings.[27] TEG may help identify hypercoagulability states resistant to traditional thromboprophylaxis after trauma or major surgery,[28,29] and as part of a point-of-care (POC) testing package with VerifyNow Aspirin (VN-ASA) may also identify occult coagulopathy that would otherwise be missed.[30]

TEG could have an important role in the detection and management of coagulopathy in patients with TBI in the acute setting. However, high-quality evidence confirming a relationship between TEG use and improved outcomes is lacking, and further data are required in this regard.

Management

There is no specific, widely used guideline for the reversal of post-TBI coagulopathy, which typically relies on the correction of coagulation abnormalities with combinations of fresh frozen plasma (FFP), recombinant factor VIIa (rFVIIa), prothrombin complex concentrate (PCC), tranexamic acid (TXA), and/or platelets according to local protocols. The reversal of anticoagulation and antiplatelet therapies in the setting of TBI are discussed separately later in the chapter.

FRESH FROZEN PLASMA

FFP is commonly administered in patients with trauma. However, there is evidence against its prophylactic use[31,32] and use in the presence of only moderate coagulopathy (INR 1.4–2.0).[33] The ratio of FFP to packed red blood cells (pRBCs) administered may be critical, with a higher FFP:pRBC ratio being associated with favorable outcomes in trauma patients with and without TBI.[34] FFP administration requires blood cross-matching and can involve large fluid volumes, which limits the speed of administration possible and is a particular issue in patients with cardiac disease, for example.

PROTHROMBIN COMPLEX CONCENTRATE

PCC is an inactivated human plasma-derived concentrate of vitamin K-dependent clotting factors II, VII, IX, and X and proteins C and S, available as 3-factor (Profilnine) or 4-factor (Octaplex, Beriplex, Kcentra) PCCs based on whether factor VII levels (3-factor) or therapeutic (4-factor) are low. Blood cross-matching is not necessary and PCC can be administered promptly due to relatively small infusion volumes. Dosage is weight-based and INR-dependent, usually determined in consultation with local hematologists. PCCs have been shown to reduce pRBC and FFP transfusion requirements and TBI-associated mortality with induced or acquired coagulopathy compared with administration of rFVIIa, irrespective of anticoagulation therapy status.[35]

RECOMBINANT FACTOR VIIA

Decreased factor VII activity has been observed in patients with isolated blunt TBI,[36] and rFVIIa may improve coagulopathies in those refractory to FFP.[37] In a large randomized controlled trial (RCT), rFVIIa reduced hematoma growth in spontaneous (nontraumatic) intracerebral hemorrhage but did not improve survival or functional outcomes in 90 days and resulted in higher risk of thromboembolic events.[38] However, data from a prospective study of 87 patients with isolated TBI found treatment with low-dose (20µg/kg) rFVIIa in combination with blood products resulted in greater INR correction, lower rates of progressive hemorrhagic injury, and no increased risk of cerebral infarction or mortality compared to those receiving blood products alone.[39] Further high-quality data are required to fully establish the role of rFVIIa in the management of post-TBI coagulopathy.

TRANEXAMIC ACID

TXA is a synthetic lysine analog that inhibits fibrinolysis through reversibly binding to lysine receptor sites on plasminogen and preventing its activation to plasmin, thereby preventing fibrin breakdown. The landmark Clinical Randomization of an Antifibrinolytic in Significant Hemorrhage 2 (CRASH-2) RCT[40] randomized 20,211 trauma patients with or at risk of significant hemorrhage to receive either TXA or placebo, finding TXA to significantly reduce all-cause mortality (14.5% vs. 16.0%, relative risk [RR]: 0.91, 95% confidence interval [CI]: 0.85–0.97, p = 0.0035) and risk of death due to bleeding (4.9% vs. 5.7%, RR: 0.85, 95% CI: 0.76–0.96, p = 0.0077). Importantly, there were no significant differences in transfusion requirements between the two arms. Subsequent analysis of the trial data found that TXA should be given as soon as possible and within 3 hours of injury, as treatment later than this is likely to be ineffective and harmful.[41]

The CRASH-2 data were not specific to TBI. In combining data from a subset of 270 patients with TBI in the CRASH-2 trial and another RCT of 240 patients with TBI,[42] a Cochrane review[43] found that TXA administration reduced all-cause mortality (RR: 0.63; 95% CI: 0.40–0.99, p = 0.05). The risk of intracranial hemorrhage expansion, defined as a 25% or greater increase in the size of total bleed relative to baseline volume, reduced following TXA administration (RR: 0.75, 95% CI: 0.58–0.98, p = 0.03), and no statistically significant increase in the incidence of vaso-occlusive events, blood transfusion, or surgical intervention was associated with TXA. However, the authors emphasize that these estimates are imprecise, not supported by evidence, and uncertain. For this reason, the CRASH-3 trial[44] was designed to evaluate the effects of TXA on mortality and disability rates specifically in TBI. Data from this study are greatly anticipated.

PLATELETS

Despite platelet deficiency and/or dysfunction being common in TBI,[16] there is relatively little guidance available for indications and thresholds for platelet transfusion in TBI-associated coagulopathy. In the presence of thrombocytopenia, many centers use a threshold of 100,000 platelets/mm^3 for transfusion, and levels below this threshold are associated with a ninefold increased risk of mortality[17] and over elevenfold increased risk of intracranial hemorrhage progression.[3]

TRANSFUSION COMPLICATIONS

The transfusion of blood products can result in a range of complications, including acute, delayed, and non-immune hemolytic reactions and pathogen transmission. In TBI, pulmonary edema resulting from transfusion-related acute lung injury (TRALI) or transfusion-associated circulatory overload (TACO) are the commonest causes of morbidity and mortality (Table 31.3).

ANEMIA

Anemia is particularly common in patients with severe TBI, affecting around 50% of patients, and may contribute to secondary injury and worsened outcomes.[8] It can activate hypoxic cell signaling pathways and adversely affect cerebral oxygen delivery, resulting in the development of cerebral ischemia/infarction. Treatment of anemia includes erythropoietin (EPO) and pRBC transfusion. Experimental evidence suggests EPO is neuroprotective, although the recent EPO-TBI RCT of 606 patients with TBI found no difference in neurologic recovery, mortality, or VTE events between the EPO and placebo groups in 6 months.[45] Around one-third of TBI patients receive a pRBC transfusion during their hospital stay.[46] Some observational studies have suggested that pRBC use is associated with worsened survival and functional outcomes in TBI patients, although a recent meta-analysis found no difference in survival between TBI patients who did and did not receive pRBCs.[46] The storage and age of transfused blood may adversely affect its efficacy, although data on this are conflicting.[47,48]

The level and duration of anemic insult necessary to cause clinically relevant cerebral ischemia is unclear, which partly explains the difficulties in establishing a threshold for transfusion in TBI. A recent RCT of 200 patients with closed head injury randomized to receive either erythropoietin or placebo with two transfusion thresholds (7 g/dL and 10 g/dL), maintained with pRBCs, found that neither the administration of erythropoietin nor maintaining a hemoglobin concentration of >10 g/dL improved neurologic outcomes in 6 months.[49] The higher (10 g/dL) transfusion threshold was associated with a higher incidence of thromboembolic events,[49] and with increased risk of severe

Table 31.3 Features of transfusion-related acute lung injury (TRALI) and transfusion-associated circulatory overload (TACO)

	TRALI	TACO
Epidemiology	• Commonest cause of major morbidity and mortality associated with blood transfusion	• Second leading cause of transfusion-related mortality
Pathophysiology	• Caused by immune complex-mediated damage to pulmonary vasculature resulting in increased permeability	• Increased hydrostatic pressure
Risk factors	• Risk of developing TRALI increases with number of blood products used • Can result from transfusions of any type of blood product, though most common with plasma transfusions	• Risk of developing TACO directly related to the transfusion volume • Can result from transfusions of any type of blood product, though most common with plasma transfusions
Clinical features/ diagnosis	• Dyspnea and bilateral pulmonary edema typically <6 h of transfusion commencing • Hypoxemia and hypotension common • Often clinically indistinguishable from ARDS	• Respiratory distress, hypoxemia, signs of fluid overload (eg, elevated JVP) • Can develop within hours of transfusion akin to TRALI • Echocardiograph or pulmonary artery catheter can facilitate diagnosis • Elevated serum BNP (normal in TRALI)
Management	• Management is supportive (supplemental oxygen, mechanical ventilation)	• Management includes urgent diuresis • Supplemental oxygen and mechanical ventilation also often required

Abbreviations: ARDS: Acute respiratory distress syndrome; BNP: B-type natriuretic peptide; JVP: jugular venous pressure.

progressive hemorrhagic injury.[50] Some have argued that a transfusion threshold of 7 g/dL, which is used in many general critical care populations, cannot be extrapolated to patients with TBI because of the increased susceptibility of the injured brain to ischemia. There is evidence from observational studies that TBI patients may benefit from pRBCs and a higher transfusion trigger of 9 g/dL,[8] below which metabolic distress is detectable by brain tissue oxygenation monitoring.[51] Despite the lack of class I evidence, it is, therefore, reasonable to recommend a transfusion threshold of 9 g/dL in patients with TBI, emphasizing the importance of avoiding aggressive transfusion practices where possible and balancing the risks of cerebral ischemia with the risks of blood transfusion. It is not clear whether anemia and blood transfusion administration are merely markers of disease severity or

independent predictors of outcome, and further research is required to elucidate on this.

SPECIFIC MANAGEMENT CHALLENGES

Anticoagulants

TBI patients on warfarin have a higher mortality rate[52] and, when requiring surgery, their management is particularly challenging. All patients on warfarin presenting to the hospital with head injury should have urgent INR evaluation, and the threshold for imaging should be low. There are several guidelines from various bodies available to guide management of warfarin reversal, but there is little consensus on the specific choice and doses of agents recommended. Intravenous phytomenadione, a naturally occurring vitamin K, is commonly used for reversing warfarin. However, this treatment when used alone takes 12–24 hours to take effect, and thus to expedite the reversal its use is often combined with PCC and/or FFP and/or rFVIIa. The British Committee for Standards in Hematology advises immediate warfarin reversal with PCC in patients with head injury prior to CT scan or the availability of INR results if there is strong suspicion of an intracerebral hemorrhage.[53] A recent meta-analysis comparing PCC to FFP for warfarin reversal in patients with major bleeding or requiring urgent surgery found that PCC significantly reduced all-cause mortality and led to more rapid INR correction and less volume overload, without an increase in thromboembolic events.[54]

The novel oral anticoagulants (NOACs), including the direct factor Xa inhibitors (apixaban, rivaroxaban) and direct thrombin inhibitors (dabigatran), are being used increasingly due to predictable pharmacokinetic and pharmacodynamic profiles allowing fixed-dose regimens and no requirement for routine monitoring. However, unlike warfarin, there is no widely available specific reversal agent or method to monitor plasma levels. Several antidotes to the NOACs are now in development, and in a recent RCT of healthy volunteers, one of these (andexanet alpha) reversed the effects of apixaban and rivaroxaban within minutes of administration.[55] No thrombotic events were observed. Further trials are required to evaluate applicability to TBI.

Antiplatelets

Platelet transfusions are commonly used in TBI patients with and without antiplatelet therapy prior to neurosurgical intervention, although the evidence base supporting this is limited and conflicting. A meta-analysis evaluating platelet transfusions in patients with intracranial hemorrhage on antiplatelet agents identified 17 retrospective cohort (and no randomized/prospective) studies,[56] finding higher in-hospital mortality in traumatic intracranial hemorrhage patients on antiplatelet therapy receiving platelet transfusion (pooled odds ratio: 1.77, 95% CI: 1.00–3.13), but the authors expressed caution regarding these findings given concerns about methodologic quality. No difference

in rates of neurosurgical intervention, length of hospital stay, or functional status at discharge was observed.[56] Clearly, this is an area that requires further study.

Venous thromboembolism prophylaxis

TBI is a significant risk factor for the development of VTE, but no popular guidelines exist to guide decision making on the initiation and timing of VTE prophylaxis. Although there exists no clear evidence of efficacy, it is generally recommended that graduation compression stockings or intermittent pneumatic compression stockings are used, unless lower limb trauma prevents their use or until the patient is ambulatory. Low molecular weight heparin or low-dose unfractionated heparin can reduce the rates of deep vein thrombosis (DVT) and mortality, respectively, but the optimal time to commence chemoprophylaxis is unclear. It is crucial to strike a balance between the associated risks of intracranial hemorrhage and the significantly higher risk of DVT if chemoprophylaxis is withheld for 7 days after injury. Based on evidence from over 5000 TBI patients, one study recommended that chemoprophylaxis should be started after 72 hours in patients at medium or high risk of hematoma expansion, and after 48 hours in those with low risk of hematoma expansion and absence of expansion (see Table 31.4 for a description of the risk groupings).[57,58]

CONCLUSION

Coagulopathy and anemia are both common following TBI and are associated with worsened outcomes. Patients on anticoagulant and/or antiplatelet agents pose particular challenges to the treating clinician, particularly if being considered for surgery. Management of coagulopathy can include the administration of FFP, PCC, rFVIIa, TXA, and platelet transfusions. Erythropoietin and pRBCs can be used in the management of anemia. There exists no single universally accepted guideline for managing coagulopathy or anemia in TBI, and management decisions should be informed by local protocols and input from hematologists. Based on the best currently available evidence, a hemoglobin treatment

Table 31.4 Risk categories for hematoma expansion

Risk group	Criteria	Risk of expansion (%)
Low risk	• (Nonoperative) extradural or subdural hematoma <9 mm • Cerebral contusion <2 cm • Single contusion per lobe • Traumatic subarachnoid hemorrhage with negative CT angiography • Intraventricular hemorrhage <2 cm in maximum diameter	25
Medium risk	• Intracranial hemorrhage to a greater degree than that described for the low risk group	43
High risk	• Patients requiring craniotomy or intracranial pressure monitoring	64

Source: Data as per Phelan HA et al., *J Trauma Acute Care Surg.* 2012;73(2 Suppl 1):S122-7.

threshold of 9 g/dL appears reasonable. Further high-quality data are required to identify optimal treatment protocols that allow the timely yet safe correction of coagulopathy and anemia in patients with TBI.

REFERENCES

1. Epstein DS, Mitra B, O'Reilly G, Rosenfeld JV, Cameron PA. Acute traumatic coagulopathy in the setting of isolated traumatic brain injury: A systematic review and meta-analysis. *Injury.* 2014;45(5):819-824.

2. Oertel M, Kelly DF, McArthur D et al. Progressive hemorrhage after head trauma: Predictors and consequences of the evolving injury. *Journal of Neurosurgery.* 2002;96(1):109-116.

3. Allard CB, Scarpelini S, Rhind SG et al. Abnormal coagulation tests are associated with progression of traumatic intracranial hemorrhage. *J Trauma.* 2009;67(5):959-967.

4. Talving P, Benfield R, Hadjizacharia P, Inaba K, Chan LS, Demetriades D. Coagulopathy in severe traumatic brain injury: A prospective study. *J Trauma.* 2009;66(1):55-61.

5. Wafaisade A, Lefering R, Tjardes T et al. Acute coagulopathy in isolated blunt traumatic brain injury. *Neurocrit Care.* 2010;12(2):211-219.

6. Franschman G, Boer C, Andriessen TMJC et al. Multicenter evaluation of the course of

coagulopathy in patients with isolated traumatic brain injury: Relation to CT characteristics and outcome. *J Neurotrauma.* 2012;29(1):128-136.

7. Stein SC, Smith DH. Coagulopathy in traumatic brain injury. *Neurocrit Care.* 2004;1(4):479-488.

8. LeRoux P. Haemoglobin management in acute brain injury. *Curr Opin Crit Care.* 2013;19(2):83-91.

9. Brain Trauma Foundation. *Guidelines for the Management of Severe Traumatic Brain Injury.* 4th ed. Campbell, CA: Brain Trauma Foundation; 2016.

10. Lustenberger T, Talving P, Kobayashi L et al. Time course of coagulopathy in isolated severe traumatic brain injury. *Injury.* 2010;41(9):924-928.

11. Mackman N. The role of tissue factor and factor VIIa in hemostasis. *Anesth Analg.* 2009;108(5):1447-1452.

12. Zhang J, Jiang R, Liu L, Watkins T, Zhang F, Dong J-F. Traumatic brain injury-associated coagulopathy. *Journal of Neurotrauma.* 2012;29(17):2597-2605.

13. Hoffman M, Colina CM, Mcdonald AG, Arepally GM, Pedersen L, Monroe DM. Tissue factor around dermal vessels has bound factor VII in the absence of injury. *J Thromb Haemost.* 2007;5(7):1403-1408.

14. Morel N, Morel O, Petit L et al. Generation of procoagulant microparticles in cerebrospinal

fluid and peripheral blood after traumatic brain injury. *J Trauma*. 2008;64(3):698-704.

15. Faille DE, El-Assaad F, Mitchell AJ et al. Endocytosis and intracellular processing of platelet microparticles by brain endothelial cells. *Journal of Cellular and Molecular Medicine*. 2012;16(8):1731-1738.

16. Davis PK, Musunuru H, Walsh M et al. Platelet dysfunction is an early marker for traumatic brain injury-induced coagulopathy. *Neurocrit Care*. 2013;18(2):201-208.

17. Schnüriger B, Inaba K, Abdelsayed GA et al. The impact of platelets on the progression of traumatic intracranial hemorrhage. *J Trauma*. 2010;68(4):881-885.

18. Jacoby RC, Owings JT, Holmes J, Battistella FD, Gosselin RC, Paglieroni TG. Platelet activation and function after trauma. *J Trauma*. 2001;51(4):639-647.

19. Auer LM, Ott E. Disturbances of the coagulatory system in patients with severe cerebral trauma II. *Acta Neurochir (Wien)*. 1979;49(3-4):219-226.

20. Awasthi D, Rock WA, Carey ME, Farrell JB. Coagulation changes after an experimental missile wound to the brain in the cat. *Surgical Neurology*. 1991;36(6):441-446.

21. Nekludov M, Bellander B-M, Blombä ck M, Wallen HKN. Platelet dysfunction in patients with severe traumatic brain injury. *Journal of Neurotrauma*. 2007;24(11):1699-1706.

22. Stein SC, Graham DI, Chen X-H, Smith DH. Association between intravascular microthrombosis and cerebral ischemia in traumatic brain injury. *Neurosurgery*. 2004;54(3):687-691.

23. Vecht CJ, Minderhoud JM, Sibinga CT. Platelet aggregability in relation to impaired consciousness after head injury. *J Clin Pathol*. 1975;28(10):814-820.

24. Brohi K, Cohen MJ, Davenport RA. Acute coagulopathy of trauma: Mechanism, identification and effect. *Current Opinion in Critical Care*. 2007;13(6):680-685.

25. Cohen MJ, Brohi K, Ganter MT, Manley GT, Mackersie RC, Pittet J-F. Early coagulopathy after traumatic brain injury: The role of hypoperfusion and the protein C pathway. *J Trauma*. 2007;63(6):1254-1261.

26. Kushimoto S, Shibata Y, Yamamoto Y. Implications of fibrinogenolysis in patients with closed head injury. *Journal of Neurotrauma*. 2003;20(4):357-363.

27. Gonzalez E, Pieracci FM, Moore EE, Kashuk JL. Coagulation abnormalities in the trauma patient: The role of point-of-care thromboelastography. *Semin Thromb Hemost*. 2010;36(7):723-737.

28. Van PY, Cho SD, Underwood SJ, Morris MS, Watters JM, Schreiber MA. Thrombelastography versus antiFactor Xa levels in the assessment of prophylactic-dose enoxaparin in critically ill patients. *The Journal of Trauma: Injury, Infection, and Critical Care*. 2009;66(6):1509-1517.

29. Dai Y, Lee A, Critchley LAH, White PF. Does thromboelastography predict postoperative thromboembolic events? A systematic review of the literature. *Anesth Analg*. 2009;108(3):734-742.

30. Gozal YM, Carroll CP, Krueger BM, Khoury J, Andaluz NO. Point-of-care testing in the acute management of traumatic brain injury: Identifying the coagulopathic patient. *Surg Neurol Int*. 2017;8(1):48.

31. Zhang L-M, Li R, Zhao X-C, Zhang Q, Luo X-L. Increased transfusion of fresh frozen plasma is associated with mortality or worse functional outcomes after severe traumatic brain injury: A retrospective study. *World Neurosurg*. 2017;104:381-389.

32. Etemadrezaie H, Baharvahdat H, Shariati Z, Lari SM, Shakeri MT, Ganjeifar B. The effect of fresh frozen plasma in severe closed head injury. *Clin Neurol Neurosurg*. 2007;109(2):166-171.

33. Anglin CO, Spence JS, Warner MA et al. Effects of platelet and plasma transfusion on outcome in traumatic brain injury patients with moderate bleeding diatheses. *Journal of Neurosurgery*. 2013;118(3):676-686.

34. Peiniger S, Nienaber U, Lefering R et al. Balanced massive transfusion ratios in multiple injury patients with traumatic brain injury. *Crit Care. BioMed Central*. 2011;15(1):R68.

35. Joseph B, Hadjizacharia P, Aziz H et al. Prothrombin complex concentrate: An effective therapy in reversing the coagulopathy of

traumatic brain injury. *J Trauma Acute Care Surg.* 2013;74(1):248-253.

36. Wu X, Du Z, Yu J et al. Activity of factor VII in patients with isolated blunt traumatic brain injury: Association with coagulopathy and progressive hemorrhagic injury. *J Trauma Acute Care Surg.* 2014;76(1):114-1120.

37. Morenski JD, Tobias JD, Jimenez DF. Recombinant activated factor VII for cerebral injury? Induced coagulopathy in pediatric patients. *Journal of Neurosurgery.* 2003;98 (3):611-616.

38. Mayer SA, Brun NC, Begtrup K et al. Efficacy and safety of recombinant activated factor VII for acute intracerebral hemorrhage. *N Engl J Med [Internet].* 2008;358(20):2127-2137. http:// www.scopus.com/inward/record.url?eid=2-s2 .0-43549087410&partnerID=40&md5 =74a0a6af5b3e0bb779d7b27de890b479

39. Yuan Q, Wu X, Du Z-Y et al. Low-dose recombinant factor VIIa for reversing coagulopathy in patients with isolated traumatic brain injury. *J Crit Care.* 2015;30(1): 116-120.

40. CRASH-2 Trial collaborators, Shakur H, Roberts I et al. Effects of tranexamic acid on death, vascular occlusive events, and blood transfusion in trauma patients with significant hemorrhage (CRASH-2): A randomised, placebo-controlled trial. *Lancet.* 2010;376 (9734):23-32.

41. CRASH-2 collaborators, Roberts I, Shakur H et al. The importance of early treatment with tranexamic acid in bleeding trauma patients: An exploratory analysis of the CRASH-2 randomised controlled trial. *Lancet.* 2011; 377(9771):1096-1101.e1-2.

42. Yutthakasemsunt S, Kittiwatanagul W, Piyavechvirat P, Thinkamrop B, Phuenpathom N, Lumbiganon P. Tranexamic acid for patients with traumatic brain injury: A randomized, double-blinded, placebo-controlled trial. *BMC Emerg Med.* 2013;13(1):2.

43. Ker K, Roberts I, Shakur H, Coats TJ. Antifibrinolytic drugs for acute traumatic injury. *Cochrane Database Syst Rev.* 2015;5 (5):CD004896-6.

44. Dewan Y, Komolafe EO, Mejía-Mantilla JH et al. CRASH-3—Tranexamic acid for the treatment of significant traumatic brain injury: Study protocol for an international randomized, double-blind, placebo-controlled trial. *Trials.* 2012;13:87.

45. Nichol A, French C, Little L et al. Erythropoietin in traumatic brain injury (EPO-TBI): A double-blind randomized controlled trial. *Lancet.* 2015;386(10012):2499-2506.

46. Boutin A, Chassé M, Shemilt M et al. Red blood cell transfusion in patients with traumatic brain injury: A systematic review and meta-analysis. *Transfus Med Rev.* 2016;30 (1):15-24.

47. Weinberg JA, McGwin G Jr., Vandromme MJ et al. Duration of red cell storage influences mortality after trauma. *The Journal of Trauma: Injury, Infection, and Critical Care.* 2010;69(6):1427-1432.

48. Yamal JM, Benoit JS, Doshi P et al. Association of transfusion red blood cell storage age and blood oxygenation, long-term neurologic outcome, and mortality in traumatic brain injury. *Journal of Trauma and Acute Care Surgery.* 2015;79(5):843-849.

49. Robertson CS, Hannay HJ, Yamal J-M et al. Effect of erythropoietin and transfusion threshold on neurological recovery after traumatic brain injury: A randomized clinical trial. 2014;312(1):36-47.

50. Vedantam A, Yamal J-M, Rubin ML, Robertson CS, Gopinath SP. Progressive hemorrhagic injury after severe traumatic brain injury: Effect of hemoglobin transfusion thresholds. 2016;125(5):1229-1234.

51. Oddo M, Levine JM, Kumar M et al. Anemia and brain oxygen after severe traumatic brain injury. *Intensive Care Med.* 2012;38 (9):1497-1504.

52. Mina AA, Bair HA, Howells GA, Bendick PJ. Complications of preinjury warfarin use in the trauma patient. *J Trauma.* 2003;54(5):842-847.

53. Keeling D, Baglin T, Tait C et al. Guidelines on oral anticoagulation with warfarin. *British Journal of Haematology.* 2011;154(4):311-324.

54. Chai-Adisaksopha C, Hillis C, Siegal DM et al. Prothrombin complex concentrates versus fresh frozen plasma for warfarin reversal. A systematic review and meta-analysis. *Thromb Haemost.* 2016;116(5):879-890.

55. Siegal DM, Curnutte JT, Connolly SJ et al. Andexanet alfa for the reversal of factor Xa inhibitor activity. *N Engl J Med.* 2015;373 (25):2413-2424.

56. Leong LB, David TKP. Is platelet transfusion effective in patients taking antiplatelet agents who suffer an intracranial hemorrhage? *J Emerg Med.* 2015;49(4):561-572.

57. Abdel-Aziz H, Dunham CM, Malik RJ, Hileman BM. Timing for deep vein thrombosis chemoprophylaxis in traumatic brain injury: An evidence-based review. *Crit Care.* 2015;19 (1):96.

58. Phelan HA, Eastman AL, Madden CJ et al. TBI risk stratification at presentation: A prospective study of the incidence and timing of radiographic worsening in the Parkland Protocol. *J Trauma Acute Care Surg.* 2012;73 (2 Suppl 1):S122-7.

PART XI

Pain management

32

Pain management

ATHIR MORAD AND SALIA FARROKH

INTRODUCTION

A force strong enough to inflict damage to neuronal tissue must penetrate through skin, fat, muscle, bone, dura, and cerebrospinal fluid (CSF) before damaging either the brain or spinal cord. As a result, neurotrauma always occurs in the context of broader tissue or organ injury that may not be identifiable during the primary and secondary examinations. Certainly, the psychological impact of trauma alone continues to be an area of great interest for study. Therefore, it is the combined effect of polytrauma that ultimately contributes to the subjective experience of pain.

While the clinician's attention to pain may come naturally for patients who sustain more visible injuries, medical staff often hesitate before administering analgesics to patients with neurologic injury for several reasons. In the setting of neurologic injury, where the overall level of sensation may be impaired, opioids specifically can depress the patient's level of consciousness and mask the neurologic examination to prevent the accurate assessment of neurologic injury. More concerning, however, is the effect of opioids on depressing respiratory drive. By decreasing minute ventilation, opioids raise blood concentrations of carbon dioxide (CO_2), thereby increasing cerebral blood flow and intracranial pressure (ICP). In the presence of an intracerebral mass effect due to hemorrhage or edema, even slight increases in blood flood can lead to catastrophic brain compression and herniation. Given the narrow safety margin that is permitted by opioids in the treatment of pain, most clinicians often ignore pain entirely in patients with neurotrauama. Alternatives to opioids carry additional risks, which will be discussed in subsequent chapters. Ultimately, in order to provide the safest and most humane care, the treatment of pain in patients with neurologic injury requires careful vigilance and thoughtful reassessment at each phase of care.

THE TRAUMA TEAM

The chief complaint of pain is a common presentation in patients presenting to emergency departments following neurotrauma. For example, headache is the most common presentation in patients with subarachnoid hemorrhage and severe back pain is most commonly reported in patients with epidural compression of the spinal cord.[1,2] The type of pain, its location, duration, and severity must be objectively recorded and reassessed at

447

regular intervals, ideally along with the neurologic exam. The Numeric Rating Scale (0–10) is a common method of quantifying pain, but other scales, such as Behavioral Pain Scale (BPS) and Critical Care Pain Observation Tool (CPOT) are available as well. In patients with neurotrauma, it is essential to assess for any evidence of increased intracranial pressure before administering analgesics (Table 32.1).[3] In the setting of increased intracranial pressure, particularly when there is a risk for expansion of a hematoma or cerebral edema, nonopioid analgesics should be the first line of therapy.

Nonopioid analgesics include the nonsteroidal anti-inflammatory drugs (NSAIDs), acetaminophen, anticonvulsants such as gabapentin or pregabalin, ketamine, and dexmedetomidine. NSAIDs work by inhibiting the cyclooxygenase (COX) enzyme. It is important to note that acetaminophen is similar to the NSAIDs in relieving mild to moderate pain and has antipyretic activity but has no anti-inflammatory properties. Gabapentin and pregabalin bind to voltage-gated calcium channels within the central nervous system (CNS) and modulate the release of excitatory neurotransmitters. Ketamine is a non-competitive N-methyl-D-aspartate (NMDA) receptor antagonist and when used in low doses, it can produce an analgesic effect. However, the dissociative state induced by ketamine often limits its use in patients with acute neurologic injury. Dexmedetomidine, a selective alpha-2 agonist, is more commonly used as a sedative as it only carries a mild analgesic effect.

The selection of nonopioid analgesics requires careful consideration of adverse side effects, such as platelet dysfunction (Table 32.2).[4] In the absence of concurrent liver disease, a single dose of intravenous acetaminophen most likely offers the best option for analgesia without affecting the level of consciousness or breathing. A recent review concluded that there is no evidence indicating the superiority of intravenous (IV) acetaminophen administration over the oral route.[5] However, the intravenous formulation is ideal in trauma patients who cannot be cleared for PO (oral) intake. Unfortunately, the cost of IV acetaminophen may prove to be prohibitive at many medical institutions. A per-rectum formulation of acetaminophen is available as an alternative route of drug delivery.[6]

Small intermittent doses (25 µg–50 µg) of short-acting IV opioids, such as fentanyl, are preferable as the first line of analgesics in patients deemed safe to receive opioids. Continuous opioid infusions should be avoided in patients with neurotrauma who are not mechanically ventilated, especially upon initial presentation to the trauma team. Patients without intracranial injury, but isolated spinal injuries, may safely tolerate longer-acting opioids (Table 32.3).[4] Caution should be exercised when using morphine as patients may experience histamine release, which may result in hypotension during a time when perfusion pressure is of critical importance. In patients requiring mechanical ventilation, infusions of short acting opioids, such as

Table 32.1 Signs and symptoms of high intracranial pressure

Early	Late
Headache	Pupillary changes; anisocoria; or bilateral, unreactive dilated pupils
Dizziness	
Loss of consciousness	Extensor or flexor posturing
Altered mental status	Absence of spontaneous venous pulsations on fundoscopy
Amnesia	
Memory loss	Cranial nerve IV and VI paralysis
Nausea and vomiting	Contralateral or ipsilateral motor paralysis
Weakness or decreased sensation of extremities	Hypertension, bradycardia, and irregular respiration (Cushing's triad)
Speech or swallowing difficulties	Apnea
	Coma

Source: Marik P et al., J Emerg Med. 1999;17(4):711-719.

Table 32.2 Nonopioid analgesics

Medication (route)	Adult dosing range	Onset of action	Duration	AE/clinical pearl
Acetaminophen, IV/PO	650 mg q4h or 1000 mg q6h	Oral <1 h IV: 5–10 min	IV/PO: 4–6 h	Nausea and vomiting, acute liver failure (do not exceed the maximum recommended daily dose (>4 g daily in adults)
Ibuprofen PO	400 mg–800 mg q6h	30–60 min	6–8 h	GI tract disturbances, renal dysfunction, prolonged bleeding time, hypersensitivity reaction
Ketorolac IV/IM/PO	15–30 mg q6h	Oral: 30–60 min IV/IM: ~30 min	IV/PO: 4–6 h	GI tract disturbances, renal dysfunction, prolonged bleeding time, hypersensitivity reaction. Maximum combined duration of treatment (for parenteral and oral) is 5 d Lower dose should be used in geriatric patients
Gabapentin PO	1800–3600 mg/d	2 hours	7–10 h	Dizziness, peripheral edema Use with caution in patients with severe renal impairment; dose adjustment is required
Pregabalin PO	75–600 mg/d in divided doses	~1 wk	>12 h	Peripheral edema, weight gain
Dexmedetomidine IV	0.2–0.7 µg/kg/h	5–10 min	1–2 h	Hypotension, bradycardia Does not cause respiratory depression Loading dose is not recommended due to hypotension and bradycardia
Ketamine IV	0.2–0.8 mg/kg bolus, may use continuous IV infusion: 2 µg/kg/min	30 sec	3–4 min	Hypertension, tachycardia, hypersalivation, hallucinations Does not cause respiratory depression

Source: Lexicomp I, American Pharmaceutical Association. Lexicomp Online, Lexi-Drugs Online. Hudson, OH: Lexicomp, Inc; 2017.

Note: Commonly used nonopioid analgesics, adult dosing range, route of administration, onset, and duration of action, and adverse effects.

fentanyl or remifentanil, can be titrated to achieve comfort and ventilator synchrony. End-tidal capnography allows for careful attention to carbon dioxide levels in patients undergoing spontaneous modes of mechanical ventilation. The necessity for continuous respiratory monitoring in nonmechanically ventilated patients will be subsequently discussed at greater length in this chapter.

Opioid allergies and opioid classification

As is required prior to the administration of any drug, a history of allergies must be captured before administering an analgesic. Many patients report allergies to opioids, particularly codeine, due to the history of nausea and vomiting that is associated

Table 32.3 Most commonly used opioids for treatment of acute pain, common adult dosing, onset of action, duration of action, and adverse effects

Medication	Adult dosing	Onset	Duration	AE/comment
Fentanyl (IV)	50–100 µg q 1–2 h CI: 0.7–10 µg/kg/h	1–2 min	1–2 h	Respiratory depression, constipation, nausea and vomiting, somnolence Preferred in hemodynamic instability Context sensitive half-life: 200 min (6 h infusion); 300 min (12 h infusion)
Hydromorphone (IV, PO)	IV: 0.2–1 mg q 2–3 h CI: 0.5–3 mg/h	IV: 5 min	4–5 h	Respiratory depression, constipation, nausea and vomiting, somnolence
Morphine (IV, PO)	IV: 2.5–5 mg q 3–4 h CI: 2–30 mg/h	10 min	3–7 h	Respiratory depression, constipation, nausea and vomiting, somnolence Higher risk of hypotension and rash due to histamine release
Methadone (IV, PO)	IV: 2.5–10 mg every 8–12 hours; titrate slowly to effect PO: Initial: 2.5 mg every 8–12 h	IV: 10–20 minutes PO: 0.5–1 h	Oral: 4–8 h increases to 22–48 h with repeated doses	ECG changes, QTc prolongation, sedation, nausea and vomiting, constipation, somnolence, respiratory depression
Oxycodone (PO)	5 to 20 mg q 4–6 h	10–15 min	3–6 h	Respiratory depression, constipation, nausea and vomiting, somnolence
Remifentanil (IV)	0.5 µg/kg CI: 0.1–0.2 µg/kg/min	1–3 min	3–10 min	Hypotension, nausea and vomiting, respiratory depression, metabolized by nonspecific plasma esterases and could be optimal choice for patients with liver and renal dysfunction Context-sensitive half-life is 3–4 min
Tramadol (PO)	50–100 mg q 4–6 h	40–60 min	6 h	Constipation, somnolence, respiratory depression

Source: Lexicomp I, American Pharmaceutical Association. *Lexicomp Online, Lexi-Drugs Online.* Hudson, OH: Lexicomp, Inc; 2017.

with the drug. While it may be prudent to avoid codeine in these patients, particularly since vomiting can exacerbate elevations in ICP, prescribing opioids from other classes of synthetic opioids rather than those of the reported drug may not necessarily protect against an allergic reaction. There are three different chemical classes of opioids: (1) Phenanthrenes, (2) Phenylpiperidine, and (3) Phenylheptane. When a patient is allergic to

an opioid from one class, prescribers often use an opioid from another class. Even though the risk of crosssensitivity is extremely low, patients who have a true allergic reaction to one opioid should be monitored carefully when a different agent from another class is substituted (Table 32.4).

Naturally occurring and semi-synthetic opioids, such as codeine, morphine, and meperidine, can cause pseudoallergies due to endogenous histamine

Table 32.4 Classifications of opioid families

Opioid chemical class	Opioid agents
Phenanthrenes	Codeine, hydromorphone, levorphanol, morphine, oxycodone, hydrocodone, and pentazocine
Phenylpiperidine	Meperidine and fentanyl
Phenylpiperidine	Methadone and propoxyphene

release from the mast cells. These symptoms include flushing, hives, itching, asthma exacerbation, and low blood pressure. A true Ig E-mediated allergy to opioids is rare.[7] Symptoms of a true opioid allergy include hives, maculopapular rash, severe hypotension, bronchospasm, and angioedema.[8]

OPERATIVE MANAGEMENT

Craniotomy surgery

The pain response in patients requiring craniotomy surgery largely depends on the location of incision. While all types of craniotomies are now recognized to result in a significant degree of postoperative pain, supratentorial surgery produces less pain than infratentorial surgery.[9–11] The reason for this difference is attributed to the greater risk of sensory nerve manipulation during suboccipital craniectomy as well as the thicker muscular layer and bone overlying the posterior fossa. For this reason, any anesthetic plan must account for the expected pain profile of the indicated surgery.

The anesthetic management of patients undergoing intracranial surgery requires careful attention to hemodynamic goals, deliberate control of cerebral edema, and rapid emergence from general anesthesia while guarding against the risk of seizure. The pharmacologic foundation of neuro-anesthesia has traditionally been based on opioids. By providing dense analgesia, the anesthesiologist is able to limit the cumulative dose of anesthetic and allow for quick emergence. The opioid reversal agent, naloxone, can be useful when patients are slow to emerge due to the residual effect of opioids. Increasingly, remifentanil infusions are used because of their favorable pharmacokinetics for a

rapid emergence. There is, however, a theoretical concern over the development of acute opioid tolerance while on remifentanil that may result in hyperalgesia postoperatively. As a result, a remifentanil infusion is often used in combination with a relatively longer-acting opioid, such as fentanyl. Fentanyl infusions carry less-favorable pharmacokinetics as the context-sensitive half-life may potentially prolong emergence from anesthesia, particularly in longer surgeries (Table 32.3).[4]

In addition to opioid analgesics, the placement of local anesthetics at specific sensory nerve sites along the scalp can significantly decrease the pain response during surgery while reducing the opioid and total anesthetic requirements.[12] A typical application involves the subcutaneous injection of 0.5% bupivacaine at the Mayfield pin sites as well as at the scalp entry points of the supratrochlear and supraorbital nerves, the zygomaticotemporal nerve, the auriculotemporal nerve, and branches of the great auricular and greater and lesser occipital nerves. The cumulative dose of bupivacaine must be limited based on the patient's body weight. Caution must also be exercised in patients with allergies to local anesthetics and those with skull defects due to either previous surgeries or trauma that may predispose them to direct cerebral puncture, wound contamination, or intravascular injection of local anesthetic.

Other medications that are routinely administered during craniotomy surgery, such as steroids and anticonvulsants, may serve as important adjuncts in mitigating the pain response. While NSAIDs are avoided during craniotomy due to concerns over causing platelet dysfunction, steroids are very commonly used to reduce cerebral edema. Concurrently, they also provide significant anti-inflammatory effects that reduce the pain response. Even a single dose of dexamethasone has proven effective in reducing postoperative pain.[13]

The routine use of anticonvulsants during a craniotomy offers additional analgesic benefits beyond their intended use. While valproate and carbamazepine have not been effective in treating acute pain, phenytoin may reduce the neuropathic pain response and result in more long-term benefits.[14] Gabapentinoids are generally avoided during craniotomies due to their relatively small effect on seizure prevention yet greater contribution to perioperative sedation and the potential for delayed emergence from general anesthesia.

Spinal surgery

The use of intraoperative monitoring, specifically evoked potentials (EP) monitoring during spinal surgery, impacts the perioperative course of patients substantially. Unlike craniotomy surgery, EP monitoring does not permit for the administration of local anesthetics into the epidural or intrathecal spaces because local anesthetics impair nerve conduction and the ability to detect any intraoperative signal changes. Therefore, the choice of analgesics for patients undergoing spinal surgery often exclude this entire class of highly effective analgesics from ordinary clinical practice.

By default, opioids serve as the foundation for analgesia during spinal surgery (Table 32.3).[5] The use of remifentanil, although potentially convenient for allowing rapid emergence from general anesthesia, can lead to a hyperalgesic state postoperatively. Other more-common choices include fentanyl, morphine, hydromorphone, and sufentanil. The cumulative dose, which patients require during surgery, varies according to multiple factors, such as age, gender, size, and, most notably, preoperative tolerance. The conversion of prehospital opioid consumption to the in-hospital requirement will be discussed in the next section. However, in the context of the operating room environment, a patient's opioid requirement can be determined prior to induction by titrating intravenous opioids in incremental doses until the patient becomes comfortable. Additionally, a single dose of intravenous methadone is most often useful in leveling the pain response during surgery, particularly when an opioid infusion is not being used.[20]

Unlike in craniotomy surgery, clinicians often permit more sedating analgesics in spine surgery since gross motor function is relatively easier to assess than subtle cranial nerve findings. Therefore, analgesics, such as the gabapentinoids, fall well within the scope of pain treatment options for patients undergoing spinal surgery. There is enough body of evidence to support the use of perioperative gabapentin and pregabalin to reduce postoperative pain and opioid consumption.[21,22] In addition, there is increasing evidence that perioperative use of these agents may provide long-term, postoperative pain relief. According to one study, pregabalin before surgery and 24 hours after surgery decreased pain at 3 months. Although there are no definite recommendations for optimal doses of these medications, a summary of selected trials that demonstrated effective pain relief, the doses used, and outcomes measured may provide further guidance (Table 32.5).

A highly effective nonopioid analgesic that is often used intraoperatively and postoperatively for patients with spine injury is ketamine. Through NMDA receptor antagonism, ketamine acts to reduce overall opioid consumption.[23] The dissoci-

Table 32.5 Summary of evidence for the use of gabapentin and pregabalin

Study (N)	Surgery	Gabapentinoid dose	Outcomes
Khan et al.[15] (175)	Laminectomy	900 mg or 1200 mg of gabapentin	Lower pain scores during the first 24 h postoperatively
Pandey et al.[16] (100)	Discectomy	600 mg, 900 mg, or 1200 mg of gabapentin given 2 h preoperatively	Lower visual analog pain scores at all time points postoperatively
Van Elstraete et al.[17] (67)	Lumbar spinal fusion	Gabapentin 21.7 mg/kg	30%–50% reduction in morphine use postoperatively
Kim et al.[18] (84)	Lumbar spinal fusion	150 mg of pregabalin preoperatively	Patient-controlled analgesia and adjuvant analgesic use were lower postoperatively in patients receiving 150 mg preoperatively
Burke and Shorten[19] (40)	Lumbar discectomy	Pregabalin 300 mg 90 minutes preoperatively and 150 mg at 12 and 24 h postoperatively	Decreased pain scores and improved function at 3 mon

ative amnesia caused by the drug, however, limits its use in cases that require careful neurologic assessment of cooperative patients. Nevertheless, the psychotropic side-effect profile of ketamine is often tolerated in exchange for the overall benefits of effective analgesia that do not interfere with evoked potential monitoring and reduced opioid consumption.

While NSAIDs are generally avoided during spine surgery due to concerns over inducing platelet dysfunction, intravenous acetaminophen remains an effective adjunct. Additionally, other routinely used agents, such as nitrous oxide and magnesium infusions, carry analgesic benefits beyond their more immediate indications.[24–26]

CRITICAL CARE MANAGEMENT

Whether arriving directly from the trauma center or postoperatively following surgery, most patients with neurotrauma require treatment in an intensive care unit (ICU). A monitored unit allows for frequent neurologic assessments as well as continuous hemodynamic surveillance using noninvasive and invasive monitors. In addition to pulse oximetry, the more recent availability of respiratory monitors, which measure the adequacy of ventilation in mechanically ventilated and nonintubated patients, plays an increasingly important role in safely providing analgesia.

Opioids are commonly used for the treatment of postoperative pain. Due to a rising incidence of opioid overdoses, providers should prescribe opioids only when the benefits are likely to outweigh the risks, such as in severe acute pain not responding to other therapies. In these cases, the lowest effective dose and a course limited to the duration of the acute pain should be prescribed. In cases in which risks outweigh benefits, such as treatment of chronic pain, opioid use should be avoided in favor of other treatments.[27]

All opioids provide their analgesic effects through activation of μ opioid receptors in the brain and spinal cord. Tramadol and methadone are exceptions as they have other pharmacologic effects. Tramadol inhibits the reuptake of norepinephrine and serotonin in addition to being a partial μ opioid agonist. Methadone is an NMDA receptor antagonist in addition to activating μ opioid receptors. It is important to note that methadone accumulates with repeated dosing, and,

therefore, dose reduction or an increase in dosing intervals may be necessary. Review of the literature has shown that, in fact, there may be up to a 20-fold interindividual variation in terminal elimination half-life and clearance (Table 32.3).[4,28]

Additionally, it is important to understand the concept of context-sensitive half-life as this is clinically relevant when lipophilic agents are given as a continuous infusion. The context-sensitive half-life measures the decrease in the drug concentration after a constant infusion of a given duration. For example, although the terminal half-life of fentanyl after one bolus injection is approximately 1 to 2 hours, the context-sensitive half-life after a 6-hour infusion is approximately 200 minutes.[29]

Opioid safety and monitoring

SEDATION

A review of the potential benefits provided to patients with neurotrauma by dedicated ICUs extends beyond the scope of this chapter. Nevertheless, several considerations that are specific to the safe delivery of analgesic therapy within the context of neurocritical care necessitate a more focused discussion.

One of the most important functions of a neurocritical care unit is to provide dedicated monitoring of neurologic function. While the continuous reporting of vital signs is a standard function of any ICU, the attention to a patient's mental state, cranial nerve function, and motor and sensory examinations is unique to neurocritical care. This becomes most important for patients who require analgesic therapy, especially in the form of opioids. Since sedation can be an early warning sign of impending neurologic catastrophe, such as brain herniation, medications with sedative properties, such as opioids, may impair the clinician's ability to detect and prevent neurologic deterioration. Commonly used sedation scales in the ICU include the Glasgow Coma Scale and the Ramsay Sedation Scale, although many other validated scales are available, even at the institutional level. Regardless of the scale, the most important factor for the safe delivery of opioids to patients with neurologic injury is the frequent assessment of mental status, by any means available.

A common misperception in medicine is that the depth of sedation is the result of excessive analgesia. However, the analgesia caused by

NSAIDs, acetaminophen, or even local anesthetics when not injected intravenously have no effect on sedation, other than allowing patients to relax from the pain relief.[30] Opioids carry additional sedative properties, which have not been well understood until recently.[31] The sedative effect of opioids is now considered to result from a central anticholinergic mechanism.[32]

Due to the fear of causing excessive sedation, opioids have historically been administered on an as-needed, *pro re nata* (PRN), basis. The theoretical advantage of nurse-delivered medication is that the patient's neurologic examination can be assessed prior to the administration of each dose of analgesic. In the case of opioids, a nurse is able to assess whether a patient is awake enough to tolerate the prescribed dose. An alternative and very common analgesic regimen in non-neurosurgical patients is intravenous patient controlled analgesia (PCA). PCAs offer patients the ability to self-deliver analgesics, usually in the form of short-acting opioids, without enduring delays caused by variable nursing response times and in drug delivery. Patients must presumably be awake enough to sense pain and engage the PCA mechanism to trigger the delivery of the drug at each permissible interval. PCAs can also reduce workload burden on nursing staff by decreasing the number of calls from patient rooms. Finally, the process of opioid reconciliation is simpler for a single opioid PCA cartridge than for individual opioid doses that a nurse must hand deliver as needed. By handling multiple doses of opioids, nurses expose patients to a higher risk of cross-contamination, and they expose themselves, collectively, to a risk of opioid diversion. Unless patients have a history of opioid dependence, continuous infusions of opioids should be avoided in nonmechanically ventilated patients.

Following the "patient knows best" approach, the superior analgesic provided by PCAs has ultimately been the drive behind the popularity of the devices for most postsurgical patients, except when it comes to neurosurgical patients, for reasons explained above. Nevertheless, increasing evidence indicates that PCAs, even in postcraniotomy patients, are more effective in reducing postoperative pain than PRN.[11,33] Thus far, studies have not been large enough in size to prove with certainty the safety of PCAs. The population size required to perform a definitive study is in itself an indication of the relative safety of PCA technology.

Respiratory depression

The relationship between plasma concentrations of carbon dioxide (PCO2) and cerebrovascular dilatation has been understood for decades.[34] Since opioids are recognized to cause respiratory depression and, thereby, increase in PCO2 and ICP, their use has historically been limited in neurotrauma. The advent of bedside respiratory monitors, such as pulse oximetry and end-tidal capnography, has substantially improved the ability of clinicians to monitor for respiratory depression while delivering opioids to patients with neurotrauma. Until recently, pulse oximetry was regarded as the gold standard for monitoring opioid-induced hypoventilation. However, several studies have shown that when patients receive supplemental oxygen, opioid-induced ventilatory depression can be masked.[35,36] Moreover, continuous assessment of oxygenation and ventilation has also proven more effective in capturing respiratory depression than intermittent monitoring.[37] While multiple technologies exist for quantifying the adequacy of ventilation in non-intubated patients, the challenge remains to accurately assess the impact of opioids on both minute ventilation and airway motor tone, especially in patients with obstructive sleep apnea (OSA).[38] Regardless of the technology used, continuous respiratory assessment in an ICU likely offers the best opportunity for the safe delivery of opioids to patients with neurologic injury.

Other adverse effects

All surgical patients receiving opioids require close monitoring, especially immediately after surgery. Opioid use is often associated with adverse effects, such as somnolence, respiratory depression, gastrointestinal (GI) adverse effects such as constipation, nausea and vomiting, and itching. Although monitoring alone may be effective, some patients may require pharmacologic interventions. Ileus associated with opioid use may increase intra-abdominal pressures, which can potentially increase ICP. Since tolerance to constipation does not occur over time, a standing regimen of stool softener and/or stimulant is recommended. More recently, newer agents, such as methylnaltrexone, naloxegol, and lubiprostone are available to treat opioid-induced constipation (Table 32.6).[4] Patients who have had a craniotomy involving posterior fossa are particularly at risk of nausea and vomiting. Emesis can be associated with substantial elevations in ICP,

Table 32.6 Opioid-related side effects and their management

Opioid-induced complications	Agent	Dose	Clinical pearl
Respiratory depression, somnolence	Naloxone (IV, IM, SubQ)	Initial: 0.4–2 mg; may repeat every 2–3 minutes. A lower initial dose (0.1–0.2 mg) should be considered for patients with opioid dependence to avoid acute withdrawal[39]	If no response is observed after 10 mg total, consider other causes of respiratory depression May use a continuous infusion (0.25–6.25 mg/h) for long-acting opioid exposure, such as methadone
Constipation	Docusate sodium	50–360 mg once daily or in divided doses	Should not be used as PRN (a standing regimen is indicated)
	Sennosides	Dose depends on formulation (8.6–34.4 mg/day)	May cause diarrhea
	Methylnaltrexone SC	Dose depends on body weight: <38 kg: 0.15 mg/kg 38 to <62 kg: 8 mg 62–114 kg: 12 mg >114 kg: 0.15 mg/kg	Should be used only if docusate and sennosides have failed Administer one dose every other day as needed; maximum: 1 dose/24 hours Methylnaltrexone is contraindicated in patients with known or suspected gastrointestinal obstruction
	Naloxegol PO	12.5 mg–25 mg daily	Use is contraindicated with strong CYP 3A4 inhibitors, such as ketoconazole, clarithromycin
	Lubiprostone PO	24 μg twice daily	Contraindicated in patients with mechanical GI obstruction
Nausea/ vomiting	Ondansetron IV, IM, PO	IM, IV: 4 mg as a single dose for prevention—if used for treatment, may use 4 mg postoperatively Oral: 16 mg as a single dose for prevention	IV, IM dose should be administered ~30 minutes before the end of anesthesia PO dose should be given 1 hour prior to induction of anesthesia Doses >16 mg are no longer recommended by the manufacturer due to the potential for QT prolongation
	Metoclopramide IV, IM, PO	10–20 mg near end of surgery for prevention 20 mg orally 2 hours prior to anesthesia for prevention	Can cause extrapyramidal symptoms (EPS) and tardive dyskinesia The risk is higher with longer duration and higher doses
	Promethazine Oral, IM, IV, rectal	12.5–25 mg every 4–6 hours, as needed	Nonspecific QT changes Anticholinergic side effects (somnolence, constipation, etc.)

Source: Lexicomp I, American Pharmaceutical Association. Lexicomp Online, Lexi-Drugs Online. Hudson, OH: Lexicomp, Inc; 2017.

therefore, postoperative nausea must be treated aggressively with agents such as ondansetron, metoclopramide, and promethazine.

Opioid use in organ dysfunction

Pregnant patients; the elderly; those with cardio-pulmonary diseases; those with renal or hepatic dysfunction; or those with neuromuscular conditions, such as myasthenia gravis, require additional attention postoperatively (Table 32.7).[40,41]

Opioid withdrawal

A physical dependence on opioids is characterized by the emergence of withdrawal syndromes such as anxiety, restlessness, mydriasis, diarrhea, diaphoresis, myalgia, arthralgia, and tachycardia if the drug is stopped abruptly, reduced in dose, or antagonized. As one may expect, these syndromes commonly complicate the care of patients in the acute-care setting (eg, postoperative, ICU) as it is extremely challenging to treat opioid withdrawal due to lack of complete history, altered mental status, and the physiologic responses of acute illness, which can be confused with withdrawal.[42,43]

The severity of opioid withdrawal depends on the consumed dose, duration of use, and route of administration.[44] The Clinical Opioid Withdrawal Scale and Objective Opioid Withdrawal Scale may be used to assess the severity of withdrawal. Withdrawal onset and duration of opioid withdrawal symptoms depend on the half-life of the opioid. For example, in patients using short-acting opioids, such as fentanyl, withdrawal begins approximately 4 hours after the last use, whereas withdrawal from methadone, a long-acting opioid, may not occur until 36 hours after the last use.[45,46] Appropriate monitoring and symptomatic management are key factors in treating opioid withdrawal. Pharmacologic agents such as opioid agonists, alpha-2 adrenergic agonists, and other nonopioid agents for symptomatic relief should be considered in these patients (Table 32.8).[47-49]

Acute pain management in patients with a history of opioid dependence

Treatment of acute pain in patients with a history of opioid abuse is challenging, mostly due to opioid tolerance; concurrent use of Opioid Abuse Treatment (OAT), such as buprenorphine or methadone; and practitioners, hesitation to treat pain in this setting due to the misconception that the patient may be seeking to abuse drugs.[45]

As a general rule, patients who are on maintenance methadone therapy should stay on their maintenance dose and providers should make every attempt to contact the treatment program to verify the dose. It is reasonable to use short-acting opioids and nonopioid agents to treat breakthrough pain in this setting. Providers should recognize that patients with a history of opioid use will most likely require higher doses of opioid to treat any acute pain.

Table 32.7 Recommendations for opioid use in renal and hepatic impairment

Opioid	Renal impairment	Hepatic impairment
Fentanyl	Appears to be safe	99% metabolized in the liver; studies have not shown alterations in PK; careful monitoring is required
Hydromorphone	Use cautiously; dose adjustment may be necessary	Use with caution (intermediate extraction ratio)
Methadone	Appears to be safe; may need to dose adjust to prevent accumulation over time	Risk of accumulation due to increased concentration of free drug
Morphine	Not recommended due to active metabolite and associated toxicity	Use with caution (high extraction ratio)
Tramadol	Not recommended	Not recommended; significant PK changes in moderate-to-severe hepatic impairment

Sources: Davis M, *Clin Pharmacokinet.* 2007;46(10):825-850; Dean M, *J Pain Symptom Manage.* 2004;28(5):497-504.

Table 32.8 Agents used in opioid withdrawal

Agent	Mechanism of action	Dose	Comment
Methadone	Opioid receptor agonist; has been shown to have NMDA receptor antagonism	10–30 mg PO daily may slowly titrate to 20–40 mg	If enteral route is not available, methadone can be administered parenterally. Doses of 1/2 to 2/3 of the total daily oral dose can be given in three to four doses by intermittent IV injection
Buprenorphine (in combination with naloxone)	Shows high-affinity binding to μ opiate receptors in the CNS; displays partial μ agonist and weak kappa antagonist activity	Initial dose: 2–4 mg daily Maintenance: 12–16 mg daily	It is important to note that early initiation of buprenorphine can precipitate withdrawal Sublingual route may limit its administration in the acute phase of care
Clonidine	Thought to produce analgesia at presynaptic and postjunctional alpha-2-adrenoceptors in the spinal cord by preventing pain signal transmission to the brain	0.1 mg–0.2 mg PO q6h	Close monitoring of blood pressure (BP) is necessary due to severe hypotension

Sources: Schug S et al., *APM:SE Working Group of the Australian and New Zealand College of Anaesthetists and Faculty of Pain Medicine (2015), Acute Pain Management: Scientific Evidence (4th edition)*, Melbourne: ANZCA & FPM; 2015:200; Shaiova L et al., *Palliat Support Care.* 2008;6(2):165-176; Kampman K, Jarvis M, *J Addict Med.* 2015;9(5):358-367.

Treating pain in patients who are on maintenance buprenorphine may be more difficult because of the pharmacology of this medication. Buprenorphine is a partial μ agonist with high affinity for the μ receptors. It is, therefore, reasonable to discontinue buprenorphine and use a full μ agonist to treat pain. Some providers have used methadone to treat opioid withdrawal as well as short-acting opioids for breakthrough pain. Alternatively, increasing the dose of buprenorphine given 3 to 4 times daily may be used to treat acute pain.[50]

Opioid conversion

It is not uncommon in the acute setting to change opioids due to loss of oral access or side effects and/or hypersensitivity reaction (this topic is covered in the previous section). The steps below should be followed to safely perform the conversion. All patients must be closely monitored and assessed for pain during the first 24 to 72 hours after changing the dose or route of administration.[51]

Appropriate steps to take for opioid conversion:

- Step 1: Determine the total daily dose of the currently prescribed analgesic.
- Step 2: Convert the currently prescribed opioid to an equivalent morphine dose (Table 32.9).[51]
- Step 3: Convert the morphine dose to the new opioid agent prescribed using the same route or convert the route using the table—consider starting at 50% of the daily morphine equivalent dose requirement.

Table 32.9 Opioid conversion table

Drug	Parenteral (mg)	Oral (mg)
Morphine	10	30
Hydromorphone	1.5	7.5
Oxycodone	–	20
Fentanyl	0.1	–
Methadone	5	10

Source: Schneider C et al., *Clin Med Res.* 2003; 1(4):337-340.

- Step 4: Determine the appropriate intervals of administration based on the opioid's pharmacokinetic properties.
- Step 5: Provide appropriate rescue or PRN dosing for breakthrough pain: short-acting agents should be prescribed in 2 to 4 hour time intervals.
- Step 6: Monitor pain and respiratory status to effectively and safely titrate baseline and as-needed doses.

MULTIMODAL ANALGESIA

The concept of multimodal analgesia incorporates the goals of analgesic therapy for all patients, particularly those with neurologic injury. The American Society of Anesthesiologists defines multimodal pain management as administration of two or more classes of analgesics to treat pain. These drugs may be administered via the same route or by different routes.[52] Based on the multimodal paradigm, no single analgesic class is relied upon to meet a patient's entire analgesic requirement. Rather, the model relies on a synergistic effect of a combination of drugs, each of which is delivered in a relatively smaller dose. By depending less on any individual class of analgesics, such as opioids, the practice of multimodal analgesia decreases a patient's risk of exposure to the associated adverse effect of the drugs, including dependency. Additional benefits have been hypothesized, such as a reduction in chronic pain.[53] Ultimately, the goal of effective analgesia is to enable patients to heal from injury to regain mobility and actively engage in rehabilitation.

REFERENCES

1. Morad AH, Tamargo RJ, Gottschalk A. The longitudinal course of pain and analgesic therapy following aneurysmal subarachnoid hemorrhage: A cohort study. Headache. 2016;56(10):1617-1625.
2. Al-Mutair A, Bednar DA. Spinal epidural hematoma. J Am Acad Orthop Surg. 2010;18 (8):494-502.
3. Marik P, Chen K, Varon J, Fromm R Jr, Sternbach GL. Management of increased intracranial pressure: A review for clinicians. J Emerg Med. 1999;17(4):711-719.
4. Lexicomp I, American Pharmaceutical Association. Lexicomp Online, Lexi-Drugs Online. Hudson, OH: Lexicomp, Inc; 2017.
5. Jibril F, Sharaby S, Mohamed A, Wilby KJ. Intravenous versus oral acetaminophen for pain: Systematic review of current evidence to support clinical decision-making. Can J Hosp Pharm. 2015;68(3):238-247.
6. van der Marel CD, van Lingen RA, Pluim MA, Scoones G, van Dijk M, Vaandrager JM et al. Analgesic efficacy of rectal versus oral acetaminophen in children after major craniofacial surgery. Clin Pharmacol Ther 2001 Jul;70 (1):82-90.
7. Nasser SM, Ewan PW. Opiate-sensitivity: Clinical characteristics and the role of skin prick testing. Clin Exp Allergy. 2001;31 (7):1014-1020.
8. Tripp DM, Brown GR. Pharmacist assessment of drug allergies. Am J Hosp Pharm. 1993;50 (1):95-98.
9. Irefin SA, Schubert A, Bloomfield EL, DeBoer GE, Mascha EJ, Ebrahim ZY. The effect of craniotomy location on postoperative pain and nausea. J Anesth. 2003;17(4):227-231.
10. Gottschalk A, Berkow LC, Stevens RD et al. Prospective evaluation of pain and analgesic use following major elective intracranial surgery. J Neurosurg. 2007;106(2):210-216.
11. Morad A, Winters B, Stevens R et al. The efficacy of intravenous patient-controlled analgesia after intracranial surgery of the posterior fossa: A prospective, randomized controlled trial. Anesth Analg. 2012;114(2):416-423.
12. Papangelou A, Radzik BR, Smith T, Gottschalk A. A review of scalp blockade for cranial surgery. J Clin Anesth. 2013;25 (2):150-159.
13. De Oliveira GS Jr, Almeida MD, Benzon HT, McCarthy RJ. Perioperative single dose systemic dexamethasone for postoperative pain: A meta-analysis of randomized controlled trials. Anesthesiology. 2011;115 (3):575-588.
14. Wiffen PJ, Derry S, Moore RA et al. Antiepileptic drugs for neuropathic pain and fibromyalgia—An overview of cochrane reviews. Cochrane Database Syst Rev. 2013;11:CD010567.
15. Khan ZH, Rahimi M, Makarem J, Khan RH. Optimal dose of pre-incision/post-incision

gabapentin for pain relief following lumbar laminectomy: A randomized study. *Acta Anaesthesiol Scand*. 2011;55(3):306-312.

16. Pandey CK, Navkar DV, Giri PJ et al. Evaluation of the optimal preemptive dose of gabapentin for postoperative pain relief after lumbar diskectomy: A randomized, double-blind, placebo-controlled study. *J Neurosurg Anesthesiol*. 2005;17(2):65-68.

17. Van Elstraete AC, Tirault M, Lebrun T et al. The median effective dose of preemptive gabapentin on postoperative morphine consumption after posterior lumbar spinal fusion. *Anesth Analg*. 2008;106(1):305-308, table of contents.

18. Kim JC, Choi YS, Kim KN, Shim JK, Lee JY, Kwak YL. Effective dose of peri-operative oral pregabalin as an adjunct to multimodal analgesic regimen in lumbar spinal fusion surgery. *Spine (Phila Pa 1976)*. 2011;36(6):428-433.

19. Burke SM, Shorten GD. Perioperative pregabalin improves pain and functional outcomes 3 months after lumbar discectomy. *Anesth Analg*. 2010;110(4):1180-1185.

20. Gottschalk A, Durieux ME, Nemergut EC. Intraoperative methadone improves postoperative pain control in patients undergoing complex spine surgery. *Anesth Analg*. 2011;112(1):218-223.

21. Hurley RW, Cohen SP, Williams KA, Rowlingson AJ, Wu CL. The analgesic effects of perioperative gabapentin on postoperative pain: A meta-analysis. *Reg Anesth Pain Med*. 2006;31(3):237-247.

22. Seib RK, Paul JE. Preoperative gabapentin for postoperative analgesia: A meta-analysis. *Can J Anaesth*. 2006;53(5):461-469.

23. Dunn LK, Durieux ME, Nemergut EC. Non-opioid analgesics: Novel approaches to perioperative analgesia for major spine surgery. *Best Pract Res Clin Anaesthesiol*. 2016;30(1):79-89.

24. Bessiere B, Laboureyras E, Chateauraynaud J, Laulin JP, Simonnet G. *A single nitrous oxide (N2O) exposure leads to persistent alleviation of neuropathic pain in rats.* J Pain. 2010;11(1):13-23.

25. Oguzhan N, Gunday I, Turan A. Effect of magnesium sulfate infusion on sevoflurane consumption, hemodynamics, and perioperative opioid consumption in lumbar

disc surgery. *J Opioid Manag*. 2008;4(2):105-110.

26. Levaux C, Bonhomme V, Dewandre PY, Brichant JF, Hans P. Effect of intra-operative magnesium sulphate on pain relief and patient comfort after major lumbar orthopaedic surgery. *Anaesthesia*. 2003;58(2):131-135.

27. Dowell D, Kunins HV, Farley TA. Opioid analgesics—Risky drugs, not risky patients. *JAMA*. 2013;309(21):2219-2220.

28. Barr J, Fraser GL, Puntillo K et al. Clinical practice guidelines for the management of pain, agitation, and delirium in adult patients in the intensive care unit. *Crit Care Med*. 2013;41(1):263-306.

29. Kapila A, Glass PS, Jacobs JR et al. Measured context-sensitive half-times of remifentanil and alfentanil. *Anesthesiology*. 1995;83(5):968-975.

30. Lentschener C, Tostivint P, White PF, Gentili ME, Ozier Y. Opioid-induced sedation in the postanesthesia care unit does not insure adequate pain relief: A case-control study. *Anesth Analg*. 2007;105(4):1143-1147, table of contents.

31. Osman NI, Baghdoyan HA, Lydic R. Morphine inhibits acetylcholine release in rat prefrontal cortex when delivered systemically or by microdialysis to basal forebrain. *Anesthesiology*. 2005;103(4):779-787.

32. Abou Hammoud H, Simon N, Urien S, Riou B, Lechat P, Aubrun F. Intravenous morphine titration in immediate postoperative pain management: Population kinetic-pharmaco-dynamic and logistic regression analysis. *Pain*. 2009;144(1-2):139-146.

33. Morad AH, Winters BD, Yaster M et al. Efficacy of intravenous patient-controlled analgesia after supratentorial intracranial surgery: A prospective randomized controlled trial. *Clinical article*. J Neurosurg. 2009;111(2):343-350.

34. Reivich M. Arterial Pco2 and cerebral hemodynamics. *Am J Physiol*. 1964;206:25-35.

35. Niesters M, Mahajan RP, Aarts L, Dahan A. High-inspired oxygen concentration further impairs opioid-induced respiratory depression. *Br J Anaesth*. 2013;110(5):837-841.

36. Fu ES, Downs JB, Schweiger JW, Miguel RV, Smith RA. Supplemental oxygen impairs

detection of hypoventilation by pulse oximetry. *Chest.* 2004;126(5):1552-1558.

37. Overdyk FJ, Carter R, Maddox RR, Callura J, Herrin AE, Henriquez C. Continuous oximetry/capnometry monitoring reveals frequent desaturation and bradypnea during patient-controlled analgesia. *Anesth Analg.* 2007;105(2):412-418.

38. Sasaki N, Meyer MJ, Eikermann M. Postoperative respiratory muscle dysfunction: Pathophysiology and preventive strategies. *Anesthesiology.* 2013;118(4):961-978.

39. Mokhlesi B, Leikin JB, Murray P, Corbridge TC. Adult toxicology in critical care: Part II: specific poisonings. *Chest.* 2003;123(3):897-922.

40. Davis M. Cholestasis and endogenous opioids: Liver disease and exogenous opioid pharmacokinetics. *Clin Pharmacokinet.* 2007;46(10):825-850.

41. Dean M. Opioids in renal failure and dialysis patients. *J Pain Symptom Manage.* 2004;28 (5):497-504.

42. Jenkins DH. Substance abuse and withdrawal in the intensive care unit. *Contemporary issues. Surg Clin North Am.* 2000;80(3): 1033-1053.

43. Zapantis A, Leung S. Tolerance and withdrawal issues with sedation. *Crit Care Nurs Clin North Am.* 2005;17(3):211-223.

44. Smolka M, Schmidt LG. The influence of heroin dose and route of administration on the severity of the opiate withdrawal syndrome. *Addiction.* 1999;94(8):1191-1198.

45. Donroe JH, Holt SR, Tetrault JM. Caring for patients with opioid use disorder in the hospital. *CMAJ.* 2016;188(17-18):1232-1239.

46. Ries RK, Fiellin DA, Miller SC, Saitz R. The ASAM principles of addiction medicine: Fifth edition. *Wolters Kluwer Health Adis (ESP)* 2014:668-684.

47. Schug S, Palmer G, Scott D, Halliwell R, Trinca J. *APM:SE Working Group of the Australian and New Zealand College of Anaesthetists and Faculty of Pain Medicine (2015), Acute Pain Management: Scientific Evidence (4th edition).* 4th ed. Melbourne: ANZCA & FPM; 2015:200.

48. Shaiova L, Berger A, Blinderman CD et al. Consensus guideline on parenteral methadone use in pain and palliative care. *Palliat Support Care.* 2008;6(2):165-176.

49. Kampman K, Jarvis M. American society of addiction medicine (ASAM) national practice guideline for the use of medications in the treatment of addiction involving opioid use. *J Addict Med.* 2015;9(5):358-367.

50. Alford DP, Compton P, Samet JH. Acute pain management for patients receiving maintenance methadone or buprenorphine therapy. *Ann Intern Med.* 2006;144(2):127-134.

51. Schneider C, Yale SH, Larson M. Principles of pain management. *Clin Med Res.* 2003;1 (4):337-340.

52. American Society of Anesthesiologists Task Force on Central Venous Access, Rupp SM, Apfelbaum JL et al. Practice guidelines for central venous access: A report by the American Society of Anesthesiologists Task Force on Central Venous Access. *Anesthesiology.* 2012;116(3):539-573.

53. Kehlet H, Jensen TS, Woolf CJ. Persistent postsurgical pain: Risk factors and prevention. *Lancet.* 2006;367(9522):1618-1625.

Palliative care

33

Health-related quality of life and palliative care issues in neurotrauma

SUPARNA BHARADWAJ AND LASHMI VENKATRAGHAVAN

INTRODUCTION

Traumatic brain injury (TBI) occurs when an external force, as a result of a fall, motor vehicle accident, or an assault injures the brain. It affects people from all walks of life. Motor vehicle accidents are the leading cause of severe TBI globally. However, the incidence varies with many sociodemographic factors. For example, TBI is more common in males than females (around 3:1), and is more likely to occur in the younger (15–24 years) and older (65+ years) age groups. Prevalence of TBI is higher in young men, likely because of motor-vehicle accidents and/or assaults. In contrast, the increased rates of TBI in the older population are usually due to falls.[1,2]

In addition, a primary brain injury may become worse because of secondary insults, such as intracranial hematomas and/or cerebral edema, which can lead to cerebral ischemia due to increased intracranial pressure (ICP).[1–3] The recovery process following a TBI is often difficult to predict, due to the effects of many heterogeneous factors, such as mechanism of injury, site of injury, presence or absence of secondary insults, aggressiveness of treatment, and, finally, characteristics of the individual patient. In patients with severe TBI, the outcome is usually poor and the neurologic deficits can be severe and long lasting.[4–6] Although the majority of people who have mild TBI can make a full recovery, having a mild injury does not mean that there will not be any long-term consequences.[2,7]

OUTCOME AFTER TBI

TBI can have a profound effect on a person's life: high levels of disability and functional impairment, difficulties in resuming social and leisure activities, relationship difficulties, and possible marriage breakdown.[8–11] Returning to work is often difficult, if it is possible at all.[12–14] There may be changes in self-perception as well as problems with emotional control and a personality change. Patients may lose their sense of "self" and have difficulty redefining themselves and their role in society; this can lead to further emotional difficulties.[14–17] TBI can also have a profound impact on the life of the person's family and others around him or her.[18,19] With the number of people affected as a result of the debilitating impact of traumatic brain injury, it is important to have a clear understanding of how the outcome can be assessed effectively and efficiently.

Factors influencing functional outcome after TBI

A wide variety of factors are known to affect outcome after TBI and despite many studies, the causes and reasons for the variance in outcome remains unexplained.[20] While the severity of the injury is consistently reported as being one of the best predictors of outcome, there are a number of patients who had a severe injury and yet made a good (or better) recovery; equally, patients who had a relatively mild injury may have a long-term negative outcome.[7,21] There are also reports that long-term morbidity following a TBI increases, regardless of the level of severity.[2] Some of the important factors affecting outcomes after TBI are discussed below.

AGE

Few studies have shown that suffering a TBI at an advanced age is generally associated with poorer outcomes.[22,23] This may be due to the differences in the flexibility between the young and the old, as the younger brain has the ability to form new connections.[22–24] In addition, increased age is also associated with long-term cognitive impairment and a higher rate of mortality.[23] On the other hand, younger children may have poorer outcomes with executive functioning (the ability to take care of oneself) compared with young adults.[25,26]

Premorbid functioning and cognitive reserve

Individuals with higher levels of cognitive ability, intelligence, and education will have a better outcome after TBI.[27,28] Higher education levels are often associated with better outcome after TBI, in terms of employment, productivity, and disability levels.[29]

GENDER

Cognitive outcomes after TBI do not vary with gender.[30] Although some studies suggest that the outcome may be poorer in women,[31–33] another study indicates that it may be better.[34]

POOR SOCIOECONOMIC STATUS

Patients from socially deprived areas are less likely to receive neurosurgical and neurointensive care treatments following TBI.[35] In addition, differences in the geographic location might also have an impact on the outcome because of variations of access to services.[36] In children, better family environments are associated with better outcomes following TBI.[37]

MEASURING OUTCOMES AFTER TBI

Conventionally, generalized Injury Severity Scores, such as the Glasgow Coma Scale (GCS) and post-traumatic amnesia (PTA), are often used for assessing the outcomes after TBI on an individual patient. Although these indicators can identify the physical impairments and limitations in the functioning of individual patients, they may not be able to capture the impairments in the personal, social, and psychological aspects of the individual patients' lives.

The GCS[1,38] is the most commonly used scale to assess the severity of injury based on levels of consciousness and to assess the severity of the injury. However, there is an ongoing debate on which GCS score most accurately reflects the severity of injury: GCS at the scene, on admission to the hospital, or the worst GCS in the first 24 hours.[39] A GCS of 13 to 15 conventionally represents a mild injury; 9 to 12, a moderate injury; and 3 to 8, a severe injury. There is increasing appreciation that while the GCS is a useful clinical tool, it does not provide a complete classification of injury severity, even when supplemented by neuroimaging results. While there is some connection between injury severity and long-term outcome, the relationship is nonlinear.

Post-traumatic amnesia (PTA) is another Injury Severity Score, which is used less frequently than GCS. It is the period of time where the patient is unable to form continuous memories. Table 33.1 demonstrates how the period of PTA corresponds with the severity of the injury. Although PTA can be assessed by a series of orientation and memory tests, it is more commonly estimated retrospectively

Table 33.1 Estimates of severity of injury based on post-traumatic amnesia (PTA) duration

Severity of injury	PTA duration
Very mild	<5 minutes
Mild	5–60 minutes
Moderate	1–24 hours
Severe	1–7 days
Very severe	1–4 weeks
Extremely severe	More than 4 weeks

by interviews.[40] However, this method of assessment may be subjected to error in recollection.

HEALTH-RELATED QUALITY OF LIFE AS AN OUTCOME MEASURE

The World Health Organization (WHO) describes quality of life (QoL)[41] as: "an individuals' perception of their position in life in the context of the culture and value systems in which they live and in relation to their goals, expectations, standards, and concerns." QoL is often used as an outcome measure in healthcare research, although it is used less often in the specific context of brain injury. QoL is a key method of measuring outcome as it addresses issues that are perhaps of greatest importance to the patient. Individuals may conceptualize and perceive QoL in very different ways, which can be problematic when trying to address this issue on a more general level.[42] It has been reported that objective measures used by healthcare professionals often bear little resemblance to a patient's functioning in day-to-day life. With patients who may appear to be similar on a functional level, they still may have very different perceptions of their daily quality of life.[43]

Historically, the TBI field has been dominated by objective measures of functional outcome; for example, patients being assessed by the Glasgow Outcome Scale. This allows individuals to be categorized into levels of disability based on the impact that their injury has on their daily lives, whether this is independence in the home, ability to work, or other ways in which their injury has affected them.

Recent interest in quality of life has made subjective measures popular. This may relate, for example, to overall satisfaction with life or satisfaction with different areas of functioning. When investigating a subjective appraisal of QoL on an individual level, there are a number of instruments that are designed to allow the individual patient to identify the domains that are important to them, and hence, it may be possible to obtain a clear picture of individual differences.

There are global measures in which the individuals rate their QoL on a simple scale from worst possible to best possible, or from delighted to terrible.[44] These global assessments of QoL have been described as being useful, because they allow the individual to rate his or her QoL in a way that is relevant to him or her rather than using an externally imposed, irrelevant concept.[44] In addition, global measures are often short and easy to complete, which may be beneficial in encouraging responses.

There are a number of disease-specific questionnaires that have been developed which are designed to examine the issues affecting different patient groups, such as cancer, asthma, epilepsy, or brain injury. This is especially useful when assessing the impact of a particular condition or comparing individuals within a specific patient group. The term health-related quality of life (HRQoL) refers to the influence of the health condition on an individual's QoL. HRQoL may also be assessed in domains that are more broadly applicable, with measures that are designed to address a large portion of the population. Examples of generic QoL measures include the WHOQoL, the Sickness Impact Profile, and the Nottingham Health Profile. These generic QoL measures are not specifically designed for people who have had a brain injury.

HRQoL MEASURES USED IN TRAUMATIC BRAIN INJURY

1. QOLIBRI Overall Scale

The QOLIBRI scales were developed as a disease-specific measure of HRQoL for TBI.[45] The original scale consists of 37 items in six domains; cognition, self, daily life and autonomy, social relationships, emotions, and physical problems.

In addition to scores for each of these domains, a total score for QoL is obtained. A shorter version of this was developed as an index measure of QoL after brain injury (the QOLIBRI-OS).[46] This is a six-item scale that addresses physical condition, cognition, emotion, functions in daily life, personal and social life, and current situations and future prospects. Satisfaction in these areas is rated on a five-point scale. The resulting score gives a measure of QoL out of a total possible score of 100.

2. Short Form 36 (SF-36)

The Short Form-36 (SF-36) is a measure of HRQoL, which has eight different subscales.[47] These can be used to calculate two component summary scales (the Physical Component Summary, PCS; and the Mental Component Summary, MCS). The eight subscales include physical functioning; role limitation due to physical problems; role limitation due to emotional problems; social functioning; mental health; energy/vitality; pain; and general health perception. Questions are given in a multiple-choice format. The SF-36 is a popular measure and has been used with a wide range of conditions. The SF-36 has been used in studies involving individuals with brain injury and its reliability and validity has been investigated in the context of TBI.

3. Glasgow Outcome Scale—Extended (GOS-E)

GOS-E[48] is a widely used measure that allows categorization of levels of disability following brain injury. The GOS-E involves questions relating to activities of daily living (shopping, travel, independence at home), ability to return to work, and participation in social and leisure activities. Respondents are also asked about any impact their injury might have had on their relationship with friends and family or on any other area of their life. Categories range from 1–8: from death to good recovery.

4. Telephone Interview for Cognitive Status

The Telephone Interview for Cognitive Status (TICS)[49] is used to assess cognitive functioning. The TICS is an 11-item test designed to give a brief assessment of cognitive status. Questions relate to orientation, and include tasks such as counting backward, serial subtraction, word memory, and recognizing an object from a verbal description. TICS manual scores of 25 or less indicates impairment. Screening tools such as the TICS are relatively insensitive to mild or moderate cognitive impairment in TBI.

5. Brain Injury Grief Inventory (BIGI)

BIGI was designed to address issues relating to loss and adjustment following brain injury.[50] The BIGI consists of 20 questions with three options: "never," "sometimes," and "mostly." Items are scored 0 to 2. There are 11 items for loss and 9 items for adjustment. Items are not weighted.

6. Other HRQoL Measures

Other QOL measures whose reliability and validity have been investigated in the context of TBI are Hardon's scale, Schedule for the Evaluation of Individual Quality of Life—Direct Weighting, Hospital Anxiety and Depression scale, Repeatable Battery for the Assessment of Neuropsychological Status, Iowa–Netherlands Social Comparison Orientation Measure, Patient Competency Rating Scale, Multidimensional Scale of Perceived Social Support, Brief-COPE, and Life Orientation Test—Revised.

The influence of cognitive impairment following TBI on the reporting of QoL measures is important. It is apparent that there will be a point at which the level of cognitive impairment may impair the ability of an individual to evaluate his or her QoL. Results from QoL measures that are not validated in a cognitively impaired population should be interpreted cautiously when applied to a TBI sample. At present, there is enough evidence to support the use of self-reported QoL measures with people with a level of cognitive impairment to justify their application in TBI. There is a view that the patient should be considered the expert in their condition, regardless of cognitive impairment.

There are many factors that influence the QoL after a brain injury; these include health perceptions and self-concept, ability to engage in day-to-day life, and the ability to return to work. There are reports of inverse or paradoxical relationships between severity of injury and QoL in the literature. Anosognosia, or a lack of awareness of deficits, can explain this inverse or paradoxical relationship. Additionally, there is evidence that patients rarely complain of their cognitive or emotional and behavioral problems, even when these difficulties are frequently observed by relatives or friends. A concept that has been developed over the past decade surrounding QoL is called "response

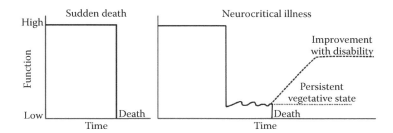

Figure 33.1 Distinctive trajectories of neurocritical illness. This figure demonstrates trajectories for patients without limitation of life-supporting therapies. Onset of neurocritical illness is often sudden, with precipitous decline from a normal baseline. However, most neurocritically ill patients do not progress to cardiovascular death or brain death, but survive with disability.

shift."[51] The theory of response shift is based on the concept that a catalyst in the form of a change in a person's circumstances leads to change in the way subjective judgment of QoL is made.

PALLIATIVE CARE IN TBI PATIENTS

Most patients with TBI have no premorbid symptoms and often suffer a sudden loss of physical and cognitive functions after TBI. In addition, following TBI, the majority of patients do not progress to death (by cardiovascular or brain death criteria); instead, they either improve slowly over several months or stagnate in a severely disabled state. Those who do not die generally have a prolonged recovery process (Figure 33.1). Brain-injured patients often make their maximal recovery in the first 3 to 6 months and improvement can continue over the coming months with aggressive rehabilitation.[52] Therefore, neurologic changes that affect their decision-making process often occur well after the initial ICU and hospital stay, necessitating the use of prognostic scales that can assist in early discussions about the goals of care. Key elements in the palliative care of patients after TBI include pain and other neurologic symptoms, patient and family support, discharge planning, and end-of-life decisions. Some of the challenges in the palliative care of patients with TBI include the difficulty in predicting the outcome in the early stages of injury, lack of knowledge about patient preferences, and their ability to cope with major disability.

HRQoL may have an outcome measure that is more relevant because it is designed to show the effect of the disease from the patient's perspective. Although increasing disability is generally associated with a reduction in QoL, there are many exceptions to this rule, with some investigators reporting fair to good QoL or happiness despite serious disability.[53] Such adjustment to illness might, in part, be caused by a response shift, which includes a change in the internal standards and values in the self-assessment of QoL. This factor is important because it shows that some patients with a poor functional outcome after acute brain injury regain a good QoL. Ideally, a combination of instruments, such as the extended GOS and the QOLIBRI or other tools, are effective outcome measures following TBI. Currently, there is considerable variability in practice regarding withholding and withdrawing of life-sustaining treatment in patients. Thus, there is a need for high-quality research to enable treatment-limiting decisions to be made within clinically relevant timeframes and to be guided by improved outcomes that are meaningful to patients.

CONCLUSION

Survivors of TBI often have a variety of physical and psychological deficits that affect their day-to-day life. Current management of TBI relies mainly on the traditional outcome measures that focus on survival and physical disability but not on functional disability and cognitive impairment. In contrast, many of the HRQoL indices focus on the outcomes, from the patient's perspective, of functional independence, mental health, and community life after TBI. Thus, HRQoL measures can provide more realistic, individualized outcome assessments, which can be useful for both the physicians and the family members for clinical and palliative care decisions.

REFERENCES

1. Hannay H, Howieson D, Loring D, Fischer J, Lezak, M. Neuropathology for neuropsychologists. In: Lezak M, Howieson D, Loring D, eds. *Neuropsychological Assesment.* New York: Oxford University Press; 2004:157-285.

2. King N, Tyerman A. Neuropsychological presentation and treatment of head injury and traumatic brain damage. In: Halligan P, Kishka U, Marshall J, eds. *Handbook of Clinical Neuropsychology.* Oxford, UK: Oxford University Press. 2003:487-505.

3. Lingsma HF, Roozenbeek B, Steyerberg EW, Murray GD, Maas AI. Early prognosis in traumatic brain injury: From prophecies to predictions. *Lancet Neurol.* 2010;9(5):543-554.

4. Ponsford J, Draper K, Schönberger M. Functional outcome 10 years after traumatic brain injury: Its relationship with demographic, injury severity, cognitive and emotional status. *J Int Neuropsychol Soc.* 2008;14(2):233-242.

5. Sloan S, Winkler D, Anson K. Long-term outcome following traumatic brain injury. *Brain Impairment.* 2007;8:251-261.

6. Colantonio A, Ratcliff G, Chase S, Kelsey S, Escobar M, Vernich L. Long-term outcomes after moderate to severe traumatic brain injury. *Disabil Rehabil.* 2004;26(5):253-261.

7. Tsushima WT, Lum M, Geling O. Sex differences in the long-term neuropsychological outcome of mild traumatic brain injury. *Brain Inj.* 2009;23(10):809-814.

8. Saatman K, Duhaime AC, Bullock R et al. Classification of traumatic brain injury for targeted therapies. *J Neurotrauma.* 2008;25(7):719-738.

9. Thornhill S, Teasdale GM, Murray GD, McEwen J, Roy CW, Penny KI. Disability in young people and adults one year after head injury: Prospective cohort study. *BMJ.* 2000;320(7250):1631-1635.

10. Dikmen SS, Machamer JE, Powell JM, Temkin NR. Outcome 3 to 5 years after moderate to severe traumatic brain injury. *Arch Phys Med Rehabil.* 2003;84(10):1449-1457.

11. Koskinen S. Quality of life 10 years after very severe traumatic brain injury (TBI): The perspective of the injured and the closest relative. *Brain Inj.* 1998;12(8):631-648.

12. Wood RL, Yurdakul LK. Change in relationship status following traumatic brain injury. *Brain Injury.* 1997;11(7):491-501.

13. Tsaousides T, Ashman T, Seter C. The psychological effects of employment after traumatic brain injury: Objective and subjective indicators. *Rehab Psychol.* 2008;(53):456-463.

14. Wehman P, Targett P, West M, Kregel J. Productive work and employment for persons with traumatic brain injury: What have we learned after 20 years? *J Head Trauma Rehabil.* 2005;20(2):115-127.

15. Tyerman A, Humphrey M. Changes in self-concept following severe head injury. *Int J Rehabil Res.*1984;7(1):11-23.

16. Kersel DA, Marsh NV, Havill JH, Sleigh JW. Psychosocial functioning during the year following severe traumatic brain injury. *Brain Inj.* 2001;15(8):683-696.

17. Yeates G, Gracey F, McGrath J. A biopsychosocial deconstruction of "personality change" following acquired brain injury. *Neuropsychol Rehabil.* 2008;18(5-6):566-589.

18. Chamberlain DJ. The experience of surviving traumatic brain injury. *J Adv Nurs.* 2005;54(4):407-417.

19. Svendsen H, Teasdale T, Pinner M. Subjective experience in patients with brain injury and their close relatives before and after a rehabilitation programme. *Neuropsychological Rehabilitation.* 2004;14:495-515.

20. Lezak M. Living with the characterologically altered brain injured patient. *J Clin Psychiatry.* 1987;39(7):592-598.

21. Ghajar J. Traumatic brain injury. *Lancet.* 2000;356(9233);923-929.

22. Cameron CM, Purdie DM, Kliewer EV, McClure RJ. Ten-year outcomes following traumatic brain injury: A population-based cohort. *Brain Inj.* 2008;22(6):437-449.

23. Senathi-Raja D, Ponsford J, Schönberger M. Impact of age on long-term cognitive function after traumatic brain injury. *Neuropsychology.* 2010;24(3):336-344.

24. Tokutomi T, Miyagi T, Ogawa T et al. Age-associated increases in poor outcomes after traumatic brain injury: A report from the Japan Neurotrauma Data Bank. *J Neurotrauma.* 2008;25(12):1407-1414.

25. Schönberger M, Ponsford J, Reutens D, Beare R, O'Sullivan R. The relationship between age, injury severity, and MRI findings after traumatic brain injury. *J Neurotrauma.* 2009;26(12):2157-2167.

26. Sonnenberg LK, Dupuis A, Rumney PG. Preschool traumatic brain injury and its impact on social development at 8 years of age. *Brain Inj.* 2010;24(7-8):1003-1007.

27. Anderson V, Catroppa C. Memory outcome at 5 years post-childhood traumatic brain injury. *Brain Inj.* 2007;21(13-14):1399-1409.

28. Sigurdardottir S, Andelic N, Roe C, Schanke AK. Cognitive recovery and predictors of functional outcome 1 year after traumatic brain injury. *J Int Neuropsychol Soc.* 2009;15(5):740-750.

29. Kesler SR, Adams HF, Blasey C M, Bigler ED. Premorbid intellectual functioning, education, and brain size in traumatic brain injury: An investigation of the cognitive reserve hypothesis. *Appl Neuropsychol.* 2003;10(3):153-162.

30. Wagner AK, Hammond FM, Sasser HC, Wiercisiewski D. Return to productive activity after traumatic brain injury: Relationship with measures of disability, handicap, and community integration. *Arch Phys Med Rehabil.* 2002;83(1):107-114.

31. Moore DW, Ashman TA, Cantor JB, Krinick RJ, Spielman LA. Does gender influence cognitive outcome after traumatic brain injury? *Neuropsychol Rehabil.* 2010;20(3):340-354.

32. Farace E, Alves WM. Do women fare worse? A meta analysis of gender differences in outcome after traumatic brain injury. *Neurosurg Focus.* 2000;8(1):e6.

33. Bounds TA, Schopp L, Johnstone B, Unger C, Goldman H. Gender differences in a sample of vocational rehabilitation clients with TBI. *NeuroRehabilitation.* 2003;18(3):189-196.

34. Wood RL. Long-term outcome of serious traumatic brain injury. *Eur J Anaesthesiol Suppl.* 2008;42:115-122.

35. Slewa-Younan S, Baguley IJ, Heriseanu R et al. Do men and women differ in their course following traumatic brain injury? *A preliminary prospective investigation of early outcome. Brain Inj.* 2008;22(2):183-191.

36. Dunn L, Henry J, Beard D. Social deprivation and adult head injury: A national study. *J Neurol Neurosurg Psychiatry.* 2003;74(8):1060-1064.

37. Spearman RC, Stamm BH, Tivis LJ. Traumatic brain injury state planning grant: Preparing for change in a rural state. *Brain Inj.* 2007;21(8):837-849.

38. Teasdale G. Jennett B. Assessment of coma and impaired consciousness: A practical scale. *Lancet.* 1974;2(7872):81-84.

39. Zuercher M, Ummenhofer W, Baltussen A, Walder B. The use of Glasgow Coma Scale in injury assessment: A critical review. *Brain Inj.* 2009;23(5):371-384.

40. Ponsford JL, Spitz G, McKenzie D. Using post-traumatic amnesia to predict outcome after traumatic brain injury. *J Neurotrauma.* 2016;33(11):997-1004.

41. Gerrard-Morris A, Taylor HG, Yeates KO et al. Cognitive development after traumatic brain injury in young children. *J Int Neuropsychol Soc.* 2010;16(1):157-168.

42. Browne JP, McGee HM, O'Boyle C. Conceptual approaches to the assessment of quality of life. *Psychology and Health.* 1997;12:737-751.

43. Sprangers M, Schwartz C. Integrating response shift into health-related quality of life research: A theoretical model. *Soc Sci Med.* 1999;48(11):1507-1515.

44. Dijkers M. Quality of life after traumatic brain injury: A review of research approaches and findings. *Arch Phys Med Rehabil.* 2004;85(4 suppl 2):S21-S35.

45. von Steinbuechel N, Peterson C, Bullinger M, QOLIBRI Group. Assessment of health-related quality of life in persons after traumatic brain injury—Development of the Qolibri, a specific measure. *Acta Neurochir Suppl.* 2005;93:43-49.

46. von Steinbuechel N, Wilson L, Gibbons H et al. QOLIBRI overall scale: A brief index of health-related quality of life after traumatic brain injury. *J Neurol Neurosurg Psychiatry.* 2012;83(11):1041-1047.

47. von Steinbuechel N, Covic A, Polinder S et al. Assessment of health-related quality of life after TBI: Comparison of disease-specific (QOLIBRI) with a generic (SF-36) instrument. *Behav Neurol.* 2016:7928014.

48. Folstein M, Folstein S, McHugh P. "Mini-mental state." A practical method for grading the cognitive state of patients for the clinician. *J Psychiatr Res.* 1975;12(3):189-198.

49. Cook SE, Marsiske M, McCoy KJM. The use of the modified telephone interview for cognitive status (TICS-M) in the detection of amnestic mild cognitive impairment. *J Geriatr Psychiatry Neurol.* 2009;22(2):103-109.

50. Ruddle JA, Coetzer BR, Vaughan FL. Grief after brain injury: A validation of the brain injury grief inventory. *Illness, Crisis & Loss.* 2005;13(3):235-247.

51. Sprangers M, Schwartz C. Integrating response shift into health-related quality of life research: A theoretical model. *Socl Sci Med.* 1999;48(11):1507-1515.

52. Diringer MN, Edwards DF, Aiyagari V, Hollingsworth H. Factors associated with withdrawal of mechanical ventilation in a neurology/neurosurgery intensive care unit. *Crit Care Med.* 2001;29(9):1792-1797.

53. McCarthy ML, Dikmen SS, Langlois JA, Selassie AW, Gu JK, Horner MD. Self-reported psychosocial health among adults with traumatic brain injury. *Arch Physl Med Rehabil.* 2006;87(7):953-961.

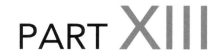
Brain death and ethical issues

34

Brain death and ethical issues

CHIARA ROBBA AND BASIL MATTA

INTRODUCTION

Brainstem death (BSD) is defined as an irreversible event with permanent cessation of cerebral function. With this condition, there are no responses from the brain, cranial nerve reflexes, or motor responses to pain stimuli (although spinal reflexes may persist); furthermore, there is no respiratory drive, and thus, there are no spontaneous breaths regardless of hypercarbia or hypoxemia.

Brain death qualifies as death, as the brain is essential for integrating critical functions of the body.[1] The main causes of BSD are trauma, subarachnoidal hemorrhage, intracerebral hemorrhage, and hypoxic ischemic encephalopathy and ischemic stroke (Figure 34.1).[2]

Brainstem death diagnosis implies the evidence of the complete and irreversible cessation of brainstem and cerebral functions, including the capacity for respiratory, brainstem, and vegetative activities. However, there is substantial variation in the criteria that are used to identify BSD; institutional

protocols in different centers for diagnosis are not universal and are often absent in some countries.[3–5]

Most institutions rely on published guidelines and have specific diagnostic mandates, especially when applied to organ donor candidates.[6]

However, a survey published in 2008 determined that there are important differences and variability in adherence to published guidelines and clinical practice.[7] Indeed, this survey reviewed the guidelines for determination of death by brain criteria in 50 institutions, and major discrepancies were found in the requirements for performance of the evaluation, prerequisites, and tests that were performed.

CRITERIA

The diagnosis of brain death is a clinical diagnosis, and the criteria for brain death require specific clinical conditions, such as evidence of absence of brain function on neurologic examination. The level and the expertise of the examiners required to

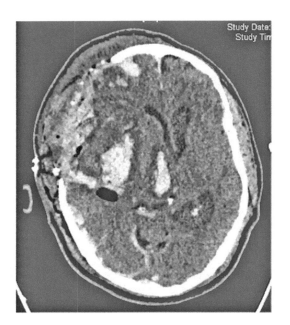

Figure 34.1 Devastating brain injury in a 43-year-old after traumatic brain injury. Brainstem death was then confirmed.

make a diagnosis of brain death varies among different countries;[3,6] there are also differences in the number of physicians required (Table 34.1).

It is commonly recommended that the examiner of brainstem criteria is not the treating physician and should not be the same physician who is a member of the transplant team or has responsibilities to the potential recipient of one or more organs.[8] Also, the examiner making the diagnosis of brain death should be familiar with the clinical criteria and comfortable with performing all aspects of the examination.

Even the length of observation required to determine brain death varies extensively from center to center. There is no sufficient evidence to determine a minimally acceptable observation period.[6,8] In general, an observation period for adults is considered optional, 6 hours of observation are often recommended, but longer periods (up to 24 hours) are recommended in cases of hypoxic ischemic encephalopathy[9] (Table 34.1) or hypothermia. In these patients, it may be advisable to perform an additional test to be sure about the diagnosis.

There is little evidence about serial examinations in this setting.[6] According to literature, the interval between the first and second examination ranges from 3 to over 50 hours in different countries.

Several prerequisites have to be met before considering a patient "brain dead."[6,10]

First, there must be clinical or neuroimaging evidence of an acute cerebral unsalvageable injury that is compatible with the clinical diagnosis of brain death (Figure 34.1). Second, there must be the certainty that no drug intoxication or poisoning has affected the clinical assessment. Arterial blood pressure (systolic blood pressure >100 mmHg) and core temperature higher than 36°C (96°F) should be ensured.

Finally, physicians must exclude any medical conditions that may affect clinical assessment, such as severe electrolyte disorders (in particular, potassium, sodium, phosphate), and endocrine disturbances.

Table 34.1 Differences among countries of brainstem criteria

Country	Number of examiners	Time of observation	Interventional tests	Apnea test
United Kingdom (UK)	2	6	Not required	Required
Switzerland	2	6	Not required	Required
Spain	1	6	Not Required	Required
Italy	1	6	Required	Required
France	2	Not specified	Required	Required
Germany	2	12	Not required	Required
Saudi Arabia	1	3	Required	Required
United States	2	6	Not required	Required
Canada	1	6	Not required	Required

Table 34.2 Reflexes to test for the diagnosis of brainstem death

Absence of pupillary light reflex

Absence of gag and reflex

Absence of cough with tracheal suctioning

Absence of oculovestibular reflexes (caloric responses)

Absence of corneal reflexes

Absence of motor response brain-originating, to pain stimulus

Absence of jaw jerk

Absence of sucking reflexes

Apnea test

CLINICAL EXAMINATION

Neurologic examination must demonstrate the absence of cerebral or brainstem function[1,11–13] (Table 34.2).

Physical examination includes the evidence of no cranial nerve reflexes, including pupillary response, oculocephalic reflex, corneal reflex, no response to tracheal suction, no spontaneous respirations, and no caloric reflex test.

Motor response

Clinical examination should demonstrate the absence of movements and motor response to pain. However, movements originating from the spinal cord or peripheral nerve may occur in brain death,[3] and can be very common. These can include semirhythmic movements of facial nerve-innervated muscles, tonic neck reflexes, passive neck displacements, upper limb pronation extension reflex, and fasciculations (twitches) of the trunk and extremities.[14,15]

Pupillary reflex

The pupillary light reflex assesses the function of the II and III cranial nerves. Pupillary reflex must be tested in each eye separately and consensual responses has to be evaluated.[16,17] Initially, the medical professional checks that the patient's pupils are the same size. Then the medical professional shines the light on each pupil and checks to see that both pupils have constricted to the same size.

Finally, the medical professional moves the penlight rapidly from the left pupil to the right several times to be sure that there are no consistent changes of the pupils.

Absence of the pupillary light reflex in comatose patients can usually occur because of herniation of mesial temporal structures from a supratentorial mass or for brainstem lesions.

Corneal reflex

The corneal reflex assesses the pathway arising from the trigeminal nerve—from small unmyelinated pain fibers in the cornea—and the dorsal parts of facial nuclei in the pons, which determines contraction of the orbicularis oculi muscles when either cornea is touched. The corneal reflex is tested by gently touching the edge of the cornea with a cotton or tissue swab and observing the absence of a responsive blink.

Oculovestibular reflex

Oculovestibular reflex is a reflex where activation of the vestibular system causes eye movement. The purpose of this reflex is to stabilize images on the retinas during head movement by producing eye movements in the opposite direction to head movement, thus preserving the image in the center of the visual field. It is usually tested through a caloric test with cold water that determines a strong stimulus for reflex eye movements sustaining turning of the head in the opposite direction and results in sustained deviation of both eyes toward the ear being stimulated. To test this reflex, the operator inclines the head of the patient 30 degrees up from the horizontal, and after inspecting the ears for obstruction or perforation, the operator injects at least 50 mL of ice water into the ear canal using a syringe.

Apnea test

The apnea test should be performed at the end of the examination, after all other criteria for brain death have been met. In cases of high cervical spinal cord lesions or neuromuscular paralysis, or in patients with severe chronic obstructive pulmonary disease with hypercapnia, the test is not considered valid.

Other prerequisites for performing the apnea test are normocapnia (partial pressure carbon dioxide (PaCO2) of 35 to 45 mmHg, absence of hypoxia, euvolemia, and hemodynamic stability.[6,18,19]

As a first step, the operator has to increase inspired oxygen before and during the test to avoid profound hypoxemia and hemodynamic instability. Preoxygenation with a fraction of inspired oxygen should be 1.0 for 10 minutes, up to a maximum oxygen partial pressure (PaO2) of 200 mmHg. After arterial blood gas is obtained and the values of PaCO2 are checked, the patient is disconnected from the ventilator. Oxygen is provided by a tracheal cannula with the tip lying at the carina.

If the test is positive, when PaCO2 increases, no respiratory response is detected; therefore, the PaCO2 increases to >60 mmHg or 20 mmHg greater than baseline values. Visual observation for detecting respiratory movements[6] for 8 to 10 minutes is recommended as a standard of observation, and PaCO2 is then measured just prior to reconnection to the ventilator to confirm that the target is achieved.

The test can be aborted if hypotension (systolic blood pressure is below 90 mmHg), hypoxemia (oxygen saturation [SaO2] below 85% for more than 30 seconds), or severe cardiac arrhythmias occur during the disconnection from the ventilator. Complications precluding the completion of the apnea test have been reported,[20–23] but with appropriate preoxygenation and hemodynamic stabilization, the apnea test can be completed in most patients.[22]

The apnea test can be challenging and requires some changes under unusual circumstances, such as patients on BSD during extracorporeal membrane oxygenation (ECMO) treatment; however, even in these situations, it has been shown to be feasible according to a number of case reports[24,25] and in a recent, larger, retrospective study.[19]

INSTRUMENTAL TESTS

In most countries, a valid clinical examination is sufficient to define and diagnose brain death in adults. However, in some cases, clinical assessment is not feasible and sometimes the clinical criteria cannot be applied.

This can happen, for example, when the cranial nerves cannot be adequately examined, when confounders make the clinical examination unreliable (the presence of a sedating or paralyzing drug that may be very slow to clear in patients with multiorgan failure), or when the tests cannot be completed or are not valid (such as the apnea test). Also, in some countries it is mandatory to use confirmatory tests to supplement the clinical examination (Table 34.1).[8]

In these cases, ancillary testing is required.[9] There are several tests that can be used to diagnose brain death (Table 34.3). The ideal test should not have "false positives"; should be accurate and suf-

Table 34.3 Instrumental tests used to diagnose brainstem death

Test	Advantages	Disadvantages
Angiography	Gold standard	Invasive, risky, may be inaccurate in some situations (such as hypotension, open cranial sutures), not easily available
EEG or SSEP	Noninvasive Included in the guidelines	Many confounding factors (hypothermia, drugs, false-positive cases), not always easily available; it detects synaptic potentials from the cerebral neocortex and does not reveal potentials from subcortical structures, such as the brainstem or thalamus
TCD	Bedside, quick, safe, easily available	Operator dependent, absence of temporal window in 10%–20% patients
CTA	Relatively accurate, not operator dependent	Poor specificity, lack of studies on patients with brain death
MRA	Relatively accurate, not operator dependent	Long procedure, not easily available
Nuclear tests	Relatively accurate	Invasive, not easily available, not quick

ficient on its own to establish that brain death is or is not present; it should be low cost, easily available, safe, and bedside applicable; and should not be susceptible to "confounders," such as drug effects.[26]

Currently, there is not an available test for brain death that meets all of these criteria; literature is lacking regarding this topic and with a limited level of evidence. Each test has different strengths and weaknesses and can be applied in different clinical situations. The main characteristics of the different tests are described in Table 34.3.

Ancillary tests can be divided in electrophysiologic tests and tests of blood flow in the brain.

Electrophysiologic tests used in the diagnosis of brain death include electroencephalogram (EEG) and evoked potentials (EPs). A flat EEG is a component of brain death declaration, and it is strongly recommended in some countries, especially for the diagnosis of brain death in very young children.[27] However, there are several anatomic and physiologic limitations of EEG for the diagnosis of brain death.

First, the EEG records totaled synaptic potentials received from the cerebral neocortex and do not assess subcortical structures, such as the brainstem or thalamus. Hence, the EEG may be flat or isoelectric in the presence of viable neurons in these structures. Second, the EEG is also vulnerable to confounding factors, in cases of sedation from medication or toxic ingestion, hypothermia, or metabolic, and there are a number of false-positive cases of flat EEG recordings in these situations.[28,29]

Somatosensory evoked potentials (SSEPs) and brainstem auditory evoked potentials (BAEPs) also have a very limited use when diagnosing brain death.[30,31]

In SSEPs, the bilateral absence of the parietal sensory cortex responses (N19-P22) in response to median nerve stimulation is supportive of brain death.

Each test activates a discrete sensory pathway and extends the electrophysiologic interrogation beyond the EEG to areas of interest in the brainstem but does not test the functional integrity of other central nervous system (CNS) structures. Also, similarly to EEG, the early components of SSEPs and BAEPs are affected by hypothermia, drugs, and metabolic derangements.[32]

Tests of blood flow to the brain are generally accepted as establishers of brain death.

Among these, angiography, transcranial Doppler, magnetic resonance angiography, computed tomographic angiography, and nuclear medicine radionuclide scanning are currently used. The advantage is that these tests are not affected by variables, such as drugs, metabolic disorders, or hypothermia; however, in severe hypotension or shock, they could be inaccurate.

Four-vessel cerebral angiography is traditionally considered the "gold standard" test for brain death. The disadvantages of this test are its invasiveness and the need to transport the patient, who is often clinically unstable, to the radiology department.

Cerebral angiography can confirm brain death, which often demonstrates absent blood flow at or beyond the carotid bifurcation or Circle of Willis.[33,34] False-negative cerebral angiograms showing normal blood flow in at least some intracranial blood vessels are reported and can occur when intracranial pressure is lowered by surgery, trauma, and ventricular shunts or in infants with pliable skulls.

Transcranial Doppler (TCD) is a safe, noninvasive, bedside, and repeatable technique. The test requires training to reduce inter- and intraobserver variability; it evaluates both anterior and posterior circulations,[35,36] and demonstrates absence of flow; however, even small systolic peaks without diastolic flow or a reverberating flow pattern suggest high vascular resistance and intracranial hypertension and support the diagnosis of brain death (Figures 34.2 and 34.3).

TCD has several limitations. In fact, 10% to 25% of patients do not present a suitable temporal window for examination that precludes evaluation of insonated intracranial arteries. Also, both false-positive and false-negative results are reported (compared with cerebral angiography or other standard),[37,38] with a sensitivity of TCD at around 70.5%, and specificity of 97.4% according to some authors.[39]

The clinical use of computed tomographic angiography (CTA) and computed tomographic perfusion in the evaluation of brain death is not clear. These tests require radiation exposure and contrast injection. Moreover, studies comparing CTA to an alternative brain death determination concluded that the sensitivities are variable, ranging from 62% to 99%.[40]

These results, and the absence of studies examining computed tomography findings in patients who are comatose, but not brain dead, preclude an assessment of this test's accuracy.[41]

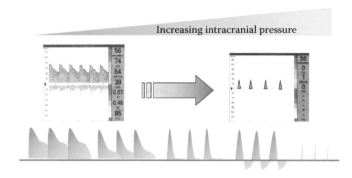

Figure 34.2 Patterns of flow velocities detected through transcranial Doppler with increasing intracranial pressure.

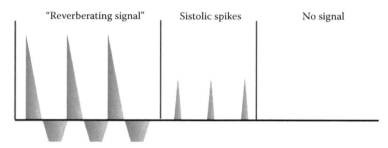

Figure 34.3 Different patterns of flow velocities compatible with brainstem death.

Magnetic resonance angiography (MRA) can be used to assess the absence of arterial blood flow and support the diagnosis of brain death. Also, MRA can show brain structures precisely, as well as cerebral edema, brainstem damage, and mass effect. MRA is a sensitive test for brain death, but it has uncertain specificity.[42] Disadvantages include the fact that patients are required to lie flat for a long time and are not easily accessible, making this somewhat problematic in unstable patients.

Finally, radionuclide modality for brain imaging can be used. Brain flow can be assessed applying a tracer, with subsequent imaging with single photon emission computed tomographic (SPECT) brain scintigraphy, which penetrates the brain parenchyma proportionally to regional blood flow.[43] In this situation, if there is no brain perfusion, there is absence of isotope uptake, and this means that the brain is not perfused and, therefore, dead.[44]

ORGAN DONATION AND ETHICAL CONSIDERATIONS

Intensive care units (ICUs) play a vital role in organ donation and transplantation.[45] The main role of intensivists is to identify and maintain potential organ donors, discuss organ donation with the relatives of the dead or dying patient, and the care for transplant recipients. Clinicians will have to carry out the wishes of the patient, providing comfort to a grieving family, and look after the donor in order to ensure that the organs are transplanted in the best possible conditions.[46] These interventions will reduce morbidity in the recipient and reduce their hospital stay, thus making the best use of scarce resources.

Organ transplants are now performed worldwide and are often the only alternative for patients with end-stage heart, lung, or liver disease. Organ transplantation is currently the treatment of choice in chronic renal failure and the only option for patients with end-stage heart, renal, liver, and lung disease.[47]

Improvements in surgical techniques, immunology, and immunosuppressive drugs increased the number of transplant candidates significantly. The advent of more effective immunosuppressive therapies resulted in improvement of the outcomes during the last two decades.

The surge in organ replacement therapy has dramatically increased the need for transplantable organs and the demand has far exceeded the supply for many years, with a growing gap between patients on the waiting list for a kidney transplant.[45] The shortage of organs for transplantation is an important medical and societal problem because transplantation is often the best therapeutic option for end-stage organ failure.[48]

In general, there are two main types of donors: the deceased donor (the heart-beating, brain dead [BDD] donor in the UK and some other countries, brain stem dead [BSD] donor), or the non–heart-beating donor. In this chapter, we will focus on brain dead donors.

Although major differences still exist between different centers with regard to the organization of organ donation, a procurement transplant coordinator is generally involved in public and professional education in the field of organs and in the organization and logistics of organs, in collaboration with critical care staff through a 24-hour, on-call service to receive referrals and subsequent organization transplant operations.[45]

All patients who become BSD should be considered as potential organ donors.

Apart from refusal to give consent, the only absolute contraindication to donation is when transplantation would result in the transfer of a potentially fatal disease for which there is no cure available, including antimicrobial-resistant infections, such as Creutzfeldt-Jakob disease, tuberculosis, malaria, malignancy, or less than a 5-year history of treated malignancy.

Relative contraindications are hepatitis C and hepatitis B surface antigen positive (unless organs are to be used for a hepatitis B surface antigen-positive patient).

COMMUNICATION AND DIFFICULT DECISIONS

It is a professional responsibility to ensure that any ethical debate is based on the best available evidence. Discussion with the family and the decision-making process should take in consideration different factors, including personal values, professional custom, practice, and ethical guidelines.[49,50]

Finally, the physician should be aware of relevant institutional and national professional rules and adherence to them. The goal as an ICU professional is to use communication skills to enhance the care of the patients. Breaking bad news is a

very difficult task to achieve as a physician, but it is necessary in the practice of critical care medicine.[51]

Typically, physicians may be afraid to add to relatives' distress, unexpected reactions, or to express their own emotions. However, the family should be made aware of the seriousness of the situation from the beginning of the patient's ICU stay.

The family should be allowed to absorb this information before beginning discussions on BSD and, eventually, organ donation.

The family's hospital experiences significantly affect whether they decide to donate organs.[52] Non-donor families have a poor understanding of brain death, are less likely to feel that they were given sufficient time to make a decision, and are more likely to feel that the person making the request was insensitive to their needs.[53]

In fact, adequate information on the process of organ donation and its benefits, as well as proper communication with the families and ensuring that they had a clear understanding of brain death, are the main factors associated with reduced rates of refusal.[53] However, there is no evidence of increase in consent rates for organ donation when relatives are approached by the clinical team and a donor transplant coordinator together rather than by the clinical team alone.[50]

Meeting the needs of a patient's family is an essential aspect of ICU care. The satisfaction of relatives is a major criterion in the assessment of quality of care and of compliance with accreditation requirements. Often, relatives are not satisfied with the emotional support they receive, with the provision of understandable, complete, and consistent information, and with the coordination of care. Poor communication is frequently cited as the main cause of dissatisfaction with care. Also, specific clinician statements during family meetings—such as assurances that the patient will not be abandoned before death, will be comfortable, and will not suffer—and the support for the family's decisions about end-of-life care, are associated with more family satisfaction.

Therefore, there are several simple recommendations to adopt in these cases; these include: the choice of a comfortable and private location, to know and use the patient's name during the discussion, introduce all people present, provide enough chairs for all attendees, ask all staff to turn off their pagers or cellular telephones, and allow time for questions.

OBTAINING CONSENT FROM THE FAMILY

Consent for organ donation can be obtained in several different ways, and this process is influenced by a multitude of factors, such as religious and cultural beliefs, public education and awareness, and a variability in ICU policies. In some countries, such as Belgium, it is assumed that you want to donate your organs after death and you have to register this wish to "opt out" if you don't wish to do so. In others countries, such as the UK, organ donation is not assumed and it has to be declared and discussed, case by case. If the patient does not record his or her wish, after death, an inquiry is made of the patient's relatives to see if they were aware of the person's wishes. If they were not aware, the relatives are asked for consent. In the UK, the registration can be on a card or electronically on the Organ Donor Registry. At the moment, even if the patient recorded his or her wish to donate while still alive, it is common practice to ask relatives for "consent" for organ donation. If they object, organ donation does not usually occur.

MANAGEMENT OF THE ORGAN DONOR

There are numerous physiologic changes after BSD and their correction may involve a significant clinical effort, including the use of invasive monitoring, blood transfusions, and drugs. Once the patient has been declared BSD, intervention strategies should change from attempts to maintain the patient and effect a "cure" or improvement in the disease process, to optimizing organs, to maintaining physiologic homeostasis, including circulation and respiration. Without this support, "brain death" occurs almost simultaneously with "cardiac death."

Efficient coordination among physicians, organ procurement organizations, and transplant centers to promote the best physiologic donor management is required to maximize the number of viable organs available for transplantation.

GENERAL PRINCIPLES

Brain death determines a number of pathophysiologic responses that can put at risk the function of potentially transplantable organs.[54] Therefore, donor management should involve a number of aggressive resuscitative efforts aimed at managing and stabilizing the donor as well as maximizing the potential viability of all organs.

The main management goals are to achieve hemodynamic stability and optimal function of all organs; and maintaining proper ventilatory support, good pulmonary toilet, and appropriate infection prophylaxis. However, this is not easy to achieve, because interventions that improve the function of one organ may be detrimental to the function of other organs.[54,55]

Temperature

Hypothermia occurs very quickly due to the absence of any spontaneous muscle movement and loss of central control of temperature. Temperature regulation in humans is controlled by the hypothalamus; after death, the hypothalamus ceases to function and preservation of normothermia in those patients who are destined to become organ donors is a fundamental part of maintaining normal physiology.

Normothermia should be maintained through invasive or noninvasive devices, including increasing the temperature of the ambient air, infrared warming lights, instillation of warmed intravenous fluids, and warm air or water blankets.

Hemodynamic

Systemic hypotension is common in brain-dead deceased donors (up to 80%) and may have different causes, such as lack of sympathetic tone central diabetes insipidus, arrhythmias, or conduction blockade. Hypotension is associated with poor organ function and should be avoided. Most centers aim to achieve a mean arterial pressure of 60 mmHg; some prefer higher values.

Restoration of intravascular volume with crystalloid solutions is the first step, and if there is no response, inotropic support should be started with measurement of cardiac output and hemodynamic monitoring to guide further management. Using the lowest dose of the least harmful agent is the preferred approach, but this is not always possible. The goal is to achieve a normotensive, euvolemic state.

Pituitary function

The posterior pituitary loses its function and no longer secretes antidiuretic hormone (ADH); therefore, the patient develops diabetes insipidus, with large hourly losses of water and dilute urine. Relative hyposmolarity of urine (<300 mOsm/L and often <200 mOsm/L) with associated high serum hyperosmolarity (>310 mOsm/L) are the mainstream for the diagnosis.

Diabetes insipidus is the most important and common endocrine problem in brain-dead donors.

Volume replacement is suggested to ensure euvolemia, but excessive diuresis is more easily managed by the administration of desmopressin or vasopressin to keep urine output in the 100 to 200 mL per hour range.

Adrenal insufficiency is also common following brain death as well as thyroid abnormalities, including the "sick euthyroid syndrome," which is also prevalent after brain death.

Respiratory

Hypocapnia may be used to reduce intracerebral pressure (ICP) and reduce brain volume. High positive-end respiratory pressure should also be avoided to reduce ICP and avoid hemodynamic compromise. Finally, hypoxemia may follow from overzealous fluid administration during resuscitation attempts, atelectasis, aspiration, pneumothorax, pulmonary contusion, or pneumonia.

PARTICULAR GROUPS OF PATIENTS

Pregnant patient

Maintenance of a BSD of a pregnant mother until delivery is challenging; however, support of pregnant patients in BSD has been reported, with the longest case being 107 days (from 15 to 32 weeks of gestation) of support.[56] The issues are clinical, legal, and ethical. According to a recent study,[56] the main

determinants of the fetus' outcome are the clinical condition of the mother and the gestational age. Clinical issues are related, as previously discussed, to the particular intensity of care necessary for long-term cardiovascular, respiratory, endocrine, metabolic, and nutritional support and to manage infections. Ethical issues may include concerns about using an ICU bed for the long-term maintenance of a BSD patient.[57,58]

The gestational age of the fetus is important to consider, since survival, *without severe complications*, is uncommon before 25 weeks. In very early pregnancy, maternal maintenance should be strongly discouraged as it is probably futile. However, it should be considered for some days when the gestational age is over 30 weeks and the condition of the mother is favorable, particularly if time is required for fetal maturation. Between 25 and 30 weeks, such a strategy may be considered. Relatives should be told that the maintenance of a BSD body is difficult and the outcome unpredictable.

Finally, there are several bioethical issues concerning the use of the body of the BSD mother as a natural incubator and the identification of who should make decisions. The previous wishes of the mother (if known) and the feelings of the partner should be carefully evaluated. The management of brain dead pregnant women requires a multidisciplinary team including obstetrics, intensive care specialists, and neurosurgeons, which should follow available guidelines and recommendations, both for organ-preserving treatment of the potential donor and supportive management of the fetus.

Children

Diagnosis and management of brain death in children presents few differences when compared with adult patients.[59] The main causes are trauma and anoxic encephalopathy, followed by infections and cerebral masses.

Similar to the adult population, there are differences among centers about the practice to adopt and the criteria for determination.[60] Additional conditions, such as hypotension, hypothermia, and metabolic disturbances, should be treated and corrected, and medications that can interfere with the neurologic examination and apnea testing should be discontinued as soon as possible. Apnea testing requires documentation of an arterial PaCO2 20 mmHg above baseline and above 60 mmHg with no respiratory effort being done during the testing period. If the apnea test cannot be completed, an instrumental test should be performed.

Supplemental studies may be used to support the diagnosis of brain death when a neurologic examination is not possible or apnea testing cannot be completed safely or if there is uncertainty about the neurologic examination.

Assessments in neonates and infants should be performed by pediatric specialists with specific critical care training; two examinations (including the apnea test) with each examination separated by an observation period are mandatory. An observation period of 24 hours for term newborns to 30 days of age, and 12 hours for infants and children (30 days to 18 years) is generally recommended, and no specific timing for the second assessment is required.

REFERENCES

1. O'Sullivan F, Miles B. *Brainstem Death. Anaesth Intensive Care Med [Internet]*. Elsevier Ltd; London, UK: 2012. Accessed June 14, 2014;13(6):249-251. http://linkinghub.elsevier.com/retrieve/pii/S1472029912000719.

2. Faul M, Coronado V. Epidemiology of traumatic brain injury. *Handb Clin Neurol*. 2015;127:3-13.

3. Wahlster S, Wijdicks EFM, Patel PV et al. Brain death declaration: practices and perceptions worldwide. *Neurology [Internet]*. 2015;84(18):1870-1879. Available from: http://ovidsp.ovid.com/ovidweb.cgi?T=JS&PAGE=fulltext&D=ovft&MODE=ovid&NEWS=N&SEARCH=0028-3878.is+and+84.vo+and+18.ip+and+1870.pg&NEWS=n.

4. Burkle CM, Pope TM. Brain death: legal obligations and the courts. *Semin Neurol*. 2015;35(2):174-179.

5. Burkle CM, Sharp RR, Wijdicks EF. Why brain death is considered death and why there should be no confusion. *Neurology*. 2014;83:1464-1469.

6. Wijdicks EFM, Varelas PN, Gronseth GS, Greer DM. Evidence-based guideline update: determining brain death in adults: report of the Quality Standards Subcommittee of the American Academy of Neurology. *Neurology [Internet]*. 2010[cited 2014 Jun 7]; 74(23):1911-1918. Available from: http://www.ncbi.nlm.nih.gov/pubmed/20530327.

7. Greer DM, Varelas PN, Haque S, Wijdicks EFM. Variability of brain death determination guidelines in leading US neurologic institutions. *Neurology*. 2008;70(4):284-289.

8. Hsieh ST. Brain death worldwide: accepted fact but no global consensus in diagnostic criteria [3]. *Neurology*. 2006;67:919.

9. Wijdicks EF, Varelas PN, Gronseth GS, Greer DM, American Academy of Neurology. Evidence-based guideline update: determining brain death in adults: report of the Quality Standards Subcommittee of the American Academy of Neurology. *Neurology*. 2010;74 (23):1911-1918.

10. Bernat JL, Capron AM, Bleck TP et al. The circulatory-respiratory determination of death in organ donation. *Crit Care Med [Internet]*. 2010. Accessed June 12, 2014. Available from: http://www.ncbi.nlm.nih.gov/pubmed/20124892.

11. Grewal A, Kaul TK, Grewal SS. Brain death. *J Anaesth Clin Pharmacol* 2006; 22(2):115–138.

12. Smith M, Citerio G. Death determined by neurological criteria: the next steps. *Intensive Care Med*. 2017;43(9):1383-1385.

13. Wijdicks EFM. The diagnosis of brain death. *N Engl J Med*. 2001;344(16):1215-1221.

14. Saposnik G, Bueri JA, Mauriño J, Saizar R, Garretto NS. Spontaneous and reflex movements in brain death. *Neurology [Internet]*. 2000;54(1):221-223. Available from: http://www.ncbi.nlm.nih.gov/pubmed/15745731.

15. Saposnik G, Basile VS, Young GB. Movements in brain death: a systematic review. *Can J Neurol Sci/J Can des Sci Neurol [Internet]*. 2009;36(2):154-160. Available from: http://www.journals.cambridge.org/abstract_S031716710000651X

16. Fugate JE, Wijdicks EFM, Mandrekar J et al. Predictors of neurologic outcome in

hypothermia after cardiac arrest. *Ann Neurol.* 2010;68(6):907-914.

17. Machado C. Diagnosis of brain death. *Neurology Int.* 2010;2:7-13.

18. Morenski JD, Oro JJ, Tobias JD, Singh A. Determination of death by neurological criteria. *J Intensive Care Med [Internet].* 2003;18(4):211-221. Available from: http://journals.sagepub.com/doi/10.1177/0885066603254359.

19. Giani M, Scaravilli V, Colombo SM et al. Apnea test during brain death assessment in mechanically ventilated and ECMO patients. *Intensive Care Med.* 2016;42(1):72-81.

20. Datar S, Fugate J, Rabinstein A, Couillard P, Wijdicks EFM. Completing the apnea test: decline in complications. *Neurocrit Care.* 2014;21(3):392-396.

21. Saposnik G, Rizzo G, Deluca JL. Pneumothorax and pneumoperitoneum during the apnea test: how safe is this procedure? *Arq Neuropsiquiatr.* 2000;58(3 B):905-908.

22. Wu XL, Fang Q, Li L, Qiu YQ, Luo BY. Complications associated with the apnea test in the determination of the brain death. *Chin Med J (Engl).* 2008;121(13):1169-1172.

23. Goudreau JL, Wijdicks EF, Emery SF. Complications during apnea testing in the determination of brain death: predisposing factors. *Neurology.* 2000;55(7):1045-1048.

24. Shah V, Lazaridis C. Apnea testing on extracorporeal membrane oxygenation: case report and literature review. *J Crit Care.* 2015;30:784-786.

25. Smilevitch P, Lonjaret L, Fourcade O, Geeraerts T. Apnea test for brain death determination in a patient on extracorporeal membrane oxygenation. *Neurocrit Care.* 2013;19(2):215-217.

26. Roberts DJ, MacCulloch KAM, Versnick EJ, Hall RI. Should ancillary brain blood flow analyses play a larger role in the neurological determination of death? *Can J Anesth.* 2010;57(10):927-935.

27. Nakagawa TA, Ashwal S, Mathur M, Mysore M. Clinical report—guidelines for the determination of brain death in infants and children: an update of the 1987 task force recommen-dations. *Pediatrics [Internet].* 2011;128(3):e720-e740. Available from: http://www.ncbi.nlm.nih.gov/pubmed/21873704.

28. Rothstein TL. Recovery from near death following cerebral anoxia: a case report demonstrating superiority of median somatosensory evoked potentials over EEG in predicting a favorable outcome after cardiopulmonary resuscitation. *Resuscitation.* 2004;60(3):335-341.

29. Heckmann JG, Lang CJG, Pfau M, Neundörfer B. Electrocerebral silence with preserved but reduced cortical brain perfusion. *Eur J Emerg Med [Internet].* 2003;10(3):241-243. Available from: http://www.ncbi.nlm.nih.gov/pubmed/12972905.

30. Ozgirgin ON, Ozcelik T, Sevimli NK. Auditory brain stem responses in the detection of brain death. *Kulak Burun Bogaz Ihtis Derg [Internet].* 2003;10(1):1-7. Available from: http://ovidsp.ovid.com/ovidweb.cgi?T=JS&PAGE=reference&D=med4&NEWS=N&AN=12529570.

31. Firsching R, Frowein RA, Wilhelms S, Buchholz F. Brain death: practicability of evoked potentials. *Neuro Surg Rev.* 1992;15(4):249-254.

32. Guérit JM. Medical technology assessment EEG and evoked potentials in the intensive care unit. *Neurophysiol Clin [Internet].* 1999;29(4):301-317. Available from: http://www.ncbi.nlm.nih.gov/pubmed/10546249.

33. Flowers WJ, Patel B. Persistence of cerebral blood flow after brain death. *South Med J.* 2000;93(4):364-370.

34. Braun M, Ducrocq X, Huot JC, Audibert G, Anxionnat R, Picard L. Intravenous angiography in brain death: report of 140 patients. *Neuroradiology.* 1997;39(6):400-405.

35. Ducrocq X, Braun M, Debouverie M, Junges C, Hummer M, Vespignani H. Brain death and transcranial Doppler: experience in 130 cases of brain dead patients. *J Neurol Sci.* 1998;160(1):41-46.

36. Kuo J, Chen C, Chio C et al. Time dependent validity in the diagnosis of brain death using transcranial Doppler sonography. *J Neurol Neurosurg Psychiatry [Internet].*

2006;77(5):646-649. Available from: http://www.pubmedcentral.nih.gov/articlerender.fcgi?artid=2117438&tool=pmcentrez&rendertype=abstract.

37. Paolin A, Manuali A, Di Paola F et al. Reliability in diagnosis of brain death. *Intensive Care Med.* 1995;21(8):657-662.

38. Vora Y, Suarez-Almazor M, Steinke D, Martin ML, Findlay J. Role of transcranial Doppler monitoring in the diagnosis of cerebral vasospasm after subarachnoid hemorrhage. *Neurosurgery.* 1999;44(6):1237-1247; discussion 1247-1248.

39. Dosemeci L, Dora B, Yilmaz M, Cengiz M, Balkan S, Ramazanoglu A. Utility of transcranial Doppler ultrasonography for confirmatory diagnosis of brain death: two sides of the coin [Internet]. *Transplantation.* 2004;77:71-75. Available from: http://ovidsp.ovid.com/ovidweb.cgi?T=JS&PAGE=reference&D=emed6&NEWS=N&AN=2004042693.

40. Taylor T, Dineen RA, Gardiner DC et al. Computed tomography (CT) angiography for confirmation of the clinical diagnosis of brain death. *Cochrane Database Syst Rev [Internet].* 2012;3:CD009694.

41. Kramer AH, Roberts DJ. Computed tomography angiography in the diagnosis of brain death: a systematic review and meta-analysis. *Neurocrit Care.* 2014;21(3):539-550.

42. Matsumura A, Meguro K, Tsurushima H et al. Magnetic resonance imaging of brain death. *Neurol Med Chir (Tokyo) [Internet].* 1996;36(3):166-171. Available from: http://ovidsp.ovid.com/ovidweb.cgi?T=JS&PAGE=reference&D=med4&NEWS=N&AN=8869153.

43. Schlake HP, Böttger IG, Grotemeyer KH, Husstedt IW, Brandau W, Schober O. Determination of cerebral perfusion by means of planar brain scintigraphy and 99mTc-HMPAO in brain death, persistent vegetative state and severe coma. *Intensive Care Med.* 1992;18(2):76-81.

44. Facco E, Zucchetta P, Munari M et al. 99m Tc-HMPAO SPECT in the diagnosis of brain death. *Intensive Care Med [Internet].* 1998;24:911-917. Available from: http://www.aomrc.org.uk/publications/reports-a-guidance/doc_download/42-a-code-of-practice-for-the-diagnosis-and-confirmation-of-death.html.

45. Citerio G, Cypel M, Dobb GJ et al. Organ donation in adults: a critical care perspective. *Intensive Care Med.* 2016;42(3):305-315.

46. Farrell A-M, Quigley M. Organ donation and transplantation. *Encycl Appl Ethics.* 2012;288-296.

47. NHS Blood and Transplant. Organ donation and transplantation. *J Tenn Med Assoc.* 2015;74(7):507-509, 515.

48. Da Silva IRF, Frontera JA. Worldwide barriers to organ donation. *JAMA Neurol [Internet].* 2015;72(1):112. Available from: http://archneur.jamanetwork.com/article.aspx?doi=10.1001/jamaneurol.2014.3083.

49. Vincent A, Logan L. Consent for organ donation. *Br J Anaesth.* 2012;108(Suppl 1):i80-i87.

50. Williams MA, Lipsett PA, Rushton CH et al. The physician's role in discussing organ donation with families*. *Crit Care Med [Internet].* 2003;31(5):1568-1573. Available from: http://content.wkhealth.com/linkback/openurl?sid=WKPTLP:landingpage&an=00003246-200305000-00041.

51. Potter JE, Herkes RG, Perry L et al. COMmunication with Families regarding ORgan and Tissue donation after death in intensive care (COMFORT): protocol for an intervention study. *BMC Health Serv Res [Internet].* 2017;17(1):42. Available from: http://bmchealthservres.biomedcentral.com/articles/10.1186/s12913-016-1964-7.

52. Bocci MG, D'Alò C, Barelli R et al. Taking care of relationships in the intensive care unit: positive impact on family consent for organ donation. *Transplant Proc.* 2016;48(10):3245-3250.

53. Ghorbani F, Khoddami-Vishteh HR, Ghobadi O, Shafaghi S, Rostami Louyeh A, Najafizadeh K. Causes of family refusal for organ donation. *Transplant Proc.* 2011;43(2):405-406.

54. Frontera JA, Kalb T. How I manage the adult potential organ donor: donation after neurological death (Part 1). *Neurocrit Care*. 2010;12:103-110.

55. Floerchinger B, Oberhuber R, Tullius SG. Effects of brain death on organ quality and transplant outcome. *Transplant Rev*. 2012;26:54-59.

56. Esmaeilzadeh M, Dictus C, Kayvanpour E et al. One life ends, another begins: management of a brain-dead pregnant mother-A systematic review-. *BMC Med [Internet]*. 2010;8(1):74. Available from: http://bmcmedicine.biomedcentral.com/articles/10.1186/1741-7015-8-74.

57. Field DR, Gates EA, Creasy RK, Jonsen AR, Laros RKJ. Maternal brain death during pregnancy. *Medical and ethical issues. JAMA [Internet]*. 1988;260(6):816-822. Available from: http://ovidsp.ovid.com/ovidweb.cgi?T=JS&PAGE=reference&D=med3&NEWS=N&AN=3392814.

58. Kosec V, Tuckar N, Gopcevic A et al. End of one life at the beginning of another (maternal brain death during pregnancy). *J Perinat Med [Internet]*. 2013;41. Available from: http://www.embase.com/search/results?subaction=viewrecord&from=export&id=L71115278%5Cnhttp://dx.doi.org/10.1515/jpm-2013-2003%5Cnhttp://sfx.library.uu.nl/utrecht?sid=EMBASE&issn=03005577&id=doi:10.1515%2Fjpm-2013-2003&atitle=End+of+one+life+at+the+beginni.

59. Banasiak KJ, Lister G. Brain death in children. *Curr Opin Pediatr*. 2003;15(3):288-293.

60. Mejia RE, Pollack MM. Variability in brain death determination practices in children. *JAMA [Internet]*. 1995;274(7):550-553. Available from: http://www.ncbi.nlm.nih.gov/pubmed/7629983.

Recent advances

35

Recent advances in anesthesia for neurotrauma

HALEY REIS, ONAT AKYOL, VADIM GOSPODAREV, CESAR REIS,
GOCKE YILMAZ, RICHARD APPLEGATE II, SHENG CHEN, AND JOHN ZHANG

INTRODUCTION

According to the International Brain Injury Association, traumatic brain injury (TBI) is the leading cause of death and disability worldwide. The Centers for Disease Control and Prevention (CDC) reported that TBI emergency room visits and hospitalizations increased from 2001 to 2010 in the United States, with emergency department visits showing the largest increase from 521.0 to 615.7 per 100,000 individuals. TBI leads to pathophysiologic events that undermine cerebral blood flow (CBF), which depends on adequate arterial blood pressure, intracranial pressure (ICP), and cerebrovascular resistance.[1] The immediate damage caused by traumatic forces includes focal, multifocal, or diffuse injury to neurons, axons, dendrites, and blood vessels.[2] Post-traumatic inflammatory responses include cytokine and metalloproteinase expression, leading to the blood–brain barrier (BBB) breakdown.[3] Damage to the BBB endothelium compromises the neurovascular unit, resulting in dysregulation of cerebrovasculature and subsequent brain edema, increased ICP, decreased cerebral perfusion pressure (CPP), hypoxia, hypotension, and even hemorrhage[4,5] (Figure 35.1). It is essential to predict development of secondary injury since finding effective prevention of these is imperative in TBI management.[4]

Spinal cord injury (SCI) is another leading cause of disability, with between 250,000 and 500,000 injuries worldwide annually, according to the World Health Organization (WHO). Mortality rates are highest during the first year after SCI due to secondary complications, including renal failure and respiratory complications, particularly for severely injured individuals. In acute SCI, vascular dysfunction occurs, including spinal and neurogenic shock, arterial hypotension, and deep-vein thrombosis (DVT). When communication between central pattern generators and spinal sympathetic neurons stops, spinal shock occurs. Hemodynamic changes include severe hypertension followed by reflex bradycardia and hypotension.[6]

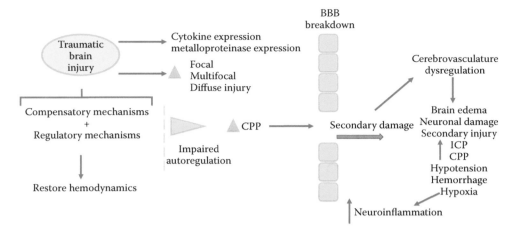

Figure 35.1 This figure demonstrates that TBI elicits compensatory and regulatory mechanisms. When those mechanisms are impaired, there will be alteration(Δ) in CPP, leading to neuronal damage, brain edema, and secondary brain injury. In addition, it leads to increased ICP, CPP, hypotension, hypoxia, and hemorrhage. TBI leads to neuroinflammation, which leads to cytokine and metalloproteinase expression. BBB integrity is lost after brain injury and contributes to secondary damage.

HEMODYNAMIC STABILITY WITH MULTIPLE TRAUMAS

In understanding neuroprotective mechanisms and properly controlling secondary insults, such as hypotension and hypoperfusion in acute TBI, it is also important to consider concomitant injuries such as hemorrhagic shock and how they can complicate neurotrauma management. To specifically evaluate outcomes of hemorrhagic shock and TBI, a post-hoc analysis of the Pragmatic Randomized Optimal Platelets and Plasma Ratios (PROPPR) trial was conducted. Eighteen percent of subjects presented with TBI + hemorrhagic shock. Hospital-free, ICU-free, ventilator-free days were lower in the TBI-only and TBI + hemorrhagic shock groups; however, adjusted 30-day mortality showed that the odds of death in TBI + hemorrhagic shock was 10.6 (95% CI 4.8–23.2) times higher than the control group. Overall, the combination of TBI and hemorrhagic shock was associated with worse coagulopathy prior to resuscitation, as well as increased morbidity and mortality compared with hemorrhagic shock alone and those having neither diagnosis.[7]

Compensatory and regulatory mechanisms are impaired following TBI, prolonging hemodynamic instability, thereby impairing CPP and making secondary damage worse (Figure 35.1).[8,9] In polytrauma, the response to hemorrhage is worsened.[10,11] Animal studies have investigated optimal fluid-resuscitation measures for combined TBI and hypovolemic shock. Brotfain and colleagues determined that survival, neurologic outcomes, and hemodynamic stability inversely correlated with aggressiveness of whole-blood resuscitation.[8] Elevated ICP impairs protective mechanisms against hemorrhagic hypotension and the type of fluid used for volume replacement impacts ICP.[12] A study showed the effectiveness of hypertonic saline solution to reduce elevated ICP caused by TBI and also found that central arterial plasma thromboxane and prostaglandin levels increased progressively at 90 minutes in the control group.[13] Thromboxane elicited a vasoconstrictive response to cerebral ischemia associated with cerebral hypoperfusion, demonstrating the influence of untreated hemorrhagic shock in the presence of ICP on the inflammatory response after TBI.[13,14]

Resuscitation with albumin-based fluid has been shown to result in increased mortality compared with normal saline (NS).[15] Fresh frozen plasma (FFP) is a more complex fluid containing many different proteins, buffers, free radical scavengers, and clotting factors.[16] Jin and colleagues looked at the use of colloids in reducing brain injury and swelling. FFP reduced the area of injury and swelling, possibly because it better preserves BBB integrity,[11] and has beneficial effects on endothelial function and permeability.[17,18] Imam and colleagues also investigated the beneficial effects of FFP compared with NS and reported neuroprotective effects of early FFP infusion with improved cerebral perfusion and brain oxygenation compared with NS-treated animals. Although this study did not assess long-term effects of FFP resuscitation, it indicated the potential role of FFP-based resuscitation in TBI and multisystem trauma.[19] Lyophilized plasma is another option for FFP and was found to be safe and effective in a polytrauma animal model.[20]

A hemoglobin-based oxygen carrier (HBOC) has been shown to stabilize hemodynamics with low-volume resuscitation to transport and unload O_2 and to increase tissue oxygenation in the presence of hemorrhage and TBI.[21] White and colleagues studied the effects of HBOC with sodium nitroglycerine to attenuate HBOC vasoconstrictive effects caused by local scavenging of nitric oxide. They found no benefit in HBOC-based fluid resuscitation over LR.[10] Investigating effects of volume resuscitation fluids may lead to improved treatment options for TBI with hemorrhagic shock.

UNDERSTANDING TEMPERATURE CONTROL

When the overall results of the National Acute Brain Injury Study: Hypothermia regarding benefits of hypothermia after SCI were negative,[22] efforts were made to understand how to improve the treatment effects of mild therapeutic hypothermia. These hypotheses included speeding up the time to reach hypothermia,[22] as well as maintaining appropriate fluid volume, cerebral perfusion pressure, and ICP.[23] Prolonged therapeutic hypothermia (32°C–34°C) starting within a median time of 3.0 hours, and lasting for at least 72 hours, followed by slow rewarming at a rate of <1°C per day under tight hemodynamic management for severe TBI did not improve neurologic outcomes, as determined by the Glasgow Outcome Scale at 6 months follow-up, or decrease the risk of mortality compared with control groups with strict temperature control (35.5°C–37°C).[24] Using therapeutic hypothermia with standard care within 10 days after injury on patients with >20 mmHg ICP despite conventional treatment after TBI did not result in better outcomes compared with those who received standard care alone.[25]

AUTOREGULATION AND ANESTHESIA

CBF and cerebral metabolic rate (CMR) are coupled in the absence of pathology or anesthetic drugs. Following TBI, regional and global changes in blood flow and metabolic rate can occur, depending on size, location, and type of tissue injury. Within the first 12 hours after the injury, changes in CBF can reach ischemic levels, falling to 18 to 20 mL/100 mL/min after severe TBI, then can uptrend to hyperemic levels.[26,27] A recent study into rheologic modulation of CBF to enhance cerebral microvascular perfusion, oxygen delivery, and metabolism used nontoxic macromolecules called drag-reducing polymers. These polymers improved CBF and ameliorated tissue hypoxia typically caused by early post-traumatic reductions in CBF.[28] Because TBI impairs autoregulation and vasoconstriction in response to increased CBF and oxygen supply, the dilatory effect was more prevalent after injection of drag-reducing polymers in the TBI group. In addition, reduced BBB damage after TBI was noted through increased vascular wall shear stress, a protective mechanism to maintain endothelium surrounding the inner vascular wall.[28,29] Another study examined CBF after TBI using an animal model using edaravone, a free radical scavenger. Edaravone significantly improved CBF (93.4 ± 5.7%) compared with the vehicle-treated group (73.7 ± 5.8%, $P < 0.05$) after TBI. It not only maintained cerebrovascular autoregulation but also reduced neuronal damage by scavenging reactive oxygen species.[30]

A family of three kinases, ERK, p38, and JNK, are critically important to hemodynamics after TBI.[31] Studies have shown activation of JNK and ERK contributed to impaired N-methyl-D-aspartate receptors (NMDA-R) cerebrovasodilation, while p38 was protective after fluid percussion injury in an animal model.[32,33] P38 inhibits upregulation of endothelin-1, which is known to antagonize NMDA-R-mediated vasodilation.[33] Activation of NMDA-Rs contributes to excitotoxic neuronal cell death and represents a mechanism in which metabolism is coupled to CBF, but these functions are impaired after TBI because of upregulation of endogenous tissue plasminogen factor (tPA).[34,35] tPA overactivates NMDA-Rs via glutamate, exacerbates exitoxicity, and impairs NMDA-R-mediated vasodilation and autoregulation during hypotension via MAPK activation.[31,32] Post-TBI administration of an inactive tPA variant, tPA-S[481] competes with endogenous tPA for binding to NMDA-R at the receptor docking site. Animal studies into the mechanism behind glutamate/NMDA-R toxicity autoregulation after TBI found neuroprotective benefits of tPA-S[481] given 30 minutes after TBI were from protected cerebrohemodynamics, blocked upregulation of ERK MAPK and upregulated p38.[36,37]

Cerebral hypoxia is most acute in the first 24 to 48 hours after injury. Cerebral oxygenation improves through increasing the fraction of inspired oxygen (Fi_{O_2}) in mechanically ventilated patients to induce hyperoxia.[38] A study investigating effects of hyperventilation or hyperoxia on cerebral hemodynamics found that normobaric hyperoxia improved brain oxidative metabolism and decreased ICP.[39] However, early hyperoxia treatment is linked to worse outcomes after TBI, possibly because of hyperoxia-induced, oxygen-free radical toxicity.[40] A study to evaluate the effect of normobaric hyperoxia on CBF velocity and cerebral oxygenation in the presence of impaired autoregulation in operated patients with severe TBI found no change in middle cerebral artery blood flow or cerebral metabolic rate of oxygen (CMRO2) with increasing Fi_{O_2} on days 3 to 6 after TBI. There were no changes in ICP across various Fi_{O_2} levels in this study, possibly due to all patients having had a craniotomy with stabilized intracranial dynamics. Increased cerebral oxygen saturation was noted in the operated side with increasing Fi_{O_2} but not observed on the nonoperated side. In addition, increased cerebral oxygen saturation in response to hyperoxia was only observed in patients with impaired cerebral autoregulation. It is thought that intact autoregulation causes vasoconstriction in response to hyperoxia, whereas without autoregulation intact, hyperoxia elicits no change in vascular resistance.[38] A phase II clinical trial examined the effect of combined treatment using hyperbaric oxygen with normobaric hyperoxia and found increased P_{aO_2} and brain tissue oxygen tension, as well as improved markers of oxidative metabolism and 26% reduction in mortality ($P = 0.048$).[41]

CO$_2$ LEVELS

It has been well established that hypercapnia is detrimental in TBI patients due to associated cerebral vasodilation, which inevitably results in increased ICP, as well as the possibility of death due to cerebral herniation.[42] Hyperventilation is a widely used technique to reduce carbon dioxide levels, thereby mitigating dangerously elevated ICP levels. However, hypocapnia-induced cerebrovascular constriction may cause significant reduction in CBF and oxygenation, which can further damage injured brain tissue through cerebral ischemia.[43] Unfortunately, excessive hyperventilation of TBI patients continues, which results in poor outcomes in this patient population.[44] The optimal partial arterial pressure of carbon dioxide (PaCO$_2$) range for TBI patients remains unclear due to the high degree of heterogeneity in values that are used to define hyper- vs. hypocapnia. Although an ideal PaCO$_2$ target range of 35 to 45 mmHg has been suggested, published TBI guidelines based on an ongoing 9-year Excellence in Prehospital Injury Care (EPIC) study recommends avoiding hyperventilating patients unless they exhibit signs of cerebral herniation.[45]

AIRWAY

Preventing cerebral herniation through careful monitoring of ICP in TBI patients is of the utmost importance, but there is also a clear association between brain tissue hypoxia and poor outcomes in this patient population.[46] TBI, in isolation, is associated with significant neuroinflammation; however, a study conducted by Yan and colleagues revealed that the neuroinflammatory state is further exacerbated by hypoxia, which has been shown to enhance cerebral cytokine production and unfavorable outcomes in TBI patients[47] (Figure 35.1). The preliminary results of an ongoing Excellence in Prehospital Injury Care (EPIC) study recommends maintaining patient oxygen saturation levels above 90%, as lower oxygenation levels have been shown to significantly increase TBI-associated mortality.[48] An obvious way to prevent brain tissue hypoxia in TBI patients is through airway management. However, there is an ongoing debate on whether endotracheal intubation is superior to basic airway management based on widely varying study findings, with some even pointing to an increased mortality in TBI patients that underwent intubation.[49] At this point in time, TBI patient outcomes following intubation vary based on the severity of TBI and other factors, such as use of sedatives, but it mainly comes down to experience of individuals performing the intubation; basic airway care performed properly results in significantly more favorable patient outcomes than a botched intubation.[50,51]

FLUIDS

Appropriate fluid resuscitation avoiding hypovolemia is crucial to maximizing CPP in TBI patients. There is a clear consensus that TBI-associated disruption of BBB makes the brain highly sensitive to changes in osmolality, but there are no clear-cut recommendations about which intravenous resuscitation fluid is best.[52] There is agreement that hypotonic solutions must be avoided, as their administration can further exacerbate cerebral edema commonly seen in TBI patients. Instead, it is common to use hypertonic solutions; hyperosmolar agents, such as mannitol and even synthetic colloid, the latter of which is thought to restore proper plasma oncotic pressure, decrease cerebral edema through minimization of extravasation, while, at the same time, expanding intravascular volume with less fluid.[52,53] Additionally, there is an ever-growing interest in understanding how fluid resuscitative efforts can be used to mitigate the neuroinflammatory state associated with TBI. An exemplary study was conducted in TBI patients by Junger and colleagues who reported that administration of 7.5% hypertonic saline restored normal activation and inhibited abnormal delayed apoptosis of polymorphonuclear neutrophils, dysfunctions of which are thought to be TBI-contributing factors.[54]

SUMMARY OF PREVENTIVE MEASURES TO AVOID SECONDARY INJURIES

- Monitor ICP in TBI → Prevent cerebral herniation
- Good airway management → Prevent brain tissue hypoxia in TBI patients
- Preserving normothermia, maintaining diuresis, avoiding hyperglycemia → Prevent neurogenic pulmonary edema
- FFP → Prevent increase in lesion size
- Hyperventilation → Prevent cerebral herniation

- Appropriate fluid resuscitation → Prevent worsening CPP
- Using hypertonic solutions → Prevent exacerbation of cerebral edema

ADVANCES IN ANESTHESIA FOR TRAUMATIC SPINAL CORD INJURY

There is no accepted evidence dictating the use of a specific anesthetic agent or technique to improve neurologic outcomes for SCI patients, either in neurocritical care or perioperative care. The crucial purpose of anesthetic management must be to preserve the maintenance of sufficient spinal cord perfusion. The anesthesiologist or neurocritical care physician should be cognizant of hyper- and hypoventilation in order to maintain normocapnia for stabilizing spinal cord perfusion. Other common concerns for spinal cord injury in the perioperative or neurocritical care setting include thromboembolic complications and maintenance of mean arterial pressure target 85 to 90 mmHg via vasopressor or inotrope administration (level III evidence). Preserving normothermia, maintaining diuresis, avoiding hyperglycemia, preventing neurogenic pulmonary edema, and awareness of autonomic dysreflexia are also important in the acute care setting. During spinal cord surgery, prone positioning might lead to impaired cerebral autoregulation, particularly in hemodynamically compromised patients. It is better for anesthesiologists to monitor cerebral oxygenation during prolonged spine surgeries. Despite supporting studies for intraoperative neurophysiologic monitoring at the time of acute SCI surgery, this is not well established in guidelines, and more clinical trials are needed.[55–57] Similarly, monitoring and analysis of intraspinal pressure during acute SCI surgery might be novel in future trials because results from small groups of patients promote safety for measurement of subdural intraspinal pressure at the spinal cord injury site.[58]

Neuroinflammation after traumatic SCI aggravates neurologic impairment. Preventing secondary injury by targeting inflammatory cascades and excitotoxicity might be an appropriate target for anesthetic neuroprotection in future experimental studies. Previous in vitro research on anesthesia and SCI revealed that methoxyflurane and propofol robustly protect motor neurons against excitotoxicity.[59,60] The potential explanation behind this neuroprotective effect is propofol's inhibitory effect on neuronal firing of organotypic spinal slices and suppression of endogenous glutamate discharge. Administration of propofol with a GABA receptor antagonist reversed neuroprotective effects on spinal networks.[59,61] An in vitro study by Kaur and colleagues found that propofol has a neuroprotective effect against excitotoxicity on spinal neurons by provoking GABA responses.[62]

Intrathecal 10 microgram dexmedetomidine administration in rabbits without injured spinal cords did not reveal any neurologic injury of the spinal cords. However, in some animals, meningeal thickening and lymphoplasmocitary infiltration in the pia-mater and arachnoid were reported.[63] He and colleagues compared the anesthesia efficacy of propofol and dexmedetomidine in the SCI rat model and found dexmedetomidine anesthesia superior for shorter anesthesia onset time, postoperative analgesia, respiratory distress, and hypotension. Propofol has more potent effects on Th1 cytokine secretion and alleviating inflammatory factors.[64] Rong and colleagues applied intrathecal dexmedetomidine before SCI in rats and demonstrated α7nAChR overexpression and TLR4 inhibition during the acute phase of SCI with an improvement of locomotor deficit and decreased apoptosis after SCI.[65]

ADVANCES IN ANESTHETICS FOR TRAUMATIC BRAIN INJURY

Management of TBI patients can be facilitated by various intravenous anesthetics in combination during neurocritical care. An important management goal in TBI patients is to reduce agitation in order to control the mechanical ventilation and cerebral hemodynamics.[66]

Intravenous anesthetics, such as propofol, thiopental, and etomidate, diminish CBF and CMRO2. Ketamine is thought to lead to unmanageable ICP with increased CBF and CMRO2. Large-vessel vasodilation then occurs due to hypercarbia in nonventilated patients and nitric oxide synthase inhibition leads to vasoconstriction. To investigate this theory, a systemic literature review in 2014 established that ketamine does not induce an increase in ICP in severe TBI when patients are intubated and sedated. Furthermore, data from

clinical trials support the acute ICP reduction effects of ketamine in patients receiving other intravenous sedatives.[67]

Previous animal studies describe the neuroprotective effects of ketamine through reduction in glutamate excitotoxicity by inhibition of NMDA receptors, thereby alleviating some inflammatory cytokines after TBI.[68,69] Additionally, ketamine has a substantial impact on preserving suppression of spreading depolarizations in TBI patients.[70]

Sedation with intravenous anesthetics can lead to a decline in mean arterial pressure (MAP). These induce peripheral vasodilatation and reductions in both CBF and metabolic rate. These systemic consequences may lead to a significant drop in cerebral perfusion pressure and oxygen distribution to the injured brain after trauma.[71,72]

A 2011 meta-analysis examined 13 randomized, controlled clinical trials and provided no reasonable proof of one sedative agent being more effective than another at regulating ICP, CPP, neurologic outcomes, and mortality in patients with severe TBI. However, in three randomized, controlled trials, boluses or short infusions of opioids caused significant increases in ICP and decreases in MAP and CPP.[73] Propofol is an intravenous, short-acting anesthetic agent and is extensively used for sedation in TBI patients. It can decrease CBF, CMR, and ICP.[74] In a rat study, propofol reduced the effects of brain edema by inhibiting IL-1β- and TNF-α-induced aquaporin-4 receptor overexpression after TBI.[75] Propofol and midazolam are intravenous agents frequently used for sedation of severe TBI patients because of their short elimination half-lives along with similar effects on cerebral hemodynamics.[76]

The main mechanisms of inhalational anesthetics involve weakening synaptic transmission by inhibiting glutamatergic neuronal excitation and activating GABAergic neuronal inhibition.[77] Common inhalational anesthetics, including isoflurane, sevoflurane, and desflurane, reduce CMR but have cerebral vasodilatory effects, particularly at more than one minimum alveolar concentration (MAC); this causes increased ICP. Nitrous oxide has no place in anesthetic management of TBI because it increases CMRO2, cerebral vasodilation, and ICP.[78,79] Rodent studies demonstrated neuroprotective effects of isoflurane pre- or post-treatment by increasing neuronal survival and decreasing neurologic impairment, hippocampal damage, cerebral glucose use, and lipid peroxidation. These neuroprotective outcomes are typically evident around 1 MAC. Higher concentrations of isoflurane, such as 1.67 MAC, triggered neurodegeneration and similar to 1.8% concentration of isoflurane, raised glutamate levels in cerebrospinal fluid, EEG activity, as well as brain water content after TBI.[80,81] An in vivo study by Thal and colleagues described the effects of isoflurane and sevoflurane on BBB integrity following TBI. They found that 3.5% sevoflurane exposure generates more definitive ZO-1 expression after TBI than 1.5% isoflurane. Nevertheless, authors did not observe any effects of these anesthetics on BBB integrity in animals without TBI.

Significant evidence exists related to neuroprotective effects of isoflurane after TBI. However, more clinical trials are necessary in order to correlate and confirm the outcomes of animal studies. Additionally, there are not enough in vivo or in vitro studies regarding the efficacy of desflurane and sevoflurane in pre- or post-treatment of TBI.

CONCLUSION

Initial management decisions for TBI and SCI impact both short- and long-term outcomes. Understanding TBI in the presence of hemorrhagic shock affects treatment parameters and requires fluid resuscitation with the additional challenge of hemodynamic stability. In isolated TBI cases, advances in fluid resuscitation include the use of hypertonic saline, while positive effects using hypertonic saline as well as FFP were seen in polytrauma studies. Maintaining CO_2 levels is important to avoid increased ICP and associated sequelae, including cerebral herniation. Careful monitoring helps to protect the injured brain from additional insults, and continued investigation into preventing secondary injury after neurotrauma is the focus of many clinical trials and animal studies.

Specific goals in management of TBI and SCI vary, yet the ultimate goal is neuroprotection and hemodynamic stability to prevent secondary injury. SCI animal studies using dexmedetomidine show improved efficacy compared with propofol, but propofol elicited more protection against an inflammatory response. Recent studies on anesthesia and TBI used isoflurane and found it to have neuroprotective effects, including maintaining BBB integrity. Investigating methods to improve acute management of neurotrauma is the goal of ongoing research. Due to the complexity of neurotrauma patients in the ICU, it is no surprise that new drugs and treatment options are slow to be accepted as beneficial or proven efficacious in decreasing mortality. Continued efforts from both basic science and clinical studies will provide continued support for advancing treatment in anesthesia for neurotrauma.

REFERENCES

1. Ursino M, Lodi CA. A simple mathematical model of the interaction between intracranial pressure and cerebral hemodynamics. *J Appl Physiol.* 1997;82(4):1256-1269.
2. McKee AC, Daneshvar DH. The neuropathology of traumatic brain injury. *Handb Clin Neurol.* 2015;127:45-66.
3. Cunningham AS, Salvador R, Coles JP et al. Physiological thresholds for irreversible tissue damage in contusional regions following traumatic brain injury. *Brain.* 2005;128 (Pt 8):1931-1942.
4. Bonds BW, Yang S, Hu PF et al. Predicting secondary insults after severe traumatic brain injury. *J Trauma Acute Care Surg.* 2015;79 (1):85-90; discussion.
5. da Fonseca AC, Matias D, Garcia C et al. The impact of microglial activation on blood-brain barrier in brain diseases. *Front Cell Neurosci.* 2014;8:362.
6. Gondim FA, Lopes AC Jr, Oliveira GR et al. Cardiovascular control after spinal cord injury. *Curr Vasc Pharmacol.* 2004;2(1):71-79.
7. Galvagno SM Jr, Fox EE, Appana SN et al. Outcomes following concomitant traumatic brain injury and hemorrhagic shock: A secondary analysis from the PROPPR trial. *J Trauma Acute Care Surg.* 2017;83(4):668-674.
8. Brotfain E, Leibowitz A, Dar DE et al. Severe traumatic brain injury and controlled hemorrhage in rats: Quest for the optimal mean arterial blood pressure after whole fresh donor blood resuscitation. *Shock.* 2012;38 (6):630-634.
9. Dennis AM, Haselkorn ML, Vagni VA et al. Hemorrhagic shock after experimental

traumatic brain injury in mice: Effect on neuronal death. *J Neurotrauma*. 2009;26(6):889-899.

10. White NJ, Wang X, Bradbury N et al. Fluid resuscitation of uncontrolled hemorrhage using a hemoglobin-based oxygen carrier: Effect of traumatic brain injury. *Shock*. 2013;39(2):210-219.

11. Jin G, DeMoya MA, Duggan M et al. Traumatic brain injury and hemorrhagic shock: Evaluation of different resuscitation strategies in a large animal model of combined insults. *Shock*. 2012;38(1):49-56.

12. Gantner D, Moore EM, Cooper DJ. Intravenous fluids in traumatic brain injury: What's the solution? *Curr Opin Crit Care*. 2014;20(4):385-389.

13. Pinto FC, Oliveira MF, Prist R, Silva MR, Silva LF, Capone Neto A. Effect of volume replacement during combined experimental hemorrhagic shock and traumatic brain injury in prostanoids, brain pathology and pupil status. *Arq Neuropsiquiatr*. 2015;73(6):499-505.

14. Gong W, Marks JA, Sanati P et al. Hypertonic saline resuscitation of hemorrhagic shock does not decrease in vivo neutrophil interactions with endothelium in the blood-brain microcirculation. *J Trauma*. 2011;71(2):275-281; discussion 81-2.

15. Brackney CR, Diaz LA, Milbrandt EB, Al-Khafaji A, Darby JM. Is albumin use SAFE in patients with traumatic brain injury? *Crit Care*. 2010;14(2):307.

16. Shuja F, Shults C, Duggan M et al. Development and testing of freeze-dried plasma for the treatment of trauma-associated coagulopathy. *J Trauma*. 2008;65(5):975-985.

17. Kozar RA, Peng Z, Zhang R et al. Plasma restoration of endothelial glycocalyx in a rodent model of hemorrhagic shock. *Anesth Analg*. 2011;112(6):1289-1295.

18. Pati S, Matijevic N, Doursout MF et al. Protective effects of fresh frozen plasma on vascular endothelial permeability, coagulation, and resuscitation after hemorrhagic shock are time dependent and diminish between days 0 and 5 after thaw. *J Trauma*. 2010;69(Suppl 1):S55-S63.

19. Imam A, Jin G, Sillesen M et al. Fresh frozen plasma resuscitation provides neuroprotection compared to normal saline in a large animal model of traumatic brain injury and polytrauma. *J Neurotrauma*. 2015;32(5):307-313.

20. Georgoff PE, Nikolian VC, Halaweish I et al. Resuscitation with lyophilized plasma is safe and improves neurological recovery in a long-term survival model of swine subjected to traumatic brain injury, hemorrhagic shock, and polytrauma. *J Neurotrauma*. 2017;34(13):2167-2175.

21. Teranishi K, Scultetus A, Haque A et al. Traumatic brain injury and severe uncontrolled haemorrhage with short delay prehospital resuscitation in a swine model. *Injury*. 2012;43(5):585-593.

22. Clifton GL, Miller ER, Choi SC et al. Lack of effect of induction of hypothermia after acute brain injury. *N Engl J Med*. 2001;344(8):556-563.

23. Clifton GL, Miller ER, Choi SC, Levin HS. Fluid thresholds and outcome from severe brain injury. *Crit Care Med*. 2002;30(4):739-745.

24. Maekawa T, Yamashita S, Nagao S, Hayashi N, Ohashi Y; Brain-Hypothermia Study G. Prolonged mild therapeutic hypothermia versus fever control with tight hemodynamic monitoring and slow rewarming in patients with severe traumatic brain injury: A randomized controlled trial. *J Neurotrauma*. 2015;32(7):422-429.

25. Andrews PJ, Sinclair HL, Rodriguez A et al. Hypothermia for intracranial hypertension after traumatic brain injury. *N Engl J Med*. 2015;373(25):2403-2412.

26. Ostergaard L, Engedal TS, Aamand R et al. Capillary transit time heterogeneity and flow-metabolism coupling after traumatic brain injury. *J Cereb Blood Flow Metab*. 2014;34(10):1585-1598.

27. Bouma GJ, Muizelaar JP, Stringer WA, Choi SC, Fatouros P, Young HF. Ultra-early evaluation of regional cerebral blood flow in severely head-injured patients using xenon-enhanced computerized tomography. *J Neurosurg*. 1992;77(3):360-368.

28. Bragin DE, Kameneva MV, Bragina OA et al. Rheological effects of drag-reducing polymers improve cerebral blood flow and oxygenation after traumatic brain injury in rats.

J Cereb Blood Flow Metab. 2017;37(3):762-775.

29. Resnick N, Yahav H, Shay-Salit A et al. Fluid shear stress and the vascular endothelium: For better and for worse. *Prog Biophys Mol Biol.* 2003;81(3):177-199.

30. Miyamoto K, Ohtaki H, Dohi K et al. Edaravone increases regional cerebral blood flow after traumatic brain injury in mice. *Acta Neurochir Suppl.* 2013;118:103-109.

31. Armstead WM, Cines DB, Bdeir KH, Bdeir Y, Stein SC, Higazi AA. uPA modulates the age-dependent effect of brain injury on cerebral hemodynamics through LRP and ERK MAPK. *J Cereb Blood Flow Metab.* 2009;29(3):524-533.

32. Armstead WM, Kiessling JW, Riley J, Cines DB, Higazi AA. tPA contributes to impaired NMDA cerebrovasodilation after traumatic brain injury through activation of JNK MAPK. *Neurol Res.* 2011;33(7):726-733.

33. Armstead WM. Age dependent endothelin contribution to NOC/oFQ induced impairment of NMDA cerebrovasodilation after brain injury. *Peptides.* 2001;22(1):39-46.

34. Nicole O, Docagne F, Ali C et al. The proteolytic activity of tissue-plasminogen activator enhances NMDA receptor-mediated signaling. *Nat Med.* 2001;7(1):59-64.

35. Faraci FM, Heistad DD. Regulation of the cerebral circulation: Role of endothelium and potassium channels. *Physiol Rev.* 1998;78(1):53-97.

36. Armstead WM, Bohman LE, Riley J, Yarovoi S, Higazi AA, Cines DB. tPA-S(481)A prevents impairment of cerebrovascular autoregulation by endogenous tPA after traumatic brain injury by upregulating p38 MAPK and inhibiting ET-1. *J Neurotrauma.* 2013;30(22):1898-1907.

37. Armstead WM, Riley J, Yarovoi S, Cines DB, Smith DH, Higazi AA. tPA-S481A prevents neurotoxicity of endogenous tPA in traumatic brain injury. *J Neurotrauma.* 2012;29(9):1794-1802.

38. Sahoo S, Sheshadri V, Sriganesh K, Madhsudana Reddy KR, Radhakrishnan M, Umamaheswara Rao GS. Effect of hyperoxia on cerebral blood flow velocity and regional oxygen saturation in patients operated on for severe traumatic brain injury—The influence of cerebral blood flow autoregulation. *World Neurosurg.* 2017;98:211-216.

39. Rangel-Castilla L, Lara LR, Gopinath S, Swank PR, Valadka A, Robertson C. Cerebral hemodynamic effects of acute hyperoxia and hyperventilation after severe traumatic brain injury. *J Neurotrauma.* 2010;27(10):1853-1863.

40. Brenner M, Stein D, Hu P, Kufera J, Wooford M, Scalea T. Association between early hyperoxia and worse outcomes after traumatic brain injury. *Arch Surg.* 2012;147(11):1042-1046.

41. Rockswold SB, Rockswold GL, Zaun DA, Liu J. A prospective, randomized Phase II clinical trial to evaluate the effect of combined hyperbaric and normobaric hyperoxia on cerebral metabolism, intracranial pressure, oxygen toxicity, and clinical outcome in severe traumatic brain injury. *J Neurosurg.* 2013;118(6):1317-1328.

42. Moppett IK. Traumatic brain injury: Assessment, resuscitation and early management. *Br J Anaesth.* 2007;99(1):18-31.

43. Curley G, Kavanagh BP, Laffey JG. Hypocapnia and the injured brain: More harm than benefit. *Crit Care Med.* 2010;38(5):1348-1359.

44. Rognas L, Hansen TM, Kirkegaard H, Tonnesen E. Anaesthesiologist-provided prehospital airway management in patients with traumatic brain injury: An observational study. *Eur J Emerg Med.* 2014;21(6):418-423.

45. Roberts BW, Karagiannis P, Coletta M, Kilgannon JH, Chansky ME, Trzeciak S. Effects of PaCO2 derangements on clinical outcomes after cerebral injury: A systematic review. *Resuscitation.* 2015;91:32-41.

46. Chang JJ, Youn TS, Benson D et al. Physiologic and functional outcome correlates of brain tissue hypoxia in traumatic brain injury. *Crit Care Med.* 2009;37(1):283-290.

47. Yan EB, Satgunaseelan L, Paul E et al. Post-traumatic hypoxia is associated with prolonged cerebral cytokine production, higher serum biomarker levels, and poor outcome in patients with severe traumatic brain injury. *J Neurotrauma.* 2014;31(7):618-629.

48. Spaite DW, Hu C, Bobrow BJ et al. The effect of combined out-of-hospital hypotension

and hypoxia on mortality in major traumatic brain injury. *Ann Emerg Med.* 2017;69 (1):62-72.

49. Karamanos E, Talving P, Skiada D et al. Is prehospital endotracheal intubation associated with improved outcomes in isolated severe head injury? *A matched cohort analysis. Prehosp Disaster Med.* 2014;29(1): 32-36.

50. Bernard SA, Nguyen V, Cameron P et al. Prehospital rapid sequence intubation improves functional outcome for patients with severe traumatic brain injury: A randomized controlled trial. *Ann Surg.* 2010;252 (6):959-965.

51. Sobuwa S, Hartzenberg HB, Geduld H, Uys C. Outcomes following prehospital airway management in severe traumatic brain injury. *S Afr Med J.* 2013;103(9):644-646.

52. Ertmer C, Van Aken H. Fluid therapy in patients with brain injury: What does physiology tell us? *Crit Care.* 2014;18(2):119.

53. Stiver SI, Manley GT. Prehospital management of traumatic brain injury. *Neurosurg Focus.* 2008;25(4):E5.

54. Junger WG, Rhind SG, Rizoli SB et al. Prehospital hypertonic saline resuscitation attenuates the activation and promotes apoptosis of neutrophils in patients with severe traumatic brain injury. *Shock.* 2013;40 (5):366-374.

55. Bao FP, Zhang HG, Zhu SM. Anesthetic considerations for patients with acute cervical spinal cord injury. *Neural Regen Res.* 2017;12(3):499-504.

56. Rand A, Litz RJ, Zahn P. Anesthesiological approach for patients with spinal cord injuries. *Anaesthesist.* 2016;65(7):553-570.

57. Babakhani B, Heroabadi A, Hosseinitabatabaei N et al. Cerebral oxygenation under general anesthesia can be safely preserved in patients in prone position: A prospective observational study. *J Neurosurg Anesthesiol.* 2017;29 (3):291-297.

58. Werndle MC, Saadoun S, Phang I et al. Monitoring of spinal cord perfusion pressure in acute spinal cord injury: Initial findings of the injured spinal cord pressure evaluation study*. *Crit Care Med.* 2014;42(3):646-655.

59. Bajrektarevic D, Nistri A. Delayed application of the anesthetic propofol contrasts the neurotoxic effects of kainate on rat organotypic spinal slice cultures. *Neurotoxicology.* 2016;54:1-10.

60. Shabbir A, Bianchetti E, Nistri A. The volatile anesthetic methoxyflurane protects motoneurons against excitotoxicity in an in vitro model of rat spinal cord injury. *Neuroscience.* 2015;285:269-280.

61. Grasshoff C, Antkowiak B. Propofol and sevoflurane depress spinal neurons in vitro via different molecular targets. *Anesthesiology.* 2004;101(5):1167-1176.

62. Kaur J, Flores Gutierrez J, Nistri A. Neuroprotective effect of propofol against excitotoxic injury to locomotor networks of the rat spinal cord in vitro. *Eur J Neurosci.* 2016;44(7):2418-2430.

63. de Pereira Cardoso HD, Fim NC, Marques MA et al. Clinical and histological effects of the intrathecal administration of a single dose of dexmedetomidine in rabbits. *Pain Physician.* 2016;19(2):E319-E327.

64. He FY, Feng WZ, Zhong J, Xu W, Shao HY, Zhang YR. Effects of propofol and dexmedetomidine anesthesia on Th1/Th2 of rat spinal cord injury. *Eur Rev Med Pharmacol Sci.* 2017;21(6):1355-1361.

65. Rong H, Zhao Z, Feng J et al. The effects of dexmedetomidine pretreatment on the pro- and anti-inflammation systems after spinal cord injury in rats. *Brain Behav Immun.* 2017;64:195-207.

66. Chang LC, Raty SR, Ortiz J, Bailard NS, Mathew SJ. The emerging use of ketamine for anesthesia and sedation in traumatic brain injuries. *CNS Neurosci Ther.* 2013;19 (6):390-395.

67. Zeiler FA, Teitelbaum J, West M, Gillman LM. The ketamine effect on ICP in traumatic brain injury. *Neurocrit Care.* 2014;21(1):163-173.

68. Woiciechowsky C, Schoning B, Cobanov J, Lanksch WR, Volk HD, Docke WD. Early IL-6 plasma concentrations correlate with severity of brain injury and pneumonia in brain-injured patients. *J Trauma.* 2002;52(2):339-345.

69. O'Shaughnessy CT, Lodge D. N-methyl-D-aspartate receptor-mediated increase in intracellular calcium is reduced by ketamine and phencyclidine. *Eur J Pharmacol.* 1988;153(2-3):201-209.

70. Hertle DN, Dreier JP, Woitzik J et al. Effect of analgesics and sedatives on the occurrence of spreading depolarizations accompanying acute brain injury. *Brain.* 2012;135 (Pt 8):2390-2398.

71. Van Hemelrijck J, Fitch W, Mattheussen M, Van Aken H, Plets C, Lauwers T. Effect of propofol on cerebral circulation and autoregulation in the baboon. *Anesth Analg.* 1990;71(1):49-54.

72. Stephan H, Sonntag H, Schenk HD, Kohlhausen S. Effect of Disoprivan (propofol) on the circulation and oxygen consumption of the brain and CO_2 reactivity of brain vessels in the human. *Anaesthesist.* 1987;36 (2):60-65.

73. Roberts DJ, Hall RI, Kramer AH, Robertson HL, Gallagher CN, Zygun DA. Sedation for critically ill adults with severe traumatic brain injury: a systematic review of randomized controlled trials. *Crit Care Med.* 2011;39 (12):2743-2751.

74. Hutchens MP, Memtsoudis S, Sadovnikoff N. Propofol for sedation in neuro-intensive care. *Neurocrit Care.* 2006;4(1):54-62.

75. Ding Z, Zhang J, Xu J, Sheng G, Huang G. Propofol administration modulates AQP-4 expression and brain edema after traumatic brain injury. *Cell Biochem Biophys.* 2013;67 (2):615-622.

76. Oddo M, Crippa IA, Mehta S et al. Optimizing sedation in patients with acute brain injury. *Crit Care.* 2016;20(1):128.

77. Belelli D, Pistis M, Peters JA, Lambert JJ. General anaesthetic action at transmitter-gated inhibitory amino acid receptors. *Trends Pharmacol Sci.* 1999;20(12):496-502.

78. Bhattacharya B, Maung AA. Anesthesia for patients with traumatic brain injuries. *Anesthesiol Clin.* 2016;34(4):747-759.

79. Sharma D, Vavilala MS. Perioperative management of adult traumatic brain injury. *Anesthesiol Clin.* 2012;30(2):333-346.

80. Tawfeeq NA, Halawani MM, Al-Faridi K, Aal-Shaya WA, Taha WS. Traumatic brain injury: Neuroprotective anaesthetic techniques, an update. *Injury.* 2009;40(Suppl 4):S75-S81.

81. Stover JF, Sakowitz OW, Kroppenstedt SN et al. Differential effects of prolonged isoflurane anesthesia on plasma, extracellular, and CSF glutamate, neuronal activity, 125I-Mk801 NMDA receptor binding, and brain edema in traumatic brain-injured rats. *Acta Neurochir (Wien).* 2004;146(8):819-830.

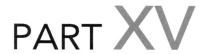

PART XV

Clinical procedures

36

Fiber-optic intubation

PRASANNA UDUPI BIDKAR AND K. NARMADHALAKSHMI

INTRODUCTION

The flexible fiber-optic endoscope was first used to perform intubation by Murphy in 1967.[1] It consists of a flexible fiber-optic bundle that works by total internal reflection (light can be totally reflected internally by the fiber-optic strand). The use of flexible fiberscopes has revolutionized the management of challenging airway cases. The flexible fiber-optic endoscope is considered the gold standard in challenging airway management. Additionally, it is included in the American Society of Anesthesiologists Difficult Airway Algorithm.[2]

COMPONENTS

Various brands of fiber-optic endoscopes are available in assorted sizes that are suitable for adults and children.

The three main components of a fiber-optic endoscope are (Figures 36.1 and 36.2):

- Control unit
- Light source
- Flexible insertion cord

- The *control unit (handle)* is composed of four essential parts:
  - A control knob, or lever, for maneuvering the distal tip, whose deflection range from 60° to 180° in the vertical plane. The entire instrument can be rotated to attain the full range of motion. The tip can be fixed at a desired angle of deflection in many fiberscopes.
  - An *eyepiece* to view the images directly or a camera can be added for viewing from a distance. A monitor screen may be attached to replace the eyepiece to visualize the projected images.

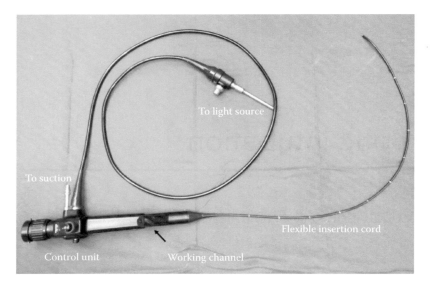

Figure 36.1 **Parts of the flexible fiber-optic bronchoscope.**

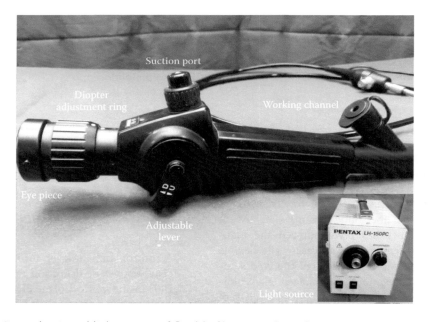

Figure 36.2 Control unit and light source of flexible fiber-optic bronchoscope.

- A *diopter adjustment ring* for focusing the image.
- A *working channel*, which allows suctioning of pooling of secretions that obscure the visualization of the airway. Additionally, this channel can also be used for insufflation of

oxygen to manage hypoxia and for administering local anesthetic agents to anesthetize the airway. Fiber-optic scopes may have either one or two ports with one working channel. When there are two ports with one working channel, both oxygen tubing and suction tubing can be connected to appropriate ports.

- A *light source* can be from an external remote source or from the one attached to the handle itself. The light source attached to the handle may be useful but the one from an external source may provide better lighting to be able to visualize more clearly.
- The *flexible insertion cord (scope)* is the one that is inserted into the patient. It consists of bundles of "coherently" arranged 10,000 to 15,000 fiber-optic glass fibers.[3] The fibers are approximately 5 to 20 microns in diameter, and they are optically insulated with a thin layer of glass. In addition to being flexible, each fiber is capable of transmitting light, thereby transmitting a clearer image. In addition to bundles, some fiberscopes possess a working channel. The entire cord is primarily protected by a wire mesh and vinyl covering. These cords vary in length and diameter and the appropriate size can be chosen for people of different ages and sizes. The diameter of cord helps to choose the tracheal tube that can be loaded over the cord. The connection between the handle and the insertion cord is usually tapered to hold a tracheal tube. There are markings on the external surface of the scope that indicate the depth of insertion. The insertion depth may vary for various purposes—oral intubation, nasal intubation, double lumen tube insertion, bronchoscopy, and adult and pediatric intubation.

INDICATIONS OF FLEXIBLE FIBER-OPTIC ENDOSCOPE

- Diagnosis
  - Diagnose diseases of the tracheobronchial tree (eg, trauma, tumor, foreign body, inhalational injury)
  - Obtain lung samples (eg, airway biopsies, bronchial washings, bronchoalveolar lavage [BAL] specimens)
- Therapies and procedures
  - Difficult intubation (eg, awake fiber-optic intubation)
  - To perform oral or nasal tracheal intubation in difficult airways (eg, small mouth opening, restricted neck mobility)
  - To perform intubation in positions other than supine (eg, sitting, semirecumbent)

- To remove foreign bodies, secretions, or blood and perform tracheobronchial toilet in case of secretions
- To guide placement and confirm the position of a percutaneous tracheostomy, double-lumen tube, bronchial blockers, and endobronchial valves
- Treatment of specific disorders (eg, control bleeding from focal lesions)

PREPARATION

The intubation using fiber-optic endoscope (FOB) calls for adequate planning and patient preparation. An experienced assistant will be required throughout the procedure to help monitor the patient's vital signs and assist the procedure. Fiberscope should be checked for adequate lighting, brightness, and clarity of the image.

- *Prevent fogging of thelens*: The tip of the insertion cord should be kept dipped in a warm water (not saline) or antifogging solution to prevent fogging of the lens when introduced into the arm milieu of the airway. A convective warming device that blows air over the tip may be used alternatively.
- *Focus adjustment*: The focus ought to be adjusted using a diopter adjustment ring by viewing the threads of gauze piece or small printed letters at 2 to 3 cm.
- *Lubrication of cord*: A water soluble lubricant should be applied over the insertion portion of the cord and care should be taken to avoid contact with the lens.
- *Oxygen/suction port*: oxygen from a central line or cylinder should be checked and attached to the port of the working channel. A suction apparatus should be checked and kept ready with tubing to attach to the port and clear secretions if required. If there are two ports with one working channel, both oxygen and suction tubing should be connected to each port and the control lever that separates the ports should be checked.
- *Tracheal tube*: It is essential to use a tracheal tube of appropriate size and type while using FOB. The internal diameter of the endotracheal tube should be 1 mm wider than the outer diameter of the insertion cord. The standard endotracheal

tube can be prewarmed to facilitate the easy passage of the tube over the cord. A spiral embedded tube or a tube with a hooded tip (eg, Parker Flex-Tip Tube) may pass more easily than a standard endotracheal tube. When the concentric gap is reduced between the scope and tracheal tube, it reduces the risk of the tube clutching the laryngeal cartilages while passing the tube into the laryngeal inlet. The tracheal tube should be threaded over the insertion cord and anchored firmly to the tapered portion, ie, the junction of the insertion cord and the handle.

- *Other essentials*: Anesthesia workstation check, monitors for vitals, the surgical face mask of appropriate size or endoscopic face mask, bite block, oral and nasopharyngeal airways, and supraglottic airway devices in the case of an emergency.

PATIENT PREPARATION

- Patient preparation is equally important as preparing the fiber-optic endoscope. Patient preparation increases the chance of success and decreases the time taken for the procedure. An explanation in detail (airway blocks, reasons for awake fiber-optic intubation, and potential complications) and ensuring that adequate sedation will be given to the patients to stay comfortable during the procedure increases patient cooperation. This discussion should ideally be done during the preop assessment period.
- *Premedication*—Sedation, antisialagogues
  - *Sedation*: Sedation of the patient before the procedure minimizes anxiety and is advantageous for anesthetizing the airway as well as the intubation. It is important to remember that sedation is advised till the patient is breathing spontaneously, is amnestic, communicative, and cooperative. This level of sedation is usually achieved using midazolam 1 to 3 mg IV in a normal adult. Short-acting opioids can be used for prevention of cough during the procedure. The sedatives and opioids should be given in a titrated manner with constant monitoring of the patient's consciousness and breathing pattern. Sedatives are contraindicated in an obstructed airway.
  - *Antisialagogues*: Antisialagogues, such as glycopyrrolate, atropine, and scopolamine, decrease the secretions, thereby facilitating clear visual passage for fiber-optic insertion. In addition, these agents allow local anesthetic drugs to act more effectively on the airway mucosa. Eight to 10 µg/kg of intramuscular glycopyrrolate administered 1 hour before the procedure is more effective than intravenous glycopyrrolate administered in the operating room. Atropine and scopolamine are rarely used as it may produce more cardiovascular and central nervous system (CNS) effects compared with glycopyrrolate.

AIRWAY ANESTHESIA

Anesthesia to the airway is accomplished by topical anesthetics and airway blocks. Anesthesia of the airway greatly reduces the dose of sedatives needed to perform intubation. It significantly boosts comfortability to the patient, thereby augmenting the success rate of intubation. The airway regions of interest for intubation include nasal and oral cavities, the pharynx (nasopharynx, oropharynx, and hypopharynx), larynx, and trachea.

Caution should be exercised with the total dose of the local anesthetic agent used when administering more than a few airway blocks. Anesthesia to the airway is not advised in patients with airway obstruction or at risk for aspiration.

Topical anesthesia

Topical anesthesia is administered either by spraying techniques or by direct application of the drug onto the target mucosa.

Spraying

Spraying local anesthetic drugs for topical anesthesia can be achieved by using atomizers, nebulizers, or commercially available spray cans.

Atomizers

Atomizers tend to convert the liquid anesthetic agent into fine spray particles, which are directed onto the mucosa of the patient by an operator.

The standard atomizer is used to construct a lignocaine atomizer. The rubber bulb in the standard atomizer is removed and replaced by connecting oxygen at a flow rate of 8 to 10 liters per minute from auxiliary oxygen outlet. This atomizer can often be used to deliver the drug to an oral, pharyngeal, and laryngeal mucosal surface. The delivery of the drug can be enhanced by asking the patient to breathe in and out heavily with an open mouth. However, it is difficult for the spray to reach the lower trachea.

Commercially, atomizer-like devices (eg, mucosal atomization device) with specially designed spray nozzles are available to spray directly over the posterior oropharyngeal cavity.

Nebulizers

Nebulizers are used to convert the local anesthetic agent to fine, cloud-like particles, which are inhaled by the patient, thereby delivering topical anesthesia to respiratory mucosa. 4 mL of 4% lignocaine can be used in a nebulizer device to anesthetize nasopharyngeal and laryngeal mucosa. Nebulization can either be done with a face mask or mouthpiece nebulizer. A face mask nebulizer allows anesthetizing both oropharyngeal and nasal mucosa, so the face mask nebulizer can be used for both oral and nasal intubation.

DIRECT APPLICATION

Topical anesthesia of airway mucosa may be accomplished by the direct application of local anesthetics using drug-soaked cotton swabs, gargling, or indirect laryngoscopy.

Relevant anatomy: Sensory innervation of the nasal cavity arises from the branches of the trigeminal nerve[4] via the sphenopalatine ganglion, which is situated in the pterygoid fossa lateral to the sphenopalatine foramen at the level of the crest of the superior turbinate. Sphenopalatine ganglion also supplies sensory fibers to the portion of the pharynx, uvula, and tonsils.

Cotton-tipped swabs or thinly rolled gauze pieces (7–9 cms in length) are soaked in 3 mL of 4% lidocaine with 5% w/v of phenylephrine (vasoconstrictor) mixture. The use of vasoconstrictor shrinks the blood vessels in the nasal cavity and enhances the cavity space. The drug-soaked swabs are placed postero-superiorly in the nasopharynx to block the branches of the trigeminal nerves.[5] The swabs are left in place for 2 to 3 minutes before removal. Caution is advised in a few cases of hypertensive patients as the use of phenylephrine may lead to an uncontrolled increase in blood pressure and produce a severe headache or related symptoms.

Nasopharyngeal airway coated with phenylephrine and viscous lidocaine can also be used to anesthetize the nasal passage. Nasal intubation with an appropriately larger-size tube can be facilitated or ensured further by inserting progressively larger airways that are coated with the mixture. This method rarely causes discomfort to the patient except for the first insertion, which may be slightly difficult.

Gargling with 5 to 7 mL of 2% to 4% lidocaine solution can be used to anesthetize oropharyngeal mucosa. But this method may not be enough to anesthetize laryngotracheal mucosa.[6] To minimize excess local anesthetic absorption, the patient is asked to expectorate the gargled solution.

Indirect laryngoscopy

With this method, the patient is made to sit with his or her mouth wide open. The oropharyngeal mucosa is made numb by spraying or gargling of lidocaine. A headlight or torch is used to see the posterior pharynx. The patient is asked to put out his tongue and retract it with a gauze piece. An indirect laryngeal mirror is positioned near the posterior pharynx to see the glottis and upper tracheal rings. Small aliquots of lignocaine are sprayed using a curved needle under indirect visualization in the mirror. This method is widely used in bronchoscopy suites.[7] The disadvantage is that this method may not cover lower tracheal rings adequately.

SAYGO TECHNIQUE

Once the oropharyngeal mucosa is anesthetized by any of the above techniques, the fiber-optic bronchoscope itself can be used to anesthetize the rest of the airway mucosa.[8] The anesthetic agent is sprayed through the working channel of the fiber-optic scope as you go further; that's why the technique is called "SAYGO" (Spray As You GO).

Spraying can be accomplished by using 1 mL of 2% lignocaine taken in a 10 mL syringe, whose piston is pulled up to the 10 mL mark to fill the rest of the syringe with air. The syringe is then attached to the working channel of the fiberscope. When the tip of the scope reaches the hypopharynx, the piston is pushed forward to inject the drug followed by air. The air is pushed to ensure that the drug is completely expelled from the working channel. After a few seconds, the fiberscope is passed through the glottis and the spraying is repeated with pauses to proceed further into the trachea.

It is essential to make sure that the suction is cut off while spraying the local anesthetic drug. Having an assistant to help with spraying and managing the suction will greatly benefit the operator.

NERVE BLOCKS

Glossopharyngeal nerve block

The glossopharyngeal nerve supplies certain areas of interest to anesthesiologists. The mucosa of the pharynx, palatine tonsil, soft palate, and posterior part of the tongue are supplied by the branches of the glossopharyngeal nerve. When the fiber-optic scope is passed through the pharynx, the gag reflex will be elicited as the scope presses the posterior part of the tongue. The glossopharyngeal nerve block will eliminate the gag reflex and allow smooth passage of the scope. This is particularly useful in spontaneously breathing awake patient with tracheal tube in situ.

LOCAL ANESTHETIC AGENT:
LIDOCAINE (0.5%)

Relevant anatomy: The distal branches of the glossopharyngeal nerve supplying the palatine tonsil and the posterior part of the tongue are lying submucosally, posterior to the palatine tonsil deep to the palatopharyngeal fold (posterior tonsillar pillar).

Gag reflex: The afferent sensory-glossopharyngeal nerve,[9] efferent motor-vagus nerve. The gag reflex is prevented by the bilateral glossopharyngeal nerve block.

The glossopharyngeal nerve can be blocked in two ways.[10]

1. *Intraoral Approach*
   The patient is made to sit and asked to open his or her mouth widely. The topical anesthesia of the tongue may allow the anesthesiologist to easily depress the tongue and facilitate needle placement. Posterior tonsillar pillar is seen clearly because the tongue is depressed with the help of a tongue depressor. A long, 8 to 10 cm, 22-gauge needle (spinal needle can be used) with the bent distal portion is inserted submucosally into the deep portion of the posterior tonsillar pillar. Five milliliters of local anesthetic are injected after careful aspiration to rule out a blood vessel. The procedure is then repeated on the other side.

   Caution: Internal carotid artery lies close to the glossopharyngeal nerve branches.

2. *Extra-oral/Peristyloid Approach*:
   This block is more comfortable for patients who will not be able to open their mouths. The patient is made to lie supine with his or her head in a neutral position. A line is drawn connecting the tip of the mastoid process and the angle of the mandible. A short, 22-gauge needle is inserted perpendicular to the midpoint of the line drawn until it hits the styloid bone underneath. Once the styloid bone is hit, the needle is withdrawn and directed posterior to the styloid bone. The needle is fixed in this position, aspirated to check any blood, and 5 to 7 mL of lignocaine is injected. The block is then repeated on the other side to achieve the bilateral glossopharyngeal block.

   Caution: Both the internal jugular vein and the internal carotid artery lies close to the glossopharyngeal nerve.

Superior laryngeal nerve block

The superior laryngeal nerve (SLN) is a branch of the vagus nerve that divides into an external and internal laryngeal nerve. The external laryngeal nerve supplies the cricothyroid whereas the internal laryngeal branch supplies the larynx from the epiglottis to the vocal cords. Thus, a superior laryngeal nerve block refers particularly to blocking the internal laryngeal nerve, which is particularly useful to patients requiring tracheal intubation before anesthetic induction.

LOCAL ANESTHETIC AGENT:
LIDOCAINE (0.5%)

Relevant anatomy. The internal laryngeal nerve is a branch of the superior laryngeal nerve that innervates airway mucosa after entering the thyrohyoid membrane just inferior to the caudal aspect of the hyoid bone between the greater and the lesser cornua of the hyoid.[11] The internal branch is blocked where it enters the thyrohyoid membrane.

Glottic closure reflex (laryngospasm): The afferent sensory-superior laryngeal nerve, efferent motor-superior laryngeal nerve, and recurrent laryngeal nerve. The superior laryngeal nerve block would relieve laryngospasm.

PROCEDURE: (FIGURE 36.3)

The patient is made to lie in a supine position with his or her neck extended. The anesthesiologist stands on the ipsilateral side of the neck to administer the SLN block. Holding the needle in the dominant hand, the anesthesiologist should feel the hyoid bone and displace it firmly toward the ipsilateral side with the nondominant hand. The displacement of hyoid produces a prominence on the ipsilateral side to guide needle insertion. The short, 22 gauge needle is inserted to hit the greater cornua of the hyoid bone, which is then walked off the caudal edge of the hyoid and advanced 2 to 3 mm. The needle tip is now resting between the thyrohyoid membrane laterally and the laryngeal mucosa medially. The needle is then checked for negative aspiration of blood before injecting 2 to 3 mL of the local anesthetic agent. An additional 1 mL is injected while the needle is withdrawn.

Caution: The needle tip is close to the laryngeal mucosa, superior laryngeal artery, and vein.

Translaryngeal block

The translaryngeal block blocks the vagal branches, providing topical anesthesia to the entire mucosal surface of the laryngotracheal airway.[12] This block is particularly useful in spontaneously breathing, awake tracheal intubation cases.

Three 3 to 4 mL of 4% lidocaine (Figure 36.4).

Relevant anatomy: The vagal nerve branch, internal laryngeal nerve innervates mucosa of the larynx from the epiglottis to the level of the vocal cords, and a recurrent laryngeal nerve innervates the distal airway mucosa.

Cough reflex: Cough receptors present in the larynx and trachea receive both afferent and efferent fibers from the vagus nerve. Cough refllex can be eliminated by the translaryngeal block.

Procedure: The patient is made to lie in a supine position with his or her neck extended adequately. The anesthesiologist should stand beside the patient to palpate the cricothyroid membrane. A 22-gauge needle or a 20 G intravenous cannula should be inserted in the midline in the caudal direction until there is no more resistance. The needle should be checked in this position for free aspiration of air. The stylet should be removed when an intravenous

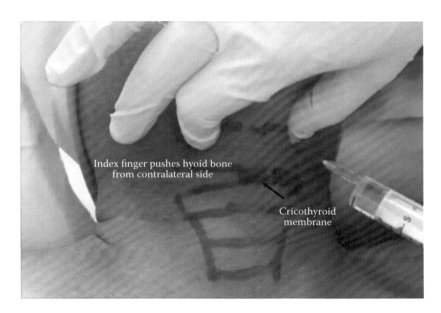

Figure 36.3 Superior laryngeal nerve block.

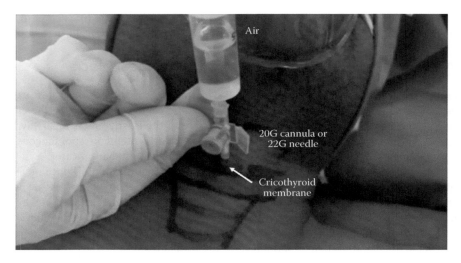

Figure 36.4 Translaryngeal block nerve field block.

cannula is used. The patient is then asked to hold his or her breath in full inspiration and 3 to 4 mL of lignocaine are injected rapidly. The injection of lignocaine through the translaryngeal space into the trachea will stimulate bouts of cough, which spread the local anesthetic to more superior laryngeal structures and to the inferior surface of the vocal cords. A cough can break the needle and lead to trauma, so the needle should be removed soon after the injection is administered. When used, the IV cannula is left in place to avoid risk of subcutaneous emphysema (through the puncture site) due to coughing.

Caution: The needle may injure vascular structures if it is inserted or deviated far off from the midline. Coughing is undesirable in few patients (eg, raised ICP). Be cautious while giving this block to patients with substantial risk of aspirating gastric contents.

THE TECHNIQUE OF FIBER-OPTIC INTUBATION

Fiber-optic intubation can be done in both awake as well as anesthetized individuals. The patient is made to lie in a supine position with his or her neck extended. The anesthesiologist stands at the head of the patient. The patient's table height is adjusted according to the requirement of the anesthesiologist. It is best to lower down the table completely in most cases.

Generally, the dominant hand of the anesthesiologist holds the proximal handle of the scope with the index finger controlling oxygen/suction port and thumb maneuvering the control knob. The distal insertion cord (scope) is held in the nondominant hand to guide the advancement. The fiber-optic endoscope is checked for orientation, tip deflection, and adjusted for white balance.

The endotracheal tube of the appropriate size is chosen, the lumen is lubricated, and its connector is removed. The endotracheal tube is then railroaded over the scope and fixed proximally to the tapered end of the handle. The choice of oral or nasal fiber-optic intubation is chosen based on the indication and expertise of the physician (Figures 36.5 and 36.6).

From here, there are certain differences between intubation of awake and anesthetized patients to be taken care of. In **an awake intubation**, the patient is asked to open his or her mouth and stick out his or her tongue or it can be held with gauze by an assistant. Asking the patient to say "eeh" opens the pharynx and brings the epiglottis into view, whereas deep inspiration opens up the glottis for scope passage.

On the other hand, in **an anesthetized patient**, loss of tone of pharyngeal muscles may obstruct the visualization and insertion of the scope via the oropharynx. This scenario calls for additional assistance to elevate the jaw and retract the tongue to facilitate the scope insertion. The tongue retractor and laryngoscope blades can be used to retract the tongue. Alternatively, specially designed airway, such as the Bermann and the Patil-Syracuse, can be used to guide the midline insertion of the scope into the oropharyngeal space. The optimal size of the

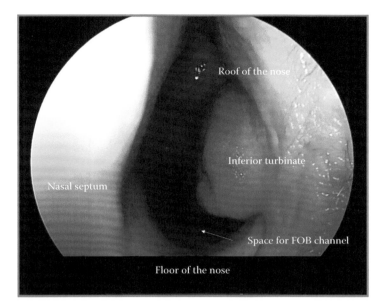

Figure 36.5 Anatomic landmarks for FOB during nasal intubation.

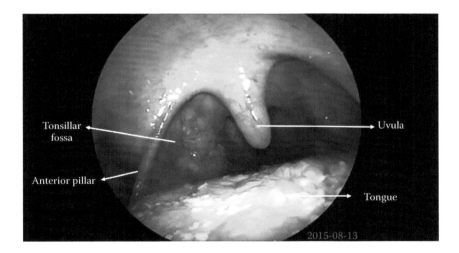

Figure 36.6 Structures seen during oral FOB.

airway should be chosen because the larger size may push the tongue backward and cause an obstruction. Occasionally, the tracheal tube is advanced into the pharynx, which can guide the endoscope tip close to the laryngeal entrance.

During insertion of the scope, the air cavity (the dark space) should constantly be kept in the center of the visual field. The image may get blurred due to secretions or blood in the passage, which can be cleared by irrigating saline and intermittent suction. If the suction is not clearing the blurred image, the lens may need to be cleaned, which can be done by advancing the scope and touching the adjacent tissue. The image may pink out as the lens touches tissue; a withdrawing of scope a little (1–2 cm) will bring an unclouded vision. Occasionally, the entire fiberscope needs to be taken out to clean the lens using warm water. Oxygenation is maintained by insufflating oxygen or by jet ventilation via a working channel.[13]

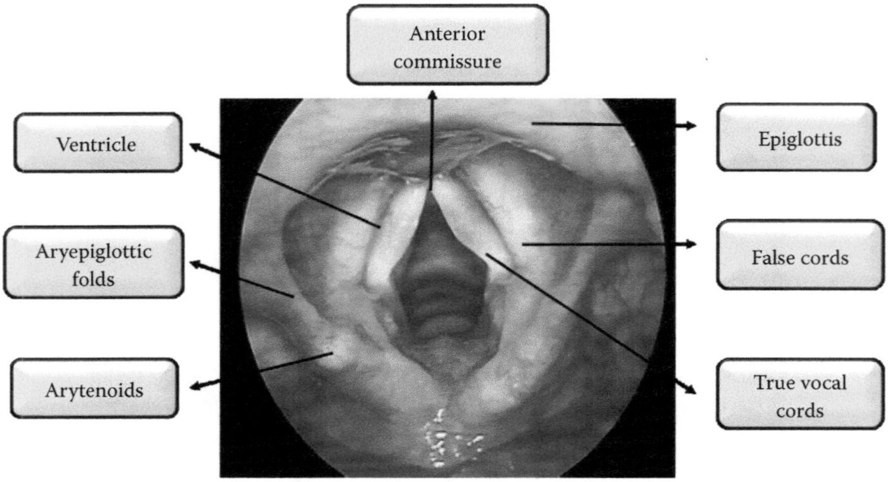

Figure 36.7 Laryngeal inlet view during fiber-optic intubation.

The landmarks for tracheal intubation are the epiglottis, glottis, tracheal rings, and carina (Figure 36.7). When the tip of the scope is just above the carina, the scope is held firmly at that position. Look at the depth mark at the level of the incisors. Ask the assistant to release the endotracheal tube and pass it over the scope. The tube is gently advanced under vision via naso/oropharynx, pharynx, and larynx. Confirm the tip of the endotracheal tube in relation to the carina and withdraw the scope. The tip of the scope should be neutral while advancing the tracheal tube and withdrawing the endoscope.

Intubation using a double-lumen tube is the same as normal endotracheal intubation except for the fact that the tip of the scope is passed until the appropriate side bronchus. The double lumen tube is then threaded over the scope into the bronchus (Table 36.1).

DISADVANTAGES

- The fiberscope is expensive and fragile; a minor blow or forceful bending can damage the glass fibers and produce irreversible damage to the insertion cord
- The procedure is time-consuming, so it is often not considered in emergency airway management (Can't Intubate Can't Oxygenate [CICO]), rapid-sequence intubation
- It requires adequate skill and experience to increase the success rate of intubation

- The flexible scope cannot be used for manipulating airway structures (eg, tongue, epiglottis), which mandate other airway accessories (tongue retractor, laryngoscope blade)
- A successful visualization of the carina is not always followed by successful intubation due to difficulties in passing the tracheal tube beyond the epiglottis, arytenoid cartilage, or pyriform fossae
- The vision may be obscured by haziness in the presence of blood and/or other secretions
- It is difficult to clean

ADVANTAGES

- A flexible fiber-optic endoscopy is a very reliable approach to difficult airway management[14] (small mouth opening, unstable cervical spine)
- It can be used for intubation of both the tracheal tube and double lumen tube
- The position of the tip of the tracheal or double lumen tube after intubation can be confirmed using a fiberscope
- Both oral and nasal intubation is possible with the fiber-optic endoscope. It allows for evaluating the airway for tumor, infections, foreign body, and tracheobronchial toilet[15]
- Patients who cannot lie in the supine position can be intubated in a sitting or semi-recumbent position using the fiber-optic scope
- In failed intubation attempts, where LMA is used to rescue the airway, subsequent intubation with

Table 36.1 Differences between oral and nasal intubation

Oral intubation	Nasal intubation
1 Oral intubation is relatively difficult as the tip of the scope has to enter the glottis at an acute angle.	Nasal intubation is comparatively easier as the tip of the scope enters the glottis at an obtuse angle.
2 May need oral airway intubators, such as the Bermann (Smiths Medical International, Watford, UK) or Patil-Syracuse airways (Anesthesia Associates, Inc., California, USA) to insert the scope in midline and to prevent the scope from getting damaged by teeth bites.	The nasopharyngeal anatomy naturally directs the tube in the midline into the trachea. The nasopharyngeal airway may be used for lubricating and dilating the nasal passage.
3 Local anesthetic sprays, atomizers, nebulizers, gargling, and lozenges are available to anesthetize the oral cavity and oropharynx.	Local anesthetic sprays, nebulizers, cotton-tipped swabs, and the nasopharyngeal airway, which is coated with viscous lignocaine, are available to anesthetize the nasal cavity and nasopharynx.
3 The scope is advanced through the oral cavity under direct vision, curving downward at the posterior pharyngeal wall, toward the epiglottis. The tip is further deflected downward as it passes beneath the epiglottis and is then turned upward to pass between the vocal cords and advanced a little to visualize the carina. For bronchial intubation, the tip is advanced into the desired mainstem bronchus. It is important that the tip is kept in the midline as it is advanced.	It is associated with less cervical spine motion. The fiber-optic scope is advanced through the nostril, into the lower nasal meatus (inferior, largest). Identify the nasal septum, the floor of the nose, and the superior turbinate. The scope is passed beyond the nasal septum to enter the nasopharynx. Steer the fiberscope into the oropharynx, before which you may need to gently part the soft palate from the posterior pharyngeal wall. The tip is advanced further between the vocal cords.
4 With the fiberscope tip in place, the lubricated tube is advanced over the scope, which functions as a stylet. The bevel should face posteriorly. The fiberscope should be used to verify that the tube tip is correctly positioned and then withdrawn, leaving the tube in place.	The fiberscope should be advanced through the tracheal tube before insertion because it may not be possible to insert a tube loaded over a fiberscope through a narrowed nasal passage after the fiberscope is successfully inserted into the trachea.

the fiber-optic scope is possible through the LMA left in place
- Oxygenation is possible during the endoscopy and intubation

COMPLICATIONS

- Sedation in excess may cause the patient to lose consciousness, stop breathing, and lead to airway obstruction
- Local anesthetic toxicity can occur due to overdose following airway anesthesia

- Bronchospasm, especially in hyperreactive airway patients
- Vessel and nerve injury during airway blocks
- Injury to the airway structures and soft tissues while advancing the tracheal tube over the fiber-optic endoscope
- Gastric distension and rupture, tension pneumothorax, and subcutaneous emphysema have all been reported after oxygen insufflation through the working channel
- Cross infection in between cases where the scope is inadequately sterilized

TROUBLESHOOTING

- The fiberscope is delicate to lift or dislodge tissues, but an air cavity or dark space at the end of the tip, it is essential to move forward. It is especially problematic in anesthetized patients where collapsed pharyngeal mucosa may contact the lens, making visualization and identification of anatomy difficult. A bite block, a Bermann airway, tongue retractor, or laryngoscope blade can be used to retract the tissues and create an air cavity.

- The image becomes foggy when the excess secretion (white out) or blood (red out) obscures the path. Irrigation with saline and suction would bring an unobstructed vision.

- If the secretions become adhered to the lens, advancing the scope to impinge on the contiguous tissue (pink out) and withdrawing the scope would clear the lens. Sometimes, the entire scope may have to be taken out to clear the lens.

- If the operator becomes disoriented in the middle of the airway, a little withdrawal of the scope and scanning of the airway by gently deflecting the tip or rotating the scope may solve the problem.

- Oxygen saturation may drop if the airway is obstructed, either by the fall of the tongue or the epiglottis. A jaw thrust followed by retraction of the tongue could clear the obstructed airway.

- Desaturation during fiber-optic endoscopy can be avoided by adequate preoxygenation before starting the procedure and continuous oxygen insufflation during the procedure. If the patient desaturates despite continuous oxygen insufflation, check whether the working channel is connected to the oxygen port or suction port. In endoscopes where two ports with one working channel are present, there are chances that the control lever that separates these two ports is left open for suction instead of oxygen.

- Difficulty is often encountered while passing the tracheal tube into the laryngeal inlet and the reason behind the resistance is claimed as the tracheal tube impinging on the epiglottis, arytenoid cartilage, or pyriform fossae. Never attempt a forceful insertion, which may injure soft tissues. The problem can be resolved by using a snugly fitting tube over the endoscope or gently rotating the tracheal tube 90° counterclockwise. Alternatively, applying a jaw thrust, applying external pressure on the larynx, or elevating the epiglottis by using a rigid laryngoscope or the fingers can help overcome the resistance to the tracheal tube passage.

- If the tip of the scope is caught in the Murphy eye of the tracheal tube, the fiberscope and tracheal tube may need to be pulled out as a unit. Threading the tracheal tube over the fiber-optic scope under direct vision to pass through the distal opening may prevent this issue.

CLEANING THE ENDOSCOPE

Proper cleaning of the endoscope involves four important steps: precleaning, leakage testing, manual cleaning, and disinfection.

Precleaning: It is done soon after the examination of the patient using an endoscope is over and taken out.

- Initially, an enzymatic detergent solution is prepared. Care should be taken that the detergent is not over- or underdiluted to prevent damage of the fiberscope.

- A clean cloth soaked in detergent solution is used to wipe off the secretions from the external surface of the flexible scope.

- The distal part of the scope is immersed in the detergent solution and it is aspirated and flushed through all channels until the fluid that comes out is clear. After that, water, and consequently, air, is aspirated.

Leakage testing

- Leakage testing is done to look for any damage prior to cleaning the endoscope, so that costly damage is avoided.

- Special leak detectors are available for this purpose.

- A leak is indicated by continuous flow of bubbles when the scope connected with the leak detector is immersed in water.

- If any leak is identified, it should immediately be referred to the manufacturer.

Manual cleaning

- A basin that is deep enough to immerse the fiberscope is used. An enzymatic detergent solution is prepared that is at the optimal temperature and concentration, as recommended by the manufacturer.

- The endoscope is immersed in the detergent solution. Before immersion, make sure that the eyepiece is submersible and cover the video connector with a water resistant cap.

- Keeping the endoscope immersed in the detergent, wipe off the debris from the external surface using a lint-free cloth.
- The working channels need to be filled with solution and allowed to rest for a recommended duration (3–5 minutes usually). Then, the channels are thoroughly cleaned to remove any debris with a special cleaning device and checked for patency. Any obstruction in the channel has to be sent for repair.
- After the recommended time of immersion in the detergent solution, immerse the endoscope in sterile water and clean it. If you use tap water, alcoholic cleaning is also recommended to prevent contamination.
- Connect the suction and aspirate water and air from all the channels. Wipe off the water droplets and excess moisture from the external surface with a dry cloth. Hanging the endoscope vertically will lead to draining of any droplet in the channels.

Disinfection
- Fiber-optic scopes are semicritical devices that carry higher risk of transmission of infections. Manual cleaning will not be sufficient; a high level of disinfection or sterilization should be performed before using it on another patient.
- Highly efficient chemical disinfectants, like glutaraldehyde and hydrogen peroxide, can be used to disinfect the endoscopes. Keep the entire scope immersed and the channels filled with the disinfectant for the recommended duration. After disinfection, clean it with sterile water and 70% alcohol.
- Gas sterilization is effective but the endoscope will not be available for a long duration of time.

REFERENCES

1. Murphy P. A fiber-optic endoscope used for nasal intubation. *Anaesthesia*. 1967;22:489-491.
2. Apfelbaum JL, Hagberg CA, Caplan RA et al. Practice guidelines for management of the difficult airway: An updated report by the American society of anesthesiologists task force on management of the difficult airway. *Anesthesiology*. 2013;118(2):251-270.
3. Laryngoscopes and tracheal intubation equipment. In: Baha Al-Shaikh, Simon Stacey, ed. Essentials of Anaesthetic Equipment. 4th ed. London, UK: Churchill Livingstone; 112-119.
4. Netter FH, Mitchell GAG. Cranial nerves. In: Brass A, Dingle RV, eds. Ciba Collection of Medical Illustrations, Volume I: The Nervous System, Part 1: Anatomy and Physiology. West Caldwell, NJ: Ciba Pharmaceuticals Company; 1983:90-109.
5. Kundra P, Kutralam S, Ravishankar M. Local anesthesia for awake fiberoptic nasotracheal intubation. *Acta Anaesthesiol Scand*. 2000; 44:511-516.
6. Simmons ST, Schleich AR. Airway regional anesthesia for awake fiberoptic intubation. *Reg Anesth Pain Med*. 2002;27(2):180-192.
7. Stubbs SE, McDougall JC. Preparation of the patient for bronchoscopy. In: Prakash UBS, ed. Bronchoscopy. 1st ed. Philadelphia, PA: Lippincott-Raven; 1997:107-108.
8. Prakash UBS, Cortese DA, Stubbs SE. Technical solutions to common problems in bronchoscopy. In: Prakash UBS, ed. Bronchoscopy. 1st ed. Philadelphia, PA: Lippincott-Raven; 1997:113.
9. Hermanowicz N, Turong DT. Cranial nerves IX (glossopharyngeal) and X (vagus). In: Goetz C, ed. Textbook of Clinical Neurology. 1st ed. Philadelphia, PA: Saunders; 1999:206-207.
10. Glossopharyngeal block. In: Brown D, ed. Atlas of Regional Anesthesia. 4th ed. Philadelphia, PA: Saunders; 2010:197-201.
11. Superior laryngeal nerve block. In: Brown D, ed. Atlas of Regional Anesthesia. 4th ed. Philadelphia, PA: Saunders; 2010:203-205.
12. Trans-laryngeal block. In: Brown D, ed. Atlas of Regional Anesthesia. 4th ed. Philadelphia, PA: Saunders; 2010:207-209.
13. Sivarajan M, Stoler E, Kil HK, Bishop MJ. Jet ventilation using fiberoptic bronchoscopes. *Anesth Analg*. 1995;80(2):384-387.
14. Thong SY, Lim Y. Video and optic laryngoscopy assisted tracheal intubation—The new era. *Anesth Intensive Care*. 2009;37:219-233.
15. Airway equipment: Laryngoscopes. In: Jerry A Dorsch, Susan E. Dorsch, eds. A Practical Approach to Anesthesia Equipment. 5th Ed. Philadelphia, PA: Lippincott Williams & Wilkins; 2008:520-560.

37

Chest drain insertion

RICHA AGGARWAL

INTRODUCTION

Chest drain placement is one of the most common surgical procedures performed in routine clinical practice. The procedure is not only performed by surgeons but also by emergency physicians, intensive care specialists, pulmonologists, interventional radiologists, and, in the emergency setting, even by nonphysician, advanced practitioners.[1]

A chest drain is a flexible, hollow, plastic tube that is inserted through the chest wall into the pleural space. It is used to drain fluid, air, blood, or pus[2] that has collected in the pleural cavity. It can also be used to instill agents to treat empyema. It helps in maintaining negative intrapleural pressure and expansion of the lungs.

APPLIED ANATOMY AND PHYSIOLOGY

The thoracic cage is formed by the vertebral column, ribs, and sternum and encloses the heart and lungs. The space between the ribs is the intercostal space.

The chest tube is generally placed in the fourth or fifth intercostal space in the midaxillary line.

The recommended site for insertion of a chest drain is the "safe triangle," which is formed anteriorly by the lateral border of the pectoralis major, laterally by the lateral border of the latissimus dorsi, inferiorly by the line of the fifth intercostal space, and superiorly by the base of the axilla (as shown in Figure 37.1). This position minimizes the risk to blood vessels (internal mammary artery), muscle and breast tissue.[3] The long thoracic nerve lies behind the midaxillary line on the surface of the serratus anterior and deep to the fascia and can be injured, if the tube is inserted posteriorly.

The intercostal space has intercostal muscles, with the vein, artery, and nerve lying in the costal groove along the inferior margin of the superior rib. It is normally advocated that the drain be located in the interspace just superior to the rib to prevent injury to this neurovascular bundle. However, injury to the collateral intercostal artery can still occur, even if one remains close to the superior margin of the inferior rib.[4]

Pressure around the lungs is lower than the atmospheric pressure outside of the body so for adequate expansion of the lungs, the intrapleural pressure should be negative. An optimal chest drain system

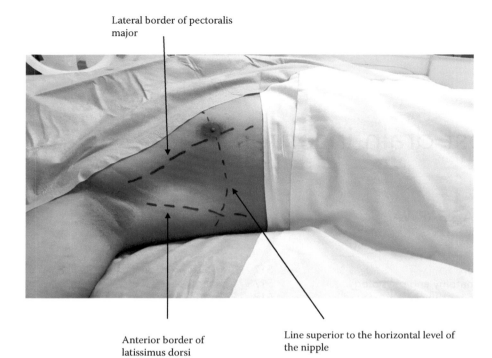

Lateral border of pectoralis major

Anterior border of latissimus dorsi

Line superior to the horizontal level of the nipple

Figure 37.1 Safe triangle.

removes fluid and air from the pleural space promptly and contains a one-way valve to prevent air and fluid from returning to the chest. This maintains the negative pressure in the pleural space.[5]

INDICATIONS FOR THE CHEST TUBE

The chest tube can be placed either electively or in an emergency situation. The various indications for a chest tube are as follows:

1. Pneumothorax
   - Spontaneous pneumothorax
   - Traumatic pneumothorax
   - Iatrogenic pneumothorax (mainly due to central line placement)
   - Tension pneumothorax
2. Hemothorax
   - Post–chest trauma
   - Postoperative
3. Pleural effusion
   - Sterile effusion
   - Infected/inflammatory effusion (empyema)
   - Malignant effusion
   - Chylothorax
4. Postoperative (after thoracotomy/esophagectomy and cardiac surgery)
5. Bronchopleural fistula (either postoperatively or due to mechanical ventilation)

CONTRAINDICATIONS OF CHEST TUBE INSERTION

There is no absolute contraindication of chest tube insertion in an emergency situation. Although there is no published evidence that abnormal clotting time or low-platelet count affect bleeding complications of a chest drain insertion, coagulopathy and platelet defect should be corrected before insertion in elective situations.[4] Prothrombin time (PT) and activated partial thromboplastin time (APTT) should be less than two times normal and platelets more than 50,000.

Other relative contraindications include

- Pulmonary bullae
- Pulmonary, pleural, or thoracic adhesions

EQUIPMENT REQUIRED FOR CHEST TUBE INSERTION

Before starting the procedure, the medical professional must ensure that he or she has the following equipment available:

- Supplemental oxygen for the patient
- Intravenous (IV) access
- Monitor (cardiac, pulse oximeter)
- Resuscitation cart
- Sterile gloves and gown
- Skin antiseptic solution, eg, betadine or chlorhexidine in alcohol
- Sterile drapes
- Surgical marker
- Lidocaine 1% with epinephrine
- Syringes, 10–20 mL (2) with needles
- Scalpel with Blade No. 10
- Large and medium Kelly clamps
- Large, curved Mayo scissors
- Large, straight, suture scissors
- Silk or nylon suture, 0 or 1–0
- Forceps and needle holder
- Vaseline gauze
- Gauze swabs
- Sterile adhesive tape
- Chest tube of appropriate size: Man: 28–32F, woman: 28F, child: 12–28F, infant: 12–16F, neonate: 10–12F
- Chest tube drainage device with underwater seal
- Suction source and tubing

PREPROCEDURE PREPARATION

Trained person: The chest tube insertion should be done either by a trained professional or supervised by an appropriate trainer. It has been determined that trained physicians can safely perform the procedure with a 3% early complication and 8% late complication rate.[6]

Exact site: The identity of the patient should be checked and side and site of insertion should be confirmed by reviewing clinical signs and radiologic information. The position of the drain is determined by the location and the nature of the collection to be drained. The preferred position in most cases is the fourth to fifth intercostal space in the midaxillary line. This area is commonly known as the "safe triangle," bordered by the anterior border of the latissimus dorsi, the lateral border of the pectoralis major, a line superior to the horizontal level of the nipple, and an apex below the axilla. If there is a loculated effusion or air, a more posterior position may be chosen. Ultrasonography may be used as a loculated pleural effusion guide in such case to determine the exact site for tube placement. Success rates of image-guided chest tube insertion vary between 71% to 86%.[7]

Bleeding diathesis: Any coagulopathy (PT and aPTT more than 2 times normal) or platelet dysfunction (platelet count less than 50,000) should be corrected in an elective situation.

Consent and premedication: Written and informed consent should be taken before the procedure. Chest drain insertion is a painful procedure and, according to a study, 50% of the patients experienced pain levels of 9 to 10 on a scale of 1 to 10[8] during the procedure. Therefore, premedication in the form of IV analgesics or mild sedation (benzodiazipines or narcotics) should be administered. Appropriate monitoring and resuscitation equipment should be available when using sedatives for the procedure.

Patient position: The patient should be positioned appropriately, which depends on the reason for insertion and the clinical state of the patient. The preferred position for drain insertion is the patient laying on the bed, head at a 45° angle, slightly rotated, with the arm raised behind the patient's head to expose the axillary area.[9] An alternative is for the patient to sit upright, leaning over an adjacent table with a pillow or in the lateral decubitus position.[10] In trauma patients, chest tube insertion is done during primary survey only and is done in the supine position.

Drain size: Chest tubes are available in a range of French (Fr) sizes from 14 to 40 (diameter in French/3 = diameters in a millimeter). A 24 Fr tube will drain about 28 L/minute for air at a suction level of −20 cm water (H_2O); however, the rate of drainage is less for liquids. The size of the drain depends on the underlying pathology. There remains intense debate about the optimum size of the drainage catheter 24 to 26 and there are no large, randomized trials directly comparing small and large bore tubes. Small bore tubes are recommended for patients with simple, spontaneous pneumothorax and nonviscous effusions, because they are better tolerated and are associated with less discomfort.[11] Large bore tubes are required for draining traumatic pneu-mothorax, hemothorax,[12] and empyema.

Antibiotic

Prophylactic antibiotics are not warranted for chest tubes placed in the setting of spontaneous pneu-mothorax or other nontraumatic indications[13] but are warranted for chest tubes placed in the setting of trauma, particularly in patients with penetrating injury.[14]

STEPWISE PROCEDURE

The steps involved in placement of a chest tube are as follows (Figures 37.2 through 37.5):

1. Give proper position to the patient as described earlier.
2. Attach cardiac monitor and pulse oximeter to the patient and start supplemental oxygen.
3. Take universal precautions and wear sterile gloves.
4. Clean the skin with 2% chlorhexidine in alcohol and drape the chest at a predetermined site of tube insertion.
5. Locally anesthetize the skin and rib perios-teum. Always anesthetize the periosteum of the rib above and below the planned intercostal

insertion site and include the muscular tissue of the intercostal space.
6. Make a 2 to 3 cm transverse (horizontal inci-sion) above and parallel to the upper border of the lower rib in the intercostal space and bluntly dissect the subcutaneous tissue.
7. Using a Kelly clamp, dissect bluntly, and create a short, subcutaneous tunnel from the incision site cephalad toward the intercostal space.
8. Push the clamp over the superior portion of the rib, keeping the clamp in the closed posi-tion and through the parietal pleura. Then open the clamp to spread the intercostal muscles and parietal pleura.
9. Insert a finger through the tract into the pleural space to confirm proper position and to make sure that there are no adhesions between the lung and the pleural surface.
10. Clamp the end of the chest tube with the Kelly clamp and guide it into the pleural space with its distal end clamped. Direct the tube anteroapical for air and inferoposterior for fluid drainage.
11. Remove the clamp and confirm the chest tube in the pleural cavity by observing the con-densation within the tube or seeing the drainage from the tube. Advance the chest tube until the last drainage hole is within the tho-racic cavity.

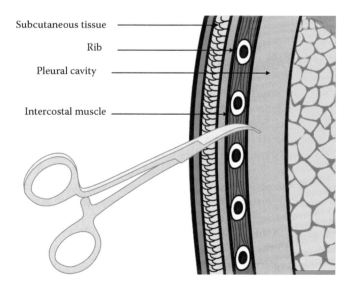

Subcutaneous tissue

Rib

Pleural cavity

Intercostal muscle

Figure 37.2 Dissection with Kelly clamp up to the intercostal space.

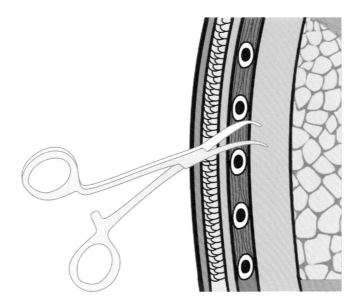

Figure 37.3 Spreading intercostal muscles with clamp open.

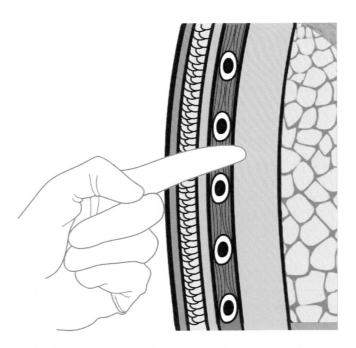

Figure 37.4 Separation of adhesions between the lung and the pleural surface.

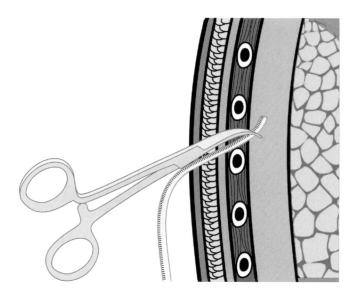

Figure 37.5 Insertion of the chest tube with the end clamped with Kelly along superior border of lower rib.

12. Attach the tube to the external drainage system. Mattress or interrupted sutures should be used on both sides of the incision to close the ends. Use the loose ends of the sutures to wrap around the tube and tie them off, anchoring the tube to the chest wall.[15] Use occlusive gauze to seal the skin around the tube.

13. After the chest tube has been inserted and connected to a drainage system, obtain a chest radiograph to confirm the tube's position. Ideally, you will want to get both the PA and lateral view. Monitor the initial drainage from the tube.

Another approach to chest drain placement is with the Seldinger technique, in which the chest tube is placed over a guidewire, as in the central venous cannulation. This technique is used for the placement of small bore tubes with the help of an ultrasound or fluoroscopy.

DRAINAGE SYSTEMS

An underwater seal chest drainage system is used to drain the pleural cavity. This maintains adequate air pressure to the lungs and reinflates a collapsed lung. The drainage system that is used can be either a one-bottle, two-bottle, or three-bottle drainage system.

One bottle drainage system: This system consists of one bottle, which serves as both a collection container and a water seal. A rigid straw is immersed into the bottle, and its tip is located 2 cm below the surface of the saline solution, which is put into the bottle. The other end of this rigid straw is connected to the thoracic drainage tube, which is placed in the pleural cavity.

The stopper of the bottle must have a vent to prevent pressure from building up when air or fluid from the pleural cavity enters the bottle. It is important to remove this valve cover before connecting the system to the patient. This system works well for uncomplicated pneumothorax but if the amount of fluid being drained is more, the fluid level in the bottle rises, and higher pressure will be required in the rigid straw to remove more fluid from the pleural cavity.[5] In such cases, a two-bottle drainage system is preferred.

Two-bottle drainage system: is preferred over a one-bottle system when large quantities of liquid are drained from the pleural cavity. With this system, the bottle that is adjacent to the patient acts as a collection bottle for the drainage and the second bottle provides the water seal and the air vent.

If the patient has a large air leak into the pleural space, gravity drainage may not be sufficient to evacuate the chest, and suction may be required. A controlled amount of suction can be readily applied to the system, if a third bottle, the suction bottle, is added to the system.

Three-bottle drainage system: The third bottle allows the application of the suction. A vent in the suction control bottle is connected to a vent on the water seal bottle. The two bottles are interconnected. The amount of negative pressure within the suction system is equal to the depth of immersion of the rigid straw below the liquid surface of the bottle.

POSTPROCEDURE CARE

Following insertion of the chest drain:

- Check that the underwater seal moves with respiration
- Order a repeat chest x-ray to confirm the position of the tube and the degree of lung reexpansion; exclude any complications
- Ensure that regular analgesia is prescribed while the chest drain is in place
- Advise the patient to keep the underwater bottle below the drain-insertion site upright and avoid compressing the tube by sitting or lying on it
- Document the procedure in the patient's medical records

Patients with chest tubes should be managed in specialist wards by staff who are trained in chest drain management.[4]

How to manage initial drainage: The amount of chest-tube drainage should be assessed on a regular basis. The rapid evacuation of large volumes of pleural effusion may lead to re-expansion pulmonary edema.[16] This has been reported to be fatal in some cases (up to 20% of subjects in one series of 53 cases).[17] Mild symptoms of re-expansion edema means that patients experience discomfort and cough. To prevent this, the chest tube should be immediately clamped and no further fluid should be removed if the patient develops a cough, chest pain, shortness of breath, or oxygen desaturation. Even without symptoms, no more than about 1.5 liters should be drained at one time and the medical professional should wait for at least 1 hour before performing any additional drainage.[18] In trauma patients, an immediate drainage of 20 mL/kg of blood or the accumulation of >3 mL/kg per hour of blood is an indication for a thoracotomy.

DAILY CARE OF THE CHEST TUBE

During the daily care of the tube, one should assess the following:

- What is the nature and the amount of drainage? Is it different from the initial drainage?
- Whether the fluid within the tube is moving with respiration. Absence of swinging indicates that either the drain is occluded or it is misplaced. If the chest tube becomes blocked because of a clot or debris, the tube can be stripped or cleared of the obstruction by maneuvers like twisting the tube 360 degrees, pulling the tube out 1 to 2 cm, passing a sterile endotracheal tube suction catheter, and injecting a small volume of sterile saline.
- Any bubbling in the tube. An air leak or bubbling in the drain may be due to a faulty connection or entrained air through the skin incision. Persistent bubbling throughout the respiratory cycle may indicate a continuing bronchopleural air leak.
- Dressings. Dressings should be changed daily to examine the site for signs of infection and to ensure that the chest drain is well placed and is properly sutured. If there are any clinical signs of infection, a swab should be taken from the chest drain site.

As a general rule, chest tubes for pneumothorax should not be clamped. Clamping a pleural drain in the presence of a continuing air leak may result in a tension pneumothorax. While changing the drain bottle, temporary clamping of the drainage tube may be necessary to prevent entry of air into the pleural cavity and the tube should be clamped between the medical professional's thumb and forefinger.

COMPLICATIONS OF CHEST TUBE INSERTION

The average complication rate after chest tube placement may vary between 5% and 10%.[19] The complications that are commonly seen:

- Bleeding
  1. Local site bleeding/hematoma
  2. Hemothorax from intercostal vessel injury
  3. Perforation of major vascular structures such as the aorta or subclavian vessels

- Misplacement of the tube
  1. Intra-abdominal placement
  2. Laceration of the lung, liver, or heart
- Pneumothorax
  1. Subcutaneous emphysema
  2. Persistent air bubbling
- Infection
  1. Insertion-site cellulitis
  2. Track infection
  3. Empyema
- Intercostal neuralgia due to trauma of neurovascular bundles

REMOVAL OF THE CHEST DRAIN

The timing of removal of the chest drain is dependent on the original reason for insertion of the tube and the clinical progress thereafter.

Removal criteria include:

- Fully expanded lung
- Resolution of air leak for 24 hours
- For pleural effusion, daily fluid output, less than 200 mL in a 24-hour period[20]

Adequate pain relief should be ensured before removal of the chest drain.

As for insertion, an aseptic technique should be used and the chest drain and drainage kit should be disposed of appropriately.

When the tube is ready to be removed, the patient should be asked to perform a Valsalva maneuver (to increase the pleural pressure and prevent air from entering the pleural cavity). The tube is withdrawn quickly. The previously placed suture is then tied to close the hole. The medical professional should be able to tie sutures securely. The wound site should be checked and an appropriate dressing should be applied.

A chest radiograph should be performed 12 to 24 hours after removal.[21] This should be done sooner if there is a clinical suspicion of a residual air leak or a new pneumothorax.

REFERENCES

1. Filosso PL, Guerrera F, Sandri A et al. Errors and complications in chest tube placement. *Thorac Surg Clin*. 2017;27(1):57-67.
2. Mattox KL, Allen MK. Systematic approach to pneumothorax, haemothorax, pneumomediastinum and subcutaneous emphysema. *Injury*. 1986;17(5):309-312.
3. Laws D, Neville E, Duff J. British thoracic society guidelines for the insertion of a chest drain. *Thorax*. 2003;58(suppl II):ii53-ii59.
4. Da Rocha RP, Vengjer A, Blanco A, de Carvalho PT, Mongon ML, Fernandes GJ. Size of the collateral intercostal artery in adults: Anatomical considerations in relation to thoracocentesis and thoracoscopy. *Surg Radiol Anat*. 2002;24(1):23-26.
5. Zisis C, Tsirgogianni K, Lazaridis G et al. Chest drainage systems in use. *Ann Transl Med*. 2015;3(3):43.
6. Collop NA, Kim S, Sahn SA. Analysis of tube thoracostomy performed by pulmonologists at a teaching hospital. *Chest*. 1997;112:709-713.
7. Reinhold C, Illescas FF, Atri M, Bret PM. The treatment of pleural effusions and pneumothorax with catheters placed percutaneously under image guidance. *Am J Roentgenol*. 1989;152:1189-1191.
8. Luketich JD, Kiss MD, Hershey J. Chest tube insertion: A prospective evaluation of pain management. *Clin J Pain*. 1998;14:152-154.
9. Tomlinson MA, Treasure T. Insertion of a chest drain: How to do it. *Br J Hosp Med*. 1997;58:248-252.
10. Boland GW, Lee MJ, Silverman S, Mueller PR. Review. Interventional radiology of the pleural space. *Clin Radiol*. 1995;50:205-214.
11. Patz EF, Goodman PC, Erasmus JJ. Percutaneous drainage of pleural collections. *J Thorac Imaging*. 1998;13:83-92.
12. Parry GW, Morgan WE, Salama FD. Management of haemothorax. *Ann R Coll Surg Engl*. 1996;78:325-326.
13. Olgac G, Aydogmus U, Mulazimoglu L, Kutlu CA. Antibiotics are not needed during tube thoracostomy for spontaneous pneumothorax: An observational case study. *J Cardiothorac Surg*. 2006;1:43.
14. Sanabria A, Valdivieso E, Gomez G, Echeverry G. Prophylactic antibiotics in chest trauma: A meta-analysis of high-quality studies. *World J Surg*. 2006;30:1843.

15. Dev SP, Nascimiento B Jr, Simone C, Chien V. Chest-tube insertion. *N Engl J Med.* 2007;357:e15.

16. Feller-Kopman D, Berkowitz D, Boiselle P, Ernst A. Large-volume thoracentesis and the risk of reexpansion pulmonary edema. *Ann Thorac Surg.* 2007;84:1656-1661.

17. Mafhood S, Hix WR, Aaron BL, Blaes P, Watson DC. Re-expansion pulmonary oedema. *Ann Thorac Surg.* 1988;45:340-345.

18. Havelock T, Teoh R, Laws D, Gleeson F. BTS Pleural Disease Guideline Group. Pleural procedures and thoracic ultrasound: British Thoracic Society Pleural Disease Guideline 2010. *Thorax.* 2010;65(Suppl 2):ii61-ii76.

19. Bailey RC. Complications of tube thoracostomy in trauma. *J Accid Emerg. Med.* 2000;17:111-114.

20. Baumann MH. What size chest tube? What drainage system is ideal? And other chest tube management questions. *Curr Opin Pulm Med.* 2003;9:276-281.

21. Tang ATM, Velissaris TJ, Weeden DF. An evidence-based approach to drainage of the pleural cavity: Evaluation of best practice. *J Eval Clin Pract.* 2002;8:333-340.

38

Bronchoalveolar lavage

MOHAN GURJAR

INTRODUCTION

The availability and advancement of the flexible bronchoscope makes bronchoscopy a routine procedure for various indications, in both noncritically ill and critically ill patients. Bronchoscopies are used to visualize proximal airways, primarily up to the third generation of branching, for diagnostic, therapeutic, or both indications simultaneously. However, we could not see beyond the subsegmental bronchi. Bronchoalveolar lavage (BAL) is used to sample the contents (cellular and acellular) of the lower respiratory tract, mainly from distal bronchiole and gas exchange units after wedging the bronchoscope. BAL is a minimally invasive and relatively safe procedure in trained hands under appropriate monitoring. It can be performed on spontaneously breathing patients as well as in mechanically ventilated patients (with an artificial airway or not [during noninvasive ventilation]).

The medical professional who performs BAL must have knowledge of airway anatomy. According to the Boyden classification of bronchi, the right main bronchus divides into the right upper lobe bronchus and right intermediate bronchus, which further divides into the right middle and right lower lobe bronchi,[1] while the left main bronchus divides into the left upper lobe bronchus, the lingular bronchus, and the left lower lobe bronchus. Each lobar bronchi further divides into segmental bronchi. The right upper lobe bronchus divides into the apical segment (B1), posterior segment (B2), and anterior segment (B3). The right middle lobe bronchus divides into the lateral segment (B4) and medial segment (B5). The right lower lobe bronchus divides into the superior segment (B6), medial segment (B7), anterior segment (B8), lateral segment (B9), and posterior segment (B10). The left lung has only eight segmental bronchi. The left upper lobe bronchus divides into the apicoposterior segment (B1/2), anterior segment (B3), superior lingular segment (B4), and inferior lingular segment (B5). The left lower lobe bronchus divides into the superior segment (B6), anteriomedial segment (B8), lateral segment (B9), and posterior segment (B10). Additionally, there are some variants that have been described in the literature.

INDICATIONS AND CONTRAINDICATIONS

BAL is indicated in various lung pathologies that involve the diffuse or localized areas.[2–7] There are better diagnostic results with BAL compared with traditional cultures and stains. BAL should be performed early in the clinical course when indicated. The BAL sample analysis can diagnose some infections precisely, like *Mycobacterium tuberculosis*, *Pneumocystis jirovecii*, *Mycoplasma*, *Legionella*, and so on, where the pathogenic organism is not considered a colonization of the respiratory tract. Also, BAL helps in the diagnosis of other lung infections, such as pneumonia, due to various bacterial and fungal organism. BAL is also useful in diagnosing noninfectious diseases, including lung malignancies, pulmonary hemorrhage, and so on (Table 38.1).

However, BAL should be avoided in some situations, such as[6,7]:

- The patient's inability to maintain oxygen saturation
- On a ventilator with high positive end-expiratory pressure (PEEP)
- Active bronchospasm
- Presence of pneumothorax
- Severe pulmonary artery hypertension
- Ongoing myocardial ischemia or recent myocardial infarction
- Presence of arrhythmias
- Severe hemodynamic instability
- Lack of adequate training and experience
- Lack of adequate infrastructure and equipment to handle complications

Table 38.1 Uses of bronchoalveolar lavage (BAL)

Infectious diseases	Noninfectious diseases
Diagnostic (colonization not known)	Diagnostic
Mycobacterium tuberculosis	Malignancies
Pneumocystis jirovecii	Histiocytosis-X
Mycoplasma	Alveolar proteinosis (milky BAL)
Legionella	Eosinophilic pneumonia
Toxoplasma gondii	
Histoplasma	
Strongyloides	
Diagnostic adjunct (colonization may be)	Diagnostic adjunct
Bacteria	Pulmonary hemorrhage
Candida	Interstitial lung disease
Aspergillus	Hypersensitivity pneumonitis
Cryptococcus	
Cytomegalovirus	Asbestosis, berylliosis, silicosis
Herpes simplex	

BEFORE THE PROCEDURE

A typical, flexible video bronchoscope has a flexible insertion tube; control handle; universal cord, which has a light guide connecter attached to a light source; and a processor and a monitor, which are usually mounted in a single tower. The insertion tube contains a biopsy/suction channel, fiber-optic light and image bundles, channels for air and water, and a tip bending control wire.

Selecting the appropriate size bronchoscope for the procedure is mainly chosen by the size of the airway as well as the outer diameter of the insertion tube of the bronchoscope (6.0 mm or less). In a spontaneously breathing adult, the bronchoscope usually occupies 10% to 15% of the cross-sectional area of the trachea; because it occupies up to two-thirds of the cross-sectional area, the patient will need a size 7.0 endotracheal/tracheostomy tube with use of 5.7 mm outer diameter of insertion tube of the bronchoscope.[6] Occupying more area of the airway by the larger bronchoscope leads to various pathophysiologic changes, including worsening of ventilator parameters, gas exchange, and hemodynamics of the patient during the procedure. The size of artificial airway for performing the procedures must be 2 mm larger than the outer diameter of the bronchoscope. For example, using a bronchoscope of 5.7 mm (outer diameter), the patient should have an airway of size 8.0 mm or larger.

The medical professional should obtain written, informed consent and review the indication and relevant chest images again before doing BAL. He or she should discontinue enteral feeding for at least 4 hours prior to the procedure and ensure that there is intravenous (IV) access, availability of all necessary drugs (including topical anesthetics, sedative, muscle relaxants, atropine, crystalloids), lubricating jelly, swivel adapter, airway carts, ventilator support, multimodal physiologic monitoring, and suction.

In the ventilated patient, the mode should be changed to volume control, FiO_2 should be increased to 1.0, positive end-expiratory pressure (PEEP) should be decreased, and arterial blood gas (ABG) should be monitored. When an endotracheal tube (ETT) is used, a mouth guard (bite-blocker) is necessary to avoid damage to the bronchoscope. Also, a shortened length of ETT should be considered so that the tip of the flexible bronchoscope reaches a more distal part of the bronchial tree.

For a patient on noninvasive ventilation (NIV), a full face mask with dual axis swivel adapter should be used. The inspiratory positive airway pressure (IPAP) should be increased up to 15 to 17 cm H_2O and the expiratory positive airway pressure (EPAP) should be decreased to 15 to 17 cm H_2O.

PROCEDURES

Ideally, the selection of the target site for doing BAL should be based on image findings; otherwise, the traditional BAL site should be considered (right side: middle lobe, left side: lingual). If biopsy or brushing is also planned, BAL should be performed first to avoid altering recovered fluid.

Personal protective equipment should be used with aseptic precautions during BAL. The distal part of the bronchoscope should be lubricated for easy insertion through the airway. The bronchoscope should be advanced toward the targeted site while viewing the video. In order to achieve optimal fluid recovery, the bronchoscope should occlude the bronchial lumen completely in the selected bronchopulmonary segment.

Twenty to 50 mL of normal saline should be instilled and recovered by negative pressure (not more than 100 mmHg). This should be repeated three to six times. At least 5% of the instilled volume should be retrieved ($\geq$30% retrieved is considered optimal). The first BAL sample mainly represents bronchial airway material rather than true alveolar return; pooling of the first BAL sample with subsequent samples depends upon the area of clinical interest.

Immediately after conducting the procedure and collecting sample, proper labeling must be ensured. There should be comprehensive documentation of the procedure; the documentation must include details of the procedure, medications used for the procedure, vitals (including ventilator parameters and ABG, if indicated) from preprocedure through postprocedure, any complication(s), an archive of important images that were saved during the procedure, and postprocedure advice.

It is preferable for the BAL sample to be transported immediately to the laboratory; if that is not possible, the sample should be kept at 4° C for up to 12 hours.[7] Diagnostic studies on BAL fluid include: gross observation, differential cell count, microbiologic studies, and cytopathology. A gross milky or opaque sample suggests pulmonary alveolar proteinosis; sequentially, more hemorrhagic fluid in each aliquot suggests the presence of an alveolar hemorrhage. In the microscopic examination, >5% epithelial cells suggests a suboptimal sample. Normally, the BAL sample from a nonsmoker adult shows >85% alveolar macrophage, 10% to 15% lymphocytes, <3% neutrophils, <1% eosinophils, and 1% epithelial cells. More than 25% lymphocytes suggests the presence of granulomatous disease (like sarcoidosis), lymphoma, cellular nonspecific or lymphoid interstitial pneumonitis, or a drug reaction, while more than 25% eosinophils strongly suggests acute or chronic eosinophilic pneumonia. Detailed microbiologic studies of the BAL sample may help to diagnose infectious etiologies; and in cytopathology, the presence of malignant cells confirms the malignancy.

Various meta-analyses favor BAL fluid analysis for diagnosing pulmonary tuberculosis in smear-negative patients, invasive aspergillosis by measuring galactomannan (optical density index cutoff value 1.5), sarcoidosis by CD4/CD8 Ratio (>3), and *P. jirovecii* by the PCR method.[8–11]

PROCEDURE-RELATED COMPLICATIONS/PROBLEMS

A flexible bronchoscopy with BAL is a relatively safe procedure in experienced hands, and incidence of complications during the procedure is very low. In a review by Geraci et al., incidences of various complications reported among 107,969 bronchoscopies were[12]:

- Hypoxemia (0.2%–21%)
- Arrhythmias (1%–10%)
- Postbiopsy bleeding (0.12%–7.5%)
- Pneumothorax or pneumomediastinitis (1%–6%)
- Fever (0.9%–2.5%)
- Complications related to local anesthesia (0.3%–0.5%)
- Death (0.1%–0.2%)

REFERENCES

1. Boyden EA. A critique of the international nomenclature on bronchopulmonary segments. *Dis Chest*. 2003;23(3):266-269.
2. Meyer KC. Bronchoalveolar lavage as a diagnostic tool. *Semin Respir Crit Care Med*. 2007;28(5):546-560.
3. Reynolds HY. Bronchoalveolar lavage and other methods to define the human respiratory tract milieu in health and disease. *Lung*. 2011;189(2):87-99.
4. Wells AU. The clinical utility of bronchoalveolar lavage in diffuse parenchymal lung disease. *Eur Respir Rev*. 2010;19(117): 237-241.
5. Brownback KR, Thomas LA, Simpson SQ. Role of bronchoalveolar lavage in the diagnosis of pulmonary infiltrates in immunocompromised patients. *Curr Opin Infect Dis*. 2014;27(4):322-328.
6. Mehta RM, and Aurangabadwalla RK. Bronchoscopy. In: Mohan Gurjar, ed. *Manual of ICU Procedures*. 1st ed. Jaypee Brothers Medical Publishers (P) Ltd.; 2016:129-145.
7. Singhal S. Bronchoalveolar lavage (BAL) and mini-BAL. In: Mohan Gurjar, ed. *Manual of ICU Procedures*. 1st ed. Jaypee Brothers Medical Publishers (P) Ltd.; 2016:146-152.
8. Tian P, Shen Y, Wang Y et al. Diagnostic value of nucleic acid amplification tests on bronchoalveolar lavage fluid for smear-negative pulmonary tuberculosis: A meta-analysis. *Biosci Rep*. 2015;35(4):e00232.
9. Heng SC, Morrissey O, Chen SC et al. Utility of bronchoalveolar lavage fluid galactomannan alone or in combination with PCR for the diagnosis of invasive aspergillosis in adult hematology patients: A systematic review and meta-analysis. *Crit Rev Microbiol*. 2015;41(1):124-134.
10. Shen Y, Pang C, Wu Y et al. Diagnostic performance of bronchoalveolar lavage fluid cd4/cd8 ratio for sarcoidosis: A meta-analysis. *EBioMedicine*. 2016;8:302-308.
11. Fan LC, Lu HW, Cheng KB, Li HP, Xu JF. Evaluation of PCR in bronchoalveolar lavage fluid for diagnosis of *Pneumocystis jirovecii* pneumonia: A bivariate meta-analysis and systematic review. *PLoS One*. 2013;8(9): e73099.
12. Geraci G, Pisello F, Sciumè C, Li Volsi F, Romeo M, Modica G. Complication of flexible fiberoptic bronchoscopy. Literature review *Ann Ital Chir*. 2007;78(3):183-192.

39

External ventricular drainage

VASUDHA SINGHAL

INTRODUCTION

Insertion of an external ventricular drain (EVD) is one of the most important life-saving procedures undertaken in the neurointensive care unit. It is the standard of care for temporarily controlling the intracranial pressure (ICP) by draining the cerebrospinal fluid (CSF) in emergency neurosurgical scenarios with severe intracranial hypertension, such as hydrocephalus, hemorrhage, tumor, meningitis, or brain trauma. It is the gold standard technique to monitor the ICP in severely brain injured patients, thereby serving as a guide for targeted resuscitation. At the same time, ventriculostomy drains also aid in the drainage of intraventricular blood and instillation of intraventricular medications when indicated.

INDICATIONS OF EVD INSERTION

External ventricular drainage is indicated to monitor and treat raised ICP in:

1. *Traumatic brain injury*: The Brain Trauma Foundation guidelines for the management of traumatic brain injury (TBI) recommend ventricular catheters, connected to an external strain gauge transducer, as the most accurate, low cost and reliable method of ICP monitoring.[1] All TBI patients with a postresuscitation Glasgow Coma Scale (GCS) score of 3 to 8 and an abnormal CT scan should be offered ICP monitoring. Patients with a normal CT scan but with ≥2 of these features—age >40 years, unilateral or bilateral posturing, or systolic blood pressure <90 mmHg—are also candidates of ICP monitoring. In recent years, both EVDs as well as intraparenchymal ICP monitors are recommended and used for the purpose of ICP monitoring.[2]

2. *Intracranial hemorrhage with intraventricular extension*: The increased ICP and the acute hydrocephalus caused by intracranial hemorrhage (ICH) is managed by placement of an EVD.[3] EVD is typically placed in the ventricle contralateral to the dominant intraventricular hemorrhage (IVH). Patients with poorer GCS, more severe IVH, and lower volumes of ICH (<30 cc) have a greater likelihood of EVD placement.[4] EVD use has been associated with a decreased mortality but poorer long-term clinical and functional outcomes.[5]

   EVDs can also be used for injecting thrombolytic agents in cases of a large IVH. Intraventricular thrombolytic therapy with low-dose tissue plasminogen activator (rtPA) has been shown to accelerate lysis and evacuation of IVH in large clinical trials.[6] However, the long-term outcome benefits of this modality is still doubtful.

3. *Subarachnoid hemorrhage (SAH)*: EVD placement has long been the standard of care in treating hydrocephalus stemming from aneurysmal SAH.[7] However, the abrupt lowering of ICP with rapid CSF drainage may lead to rebleeding in these patients, due to decreased transmural pressure across the aneurysmal wall or removal of the clot sealing the previously ruptured aneurysm.[8] Also, the administration of antiplatelets and anticoagulants during endovascular coiling of ruptured aneurysms may increase the risk of EVD-related hemorrhage.[9]

4. *Acute cerebellar ischemic stroke*: In patients with cerebellar stroke with early swelling, placement of an EVD is indicated for the treatment of acute symptomatic hydrocephalus. This is usually accompanied by an urgent suboccipital decompressive craniectomy, to avoid deterioration from upward cerebellar displacement.[10]

5. *Bacterial meningitis*: EVD insertion for CSF drainage has been shown to improve outcome in patients with community-acquired acute bacterial meningitis presenting with altered sensorium, by lowering the ICP, and thus, improving the cerebral perfusion pressure in the brain and preventing brain herniation.[11]

   EVD is also used for the intraventricular instillation of antibiotics in cases of CSF infections not responding to systemic therapy. The intraventricular route allows controlled, localized delivery of the antibiotic directly to the brain, thereby achieving higher concentrations and more reliable bactericidal action.[12] The antibiotics commonly given via the intraventricular route are vancomycin, gentamicin, amikacin, and colistin.[13–18]

6. *Acute hydrocephalus due to tumor or shunt failure*: Perioperative ventriculostomy has been used in the management of obstructive hydrocephalus associated with infratentorial tumors, avoiding the need for indwelling shunts and their associated problems, such as shunt dysfunction, tumor deseeding, and upward herniation.[19] The presence of an EVD also facilitates postoperative ICP monitoring and drainage of CSF mixed with blood and tumor debris.

   EVD insertion may also be taken up as an urgent short-term treatment in cases of ventriculoperitoneal shunt malfunction and blockage, causing an acute hydrocephalus and rise in ICP.

TECHNIQUE OF INSERTION

The right, nondominant frontal hemisphere is the preferred site for twist drill ventriculostomy placement in most patients, as it does not control language in >90% of patients. The site of incision selected for placing the intraventricular catheter is the Kocher's point (Figure 39.1), so as to avoid the superior sagittal sinus and the frontal cortex motor strip.[20] This point is located approximately 11 to 12 cm posterior to the nasion, and 3 cm lateral to the midline, at approximately the mid-pupillary line. The point of entry should be 1 cm anterior to the coronal suture, to avoid the eloquent area of the brain.

The patient is adequately sedated and placed in a supine position, with the head of the bed elevated to 45°. The incision area is prepared by clipping the head, painting with chlorhexidine, and draping appropriately. The scalp is infiltrated with 1% lidocaine around the planned incision site. A linear incision is taken at the Kocher's point with a scalpel and carried down to the skull. The periosteum is scraped and a burr hole made with a drill placed perpendicular to the skull, to penetrate the outer and inner tables of the skull. The dura is pierced with a scalpel and the ventricular catheter introduced with the stylet, up to 5 cm below the dura or 6 to 7 cm below the skull surface, to place the catheter just above the ipsilateral foramen of Monroe. The catheter trajectory is directed toward the contralateral medial canthus in the coronal plane[21,22] and just anterior to the ipsilateral tragus in the sagittal plane. Once a spontaneous CSF flow is obtained after removal of the catheter stylet, the opening ICP may be obtained by transducing the pressure to an external gauge. The catheter is secured externally by tunnelling through the scalp 5 to 7 cm posteriorly and laterally to prevent infection. It is then connected to an external drainage system and an ICP measuring transducer.

The accuracy of EVD insertion has further increased with technological advancements, such as CT and intraoperative ultrasound guidance, stereotactic neuronavigation, and electromagnetic navigation.[23–27] Image guidance may be

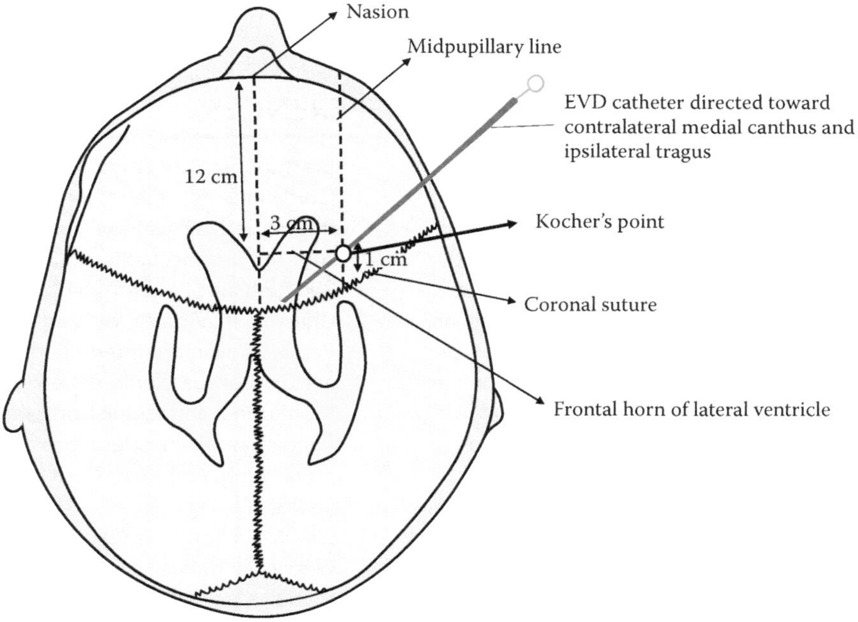

Figure 39.1 Surface anatomy of Kocher's point.

particularly indicated in cases where the ventricular anatomy is distorted or the ventricles are mere slits.

MANAGEMENT OF EVD

EVD is calibrated at the level of the foramen of Monroe, which lies at the level of the external auditory meatus in the supine position and at the midsagittal line (between the eyebrows) in the lateral position.[28] Leveling needs to be done every time the position of the patient is changed, in order to avoid erroneous ICP readings and CSF over/ underdrainage.

The mean opening CSF pressure and the underlying pathology of the patient determines the desired height of the collecting system. In cases of an unsecured aneurysmal SAH, the initial height of the collecting system is set high, to avoid rapid CSF drainage, which may lead to rebleeding. The height may be kept low in cases of massive intraventricular bleed and negative pressure hydrocephalus.[29]

If clinically indicated, the EVD drainage system may be accessed by the physician under all aseptic precautions to withdraw CSF for analysis or to instill medications. CSF samples should be aspi-

rated from the proximal port of the EVD (closest to the head) at a rate not exceeding 1 mL/min. Sampling from collection bags or the distal ports is discouraged as the cellular components degrade rapidly. When instilling medications, such as rtPA in IVH or antibiotics in meningitis, the EVD should be clamped for an hour postadministration.

COMPLICATIONS OF EVD INSERTION

Hemorrhage, infections, and catheter malfunction are the most common complications occurring after the insertion of EVDs.

1. *Hemorrhage*: EVDs may be associated with imaging evidence of hemorrhage, after either placement or removal.[30,31] Coagulopathy and overdrainage of CSF seem to be the most important risk factors associated with hemorrhagic complications.[32] The incidence of hemorrhage with EVD ranges from 0% to 41%, but most of these hemorrhages are small and insignificant and rarely require surgical evacuation. Interestingly, early pharmacologic venous

thromboembolism prophylaxis, initiated within 24 hours of EVD placement, is not associated with an increased risk of hemorrhage.[33]

2. *Infection*: EVD-related infections remain a primary concern that prolong the hospital stay, increase costs, and negatively impact the patient's outcome. The incidence of these range from <5% to 23%, most commonly 10%.[34–36]

The Neurocritical Care Society (NCS) recently published evidence-based guidelines for the management of EVDs to reduce the risk of infections.[37] They recommend keeping the EVDs for the minimum time necessary and removing them as soon as the clinical situation allows.[37,38] If the patient, however, needs continued monitoring, routine change of catheters is not recommended.[39] Only one dose of antimicrobials prior to EVD insertion is sufficient, as the use of prophylactic antibiotics increases the risk of resistant organisms and *Clostridium difficile* colitis.[40,41] Antimicrobial-impregnated catheters may reduce the risk of infection.[42–44] Routine CSF sampling should be avoided and CSF analysis should be done only when clinically indicated.[45,46] A bundled approach to the insertion and care of the patient with a ventricular drain helps in reduction of ventriculostomy-related infections, which includes aseptic insertion, tunneling of the catheter, use of impregnated catheters, minimal manipulation of the closed system, sterile dressings, and early weaning.[47–49]

3. *Catheter-related complications*: Obstruction of the catheter due to blood clots/cellular debris or tube kinking may occur. Catheter adjustment or irrigation with a small volume of sterile isotonic saline under aseptic conditions may help restore the patency.[50] Catheter malfunction may warrant change of the entire system.

CONCLUSION

EVD catheters are a relatively safe and reliable method of ICP monitoring and ventricular decompression. Institutional EVD management bundles can help to improve the care and outcome of patients by reducing ventriculostomy-related infection rates to a minimum. Current guidelines strongly support thromboembolism prophylaxis and antibiotic-impregnated catheters in these patients. Finally, good and accountable nursing care is the harbinger of better outcomes in patients with EVDs.

REFERENCES

1. Bratton SL, Chestnut RM, Ghajar J et al. Guidelines for the management of severe traumatic brain injury. VII. Intracranial pressure monitoring technology. *J Neurotrauma.* 2007;24(suppl 1):S45-S54.
2. Chesnut R, Videtta W, Vespa P, Le Roux P. Participants in the International Multidisciplinary Consensus Conference on Multimodality Monitoring. Intracranial pressure monitoring: Fundamental considerations and rationale for monitoring. *Neurocrit Care.* 2014;21(suppl 2): S64-S84.
3. Dey M, Jaffe J, Stadnik A, Awad IA. External ventricular drainage for intraventricular hemorrhage. *Curr Neurol Neurosci Rep.* 2012;12 (1):24-33.
4. Herrick DB, Ullman N, Nekoovaght-Tak S et al. Determinants of external ventricular drain placement and associated outcomes in patients with spontaneous intraventricular hemorrhage. *Neurocrit Care.* 2014;21(3): 426-434.
5. Lovasik BP, McCracken DJ, McCracken CE et al. The effect of external ventricular drain use in intracerebral hemorrhage. *World Neurosurg.* 2016;94:309-318.
6. Ziai WC, Tuhrim S, Lane K et al. A multicenter, randomized, double-blinded, placebo-controlled phase III study of Clot Lysis Evaluation of Accelerated Resolution of Intraventricular Hemorrhage (CLEAR III). *Int J Stroke.* 2014;9(4):536-542.
7. Gigante P, Hwang BY, Appelboom G et al. External ventricular drainage following aneurysmal subarachnoid haemorrhage. *Br J Neurosurg.* 2010;24(6):625-632.
8. Fountas KN, Kapsalaki EZ, Machinis T et al. Review of the literature regarding the relationship of rebleeding and external ventricular drainage in patients with subarachnoid hemorrhage of aneurysmal origin. *Neurosurg Rev.* 2006;29(1):14-18.
9. Zhu X. The hemorrhage risk of prophylactic external ventricular drain insertion in aneurysmal subarachnoid hemorrhage patients requiring endovascular aneurysm treatment:

A systematic review and meta-analysis. *J Neurosurg Sci.* 2017;61(1):53-63.

10. Wijdicks EF, Sheth KN, Carter BS et al. Recommendations for the management of cerebral and cerebellar infarction with swelling: A statement for healthcare professionals from the American Heart Association/American Stroke Association. *Stroke.* 2014; 45(4):1222-1238.

11. Glimåker M, Johansson B, Halldorsdottir H et al. Neuro-intensive treatment targeting intracranial hypertension improves outcome in severe bacterial meningitis: An intervention-control study. *PLoS One.* 2014;9(3):e91976.

12. Wen DY, Bottini AG, Hall WA, Haines SJ. Infections in neurologic surgery. The intraventricular use of antibiotics. *Neurosurg Clin N Am.* 1992;3(2):343-354.

13. Bayston R, Hart CA, Barnicoat M. Intraventricular vancomycin in the treatment of ventriculitis associated with cerebrospinal fluid shunting and drainage. *J Neurol Neurosurg Psychiatry.* 1987;50(11):1419-1423.

14. Tangden T, Enblad P, Ullberg M, Sjolin J. Neurosurgical gram-negative bacillary ventriculitis and meningitis: A retrospective study evaluating the efficacy of intraventricular gentamicin therapy in 31 consecutive cases. *Clin Infect Dis.* 2011;52(11):1310-1316.

15. Wang JH, Lin PC, Chou CH et al. Intraventricular antimicrobial therapy in postneurosurgical gram-negative bacillary meningitis or ventriculitis: A hospital-based retrospective study. *J Microbiol Immunol Infect.* 2014; 47(3):204-210.

16. Karaiskos I, Galani L, Baziaka F, Giamarellou H. Intraventricular and intrathecal colistin as the last therapeutic resort for the treatment of multidrug-resistant and extensively drug-resistant *Acinetobacter baumannii* ventriculitis and meningitis: A literature review. *Int J Antimicrob Agents.* 2013;41(6): 499-508.

17. Fotakopoulos G, Makris D, Chatzi M et al. Outcomes in meningitis/ventriculitis treated with intravenous or intraventricular plus intravenous colistin. *Acta Neurochir (Wien).* 2016;158(3):603-610.

18. De Bonis P, Lofrese G, Scoppettuolo G et al. Intraventricular versus intravenous colistin for the treatment of extensively drug resistant *Acinetobacter baumannii* meningitis. *Eur J Neurol.* 2016;23(1):68-75.

19. Rappaport ZH, Shalit MN. Perioperative external ventricular drainage in obstructive hydrocephalus secondary to infratentorial brain tumours. *Acta Neurochir.* 1989;96(3–4):118-121.

20. Huyette DR, Turnbow BJ, Kaufman C et al. Accuracy of the freehand pass technique for ventriculostomy catheter placement: Retrospective assessment using computed tomography scans. *J Neurosurg.* 2008;108 (1):88-91.

21. Muirhead WR, Basu S. Trajectories for frontal external ventricular drain placement: Virtual cannulation of adults with acute hydrocephalus. *Br J Neurosurg.* 2012;26(5):710-716.

22. Kirkman MA, Muirhead W, Sevdalis N. The relative efficacy of 3 different freehand frontal ventriculostomy trajectories: A prospective neuronavigation-assisted simulation study. *J Neurosurg.* 2017;126(1):304-311.

23. Krötz M, Linsenmaier U, Kanz KG et al. Evaluation of minimally invasive percutaneous CT controlled ventriculostomy in patients with severe head trauma. *Eur Radiol.* 2004;14(2):227-233.

24. Mahan M, Spetzler RF, Nakaji P. Electromagnetic stereotactic navigation for external ventricular drain placement in the intensive care unit. *J Clin Neurosci.* 2013;20(12):1718-1722.

25. Greenfield JP, Schwartz TH. Catheter placement for Ommaya reservoirs with frameless surgical navigation: Technical note. *Stereotact Funct Neurosurg.* 2008;86(2):101-105.

26. Crowley RW, Dumont AS, Asthagiri AR et al. Intraoperative ultrasound guidance for the placement of permanent ventricular cerebrospinal fluid shunt catheters: A single-center historical cohort study. *World Neurosurg.* 2014;81(2):397-403.

27. Banerjee PP, Luciano CJ, Lemole GM, Jr, Charbel FT, Oh MY. Accuracy of ventriculostomy catheter placement using a head and hand-tracked high-resolution virtual reality simulator with haptic feedback. *J Neurosurg.* 2007;107(3):515-521.

28. Bisnaire D, Robinson L. Accuracy of levelling intraventricular collection drainage systems. *J Neurosci Nurs.* 1997;29(4):261-268.

29. Hunn BH, Mujic A, Sher I et al. Successful treatment of negative pressure hydrocephalus using timely titrated external ventricular drainage: A case series. *Clin Neurol Neurosurg.* 2014;116:67-71.

30. Miller C, Tummala RP. Risk factors for hemorrhage associated with external ventricular drain placement and removal. *J Neurosurg.* 2017;126(1):289-297.

31. Gardner PA, Engh J, Atteberry D, Moossy JJ. Hemorrhage rates after external ventricular drain placement. *J Neurosurg.* 2009;110 (5):1021-1025.

32. Lele AV, Hoefnagel AL, Schloemerkemper N et al. Perioperative management of adult patients with external ventricular and lumbar drains: Guidelines from the Society for Neuroscience in Anesthesiology and Critical Care. *J Neurosurg Anesthesiol.* 2017;29 (3):191-210.

33. Tanweer O, Boah A, Huang PP. Risks for hemorrhagic complications after placement of external ventricular drains with early chemical prophylaxis against venous thromboembolisms. *J Neurosurg.* 2013;119(5): 1309-1313.

34. Lozier AP, Sciacca RR, Romagnoli MF, Connolli ES, Jr. Ventriculostomy-related infections: A critical review of the literature. *Neurosurgery.* 2008;62(suppl 2):688-700.

35. Camacho EF, Boszczowski I, Basso M et al. Infection rate and risk factors associated with infections related to external ventricular drain. *Infection.* 2011;39(1):47-51.

36. Kim JH, Desai NS, Ricci J et al. Factors contributing to ventriculostomy infection. *World Neurosurg.* 2012;77(1):135-140.

37. Fried HI, Nathan BR, Rowe AS et al. The insertion and management of external ventricular drains: An evidence-based consensus statement: A statement for healthcare professionals from the Neurocritical Care Society. *Neurocrit Care.* 2016;24(1):61-81.

38. Chi H, Chang KY, Chang HC, Chiu NC, Huang FY. Infections associated with indwelling ventriculostomy catheters in a

teaching hospital. *Int J Infect Dis.* 2010;14(3): e216–e219.

39. Lo CH, Spelman D, Bailey M et al. External ventricular drain infections are independent of drain duration: An argument against elective revision. *J Neurosurg.* 2007;106:378-383.

40. Dellit TH, Chan JD, Fulton C et al. Reduction in *Clostridium difficile* infections among neurosurgical patients associated with discontinuation of antimicrobial prophylaxis for the duration of external ventricular drain placement. *Infect Control Hosp Epidemiol.* 2014;35(5):589-590.

41. Saini NS, Dewan Y, Grewal SS. Efficacy of periprocedural vs extended use of antibiotics in patients with external ventricular drains— A randomized trial. *Indian J Neurotrauma.* 2012;9:30-32.

42. Zabramski J, Whiting D, Darouiche R et al. Efficacy of antimicrobial-impregnated external ventricular drain catheters: A prospective, randomized, controlled trial. *J Neurosurg.* 2003;98(4):725-730.

43. Pople I, Poon W, Assaker R et al. Comparison of infection rate with the use of antibiotic-impregnated vs standard extraventricular drainage devices: A prospective, randomized controlled trial. *Neurosurgery.* 2012;71 (1):6-13.

44. Muttaiyah S, Ritchie S, John S, Mee E, Roberts S. Efficacy of antibiotic-impregnated external ventricular drain catheters. *J Clin Neurosci.* 2010;17(3):296-298.

45. Williams TA, Leslie GD, Dobb GJ, Roberts B, van Heerden PV. Decrease in proven ventriculitis by reducing the frequency of cerebrospinal fluid sampling from extraventricular drains. *J Neurosurg.* 2011;115(5): 1040-1046.

46. Williamson RA, Phillips-Bute BG, McDonagh DL et al. Predictors of extraventricular drain-associated bacterial ventriculitis. *J Crit Care.* 2014;29(1):77-82.

47. Harrop JS, Sharan AD, Ratliff J et al. Impact of a standardized protocol and antibiotic-impregnated catheteis on ventriculostomy

infection rates in cerebrovascular patients. *Neurosurgery.* 2010;67(1):187-191.

48. Dasic D, Hanna SJ, Bojanic S, Kerr RS. External ventricular drain infection: The effect of a strict protocol on infection rates and a review of the literature. *Br J Neurosurg.* 2006;20(5):296-300.

49. Leverstein-van Hall MA, Hopmans TE, van der Sprenkel JW et al. A bundle approach to reduce the incidence of external ventricular and lumbar drain-related infections. *J Neurosurg.* 2010;112(2):345-353.

50. Muralidharan R. External ventricular drains: Management and complications. *Surg Neurol Int.* 2015;6(suppl 6):S271-S274.

40

Lumbar drain

KIRAN JANGRA

INTRODUCTION

Lumbar drain insertion is the procedure of placement of a small flexible catheter in the lumbar subarachnoid space to either drain cerebrospinal fluid (CSF) or to monitor CSF pressure. It is considered as one of the commonly performed procedure in neurosurgical patients. Anesthesia providers might have a limited experience in managing the patients with lumbar drain. Mismanagement of lumbar drain and lack of vigilance can lead to catastrophe. This chapter describes in brief about the procedure, commonly encountered problems related to it, and recent guidelines to manage the patients with lumbar drain.

APPLIED ANATOMY (FIGURE 40.1)

The spinal cord is a continuation of the brainstem proximally that terminates in conus medullaris distally. The meninges covering the brain are continued with spinal cord, including (from inside to outside) pia mater, arachnoid mater, and duramater. The CSF runs in the space between the pia mater and the arachnoid mater, known as the subarachnoid (or intrathecal) space.[1] In young children, it terminates at the upper border of L3 vertebral body, whereas in adults it terminates at the upper border of L2 or the lower border of L1 vertebra. This is due to the differential growth rates of bony vertebral canal and spinal cord. As the spinal cord falls short of the vertebral column, lower lumbar and sacral nerve roots traverse the spinal canal below the level of spinal cord as cauda equina. The dural sac extends beyond the spinal cord till the S2 vertebral body. The meninges extend from conus medullaris as the filum terminale (fibrous extension) till coccyx. The subarachnoid space is approached between L2–S1 intervertebral spaces to avoid injury to the spinal cord.

Planes between the surface of the skin and subarachnoid space

To approach the subarachnoid space, the needle penetrates through the skin, subcutaneous tissue, supraspinous ligament, interspinous ligament, ligamentum flavum, duramater, and arachnoid (Figure 40.1). Supraspinous ligament attaches the tip of each spinous process. Interspinous ligament runs in between the spinous processes. The ligamentum flavum runs in between the vertebral lamina inside the vertebral canal and forms the roof of the vertebral canal.

Anatomic landmarks

The most important landmark is the line joining the highest points of iliac crests (intercristine or Tuffier's line; Figure 40.2). It corresponds to the L4/L5 interspinous space or L4 spinous process. The vertebral spaces can also be counted down from the C-7 vertebral spine, which is the most prominent cervical spine, or line joining the tips of scapulae that lies at the level of D-7 vertebra. Any of these landmarks may be used to identify the vertebral spaces to localize the L2–S1 intervertebral spaces.

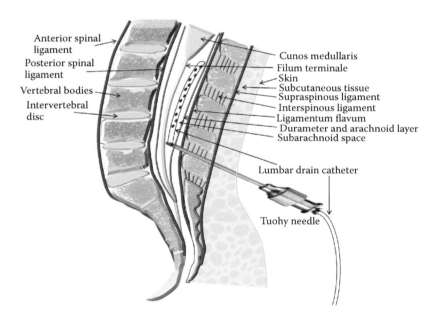

Figure 40.1 Diagrammatic representation of anatomy of spinal cord.

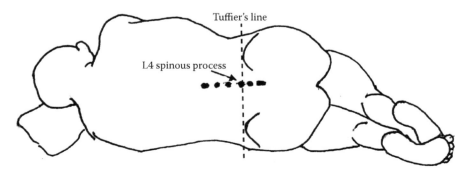

Figure 40.2 External landmarks for insertion site.

INDICATIONS OF LUMBAR DRAIN PLACEMENT

There are diverse indications of inserting lumbar drain in neurologic, neurosurgical, and nonneurosurgical patients. Table 40.1 enumerates various indications for the insertion of lumbar drain.

CONTRAINDICATIONS

1. Thrombocytopenia, platelet count <50,000/mm^3.[2]
2. Patients receiving anticoagulants or who are known to have a bleeding diathesis.
3. Infection present at the insertion site, including skin, subcutaneous tissue, bone, or epidural space.

Table 40.1 Indications for lumbar drain insertion

I. To control ICP
Acute hydrocephalus in SAH[3]/IVH/infection/
   perioperatively

II. Spinal cord protection in high risk surgeries
Thoracoabdominal aortic surgery[4–8]

III. Active CSF leak
Otorrhea
Rhinorrhea[9]
Where CSF leak is anticipated in postoperative
   period:
   During skull base procedures[10–12]
   Spinal surgeries

IV. Facilitate intraoperative brain relaxation by
   decreasing intracranial brain volume
Skull base surgeries[13]
Transcranial pituitary resection
Aneurysm surgery

V. Facilitate trans-sphenoidal pituitary resection
   by increasing the intracranial brain volume by
   injecting the saline or air through lumbar drain
   to push the suprasellar component in the salla

VI. Facilitate monitoring of intracranial pressure
Evaluation of normal pressure hydrocephalus

VII. Access for intrathecal medication adminis-
   tration and/or CSF sampling

Abbreviations: CSF: Cerebrospinal fluid; ICP: intracranial
   pressure; IVH: intraventricular hemorrhage;
   SAH: subarachnoid hemorrhage.

4. If trained personnel are not available to supervise monitoring and drainage on a 24 hour-a-day basis.
5. High rostral-caudal CSF pressure gradient, patients with noncommunicating hydrocephalus such as in the presence of large intracranial mass lesions, tumors, hematomas, or cysts.

EQUIPMENT

Equipment to maintain sterility: Sterile drape, gloves, gown, mask, sterile cap, cleaning agents such as betadine or chlorhexidine

Pressure monitoring equipment: Column-type manometer or fluid-filled pressure transducer system

CSF drainage set including (Figures 40.3 and 40.4):

- 14 G Tuohy needle (with a curved end, cutting bevel, stylet)
- Guidewire to facilitate the intrathecal catheter by stiffening it
- 16-gauge silicone catheter (the catheter is made from kink resistant, translucent silicone elastomer tubing)
- Luer-lock connector to be attached at the end of the catheter
- Collection bag for CSF

PREPROCEDURE PREPARATION

A detailed preanesthetic evaluation of the patient is mandatory. The components of preoperative assessment including history, physical evaluation, laboratory investigations, and imaging are described in Table 40.2.[14]

Written informed consent must be obtained. Adequate intravenous access should be secured and monitoring including pulse oximetry, noninvasive blood pressure, and electrocardiogram should be initiated. Sterile packs containing fenestrated drapes, swabs and towels, syringes, needles, sterilizing solution, and local anesthetic for skin infiltration should be used. Lumbar drain set should be opened under aseptic conditions. A variety of cleansing solutions are used such as chlorhexidineor alcohol and iodine solutions. Chlorhexidine with alcohol is an effective solution as a skin disinfectant,

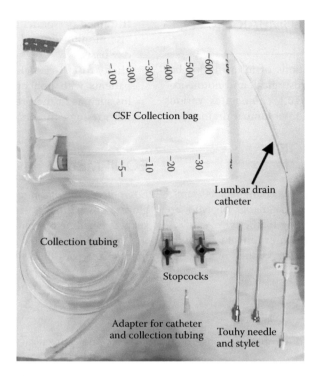

Figure 40.3 Lumbar drain kit and collection system.

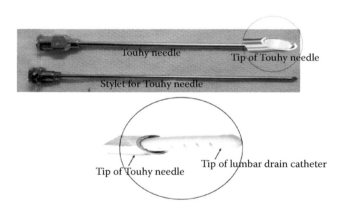

Figure 40.4 Touhy needle and epidural catheter.

but should be allowed to dry completely before skin puncture as it is neurotoxic.[15]

TECHNIQUE OF INSERTION

It is inserted at bedside, in the operation theater, or in the radiology suite. There are two techniques described in the literature—blind and fluoroscopic or computer tomography guided.

Step 1: Positioning

Patients are placed in a lateral (preferable) decubitus position with back parallel to the edge of the operating table, thighs flexed onto the abdomen, and

Table 40.2 Preprocedural evaluation for lumbar drain insertion

History
- To evaluate the need of placement such as intracranial pathologies or aortic aneurysm and others (Table 40.1)
- Medications: Anticoagulants, antiplatelets
- Other systemic diseases affecting coagulation such as hematological disorders, malignancies, and hepatic diseases
- History of prior spine surgery

Physical examination
- Focused neurologic examination
- Vital signs: To evaluate MAP and CPP
- Local site inspection to rule out any infection
- Spine examination to assess the obvious deformity and other anticipated difficulties for lumbar space access

Laboratory examinations
- Complete hemogram with platelet counts
- Coagulation profile

Imaging
- CT or MRI (optional, depending upon indication) to rule out obstructive hydrocephalous

Abbreviations: CPP: Cerebral perfusion pressure; CT: computed tomography; MAP: mean arterial pressure; MRI: magnetic resonance imaging.

neck flexed to allow the forehead to be as close as possible to the knees in an attempt to "open up" the vertebral spaces. The success of midline approach lies on the ability of patients and assistants to minimize lumbarlordosis.

Landmarks

The intercristal line is drawn between the highest points of the two iliac crests, which traditionally corresponds to the level of the L4 vertebral body or the L4–L5 interspace.[1] For inserting the lumbar drain catheter, L3–L4, L4–L5, or L5–S1 interspace is chosen.

Step 2: Techniques of needle insertion

After appropriate space has been chosen, a subcutaneous skin wheal of local anesthetic is raised over this space.

During a blind midline technique, the needle bevel is kept parallel to the midline and is advanced slowly with the sense of tissue planes traversed until the characteristic change in resistance is felt as the needle passes through the ligamentum flavum and dura. After piercing the dura, there is often a slight "click" or "pop" sensation. The stylet is then removed and CSF should drain freely through the needle hub.

The paramedian approach may be useful in patients with diffuse calcification of the interspinous ligament. The needle is inserted 1 cm lateral and 1 cm caudad to the corresponding spinous process at 10–15 degrees off the sagittal plane in a cephalomedial plane. The feel of the ligaments and dura is possible (similar to the midline approach), but only once when the ligamentum flavum is reached, as the needle is not passing through the supraspinous and interspinous ligaments.

During the fluoroscopy-guided technique, the patient is positioned on a radiolucent operating table and the puncture site confirmed using a standard angiography system with a rotatable C-arm. Positioning, landmarks, and skin preparation is done in a similar way as during the blind technique. Once CSF is encountered, contrast media is infused to confirm access to the subarachnoid space after removing the stylet. Diffuse spreading of the contrast media is observed after a successful puncture. An irregularly shaped contrast pattern is observed if the needle is in the epidural space and a typical "railroad track appearance" is seen if the needle is in the subdural space.[16] This technique is useful in situations where CSF is flowing through the Tuohy needle, but the catheter negotiation is a problem. This scenario is encountered when needle bevel is partially inside the intrathecal space and partially in the epidural space.[17]

After the placement of needle in the CSF space, it is vital to minimize the CSF leak even in patients with normal ICP.

Step 3: Insertion of catheter

The Tuohy needle is now rotated to orient the bevel in the cranial direction, and the catheter is advanced 5–8 cm past the needle into the subarachnoid space.[14] The stylet is removed once an appropriate depth is inserted. If there is resistance in inserting the catheter, it should be withdrawn along with the needle to avoid shearing the catheter. If the resistance is encountered while removing the stylet, full flexion position is made to open the spaces that allow the smooth removal of the stylet. The catheter should be secured on the skin or tunneled in the subcutaneous track and should be covered with clear dressings that allows the inspection of the underling insertion site. The CSF drainage kit is assembled as a closed collection system. The monitoring system should not be connected to the pressure flush system and should ensure a continuous fluid column in the collection and monitoring system. Stopcocks should be kept closed to prevent unplanned CSF drainage. **In traumatic insertions, anticoagulants should be initiated only after 24 hours**.

Protocols for CSF drainage from the lumbar drain

Depending on the patient's condition, it is advisable to drain the CSF at not more than 10–20 mL/ hour to avoid the complications related to over-drainage.[18] If the CSF pressure is persistently elevated despite draining a significant amount of CSF, the drainage system should be assessed for kinking or blockage and the transducer should be rezeroed.

POSTPROCEDURE CARE

Keep the insertion site dry and covered with transparent sterile dressing. Inspect daily for infection and/or CSF leakage around the catheter. Box 40.1 enumerates the various points to be assessed periodically after placement of lumbar drain. Box 40.2 enumerates a few common problems encountered during the routine use of lumbar drain catheter. The catheter should be removed using a slow and steady pull, as an improper technique can break the catheter and fragments may be retained within the subarachnoid space. If there is a significant resistance, the catheter should not be pulled. To overcome this problem, the patient should be placed in a curl-up (flexion) position that opens up the vertebral interspaces and facilitates the catheter removal. If the catheter breaks while pulling it, a CT scan of the spine should be performed to determine the track and location of the retained fragments. The decision to remove the retained fragments should be individualized.[19]

BOX 40.1 Checklist after the insertion of lumbar drain

- Integrity of drainage system
- Insertion site assessment through the clear dressing for signs of infection or CSF leaks
    - Avoidance of activities that promote "bearing down" is crucial to prevent recurrent leakage
- Motor/sensory examination for injuries for neuronal structures
- Neurological examination of CSF leak to rule out complications secondary to overdrainage
- Vital signs
    - As multimodal tools for targeting appropriate CPP of brain and spinal cord
    - Early warning signs for impending neurological complications
- Drain function: Rule out obstruction/ overdrainage
- Evaluate medications such as anticoagulants
- All staff members should be aware that lumbar CSF drainage is in use
    - Report changes in assessment findings

BOX 40.2 Lumbar drain troubleshoot

- Not draining enough CSF: reposition patient, check tubings for kinks
    - If no change: lower collection chamber, raise bed
    - If no change: notify the appropriate provider as system may need to be flushed
    - Flush toward drainage system first, patient last
- Draining too much CSF: raise collection chamber, use volume limiting drainage system
- Radicular pain: steroids, gabapentin, slower drainage
- Neurologic change: CT scan/MRI, possible removal of drain
- Fever/confusion: evaluate for infection, check insertion site, look for meningeal signs

SPECIAL SCENARIO PLACEMENT OF LD IN PATIENTS REQUIRING SYSTEMIC ANTICOAGULATION

It is safe to insert lumbar drain during surgeries requiring subsequent systemic heparinization.[20,21] The risk of neuraxial hematoma and neurologic injuries are rare and can be further lowered by following certain guidelines such as delaying surgery for 24 hours in the event of a traumatic instrumentation or bloody tap, heparinization should be delayed for more than 60 minutes after catheter insertion, and anticoagulation should be tightly controlled perioperatively.[22] American Society of Regional Anesthesia and Pain Medicine (ASRA) has provided guidelines for the neuraxial blockade in patients with anticoagulants and antiplatelets.[23] These guidelines should be followed while inserting lumbar drain also, as the violation of these guidelines increases the risk of neuraxial hematoma formation.[24] Adequate reversal of coagulopathy and optimum surgical hemostasis should be assured prior to the removal of the lumbar drain.[23]

COMPLICATIONS/PROBLEMS

Complications of lumbar CSF drainage include those related to lumbar puncture, the presence of an indwelling catheter, and the drainage of CSF (Box 40.3). Out of these complications, hematoma formation, infection, and overdrainage are the most serious.

BOX 40.3 Complications of lumbar drain placement

Related to Lumbar Puncture

- Neural injury
- Neuraxial hematoma

Related to Indwelling Catheter

- Infections
- Fracture of catheters with retained fragment of catheter
- Occlusion and malfunction
- Malposition

Related to Drainage of CSF

- Subdural or epidural or intracerebral hemorrhage
- Rebleeding from ruptured intracranial aneurysm
- Cerebral tonsillar herniation
- Paradoxical herniation
- Pneumocephalus
- Postdural puncture headache

Complications related to lumbar puncture

There are various reports of direct spinal cord trauma or nerve root injuries after needle placement in the subarachnoid space.[25–27] These complications can be minimized by choosing the lower lumbar spine from L3–L5 for lumbar drain insertion.

One of the dreaded complications of needle insertion in the lumbar space is neuraxial hematoma formation. Incidence varies from 0% to 3.2% and might increase up to 50% in traumatic instrumentation.[27,28] A bloody tap through the catheter is an insensitive marker for epidural hematoma formation as blood in the epidural space does not communicate with the subarachnoid space.[27] Careful assessment of neurologic examination will help in early recognition and timely management. The most important risk factor for hematoma formation is deranged coagulation or platelet functions. A larger needle (14-gauge Tuohy for lumbar drain) also adds on to the risk of bleeding. To prevent this complication, a detailed preoperative assessment and optimization is advised.

Complications related to indwelling catheter

After a lumbar drain insertion, infections are the most feared complication, with incidence varying from 0% to 50%.[25,29–31] Factors that increase the risk of infections include catheter placement and handling under nonsterile conditions, nontunneled catheters, intraventricular hemorrhage, repeated sampling and irrigation of catheters, and longer duration of indwelling catheter.[31] These infections can be minimized by strict adherence to the aseptic techniques such as cleansing the insertion site using an antimicrobial agent, using sterile dressing as a part of a management bundle, using antimicrobial-impregnated catheters, avoiding routine CSF sampling, and limited manipulation of the CSF collecting system.[14]

There are no guidelines or consensus statements regarding periprocedural administration of antibiotics prior to lumbar drain placement, but guidelines for EVD placement are being followed for lumbar drain insertion also. These guidelines state that routine use of antibiotic prophylaxis is not recommended.[32]

Complications related to drainage of CSF

Rapid drainage of large volumes of CSF leads to the collapse of ventricles causing shrinking of cerebral hemispheres away from the skull and dura. This leads to rupture of bridging veins and can cause acute subdural hematomas, intraventricular or intracerebral hemorrhage.[33] If the patient has an unsecured intracranial aneurysm, rapid drainage of CSF while the dura is closed can cause acute rise in transmural pressure of the aneurysm and provoke rebleeding.[34] Overdrainage might occur with the change of posture such as in a head-up position or if the drainage bag hangs down much below the insertion point.[35] If blood starts mixing in the CSF, it should raise the suspicion of intracranial hemorrhage. In such a situation, a quick neurologic assessment is done. If there is a change in neurologic status, urgent imaging (CT/MRI) should be done.

The devastating complication of CSF drainage is herniation,[36–38] which is more common when there is pressure gradient between intracranial and spinal CSF, and in patients with raised intracranial pressure.[39] It causes cranial nerve palsies, bradycardia or hypertension,[40] and might also cause brainstem hemorrhage.[41] This complication can often be managed by placing the patient in a Trendelenburg position.[42] Injection of sterile isotonic saline solution through the lumbar drain can also be used as an emergency measure. In patients with decompressive hemicraniectomy, there is a risk of paradoxic herniation after lumbar drainage of the CSF. In these patients, even smaller decreases in CSF pressure can cause a significant brain sag and herniation ("trephined syndrome").[43,44] Other complications, such as tension pneumocephalus and subdural hematoma from brain sag, are also described in the literature after lumbar drains placement.[45,46]

Post-dural puncture headache may develop with catheter in situ or after removal of the catheter. This headache is worse while sitting or standing, but gets relieved in a supine position. If the catheter is in place, then fluid drain can be occluded for a few minutes, which usually alleviates the headache. If headache develops after the tube is removed, drinking plenty of water and analgesics such as acetaminophen and caffeine-containing drinks might alleviate the headache.[20,47] In severe cases, epidural blood patch can be tried to seal the CSF leak.

GUIDELINES FOR PERIOPERATIVE MANAGEMENT OF PATIENTS WITH LUMBAR DRAIN

The Society for Neuroscience in Anesthesiology & Critical Care (SNACC) has generated the evidence-based guidelines for clinicians involved in the management of perioperative care of patients with indwelling external ventricular catheter and lumbar drains (Table 40.3).

Table 40.3 Summary of guidelines for perioperative management of the external ventricular and lumbar drain

Parameters discussed	Guidelines or consensus statements/level of recommendation
Prevention of hemorrhagic and infectious complications associated with EVD and LD	Prompt diagnosis and correction of coagulopathy prior to insertion ***Class I Recommendation; Level of Evidence E*** Perioperative anticoagulation management should be performed within the framework of the current ASRA guidelines ***Class I Recommendation; Level of Evidence E*** Antibiotics should only be administered prior to placement of an EVD and LD, with the choice based on institutional practice ***Class I Recommendation; Level of Evidence E*** Strict aseptic technique is recommended for insertion and handling based on national and institutional guidelines ***Class I Recommendation; Level of Evidence E***
Preoperative evaluation of patient with EVD and LD	A thorough preoperative evaluation should be performed in all patients with an indwelling EVD and LD ***Class I Recommendation; Level of Evidence E*** Preoperative evaluation should include: a. CSF color and consistency b. ICP values, ICP trends, autoregulation indices, and relationship with CPP and other multimodal monitoring data c. Clinical (worsening headache, depressed level of consciousness, cranial nerve deficits, ICP elevation) and radiographic evidence of clamp trial tolerance (worsening hydrocephalus) ***Class I Recommendation; Level of Evidence E*** All information pertinent to the EVD and LD should be incorporated into a standardized preoperative handoff ***Class I Recommendation; Level of Evidence E***
Transporting patients with EVD and LD	It is recommended to use a dedicated intravenous pole to mount the transducer and drainage system ***Class I Recommendation; Level of Evidence E*** Do not routinely clamp EVD during intrahospital transport. The decision whether to open or clamp EVD for intrahospital transport should be individualized Factors in pretransport evaluation that may influence decision to travel with EVD open or clamped include: 1. Hourly and daily CSF output and setting of EVD 2. EVD clamp status in the intensive care unit 3. Patient's tolerance to clamping 4. Reason transport is undertaken (diagnostic versus therapeutic procedure) Test tolerance to clamping prior to making clamping decision as patients at high risk for high ICP may benefit from opening of EVD ***Class I Recommendation; Level of Evidence B-NR*** If the EVD is clamped during transport, clamping should be undertaken at two sites: (1) proximal port on the EVD/LD and (2) distal port on the collecting system of EVD/LD ***Class I Recommendation; Level of Evidence E***

(Continued)

Table 40.3 (Continued) Summary of guidelines for perioperative management of the external ventricular and lumbar drain

Parameters discussed	Guidelines or consensus statements/level of recommendation
	Continue all pretransport monitoring, including ICP monitoring and other vital signs including end-tidal carbon dioxide during intrahospital transport *Class I Recommendation; Level of Evidence B-NR*
	Transport personnel should be prepared to treat intracranial hypertension during intrahospital transport *Class I Recommendation; Level of Evidence E*
Intraoperative management of EVD and LD	Anesthesia providers should be knowledgeable about the specific EVD and LD device in use locally as details vary *Class I Recommendation; Level of Evidence E*
	Set up your anesthetizing location following the standards of your institution, including a consistent choice of reference level and measurement scale *Class I Recommendation; Level of Evidence E*
	Level EVD or LD using a carpenter's (bubble) or laser level rather than by visual inspection *Class I Recommendation; Level of Evidence B-NR*
	Close the EVD/LD to drainage during any changes in position if clinically feasible *Class I Recommendation; Level of Evidence C*
	Relevel the transducer after changing patient position *Class I Recommendation; Level of Evidence C*
	Monitor intracranial or intraspinal pressure with an attached transducer that is appropriately leveled and zeroed according to manufacturer guidelines *Class I Recommendation; Level of Evidence E*
	A pressure bag and pressurized flush system should not be attached to the EVD/LD *Class III Recommendation; Level of Evidence E*
	Pressure measurements should not be made while simultaneously draining *Class III Recommendation; Level of Evidence B-NR*
	If open for continuous drainage, it is recommended to close the EVD or LD to measure pressure at least once per hour or more often if clinically indicated *Class I Recommendation; Level of Evidence E*
	The decision for either continuous drainage or continuous monitoring should be made in consultation with the surgical team. Continuous monitoring with intermittent drainage may be considered in patients with aneurysmal SAH and continuous drainage may be considered for adults with severe TBI *Class IIb Recommendation: Level of Evidence B-R*
	It is recommended to document the following information pertinent to EVD and LD on the anesthesia record at least hourly: 1. Pressure = ICP/CPP orintraspinal pressure/spinal cord perfusion pressure 2. Amount of CSF drainage (expressed in mL) 3. Color of CSF and any change in color of CSF observed during the procedure 4. Drain height relative to the reference level

(Continued)

Table 40.3 (Continued) Summary of guidelines for perioperative management of the external ventricular and lumbar drain

Parameters discussed	Guidelines or consensus statements/level of recommendation
	5. EVD/LD status (open or clamped) as set by the stopcocks in the device *Class I Recommendation; Level of Evidence E*
Management of EVD and LD in special clinical scenarios	EVD or LD tubing that is accidently disconnected should be clamped immediately to prevent overdrainage of cerebrospinal fluid *Class I Recommendation; Level of Evidence C*
	If the EVD or LD systems are contaminated by disconnection, all distal parts should be replaced with new sterile tubing *Class IIa Recommendation; Level of Evidence E*
	Routine flushing of the EVD or LD catheter should not be performed *Class III Recommendation; Level of Evidence E*
	In patients with ruptured cerebral aneurysm, sudden excessive drainage of cerebrospinal fluid prior to securing the aneurysm can provoke aneurysm re-rupture and should be avoided *Class III Recommendation; Level of Evidence C*
	Identification of EVD or LD tubing by appropriate labels and use of other visual aids is recommended to prevent confusion with intravenous ports *Class I Recommendation; Level of Evidence E*
	Accidental intrathecal injection should be recognized and reported to the neurosurgeon *Class IIa Recommendation; Level of Evidence E*
	Lavage of the intrathecal space after accidental injection is not recommended *Class III Recommendation; Level of Evidence C*
	Establish institutional standards to ensure safe intrathecal injection of fluorescein dye via lumbar drain in patients with suspected cerebrospinal fluid leak *Class I Level Recommendation; Level of Evidence E*
Perioperative checklist, developing clinical competencies for EVD/LD and continued medical education	Clinicians involved in perioperative care of patients must familiarize themselves with information regarding indications, contraindications, leveling, zeroing of transducer, and current standards related to transporting and intraoperative care of patients with EVD or LD *Class I Recommendation; Level of Evidence E*
	It is reasonable to provide educational material aimed at perioperative management of EVD and LD in the form of text and/or multimedia to all clinicians involved in perioperative care of patients *Class IIa Recommendation; Level of Evidence E*
	To standardize care of patients with EVD and LD, and to promote a shared mental model, use of a perioperative checklist is recommended *Class I Recommendation; Level of Evidence E*
	It is recommended that institutions set up competency standards for clinicians involved in perioperative care of patients with EVD and LD *Class I Recommendation; Level of Evidence E*

Abbreviations: ASRA: American Society of Regional Anesthesia and Pain Medicine; CPP: cerebral perfusion pressure; CSF: cerebrospinal fluid; EVD: external ventricular drain; ICP: intracranial pressure; LD: lumbar drain; SAH: subarachnoid hemorrhage.

REFERENCES

1. Brull R, Macfarlane AJ, Chan VW. Spinal, epidural, and caudal anesthesia. In: Miller RD, Cohen NH, Erikson LI et al., eds. *Miller's Anesthesia*. Philadelphia, PA: Elsevier Saunders; 2015:1684-1720.

2. Smith DS. Lumbar cerebrospinal fluid drain. *Procedures consult (Anaesthesia Speciality)*. ©2014 Elsevier Inc. http://www.procedures consult.com/medical-procedures/lumbar -cerebrospinal-fluid-drain-AN-010-proce dure.aspx. Accessed on June 2017.

3. Connolly ES, Jr., Rabinstein AA, Carhuapoma JR et al. Guidelines for the management of aneurysmal subarachnoid hemorrhage: A guideline for healthcare professionals from the American Heart Association/American Stroke Association. *Stroke*. 2012;43(6):1711-1737.

4. Hiratzka LF, Bakris GL, Beckman JA et al. 2010 ACCF/AHA/AATS/ACR/ASA/SCA/SCAI/SIR /STS/SVM guidelines for the diagnosis and management of patients with thoracic aortic disease: Executive summary: A report of the American College of Cardiology Foundation/ American Heart Association Task Force on Practice Guidelines, American Association for Thoracic Surgery, American College of Radi- ology, American Stroke Association. *Circula- tion*. 2010;121(13):e266-e369.

5. Basauri LT, Concha-Julio E, Selman JM, Cubillos P, Rufs J. Cerebrospinal fluid spinal lumbar drainage: Indications, technical tips, and pitfalls. *Crit Rev. Neurosurg*. 1999;9 (1):21-27.

6. Coselli JS, LeMaire SA, Koksoy C, Schmittling ZC, Curling PE. Cerebrospinal fluid drainage reduces paraplegia after thoracoabdominal aortic aneurysm repair: Results of a random- ized clinical trial. *J Vasc Surg*. 2002;35(4): 631-639.

7. Ling E, Arellano R. Systematic overview of the evidence supporting the use of cerebro- spinal fluid drainage in thoracoabdominal aneurysm surgery for prevention of paraple- gia. *Anesthesiology*. 2000;93(4):1115-1122.

8. Mancio J, Pires-Morais G, Bettencourt N et al. Meningeal haemorrhage secondary to cerebrospinal fluid drainage during thoracic endovascular aortic repair. *Oxf Med Case Reports*. 2014;2014(3):56-59.

9. Albu S, Florian IS, Bolboaca SD. The benefit of early lumbar drain insertion in reducing the length of CSF leak in traumatic rhinorrhea. *Clin Neurol Neurosurg*. 2016;142:43-47.

10. Bell RB, Dierks EJ, Homer L, Potter BE. Management of cerebrospinal fluid leak associated with craniomaxillofacial trauma. *J Oral Maxillofac Surg*. 2004;62(6):676-684.

11. Crowson MG, Cunningham CD, 3rd, Moses H, Zomorodi AR, Kaylie DM. Preoperative lumbar drain use during acoustic neuroma surgery and effect on CSF leak incidence. *Ann Otol Rhinol Laryngol*. 2016;125(1): 63-68.

12. Bakhsheshian J, Hwang MS, Friedman M. What is the evidence for postoperative lumbar drains in endoscopic repair of CSF leaks? *Laryngoscope*. 2015;125(10):2245-2246.

13. Andrews RJ, Bringas JR. A review of brain retraction and recommendations for minimizing intraoperative brain injury. *Neu- rosurgery*. 1993;33(6):1052-1063; discussion 1063.

14. Lele AV, Hoefnagel AL, Schlomerkemper N et al. Perioperative management of adult patients with external ventricular and lumbar drains: Guidelines from the Society for Neu- roscience in Anesthesiology and Critical Care. *J Neurosurg Anesthesiol*. 2017;29 (3):191-210.

15. O'Grady NP, ALexander M, Dellinger EP et al. Guidelines for the prevention of intravas- cular catheter-related infections. *Am J Infect Control*. 2002;30:476-489.

16. Chee CG, Lee GY, Lee JW et al. Fluoroscopy- guided lumbar drainage of cerebrospinal fluid for patients in whom a blind beside approach is difficult. *Korean J Radiol* 2015;16 (4):860-865.

17. Qureshi AL, Khan AA, Malik AA et al. Lumbar catheter placement using paramedian approach under fluoroscopic guidance. *J Vasc Interv Neurol*. 8(5)(5):55-62.

18. Cardillo SM, Bernstein WK. Controversies in the anesthetic management of lumbar drains for aortic surgery. *J Vasc Med Surg*. 2015;3:189.

19. Olivar H, Bramhall JS, Rozet I et al. Subarachnoid lumbar drains: A case series of fractured catheters and a near miss. *Can J Anaesth.* 2007;54(10):829-834.

20. Grady RE, Horlocker TT, Brown RD, Maxson PM, Schroeder DR. Neurologic complications after placement of cerebrospinal fluid drainage catheters and needles in anesthetized patients: Implications for regional anesthesia. Mayo Perioperative Outcomes Group. *Anesth Analges.* 1999;88(2):388-392.

21. Safi HJ, Hess KR, Randel M et al. Cerebrospinal fluid drainage and distal aortic perfusion: Reducing neurologic complications in repair of thoracoabdominal aortic aneurysm types I and II. *J Vasc Surg.* 1996;23(2):223-229.

22. Chaney MA. Intrathecal and epidural anesthesia and analgesia for cardiac surgery. *Anesth Analg.* 2006;102(1):45-64.

23. Horlocker TT, Wedel DJ, Rowlingson JC et al. Regional anesthesia in the patient receiving antithrombotic or thrombolytic therapy: American Society of Regional Anesthesia and Pain Medicine Evidence-Based Guidelines (3rd ed.). *Reg Anesth Pain Med.* 2010;35(1):64-101.

24. Bateman BT, Mhyre JM, Ehrenfeld J et al. The risk and outcomes of epidural hematomas after perioperative and obstetric epidural catheterization: A report from the Multicenter Perioperative Outcomes Group Research Consortium. *Anesth Analg.* 2013;116(6):1380-1385.

25. Estrera AL, Sheinbaum R, Miller CC et al. Cerebrospinal fluid drainage during thoracic aortic repair: Safety and current management. *Ann Thorac Surg.* 2009;88(1):9-15.

26. Puchakalaya MR, Tremper KK. BrownSéquard syndrome following removal of a cerebrospinal fluid drainage catheter after thoracic aortic surgery. *Anesth Analg.* 2005;101(2):322-324.

27. Weaver KD, Wiseman DB, Farber M et al. Complications of lumbar drainage after thoracoabdominal aortic aneurysm repair. *J Vasc Surg.* 2001;34(4):623-627.

28. Vandermeulen EP, Van Aken H, Vermylen J. Anticoagulants and spinal-epidural anesthesia. *Anesth Analg.* 1994;79(6):1165-1177.

29. Scheithauer S, Burgel U, Bickenbach J et al. External ventricular and lumbar drainage-associated meningoventriculitis: Prospective analysis of time-dependent infection rates and risk factor analysis. *Infection.* 2010;38(3):205-209.

30. Grady RE, Horlocker TT, Brown RD, Maxson PM, Schroeder DR. Neurologic complications after placement of cerebrospinal fluid drainage catheters and needles in anesthetized patients: Implications for regional anesthesia. Mayo Perioperative Outcomes Group. *Anesth Analg.* 1999;88(2):388-392.

31. Liang H, Zhang L, Gao A et al. Risk factors for infections related to lumbar drainage in spontaneous subarachnoid hemorrhage. *Neurocrit Care.* 2016;25(2):243-249.

32. Fried HI, Nathan BR, Rowe AS et al. The insertion and management of external ventricular drains: An evidence-based consensus statement: A statement for healthcare professionals from the Neurocritical Care Society. *Neurocrit Care.* 2016;24(1):61-81.

33. Civelek E, Cansever T, Karasu A et al. Chronic subdural hematoma after endoscopic third ventriculostomy: Case report. *Turk Neurosurg.* 2007;17(4):289-293.

34. Fountas KN, Kapsalaki EZ, Machinis T et al. Review of the literature regarding the relationship of rebleeding and external ventricular drainage in patients with subarachnoid hemorrhage of aneurysmal origin. *Neurosurg Rev.* 2006;29(1):14-20.

35. Muraskin SI, Roy RC, Petrozza PH. Overdrainage of cerebrospinal fluid during central venous catheter exchange in a patient with an external ventricular drain. *Anesth Analg.* 2007;105(5):1519-1520.

36. Bloch J, Regli L. Brain stem and cerebellar dysfunction after lumbar spinal fluid drainage: Case report. *J Neurol Neurosurg Psychiatry.* 2003;74(7):992-994.

37. Dagnew E, van Loveren HR, Tew JM, Jr. Acute foramen magnum syndrome caused by an acquired Chiari malformation after lumbar drainage of cerebrospinal fluid: Report of three cases. *Neurosurgery.* 2002;51(3):823-828; discussion 828-829.

38. Manley GT, Dillon W. Acute posterior fossa syndrome following lumbar drainage for treatment of suboccipital pseudomeningocele. Report of three cases. *J Neurosurg.* 2000;92(3):469-474.

39. Borire AA, Hughes AR, Lueck CJ. Tonsillar herniation after lumbar puncture in idiopathic intracranial hypertension. *J Neuroophthalmol.* 2015;35(3):293-295.

40. Komotar RJ, Mocco J, Ransom ER et al. Herniation secondary to critical postcraniotomy cerebrospinal fluid hypovolemia. *Neurosurgery.* 2005;57(2):286-292.

41. Yuan X, Zhao H, Zhao C et al. Duret hemorrhage after lumbar drainage. *J Craniofac Surg.* 2014;25(4):1551-1552.

42. Kawahara I, Tsutsumi K, Matsunaga Y et al. Early awareness of cerebrospinal fluid hypovolemia after craniotomy for microsurgical aneurysmal clipping. *Acta Neurochir.* 2013; 155(8):1543-1548.

43. Fields JD, Lansberg MG, Skirboll SL, Kurien PA, Wijman CA. "Paradoxical" transtentorial herniation due to CSF drainage in the presence of a hemicraniectomy. *Neurology.* 2006;67(8):1513-1514.

44. Zhao J, Li G, Zhang Y, Zhu X, Hou K. Sinking skin flap syndrome and paradoxical herniation secondary to lumbar drainage. *Clin Neurol Neurosurg.* 2015;133:6-10.

45. Saito K, Inamasu J, Kuramae T, Nakatsukasa M, Kawamura F. Tension pneumocephalus as a complication of lumbar drainage for cerebral aneurysm surgery: Case report. *Neurol Med Chir (Tokyo).* 2009;49(6):252-254.

46. Tan VE, Liew D. A case of chronic subdural hematoma following lumbar drainage for the management of iatrogenic cerebrospinal fluid rhinorrhea: Pitfalls and lessons. *Ear Nose Throat J.* 2013;92(10-11):513-515.

47. McLeod AD, Hirsch NP, Scrutton MJ. Neurologic complications of cerebrospinal fluid drainage catheters. *Anesth Analg.* 2000;90(1):228-229.

41

Cranial burr hole

SRILATA MONINGI

INTRODUCTION

Burr hole or trephination is the basic neurosurgical intervention to access the cranial cavity for various anatomical targets and pathologies. As of date, burr holes are the first step for cranial flap for any craniotomy/craniectomy. The placement of a burr hole on the skull takes into consideration important factors like the site of the surgical pathology, surgical approach, skull anatomy, and nearby vascular structures.

APPLIED ANATOMY/PHYSIOLOGY

Anatomy of the scalp, cranial bone, and of the meninges is important for understanding the steps involved in the creation of a burr hole. The structures traversed during a burr hole procedure from outside to inside include: skin, subcutaneous tissue containing scalp vessels, galea aponeurotica, loose areolar tissue, pericranium, cranial bone, and dural meninges.[1] Each layer with its own implications is described in Table 41.1.

The flat calvarial cranium bone formed by membranous ossification has three layers: the inner table and outer table with a diploic space interposed between the two tables. First, both tables are made up of compact cancellous bone, whereas the diploic space is made up of spongy bone. Second, the diploic space is aerated at places forming air sinuses and at places it is absent like in suture lines. It contains diploic veins, which communicate with the extracalvarial emissary veins. Bleeding from diploic vessels may arise at the time of traversing the skull bone during burr hole surgery. And, opening of diploic veins communicating to the major venous sinuses may lead to air embolism.[2]

Indications: It has varied applications both for diagnostic and therapeutic purposes, and as a simple burr hole or as a preliminary step to major craniotomy/craniectomy.[3,4]

A. Simple burr hole
   a. Diagnostic
      i. Placement of intracranial pressure (ICP) monitor: Continuous monitoring of ICP[5]
      ii. Brain biopsy (either with frame or frameless stereotaxy or by landmark approach)[6]
   b. Therapeutic
      i. Drainage of brain abscess or intracranial hematoma (subdural/extradural/intraparenchymal)[7,8]
      ii. Drainage of CSF (ventricular drain or shunt procedures or endoscopic third ventriculostomy)[9-11]
      iii. For growth of granulation tissue in cases with extensive scalp loss due to trauma[12]

Table 41.1 Structures traversed during burr hole procedure with applied aspects

Layers of scalp	Implications	Applications
Skin	Painful structure	Local infiltration anesthesia/regional nerve block/ multimodal analgesia.
Subcutaneous tissue	Contains scalp vessels and free nerve endings	Infiltration of this layer with local anesthetics and vaso-spastic agents takes care of analgesia and bleeding.
Galea aponeurotica	Tough structure	Bleeding from the scalp vessels are controlled either by application of Raney clips or by Dandy arterial forceps at the cut margin of the galea and everting it. This helps in compression of the scalp vessels in the connective tissue and controls bleeding. Proper closure of the scalp in two layers prevents cerebrospinal fluid leakage from the wound.[1]
Loose areolar tissue	Area of dissection	Potential space that can be utilized for mobilizing the scalp and for drainage procedures connecting the cranial cavity to the systemic circulation.
Pericranium	Important structure for bone growth	Painful structure and needs to be anesthesized. Can be harvested and used as an autologus, local dural substitute.
Cranial bone: Outer and inner table with inter-posed diploic space	This is perforated or drilled to access the cranial cavity	The varying nature of the tables and diploic space gives a give way feel to the surgeon once the inner table is penetrated at the time of creation of burr hole; air embolism is a rare occurrence.
Meninges	For the traditional burr hole approach, a crisscross cruciate incision of the dural meninges is given	The dural incision should not extend to the edge of the bone; some dura should be left to control bleeding if it occurs.

iv. For elevation of a depressed fragment of skull fracture[13]

v. Deep brain stimulation surgery for electrode placement[14,15]

vi. For access to dural venous sinus for transvenous endovascular procedures like glue or coil embolization[16]

B. Preliminary step to craniotomy/craniectomy: to access intracranial pathologies (brain parenchyma, ventricles, and meninges[4,17,18]

C. Preliminary step to keyhole surgeries and minimally invasive endoscopic procedures[19,20]

Emergency targeted burr hole placement for evacuation of an extra-axial hematoma with GCS <9 by a non-neurosurgeon can be safely accomplished with the help of clutch drill bits.[21,22] The relative contraindication includes lack of imaging facilities. Once the inner table is penetrated, the drill disengages and minimizes the risk of "plunging," making it a safe procedure. Acceptable outcomes were seen when these emergent neurosurgical procedures were performed by non-neurosurgeons.[23,24] Emergent burr holes should be performed by general surgeons or physicians who are formally trained by neurosurgeons and should be performed in places where it is accessible to a neurosurgeon in cases of need.[3]

Stereotaxy and neuronavigation have been successfully used for burr hole evacuation of spontaneous cerebellar hemorrhage, thus avoiding the prolonged operating time of suboccipital craniectomy and its complications.[25] Neuronavigation was used to simulate the site of burr hole for DBS to be performed later in a patient who underwent frontal craniotomy for aneurysm clipping in order to avoid overlapping of the surgical approaches.[26] Thus, it is important for proper planning of the surgical approach in patients with multiple pathologies.

Burr hole procedure in pediatrics: Special precautions should be considered at the time of burr hole procedure in children. In neonates and young infants, the skull thickness rarely exceeds 3 mm and the fontanelles and sutures are open. It is dangerous to use heavy instruments requiring force, like perforators and drill, as the individual bones are not anchored securely to each other.[27]

The delayed development of the frontal sinuses in early childhood dictates careful selection of the target area for burr hole placement. Burr holes near the parasagittal area has important points to ponder: They should be placed in such a way that the medial aspect should border upon the lateral aspect of the superior sagittal sinus (SSS). Cerebral angiography gives a clue about the caliber, number, and the site of entry for bridging cortical veins into the SSS. And, powered instruments to create a burr hole is again avoided even in adolescents, since the clutch-driven perforator is available in adult size only.[27]

The cranial bone is too soft, hence slow and steady movement of the perforator and drill is done to avoid any mishaps. The skin is too thin and is closed in layers with good apposition to prevent cerebrospinal fluid leak.

Contraindications:

1. Active infection at the suggested site of burr hole
2. Coagulopathies

Equipment (Figure 41.1):

1. Sterile drapes
2. Antiseptic solution
3. Scalpel blade for the incision of the scalp
4. Self-retaining retractors/Manual retractors help in bone exposure by keeping the skin margins away
5. Arterial forceps/clips to control bleeding
6. Periosteal elevator
7. Perforator for bone penetration
8. Burr mounted on the Hudson's brace or drill for bone penetration
9. Drill bits of appropriate size; always check for appropriate size drill bits that fit the drill

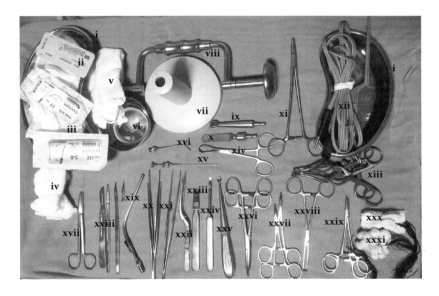

Figure 41.1 Paraphernalia for burr hole procedure. (i) Kidney tray; (ii) bone wax; (iii) sutures; (iv) gauze pieces; (v) swab; (vi) bowl; (vii) sterile light handle; (viii) Hudson's brace; (ix) drill; (x) perforator; (xi) needle holder; (xii) cautery cable with forceps; (xiii) Langenbeck self-retaining retractors; (xiv) towel clip; (xv) brain cannula; (xvi) saline cannula; (xvii) suture cutting scissors; (xviii) scalpel handle with blades; (xix) suction cannula; (xx) toothed forceps; (xxi) straight forceps; (xxii) bayonet; (xxiii) periosteal elevator; (xxiv) Adson dissector and elevator; (xxv) bone scoop/curette; (xxvi) Robert's long curved artery forceps; (xxvii) mosquito curved artery forceps; (xxviii) Allis forceps; (xxix) mosquito straight artery forceps; (xxx) swabs; (xxxi) cottonoids.

10. Bone curette or scoop/blunt hook to remove thin shells of bone
11. Swabs
12. Bipolar diathermy
13. Gel foam/Bone wax
14. Dural hook
15. Scissors for cutting sutures
16. Absorbable suture and monofilament 3–0 silk suture
17. Suction apparatus
18. Drain
19. Normal saline

Preprocedure preparation:

1. Like any other major surgery, preanesthetic checkup with relevant investigations is a must for craniotomy under general anesthesia. Basic investigations, like hemogram and coagulation profile, are required for a simple burr hole placement under local anesthesia.[28]
2. Next is an informed and written consent. The indications of this procedure, steps of procedure, administration of local or general anesthesia, or local with monitored anesthesia care, its complications like hematoma, infection, and meningitis are explained to the patient or patient's relatives, whichever is applicable.[28]
3. The whole head or the specific site of surgery and around it (approximately a strip of 5 cm) is shaved on the day prior to surgery or on the day of surgery.
4. The patient is kept nil orally for at least 6 hours prior to surgery, especially for patients undergoing the procedure under general anesthesia. Patients undergoing emergency burr hole surgery and or under local anesthesia may be shifted to the operation theater without any nil oral protocols.
5. Patients with low GCS are not given any premedication. Normal, healthy, anxious patients may be given short-acting benzodiazepines like alprazolam.
6. All patients are shifted to the operation theater on a trolley.
7. Basic standard monitoring like oxygen saturation by pulse oximetry, heart rate, and noninvasive blood pressure are mandatory for procedures, both under local and general anesthesia. End-tidal carbon dioxide monitoring is an additional mandatory monitoring for patients under general anesthesia and for patients undergoing transvenous interventional procedures. This also helps in early detection of intraoperative air embolism, especially in posterior fossa surgery and surgery around major venous sinuses. Patients with limited cardiorespiratory reserve and requiring general anesthesia would need invasive monitoring like arterial blood pressure and central venous pressure.
8. Prophylactic antibiotics are administered prior to the procedure. Patients with steroid or antiepileptic cover would receive their prophylactic dose before the procedure.

Technique for simple burr hole procedure (Figure 41.2):

Step 1: Proper positioning of the head is planned as per the surgical lesion and approach. Usually, burr holes are preferred on the right side to access ventricles as a majority of them are left hemisphere dominant. There are some important landmark points for placement of burr holes to access the cranial cavity and its ventricles, either via a burr hole or for craniotomy/craniectomy (Table 41.2; Figure 41.3). If hematoma, burr holes are placed over the thickest aspect of hematoma, ideally at the superior temporal line (above the temporalis muscle). Usually, more than one burr hole is done in such cases for proper irrigation of the lesion.

Step 2: The head may be positioned on a horseshoe frame or fixed with skull pins or immobilized with adhesive tapes. The head is elevated to at least 30° C above the level of the heart to avoid venous pooling in the venous sinuses. The head is rotated to the opposite side (as needed) and padding placed under the ipsilateral shoulder to gain access to the frontal, temporal, or parietal area. The patient is placed prone with head flexed, to provide access to posterior fossa or occipital lesions.

Hemodynamic perturbations due to pin insertion would be attenuated with specific nerve blocks of the scalp or local infiltration of the skin at the site of pin insertion. A 0.5% bupivacaine in combination with or without 2% lignocaine is used for administration of the block. Adjuvants like fentanyl and dexmedetomidine are added to prolong the duration of the block.

Step 3: All instruments required for the procedure should be checked for and kept ready.

Step 4: The surgical site is properly cleaned at least twice, povidone iodine/chlorhexidine applied, and draped.

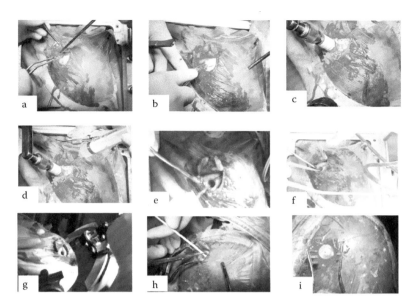

Figure 41.2 Steps of burr hole procedure. (a) Elevation of the scalp flap. (b) Periosteal elevation. (c) Burr hole with Hudson's brace and perforator. (d) Scoop for removal of bony edges. (e) Incision of the dura with scalpel and no. 15 blade. (f) Bipolar cauterization of the dura matter. (g) Placement of DBS needles through the burr hole. (h) Shunt placement via a burr hole. (i) EVD placement via a burr hole.
Abbreviations: DBS: Deep brain stimulation; EVD: External ventricular drain.

Step 5: Local anesthetic solution (2% lignocaine with 1:200,000 adrenaline) is infiltrated into the proposed skin site, size around 3 cm. After 10 minutes, the scalp skin is incised with a No. 15 blade up to the pericranium. Bipolar cautery is used to control skin bleeding. Further, bleeding from the scalp vessels is controlled either with clips or arterial forceps and by everting the galea. The pericranium is separated from the underlying bone and self-retaining retractors are used to expose the bone before creating a burr hole.

Step 6: Initially, a perforator mounted on the Hudson's brace is used to make a hole in the cranium till the inner table is reached. This is indicated by the clinical sense and feeling of "give away" to the surgeon, and he should stop at this point of time. Next, a burr is mounted on the Hudson's brace and is used to widen the opening till the inner table is thinned out and the underlying dura is visible. At this point, the burr is withdrawn and the rest of the left-out bone can be scooped with a bone curette or a blunt hook. On the other hand, if a drill is available, it can be used for both perforating the bone and widening the burr hole. The drill is applied perpendicular to the bone and pushed firmly for drilling. The head should be stabilized by an assistant at the time of drilling and

continuous saline irrigation done as drilling continues. The drilling should not be stopped in between and should be continued till the drill stops spinning once it breaches the inner table. Figure 41.4 depicts the gentle perforation and nibbling of the bone for creating a burr hole in an infant.

Step 7: In cases where the burr hole needs to be enlarged, it is done with Kerisson ronguers.

Step 8: Once the dura is visible, it is cauterized with bipolar cautery before and after placing a cruciate-fashioned incision over it to control bleeding from meningeal vessels. This is done in patients requiring a burr hole for shunt or reservoir placement, stereotactic biopsy, DBS, ETV and key burr hole surgery.

Evacuation of hematoma (in cases of extra-axial hematoma): The depth of hematoma is estimated by counting the number of slices of the hematoma as seen in the computed tomography (CT) scan and multiplying by the slice thickness. Once the dura is separated from the bone, the blood in the extradural hematoma (EDH) is visible and can be gently suctioned out. The subdural hematoma (SDH) appears as a dural tent and blood may be clotted. Here, the dura is lifted with a hook and is incised in a cruciate manner with a No. 11 or No. 15 scalpel blade to drain the hematoma.[22]

Table 41.2 Landmarks for burr hole placement and its applied aspects

Burr hole designation	Approach	Landmarks	Special precautions
Kocher's point	Frontal burr hole	1 cm anterior to the coronal suture and 2 cm lateral to the midline; approximately at the mid pupillary line	This is placed anterior to the coronal suture to avoid any damage to the motor cortex. External ventricular drain is usually placed at this point; the goal is to place the catheter in the frontal horn of the lateral ventricle or third ventricle.
Keen point	Temporal burr hole: The incision penetrates the temporalis muscle that should be scraped off the temporalis bone with the back of the scalpel	3 cm above and behind top of pinna	The superficial temporal artery is palpated and damage to the artery should be avoided.
Dandy point	Occipital/posterior fossa burr hole	3 cm above the inion and 2 cm lateral to the midline	The burr hole placement is avoided high up to prevent injury to the transverse sinus.
Double Dandy point	Parietal burr hole	6 cm above the inion and 4 cm lateral to the midline	
Endoscopic third ventriculostomy burr hole	Slightly anterolateral to the conventional frontal burr hole	1–2 cm anterior to the coronal suture and 2–3 cm lateral to the midline	Preoperative magnetic resonance imaging delineates the anatomy of the ventricles.
Key burr hole procedure	Burr hole for a pure supraorbital or fronto-temporal/pterional craniotomy McCarty's keyhole includes the orbitozygomatic component	At the junction of the supraorbital ridge and the superior temporal crest	Traditional key burr hole: The trajectory and the angle of drilling is directed more posterosuperiorly to avoid entry into the orbital contents. McCarty's hole: The angle of drilling is directed more anteroinferiorly to enable an approach to the orbital rim and the zygomatic component.

Note: The burr hole placement is avoided in the midline to prevent damage to the SSS. Accidental penetration of any sinus may cause uncontrolled bleeding with catastrophic results.

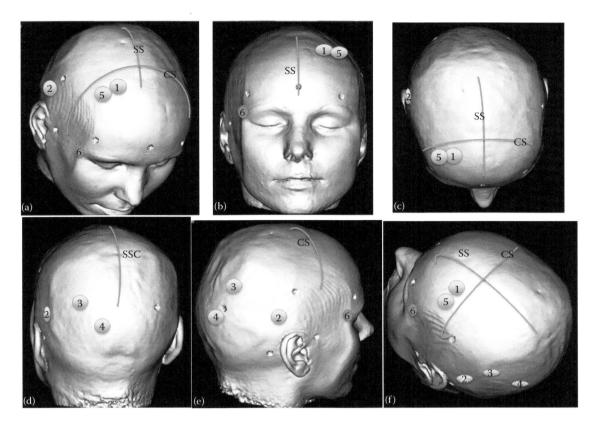

Figure 41.3 Landmarks for burr holes in a three-dimensional image of the head in different views. (a) Right anterosuperior oblique view. (b) Anterior view. (c) Superior view. (d) Posterior view. (e) Right lateral oblique view. (f) Right posterosuperior oblique view. (1) Kocher's point; (2) Keen's point; (3) double Dandy's point; (4) Dandy's point; (5) burr hole for ETV placement; (6) key burr hole.
Abbreviations: ETV: Endoscopic third ventriculostomy.

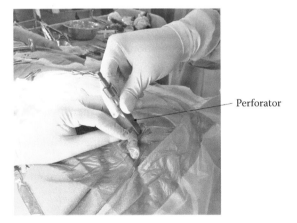

Figure 41.4 Gentle use of a perforator manually for creation of a burr hole trephination in an early infant.

Step 9: Application of suction: Suction should be applied in lower pressures for evacuation of SDH. Extra care is taken to avoid direct application of suction to the brain.[29]

Step 10: The galeal layer is closed with 2–0 absorbable sutures and the skin with staples or monofilament sutures like nylon.[29]

Postprocedure care:

1. Antibiotics are continued at least for 2 days along with analgesics and antiepileptic agents, depending upon the type of insult and the type of procedure.
2. Change of dressings should be done on the first and third postoperative day and be removed on the seventh postoperative day, unless a CSF leak develops.

3. Closure of the burr hole defect: The bony defect is either left as such or packed with bone dust, with burr hole buttons or bone substitutes like polymethylmethacrylate (PMMA).
4. Patients are nursed in the supine and slight head down position, especially in cases of traumatic chronic SDH, and good hydration is maintained to allow expansion of the brain. Bilateral SDH and nursing in propped up position are associated with recurrence of bleed in chronic SDH cases.[30,31]
5. CT imaging in the postoperative period is helpful in evaluating a patient's condition following surgery. Sometimes, removal of drains causes intracranial injury. Hence, CT imaging is done after removal of drains to exclude any injury during drain removal.[32]

Complications/Problems:

a. Common complications. The incidence is around 5%.
   1. Local skin infection: Antibiotics are the first line of treatment. Refractory cases may develop osteomyelitis of the bone. This requires bone curettage and sometimes bone flap removal and cosmetic remodeling of the calvarium.
   2. Minor pain: Treated with analgesics like tramadol and diclofenac.
   3. Inadvertent injury to the underlying dura, brain, or ventricles due to accidental entry of the perforator, burr, or the drill bit leading to hematoma or brain contusion.[33,34] Other mechanics for causation include over drainage and intracranial hypotension, sudden decompression, cerebral venous outflow obstruction, acute loss of CSF, vascular dysregulation and shift of intracranial contents. Rare bleeds include brain stem, contralateral SDH, and cerebellar hemorrhage.[35–37]

      Increased postoperative bleeding is also associated with previous history of hematologic disorders and prior shunt surgery.[38] Injury to the dural venous sinus or diploic veins, sometimes leading to air embolism. Timely identification and proper management ameliorates this condition.
   4. Improper control of bleeding from scalp or diploic vessels leading to EDH may require re-exploration. Bleeding may also result

from the use of drugs like anticoagulants and antiplatelets.[31]
   5. Failure of the brain to re-expand: Patients are nursed in head low position and are well hydrated to allow re-expansion of the brain.
   6. Pneumocephalus.[39]
   7. Incomplete evacuation of hematoma.
   8. Increased possibility of recurrence, especially seen after evacuation of SDHs in patients with diabetes.[38,40] Glycemia management in the perioperative period may help in prevention of recurrence.
   9. Cosmetic deformity: Different techniques and marking materials like autologous bone dust and bone grafts are used to correct the deformity.[41,42]
   10. Trephination syndrome: Rarely seen after major craniectomies and results due to dynamic movements of the brain through the bony defect; usually characterized by headache, which is progressive in nature and sometimes with neurologic deficits that include motor (57%), cognitive (41%), and language deficits (28%). This is more common in males and the incidence is around 60%. Cranioplasty may result in reversal of the symptoms within 4 days.[43]

b. Uncommon complications. Incidence is around 1% to 5%.
   1. Increased stress and anxiety may lead to myocardial infarction, especially in elderly patients. Hypertensive and embolic episodes are common and may result in stroke with neurologic deficits, which may be temporary or permanent.
   2. The clinical condition of the patient may not improve or further decline after evacuation of the hematoma due to the presence of the initial clot and its severity.
   3. Others include collapse of the lungs, deep vein thrombosis, and hyponatremia.
   4. Obese patients may have increased risk of local infections, respiratory and cardiac complications, and thrombosis.

c. Rare complications. The incidence is around <1%.
   1. CSF leak may be prevented by proper closure of the scalp in layers.
   2. Meningitis: Rarely seen in some complicated cases.
   3. Epilepsy may occur.

CONCLUSION

Burr hole procedure is the main armamentarium of any neurosurgical procedure. Basic knowledge of the applied anatomy, its implications, stepwise approach, and management of the perioperative complications helps not only the neurosurgeon, but also a basic critical care physician or surgeon to intervene at least in emergency lifesaving conditions like extra axial hematomas and increased ICP.

REFERENCES

1. Ellis H, Mahadevan V. The surgical anatomy of the scalp. *Surgery (Oxford)*. 2014;32:e1-e5.
2. García-González U, Cavalcanti DD, Agrawal A et al. The diploic venous system: Surgical anatomy and neurosurgical implications. *Neurosurg Focus*. 2009;27(5):E2.
3. Donovan DJ, Moquin RR, Ecklund JM. Cranial burr holes and emergency craniotomy: Review of indications and technique. *Mil Med*. 2006;171(1):12.
4. Winn HR, Youmans JR. Basic principles of cranial surgery for brain tumours. In: Winn HR, ed. *Youmans Neurological Surgery*, 6th. ed. New York: Saunders/Elsevier; 2011:899.
5. Pattinson K, Wynne-Jones G, Imray CH. Monitoring intracranial pressure, perfusion and metabolism. *Continuing Education in Anaesthesia, Critical Care & Pain*. 2005;5(4):130-133.
6. Manoj N, Arivazhagan A, Bhat D et al. Stereotactic biopsy of brainstem lesions: Techniques, efficacy, safety, and disease variation between adults and children: A single institutional series and review. *Journal of Neurosciences in Rural Practice*. 2014;5(1):32.
7. Mark W, Ian S. Acute neurosurgical emergencies. In: William E, Thomas G, Malcolm W, Reed R, Michael GW, eds. *Oxford Textbook of Fundamentals of Surgery*. 1st ed. New York: Oxford University Press; 2016:451.
8. Karibe H, Hayashi T, Hirano T et al. Surgical management of traumatic acute subdural hematoma in adults: A review. *Neurologia Medico-Chirurgica*. 2014;54(11):887-894.
9. Huh J. Burr hole drainage: Could be another treatment option for cerebrospinal fluid leakage after unidentified dural tear during spinal surgery? *J Korean Neurosurg Soc*. 2013;53(1):59-61.
10. Ling JM, Tiruchelvarayan R. A review of endoscopic treatment of hydrocephalus in paediatric and adult patients. *Proceedings of Singapore Healthcare*. 2013;22(3):203-212.
11. Tandon PN, Ramamurthi R. Basic surgical principles in craniotomy. In *Textbook of Neurosurgery*, 3rd ed. Three volume set. New Delhi, India: Jaypee Brothers, Medical Publishers Pvt. Limited; 2012:183.
12. Furlanetti LL, de Oliveira RS, Santos MV et al. Multiple cranial burr holes as an alternative treatment for total scalp avulsion. *Childs Nerv Syst*. 2010;26(6):745-749.
13. Bullock MR, Chesnut R, Ghajar J et al. Surgical management of depressed cranial fractures. *Neurosurgery*. 2006;58(3):S2-S56.
14. Machado A, Rezai AR, Kopell BH et al. Deep brain stimulation for Parkinson's disease: Surgical technique and perioperative management. *Mov Disord*. 2006;21(suppl 14) S247-S258).
15. Toyoda K, Urasaki E, Umeno T et al. The effectiveness of the stereotactic burr hole technique for deep brain stimulation. *Neurol Med Chir (Tokyo)*. 2015;55(9):766-772.
16. McLaughlin N, Martin NA. Effectiveness of burr holes for indirect revascularization in patients with moyamoya disease—A review of the literature. *World Neurosurg*. 2014;81 (1):91-98.
17. Gordon TS, Lawrence MS, Steven DC. Craniotomy for tumor. In: Richard AJ, Brenda G, Clifford AS. eds. *Anesthesiologist's Manual of Surgical Procedures*, 5th ed. Monsey, NY: Wolters Kluwer Health; 2012:29.
18. Tandon P. Basic Surgical Principles in Craniotomy. In *Textbooks of Operative Neurosurgery* (2 Vol.). Ramamurthi R, Sridhar K. eds. Vasudevan MC: B.I. Publications Pvt. Limited; 2005.
19. Hellwig D, Tirakotai W, Riegel T et al. Endoscopy in neurosurgery. *Deutsches Arzteblatt-Koln-*. 2007;104(4):161.
20. Hafez MME, Bary THA, Ismail AS, Mohammed MAM. Frontolateral key hole craniotomy approach to anterior cranial base. *ZUMJ*. 2015;19(1):91-99.
21. Wilson MH, Wise D, Davies G, Lockey D. Emergency burr holes: How to do it. *Scand J Trauma Resusc Emerg Med*. 2012;20 (1):24.

22. Ganti L. *Burr Hole Craniotomy. Atlas of Emergency Medicine Procedures.* Berlin, Germany: Springer; 2016.

23. Treacy PJ, Reilly P, Brophy B. Emergency neurosurgery by general surgeons at a remote major hospital. *ANZ J Surg.* 2005;75 (10):852-857.

24. Gilligan J, Reilly P, Pearce A, Taylor D. Management of acute traumatic intracranial haematoma in rural and remote areas of Australia. *ANZ J Surg.* 2017;87(1-2):80-85.

25. Lee JH, Kim DW, Kang SD. Stereotactic burr hole aspiration surgery for spontaneous hypertensive cerebellar hemorrhage. *J Cerebrovasc Endovasc Neurosurg.* 2012;14 (3):170-174.

26. Kobayashi K, Nakamura S, Watanabe M et al. Simulation to locate burr hole sites in a patient for deep brain stimulation surgery and clipping of intracranial aneurysm. *Neuromodulation.* 2013;16(1):51-54.

27. Raimondi AJ, Ishak BA, Noah ZL. Burr holes and flaps. In: *Pediatric Neurosurgery: Theoretical Principles. Art of Surgical Techniques,* Illustrated ed. New York: Springer; 2013:73.

28. Rabi NS, Kuntal KD, Arun KS. Cranial burr hole. In: Gurjar M, ed. *Manual of ICU Procedures,* 1st ed. New Delhi, India: Jaypee Brothers, Medical Publishers Pvt. Limited; 2015:430.

29. Loukas M, Tubbs RS, Feldman J. Burr hole craniotomy. In: *Netter's Introduction to Clinical Procedures e-book,* 1st ed. New York: Elsevier Health Sciences; 2016.

30. Abouzari M, Rashidi A, Rezaii J et al. The role of postoperative patient posture in the recurrence of traumatic chronic subdural hematoma after burr-hole surgery. *Neurosurgery.* 2007;61(4):794-797.

31. Torihashi K, Sadamasa N, Yoshida K et al. Independent predictors for recurrence of chronic subdural hematoma: A review of 343 consecutive surgical cases. *Neurosurgery.* 2008;63(6):1125-1129.

32. Deliği KSHİB, Sonrasında T. Routine postoperative CT-scans after burr hole trepanation for chronic subdural hematoma—Better before or after drainage removal? *Turkish Neurosurgery.* 2013;23(4):458-463.

33. Rusconi A, Sangiorgi S, Bifone L, Balbi S. Infrequent hemorrhagic complications following surgical drainage of chronic subdural hematomas. *J Korean Neurosurg Soc.* 2015;57 (5):379-385.

34. Rohde V, Graf G, Hassler W. Complications of burr-hole craniostomy and closed-system drainage for chronic subdural hematomas: A retrospective analysis of 376 patients. *Neurosurg Rev.* 2002;25(1):89-94.

35. Sun H-L, Chang C-J, Hsieh C-T. Contralateral acute subdural hematoma occurring after evacuation of subdural hematoma with coexistent contralateral subdural hygroma. *Neurosciences (Riyadh).* 2014;19(3):229.

36. Rojas-Medina LM, Goel A. Brainstem hemorrhage secondary to evacuation of chronic subdural hematoma. *Neurology India.* 2014;62 (4):435.

37. Kollatos C, Konstantinou D, Raftopoulos S et al. Cerebellar hemorrhage after supratentorial burr hole drainage of a chronic subdural hematoma. *Hippokratia.* 2011;15(4):370.

38. Pang CH, Lee SE, Kim CH et al. Acute intracranial bleeding and recurrence after bur hole craniostomy for chronic subdural hematoma. *J Neurosurg.* 2015;123(1):65-74.

39. Ihab Z. Pneumocephalus after surgical evacuation of chronic subdural hematoma: Is it a serious complication? *Asian J Neurosurg.* 2012;7(2):66.

40. Shakal AAS, El Gamal EE, Farid AM. Chronic subdural hematoma: Complication avoidance. *Tanta Medical Journal.* 2014;42(1):6.

41. Cokluk C, Şenel A, İyigün Ö et al. Reconstruction of burr hole by using autologous button-shaped graft harvested from inner table of craniotomy flap: Technique and clinical result. *Minim Invasive Neurosurg.* 2003;46(06):372-373.

42. Worm PV, Ferreira NP, Faria MB et al. Comparative study between cortical bone graft versus bone dust for reconstruction of cranial burr holes. *Surg Neurol Int.* 2010;1:91.

43. Ashayeri K, Jackson EM, Huang J, Brem H, Gordon CR. Syndrome of the trephined: A systematic review. *Neurosurgery.* 2016;79 (4):525-534.

42

Percutaneous tracheostomy

ANKUR LUTHRA

INTRODUCTION

Tracheostomy is defined as the creation of an opening in the trachea by suturing the skin of the neck to the tracheal mucosa. **Asclepiades**, in the first century BC, clearly described the use of tracheostomy for the relief of the upper airway obstruction. **Fabricius** wrote in the seventeenth century: "This operation redounds to the honor of the physician and places him on a footing with the Gods."

The percutaneous approach to tracheostomy was first described in 1955 when Shelden et al. performed the first modern percutaneous tracheotomy.[1] However, the complication rate was very high because of traumatic lacerations of the surrounding structures by the trocar.[2–4]

Ciaglia et al. used an innovative technique in 1985 that was based on serial dilatations with sequentially larger dilators placed over a needle guidewire after the creation of midline puncture in the neck.[5] Additionally, many different variations of the Seldinger technique have evolved, including

the use of dilating forceps, screw action dilators (corkscrew type), and a translaryngeal approach. The consistent feature of all these techniques is the use of the Seldinger guidewire to provide a safe, controlled approach to dilation of the tracheal opening.

RELEVANT ANATOMY

The trachea is a fibrocartilaginous structure, which lies in the midline of the neck. It begins from the cricoid cartilage (C6) to the tracheal bifurcation (T5), and has 18 to 22 C-shaped rings, which are formed of rigid cartilage anteriorly and laterally, and a membranous posterior portion to allow for expansion of the esophagus during deglutition. It is 11 cm in length, with a range of 10 to 13 cm and has a width of 2.3 cm. The second to the fourth cartilaginous rings are covered by the isthmus of the thyroid.

The trachea in children is more deeply placed and is smaller in diameter. The left brachiocephalic vein and artery may cross in front of the trachea (in children up to the age of 2 years) and the thymus of the thyroid gland is large and is connected on the anterior aspect of the trachea.

PHYSIOLOGY OF TRACHEOSTOMY

There are many advantages of performing a tracheostomy (Table 42.1). When compared with the endotracheal tube, the tracheostomy tube has the potential to decrease both the **resistive and elastic work of breathing**. They are more rigid, shorter, and less likely to deform in the upper airway; and by reducing resistance, expiratory flow can be enhanced. Also, the potential to dynamic hyperinflation and development of intrinsic positive end-expiratory pressure (PEEP) is decreased.

The advantages specific to the percutaneous technique include:

- Ability to perform it at the bedside in the ICU, thus avoiding a potentially hazardous transfer of critically ill patients to the operating room
- Avoids long waiting lists for operating room scheduling
- Significant reduction in the cost of tracheostomy

Table 42.1 Advantages of tracheostomy

1. Improved patient comfort
2. Less need for sedatives
3. Reduced work of breathing
4. Improved oral hygiene and early oral intake
5. Early ability to speak and better long-term laryngeal function (controversial)
6. Faster weaning from mechanical ventilation
7. Shorter ICU and hospital stay

Table 42.2 Indications of percutaneous tracheostomy

1. Need for prolonged intubation for respiratory failure
2. Airway obstruction due to foreign body, neoplasms, and laryngeal trauma
3. Bilateral vocal cord paralysis
4. Congenital airway lesions (vascular web, laryngeal hypoplasia)
5. Prophylaxis for extensive head and neck procedures

However, there are some pitfalls, too. Because the creation of a tracheostomy stoma bypasses the nasal airways, it disturbs the natural humidification and warming of inspired air, which leads to early dessication of tracheal mucosa with the consequent development of squamous metaplasia and reduced ciliary function, making the patient more prone to recurrent respiratory tract infections.

Various indications of percutaneous tracheostomy are listed in Table 42.2.

CONTRAINDICATIONS AND LIMITATIONS

Although percutaneous tracheostomy has gained widespread acceptance, recognizing the contraindications is imperative. Absolute contraindications include the need for an emergent airway or inability to intubate the patient in an emergency situation. Preadolescent patients are also not ideal candidates for percutaneous tracheostomy.[6,7]

Relative contraindications include thyroid mass, poorly demarcated or obstructed landmarks, or severe coagulopathy (INR >1.5 or platelets <50,000). The presence of infection at or near the tracheostomy site should also preclude a percutaneous approach. Morbid obesity, previously considered a relative contraindication, may be overcome now by use of specific percutaneous tracheostomy kits designed specifically for such patients. Additionally, percutaneous tracheostomy generally should not be done in patients where a difficult reintubation is anticipated or in patients with PEEP >15 cm H_2O and peak airway pressures >45 mmHg, or a PaO_2/FiO_2 <200.[7,8]

PREOPERATIVE WORKUP AND PREREQUISITES

In general, a coagulation panel and complete blood count should be obtained to assess bleeding risk. Platelets should be >50,000 and bleeding time <10 min. Informed consent should be obtained from the relatives and they should be well explained about the operating procedure, loss of voice, and complications of the procedure. Routine ASA monitoring including ECG, pulseoximetry, endtidal CO_2, and noninvasive BP should be monitored while the procedure is being carried out. It is vital that an experienced person administers the necessary sedative and hypnotic drugs and also monitors physiological parameters. Expertise in airway management is extremely valuable when unanticipated difficulties and complications arise.

Two important issues that may arise during the procedure are accidental penetration of the endotracheal tube cuff with the introducer needle during the initial puncture of the anterior tracheal wall and possible dislocation of the endotracheal tube. These should be addressed timely so that possible complications can be avoided.

The patient is mechanically ventilated before beginning the procedure with the fraction of inspired oxygen at 1.0. The patient's neck should be slightly hyperextended by placing a sandbag underneath the shoulder blades and the part should be adequately cleaned and draped before beginning the procedure.

TECHNIQUES FOR PERCUTANEOUS TRACHEOSTOMY

The Ciaglia method is currently the most commonly used percutaneous technique. Originally, it was described as using serial dilations with progressively larger hydrophilic-coated dilators; however, now the technique has been modified and adapted in commercially available kits to use a single conicaldilator (Ciaglia Blue Rhino Tracheostomy Introducer Kit, Cook Critical Care, Bloomington; Figure 42.1).

After the neck is prepped and draped in a sterile fashion, Lidocaine 1% with 1:100,000 epinephrine is locally infiltrated. The initial incision can be made vertically or horizontally along the midline at the level of the inferior border of the cricoid cartilage. The typical incision is about 2 to 3 cm in length. Dissection of the pretracheal tissue is performed to push the thyroid isthmus inferiorly.

The introducer needle along with the cannula is then advanced through the anterior tracheal membrane with care not to advance the needle too much into the posterior tracheal wall.[6,9] A flexible fiber-optic bronchoscope may be used to visualize the entrance of the needle and prevent a posterior tracheal wall puncture. The needle is then

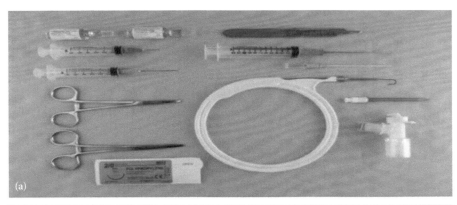

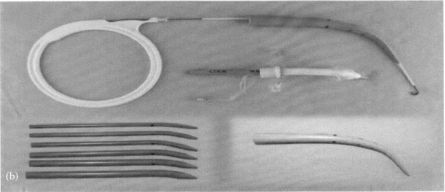

Figure 42.1 (a) Ciaglia Blue Rhino Tracheostomy Introducer Kit, Cook Critical Care, Bloomington. (b) Ciaglia Blue Rhino dilators and guidewire.

withdrawn, maintaining the cannula within the lumen of the trachea. A J-tipped guidewire is then introduced through the cannula into the tracheal lumen. The cannula is then removed and the dilator is inserted over the guidewire and advanced through the anterior wall of the trachea (Figure 42.2). Following dilation, a tracheostomy tube is placed over the guidewire and advanced toward the trachea. After placement of the tracheotomy tube, the guidewire is removed and the cuff of the tracheotomy tube is inflated and CO_2 return is confirmed by continuous waveform capnography.[6] The tube should be secured with four nonabsorbable sutures and a tracheotomy collar.

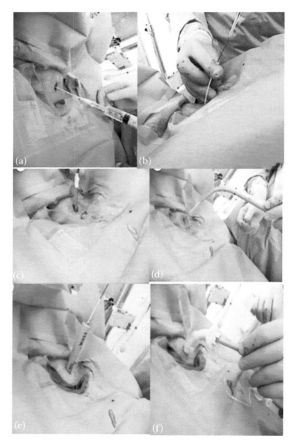

Figure 42.2 Introduction of needle into tracheal lumen and its confirmation through aspiration into saline filled syringe (a), insertion of guidewire through the cannula (b), passage of dilator over the guidewire (c and d), insertion of dilator to sufficient length into tracheal lumen (e), and passage of tracheostomy tube over the guidewire and dilated track (f).

This single dilator technique (Blue Rhino) is associated with lesser airway injury and the hydrophilic coating of the Blue Rhino dilator allows it to pass through the pretracheal tissues with greater ease than with other percutaneous devices. It is associated with less procedure time and is less expensive than the multiple dilator kit.

BALLOON DILATATIONAL TECHNIQUE

The balloon dilatational technique was first described by Zgoda and Berger in 2005. A balloon cannula apparatus (Figure 42.3) is passed over a guidewire until the balloon tip mounted at the distal end of the apparatus is seen in the trachea. The balloon is inflated with saline solution to 11 atmospheres for a few seconds and deflated, and the 8.0 mm ID tracheostomy tube preloaded onto a customized stylet, which forms the proximal portion of the apparatus that is inserted. The advantage of this modified technique is that rather than applying pressure inward toward the tracheal lumen using a tapered dilator, radial force is applied to the tracheal wall using a balloon, which is reported to have lesser incidence of posterior tracheal wall perforation than the conventional Ciaglia technique.

GRIGGS TECHNIQUE (GUIDEWIRE DILATING FORCEPS TECHNIQUE)

The Griggs technique uses guidewire dilator forceps (GWDF) against the serial dilators or one-step dilator of the Ciaglia technique.

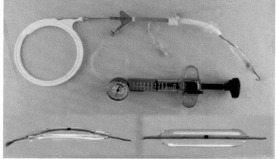

Figure 42.3 Balloon cannula apparatus (Ciaglia Blue Dolphin Tracheostomy Introducer Kit).

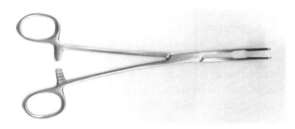

Figure 42.4 Griggs forceps.

The GWDF has a curved design (Figure 42.4), which decreases the risk of damage to the posterior tracheal wall when inserted. GWDF is used to enlarge the hole in the anterior tracheal wall to allow tracheotomy tube placement. The initial part of the procedure is similar to the Ciaglia technique, including positioning and incision.

Next, a 14-gauge intravenous cannula with an attached syringe is inserted along the midline incision and is advanced until air bubbles are seen on aspirating with the syringe, confirming placement in the lumen of the trachea. The needle is then removed while the cannula remains in situ. The J-tipped Seldinger wire is introduced through the cannula into the tracheal lumen. The cannula is removed while the guidewire in left in place. Then, the wire tip is passed through the bore at the end of the closed GWDF to advance through the soft tissues of the anterior neck. The handles of the forceps are lifted vertically to allow penetration into the anterior tracheal wall and further advanced till the tip lies longitudinally within the tracheal lumen. The forceps are then opened so as to dilate the tracheotomy hole in the anterior wall. After the forceps are withdrawn, the tracheotomy tube is seated over the guidewire and advanced into the tracheal lumen. Its placement is confirmed by capnography. The cuff is inflated appropriately and the tube is secured with nonabsorbable sutures and a tracheotomy collar.

FANTONI'S TECHNIQUE (TRANSLARYNGEAL APPROACH)

Fantoni and Ripomonti described the translaryngeal approach for tracheotomies for the first time in 1997.[10] After positioning and draping, the endotracheal tube is retracted back to the glottis under direct laryngoscopy. Through this endotracheal tube, a flexible bronchoscope is advanced so as to allow visualization of the tracheal lumen. A needle is then inserted into the anterior trachea, following which a Seldinger guidewire is advanced upwards in the trachea in a retrograde fashion out of the patient's mouth. A unique device made up of a flexible plastic cone with a metal tip attached to an armored tracheal cannula is adhered to the guidewire and advanced through the oral cavity into the trachea.

Once the cannula advances to the site of the guidewire in the tracheal lumen piercing the anterior trachea, a moderate amount of force is applied anteriorly by the operator on the cone and cannula so as to penetrate the tracheal wall.[11] Simultaneously, a counterpressure is held by the operator's other hand on the anterior neck, ensuring maximal control. Once it has emerged through the skin, the cone is then advanced to its final placement.[11,12] By stabilizing the anterior trachea, soft tissue injury is minimized and counterforce is applied meticulously, as the metal tip and cone are advanced through the anterior trachea.[12]

PERCTWIST (SCREW ACTION DILATOR)

The PercTwist is a dilator (Figure 42.5) with its inherent screw action that is designed to address the issues of excessive force that may be exerted on the tracheal wall, which is different from the traditional percutaneous tracheostomy techniques. The concept behind its development is to avoid excessive downward force on the trachea by using a screw action, which lifts the trachea upwards on the dilating device as against the forcing of dilator downwards into the trachea. The procedure begins, similar as described earlier, with the insertion of the needle and guidewire. Instead of using serial dilators, the PercTwist is inserted up to the level of the trachea over the guidewire. It is then advanced with a rotational action, which lifts up the trachea instead of exerting downward pressure. The remaining procedure proceeds in a parallel fashion

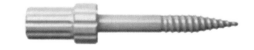

Figure 42.5 PercTwist dilator.

to that of the already mentioned Ciaglia technique.[4,13,14]

PROCEDURAL ADJUNCTS

Flexible fiber-optic bronchoscopy-guided tracheostomy (Figure 42.6)

Various advantages of flexible fiberoptic-guided tracheostomy include

- Real-time visual guidance
- Confirmation of appropriate ETT positioning
- Midline placement of the introducer needle and catheter
- Guidance on the direction of the guidewire
- Proper placement of the tracheal cannula
- Prevention of injury to the posterior tracheal wall
- Lower rates of accidental extubation, false passage, pneumomediastinum, and pneumothorax

The use of bronchoscopy is not without its drawbacks. It may contribute to oxygen desaturation and retention of CO_2 during the procedure and could be contraindicated in patients who cannot tolerate hypercapnia (eg, raised ICP in traumatic brain injury).[7,15]

In 2005, Kost reported (in a series of 500 consecutive patients undergoing percutaneous tracheostomy with bronchoscopic guidance) that the potential complications associated with simultaneous use of bronchoscopy were very few compared with its benefits.[16] Only 2.8% of the patients experienced transient oxygen desaturation.

ULTRASOUND-GUIDED PERCUTANEOUS TRACHEOSTOMY

The ultrasound has come a long way since it was introduced into the medical practice. It well defines the anatomy of the airway and helps in

- Accurate placement of the introducer needle into the trachea
- Estimating the distance from the skin to the trachea
- Identifying anomalous vascular anatomy
- Preventing damage to vascular and adjacent structures

However, training in ultrasound (a definitive learning curve is required) and difficulty in identifying the endotracheal tube cuff in ultrasound are two major limitations that preclude its use.

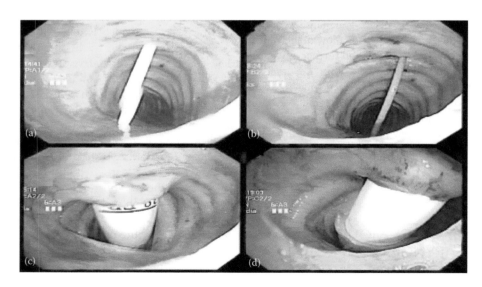

Figure 42.6 Flexible fiber-optic bronchoscopy-guided percutaneous tracheostomy. (a) Introducer needle visualized in trachea. (b) Guidewire through introducer visualized in trachea. (c) The dilator as visualized inside the trachea. (d) The actual tracheostomy tube visualized in the trachea.

Table 42.3 Complications of percutaneous tracheostomy

Early complications	Late complications
Bleeding	Tracheal stenosis
Tracheal ring fracture	Tracheomalacia
Incorrect placement of tracheostomy tube	Tracheo-innominate fistula
Accidental extubation and hypoxia	Tracheo-esophageal fistula
Damage to mediastinal structures	Wound infections
Pneumothorax and pneumomediastinum	Subglottic stenosis
Cardiac dysarrhythmias	Decannulation problems

PERIOPERATIVE COMPLICATIONS

The complications of percutaneous tracheostomy are divided into **early** and **late** complications (Table 42.3).

Bleeding

It is the most common complication that occurs during or immediately after the procedure. Mostly, minor bleeding occurs, which has 20% incidence and resolves on its own. In most cases, bleeding usually stops by digital pressure or pressure by tracheostomy tube. Major bleeding that mainly occurs due to vascular injury (mostly venous) may be seen in 5% of the cases.[8] Thrombocytopenia is the strongest single risk factor for chronic bleeding.

Prophylactic doses of heparin do not increase the risk of bleeding if APTT and platelet counts are normal.

Tracheal wall injury

Injury to tracheal rings may occur due to use of excessive pressure by a dilator or tracheostomy tube that deforms the anterior wall leading to stress fractures.

In one study, percutaneous tracheostomy was performed on cadaveric specimens, which demonstrated significant peristomal mucosal tear and cartilaginous fractures.[17] Tracheal ring fractures have also been demonstrated during a PercuTwist tracheostomy procedure.[18] Most of the cases heal spontaneously with consequent tracheal stenosis.

INCORRECT PLACEMENT OF TRACHEOSTOMY TUBE

The incidence of insertion of the cannula outside the tracheal lumen is below 1%, while the incidence of a false route during dilatational steps is slightly higher. Incorrect placement of the cannula is prevented by the use of a guidewire and a guiding catheter. During dilatation of the tract, it should be possible to move the guidewire freely.

Other, rare, short-term complications include pneumothorax, esophageal injury, and tracheal-wall penetration.[7]

LONG-TERM COMPLICATIONS

Long-term complications have been extensively reported in a number of studies and meta-analyses. Steele and coworkers followed up patients with spiral CT scans and observed tracheal dilation in eight out of 25 patients but no case of stenosis. They reported voice change as the most common complaint occurring in 11 patients.[19] In addition, Sviri and colleagues observed that the most common complications were voice change (38%) and chronic, severe cough (12%). Also, eight out of 41 patients (19.5%) had an obstruction based on spirometry, but only two patients were symptomatic with stridor or shortness of breath (5%).[20]

Another study demonstrated that 89.5% of patients developed tracheal stenosis but fewer than 25% were actually symptomatic and only one patient experienced clinically relevant stenosis. It was also reported that this stenosis was due to the puncture site and tracheal ring fracture while inserting the dilator. Consequently, this group advocated careful dilation under endoscopic guidance.[21]

Tracheal stenosis most commonly occurs at the stomal level or above the stoma (suprastomal) but below the vocal cords (subglottic). Only 3% to 12% of patients demonstrate clinically important stenosis that ultimately requires intervention.[21] Multiple risk factors are associated with stomal stenosis, including sepsis, stomal infection, hypotension, advanced age, male sex, steroids, a tight-fitting or oversized cannula, excessive tube motion, prolonged placement, and disproportionate excision of anterior tracheal cartilage.

Suprastomal injury occurs whenever there is guidewire-related injury to the posterior tracheal wall and further development of granulation tissue. Additionally, the dilators that are used to enlarge the percutaneous dilatational tracheostomy stoma can injure the anterior tracheal cartilage, including tracheal ring fracture, causing these deformed structures to invaginate and protrude into the tracheal lumen, causing obstruction.

The third location for tracheal stenosis is at the site of the tracheal tube cuff, where ischemic injury to the tracheal mucosa can take place. Generally, the incidence of tracheal stenosis post percutaneous tracheostomy is lower than for the surgical procedure and quoted as 6% to 7%.[22]

In 2007, Higgins and Punthakee[22] published a large meta-analysis of 15 prospective trials, including 973 patients, where they demonstrated the most common long-term complications were decannulation/obstruction, minor hemorrhage, wound infection, unfavorable scarring, and subglottic stenosis. There was no significant difference in these complication rates between open and percutaneous techniques.[22]

One of the most feared complications is Tracheo-innominate artery erosion. Risk factors for the development of trachea-innominate fistula include excessive movement of the tracheostomy, high pressure (or overinflated) cuff, or a tube that has been placed too low. The innominate artery lies adjacent to the trachea and crosses it at approximately the ninth tracheal ring. If the tracheostomy tube is placed too low (below the third tracheal ring), the inferior concave surface of the cannula may erode into the artery and may result in torrential bleeding. It occurs in less than 1% of patients. Approximately, 75% will occur within 3 to 4 weeks of placement of tracheostomy. The mortality rate is as high as 100%, even when surgical intervention is undertaken. The most common clinical presentations are bleeding around the tracheostomy tube or massive hemoptysis.

Another less common complication is tracheoesophageal fistula. It occurs in less than 1% of patients undergoing tracheostomy. It is an iatrogenic complication resulting from injury to the posterior tracheal wall during the procedure. Alternatively, excessive cuff pressure or the tip of the tracheostomy tube can cause posterior wall injury. The manifestations include recurrent aspiration of food, increasing dyspnea, a persistent cuff leak, or severe gastric distention. Treatment includes placement of a double stent (in esophagus and trachea) in nonoperative patients or surgical repair in patients capable of tolerating thoracic surgery.

TRACHEOMALACIA

It results from ischemic injury to the trachea, followed by chondritis and subsequent destruction and necrosis of supporting tracheal cartilage wall. Compliant tracheal airway collapses during expiration. This can result in expiratory airflow limitation, air trapping, and retained respiratory secretions.

Tracheomalacia may present as failure to wean from mechanical ventilation or it may present as dyspnea in a patient with previous tracheostomy. With more severe cases, therapeutic options include placement of a longer tracheostomy tube, stenting, tracheal resection, or tracheoplasty.

SURGICAL VERSUS PERCUTANEOUS TRACHEOSTOMY

The debate of surgical vs. percutaneous approaches to tracheotomy has been widely discussed. Percutaneous techniques were developed originally out of interest in minimally invasive procedures that could be performed outside of the operating room with minimal personnel and cost. Generally speaking, the percutaneous technique is as safe as the open technique in properly selected patients. Percutaneous approach requires fewer personnel, less time, and less money.

Overall, the rates of significant hemorrhage have been shown to be less common with percutaneous when compared to surgical tracheostomy. A retrospective study of 794 patients with surgical open tracheostomy by Arola showed that bloody secretions occurred in 22% and tracheoarterial fistula occurred in 0.6% of the patients.[23] A meta-analysis by Cheng and Fee in 2000 compared outcomes in percutaneous versus standard surgical tracheotomy, demonstrating that percutaneous tracheostomy produced less intraoperative minor bleeding (9% vs. 25%), less postoperative bleeding (7% vs. 18%), and resulted in fewer overall complications (14% vs. 60%).[24]

PROCEDURAL TRAINING AND GUIDELINES

Specific training is required to perform percutaneous dilatational tracheostomy with most guidelines using expert opinions to determine a recommended number of procedures to be used as a surrogate marker. The *American College of Chest Physicians* recommends a minimum of 20 procedures, whereas the *American Thoracic Society* and the *European Respiratory Society* recommends 5–10 procedures before performing percutaneous tracheostomy independently, with a minimum of 10 procedures per year to maintain proficiency while doing this procedure.[25]

In addition, it is recommended that physicians performing percutaneous tracheostomy have extensive experience in airway management and the treatment of critically ill patients.

REFERENCES

1. Shelden CH, Pudenz RH, Freshwater DB et al. New method for tracheotomy. *J Neurosurg.* 1955;12:428-431.
2. Goldenberg D, Golz A, Netzer A et al. Tracheotomy: Changing indications and a review of 1,130 cases. *J Otolaryngol.* 2002;31:211-215.
3. Seldinger SI. Catheter replacement of the needle in percutaneous arteriography. *Acta Radiol.* 1953;39:368-376.
4. Durbin C. Techniques for performing tracheostomy. *Respir Care.* 2005;50(4):488-496.
5. Ciaglia P, Firsching R, Syniec C. Elective percutaneous dilatational tracheostomy: A new simple bedside procedure; preliminary report. *Chest.* 1985;87(6):715-719.
6. Bhatti N. Percutaneous dilational tracheotomy: Ciaglia method. In: Goldenberg D, Friedman M, eds. *Operative Techniques in Head and Neck Surgery.* New York: Elsevier; 2007;18:90-94.
7. Park S, Goldenberg D. Percutaneous tracheotomy: Griggs technique. In: Goldenberg D, Friedman M, eds. *Operative Techniques in Head and Neck Surgery.* New York: Elsevier; 2007;18:95-98.
8. Goldenberg D, Golz A, Huri A et al. Percutaneous dilation tracheotomy versus surgical tracheotomy: Our experience. *Otolaryngol Head Neck Surg.* 2003;128:358-363.
9. Westphal K, Byhahn C, Hans-Joachim W, Lischke V. Percutaneous tracheostomy: A clinical comparison of dilational (Ciaglia) and translaryngeal (Fantoni) techniques. *Anesth Analg.* 1999;89:938-943.
10. Fantoni A, Ripamonti D. A non-derivative, non-surgical tracheostomy: The translaryngeal method. *Intensive Care Med.* 1997;23(4):386-392.
11. Fantoni A, Ripamonti D, Lesmo A, Zanoni CI. Translaryngeal tracheostomy. A new era? *Minerva Anestesiol.* 1996;62(10):313-325.
12. Meininger D, Byhahn C. Translaryngeal tracheotomy. In: Goldenberg D, Friedman M, eds. *Operative Techniques in Head and Neck Surgery.* New York: Elsevier; 2007;18:99-104.
13. Westphal K, Maeser D, Scheifler G, Lischke V, Byhahn C. PercuTwist: A new single dilator technique for percutaneous tracheostomy. *Anesth Analg.* 2003;96:229-232.
14. Frova G, Quintel M. A new simple method for percutaneous tracheostomy: Controlled rotating dilation: A preliminary report. *Intensive Care Med.* 2002;28(3):299-303.
15. Paran H, Butnaru G, Hass I et al. Evaluation of a modified percutaneous tracheostomy technique without bronchoscopic guidance. *Chest.* 2004;126(3):868-881.
16. Kost K. Endoscopic percutaneous dilational tracheotomy: A perspective evaluation of 500 consecutive cases. *The Laryngoscope.* 2005;115(10 pt 2):1-30.
17. Hotchkiss KS, McCaffery JC. Laryngotracheal injury after percutaneous dilatational tracheostomy in cadaver specimens. *Laryngoscope.* 2003;113(1):16-20.
18. Scherrer E, Tual L, Dhonneur G. Tracheal ring fracture during a PercuTwist tracheostomy procedure. *Anesth Analg.* 2004;98(5):1451-1453.
19. Steele AP, Evans HW, Afaq MA et al. Long-term follow-up of Griggs percutaneous tracheostomy with spiral CT and questionnaire. *Chest.* 2000;117(5):1430-1433.
20. Sviri S, Samie R, Roberts BL et al. Long-term outcomes following percutaneous tracheostomy using the Griggs technique. *Anaesth Intensive Care.* 2003;31(4):401-407.

21. Dollner R, Verch M, Schweiger P et al. Long-term outcome after Griggs tracheostomy. *J Otolaryngol.* 2002;31(6):386-389.

22. Higgins KM, Punthakee X. Meta-analysis comparison of open versus percutaneous tracheostomy. *The Laryngoscope.* 2007;117 (3):447-454.

23. Arola MK. Tracheostomy and its complications. A retrospective study of 794 tracheostomized patients. *Annales Chirurgiae Et Gynaecologiae.* 1981;70(3):96-106.

24. Cheng E, Fee W. Dilational versus standard tracheostomy: A meta-analysis. *Annals of Otology, Rhinology and Laryngology.* 2000;109(8):803-807.

25. Ernst A, Gerard A, Johnstone D. Interventional pulmonary procedures: Guidelines from the American College of Chest Physicians. *Chest.* 2003;123(5):1693-1717.

43

Immobilization of spine

RAJEEB K. MISHRA

INTRODUCTION

Spinal immobilization is an integral part of management and is advocated not only for patients with potential spinal injury, but also for stabilizing the spinal column to aid in the healing process or controlling pain. Risk of secondary neurologic deterioration as a result of motion of the injured vertebrae can happen in cases of spinal injury. Approximately 3% to 25% of spinal cord injuries can occur after the initial traumatic insult, mostly attributable to improper care while in transit or early management.[1] It is estimated that 20% of spinal column injuries involve multiple noncontinuous vertebral levels; which implies, the entire spinal column is potentially at risk.[2] For that reason, whole spinal immobilization has been proposed in prehospital spinal care algorithm to counter any motion until injury has been ruled out.[2,3]

INDICATIONS FOR SPINAL IMMOBILIZATION

Reasons of injury, associated with a high risk of cervical spine injury, are severe force (eg, motor vehicle accident or fall), acceleration deceleration injuries, sports injury (particularly hockey, football, and horseback riding).

Physical examination features suggestive of cervical spine injury include[4] altered mental status (including intoxication or drowsiness), tenderness at the posterior midline of the cervical spine, decreased cervical range of motion, neurologic deficits and polytrauma, and distracting injuries.

METHODS OF SPINAL IMMOBILIZATION

Neutral position

Neutral position is meant to maximize cervical spine protection but is not well defined. The most frequently cited definition is "the normal anatomic position of the head and torso that one assumes when standing and looking straight ahead."[5] Some authors suggest that neutral position is maintained when the external auditory meatus is in line with the shoulder in the coronal plane.[6] The Advanced Trauma Life Support (ATLS) program defines the neutral position as "supine without rotating or bending the spinal column."[7]

Adults require occipital elevation to maintain the neutral position. No consensus regarding the amount of elevation exists; the range described in the literature varies from 1.3 to 9.5 cm, with most authors favoring approximately 2 cm.[5,8] Correlation with spinal magnetic resonance imaging suggests that 2 cm of occipital padding provides a favorable ratio of spinal canal to spinal cord cross-sectional area.[9]

IMMOBILIZATION DEVICES

Various devices and techniques exist to provide immobilization of the cervical spine; however, the optimal device has not yet been identified. In general, for effective spinal immobilization, cervical collars, lateral head supports, and backboards with straps to attach are essential. It is imperative to immobilize the entire patient's body to the board. The use of one of these devices without the other does little to prevent exacerbation of cervical cord injury.[10] Present recommendations call for selective spinal immobilization to decrease unnecessary application and potential harm (see recommendations).

Cervical collars

Cervical collars should be rigid (Philadelphia collar and the Miami J collar) and appropriately sized, and should not interfere with management of the airway. As a general rule, high-cut collars are optimal because they provide points of support at the chin, angle of the jaw, and the mastoid processes. Decreased mouth opening while in a C-collar can lead to increased difficulty with airway management.[11] Several studies have shown a positive association between cervical collar application and rise in intracranial pressure (ICP).[12,13] Although the mechanism for this increase in ICP is unclear, it may be attributable to venous congestion in the neck.[14] Cervical collars may aggravate existing spinal cord injury in certain situations. A cadaveric study where researchers divided the anterior-posterior ligamentous support to simulate ligament injury resulted in a 7.3 mm separation of C1 and C2 following application of a cervical collar.[15] In a study it was found that there was less motion with a cervical collar in place than without,[16] whereas others found that the use of a cervical collar did not effectively reduce motion in an unstable spine.[17]

Spine boards

Traditionally, patients with cervical spine injury are secured to a backboard in order to fully immobilize the cervical spine. Two biomechanical studies demonstrated increased neck motion when using conventional extrication techniques (cervical collar with backboard) versus controlled self-extrication with cervical collar only.[18,19] Patients immobilized with a backboard are more likely to complain of occipital pain and lumbosacral pain.[20] Hence, it is advisable to adequately pad all of the pressure points, such as the occiput, scapulae, sacrum, and heels while transporting on spine boards.

Use of backboards for spinal immobilization is indicated in blunt trauma and altered level of consciousness, spinal tenderness, neurologic symptoms, high-energy mechanism of injury and drug or alcohol intoxication, inability to communicate, and/or distracting injury.[21,22]

Cervicalthoracic braces (Minerva jacket)

Injuries involving cervico-thoracic spine require a special brace to restrict movement of the neck and upper back after an injury or neck fusion surgery. A plastic padded chest jacket in two pieces (a front and a back piece), fastened with Velcro straps, is an effective method of immobilization. Supports for the chin and back of the head arise from the chest jacket.

Halo ring braces

These are used to restrict head and neck movement after a fracture or neck fusion. It consists of a fleece-lined plastic jacket that is worn on the chest, a lightweight metal ring (halo) that is fastened to the head with pins and rods that attach the vest to the head-ring.

RECOMMENDATIONS[1]

Level II

1. Spinal immobilization of all trauma patients with a cervical spine or spinal cord injury or with a mechanism of injury having the potential to cause cervical spinal injury is recommended.

2. Triage of patients with a potential spinal injury at the scene by trained and experienced emergency medical services (EMS) personnel to determine the need for immobilization during transport is recommended.

3. Immobilization of trauma patients who are awake, alert, and are not intoxicated; who are without neck pain or tenderness; who do not have an abnormal motor or sensory examination; and who do not have any significant associated injury that might detract from their general evaluation is not recommended.

Level III

1. A combination of a rigid cervical collar and supportive blocks on a backboard with straps is effective in limiting motion of the cervical spine and is recommended.

2. The longstanding practice of attempted spinal immobilization with sandbags and tape is insufficient and is not recommended.

3. Spinal immobilization in patients with penetrating trauma is not recommended because of increased mortality from delayed resuscitation.

Spinal immobilization can diminish untoward movement of the cervical spine and can decrease the possibility of the secondary neurologic deterioration in patients with unstable cervical spinal after trauma. The medical professional should consider that not all trauma patients require spinal immobilization during prehospital resuscitation and transport. A combination of a rigid cervical collar with support on a rigid backboard secured with straps and tape to immobilize the entire spine is efficient for safe transport. The traditional practice of attempted spinal immobilization with sandbags and tape with the patient strapped to a rigid backboard is not sufficient and strongly discouraged.

Cervical spine immobilization devices are efficient but can result in patient morbidity. Spinal immobilization devices should be used to accomplish the goals of spinal stability for safe extrication and transportation. They should be removed as soon as a definitive assessment is achieved and/or definitive management is initiated. The development of precise selection criteria for patients who require immobilization remains an area of exploration. Current publications on the use of contemporary, well-defined EMS triage protocols provide level II medical evidence for their utility. The wide variety of techniques used and the lack of substantial evidence to advocate a uniform device for spinal immobilization make immobilization techniques and device recommendations difficult.

REFERENCES

1. Theodore N, Hadley MN, Aarabi B et al. Prehospital cervical spinal immobilization after trauma. *Neurosurgery.* 2013;72:22-34.
2. Muhr MD, Seabrook DL, Wittwer LK. Paramedic use of a spinal injury clearance algorithm reduces spinal immobilization in the out-of-hospital setting. *Prehosp Emerg Care.* 1999;3:1-6.
3. De Lorenzo RA. A review of spinal immobilization techniques. *J Emerg Med.* 1996;14: 603-613.
4. Hoffman JR, Mower WR, Wolfson AB et al. Validity of a set of clinical criteria to rule out injury to the cervical spine in patients with blunt trauma. National Emergency XRadiography Utilization Study Group. *N Engl J Med.* 2000;343:94.
5. Schriger DL, Larmon B, LeGassick T, Blinman T. Spinal immobilization on a flat backboard: Does it result in neutral position of the cervical spine? *Ann Emerg Med.* 1991;20:878.
6. Herzenberg JE, Hensinger RN, Dedrick DK, Phillips WA. Emergency transport and positioning of young children who have an injury of the cervical spine. The standard backboard may be hazardous. *J Bone Joint Surg Am.* 1989;71:15.
7. Spine and spinal cord trauma. In: American College of Surgeons, eds. *Manual of Advanced Trauma Life Support*, 7th ed, Chicago 2004:177.
8. De Lorenzo RA. A review of spinal immobilization techniques. *J Emerg Med.* 1996; 14:603.
9. De Lorenzo RA, Olson JE, Boska M et al. Optimal positioning for cervical immobilization. *Ann Emerg Med.* 1996;28:301.

10. Perry SD, McLellan B, McIlroy WE et al. The efficacy of head immobilization techniques during simulated vehicle motion. *Spine (Phila Pa 1976)*. 1999;24:1839.

11. Goutcher CM, Lochhead V. Reduction in mouth opening with semi-rigid cervical collars. *Br J Anaesth*. 2005;95(3):344-348.

12. Dunham CM, Brocker BP, Collier BD, Gemmel DJ. Risks associated with magnetic resonance imaging and cervical collar in comatose, blunt trauma patients with negative comprehensive cervical spine computed tomography and no apparent spinal defcit. *Crit Care*. 2008;12(4):R89.

13. Mobbs RJ, Stoodley MA, Fuller J. Effect of cervical hard collar on intracranial pressure after head injury. *ANZ J Surg*. 2002;72(6):389-391.

14. Stone MB, Tubridy CM, Curran R. The effect of rigid cervical collars on internal jugular vein dimensions. *Acad Emerg Med*. 2010;17(1):100-102.

15. Ben-Galim P, Dreiangel N, Mattox KL, Reitman CA, Kalantar SB, Hipp JA. Extrication collars can result in abnormal separation between vertebrae in the presence of a dissociative injury. *J Trauma*. 2010;69(2):447-450.

16. Conrad BP, Rechtine G, Weight M, Clarke J, Horodyski M. Motion in the unstable cervical spine during hospital bed transfers. *J Trauma*. 2010;69,432-436.

17. Horodyski M, DiPaola CP, Conrad BP, Rechtine GR. Cervical collars are insufficient for immobilizing an unstable cervical spine injury. *J Emerg Med*. 2011;41(5):513-519.

18. Engsberg JR, Standeven JW, Shurtleff TL, Eggars JL, Shafer JS, Naunheim RS. Cervical spine motion during extrication. *J Emerg Med*. 2013;44(1):122-127.

19. Dixon M, O'Halloran J, Cummins NM. Biomechanical analysis of spinal immobilization during prehospital extrication—A proof of concept study. *Emerg Med J*. 2014;31(9):745-749.

20. Chan D, Goldberg RM, Mason J, Chan L. Backboard versus mattress splint immobilization: A comparison of symptoms generated. *J Emerg Med*. 1996;14(3):293-298.

21. White CC, Domeier RM, Millin MG. EMS spinal precautions and the use of the long backboard—Resource document to the position statement of the National Association of EMS Physicians and the American College of Surgeons Committee on Trauma. *Prehosp Emerg Care*. 2014;18(2):306-314.

22. American College of Emergency Physicians. Policy Statement—EMS Management of Patients with Potential Spinal Injury. 2015. http://www.acep.org/Physician-Resources/Policies/Policy-Statements/EMS-Management-of-Patients-with-PotentialSpinal-Injury. Accessed June 22, 2017.

44

Nasogastric tube insertion

ZULFIQAR ALI

INTRODUCTION

A nasogastric tube, often referred to as an NG tube, is a flexible tube that is inserted transnasally through the back of the throat into the esophagus and into the stomach. It is used for enteral feeds, medication, or aspiration of the gastric contents.

The nasogastric tubes are made of polyurethane. They have a radio-opaque marking throughout their length with external visible length markings that help in the insertion. A guidewire may be associated with them that facilitates their insertion. Nasogastric feeds are used when the feeding is needed for more than 14 days. They usually need to be changed every 30 to 90 days.[1]

Nonfeeding nasogastric tubes (e.g., Ryles tubes) are mainly made of polyvinyl chloride. They can be used for a maximum duration of 7 to 10 days. They are not recommended for feeding as there may be leaching of plasticizers from PVC tubes when it comes in contact with fats in nutritional formulae. However, they may be used for administration of essential drugs and initial feeding in the critical care setting.

The two commonly used NG tubes are the Levin tube and the Salem sump. They have a diameter which ranges from 12 to 18 French Guage (Fr) and a length of 42–50 inches. The Levin tube has a single lumen with holes at the tip and the distal end. It is mainly used for nasogastric feeding, gastric lavage, and decompression of the gastric contents.

It should not be used for suctioning as it may adhere to the mucosal surface and cause mucosal injury.[2]

The Salem sump is a dual lumen tube. It allows for safer continuous and intermittent gastric suctioning. The large lumen allows for easy suction of gastric contents, decompression, irrigation, and medication. The smaller vent lumen allows for atmospheric air to be drawn into the tube and equalizes the vacuum pressure in the stomach once the contents have been emptied. This prevents the suction eyelets from adhering to and damaging the stomach lining. The silicone Salem Sump tube provides the patient with optimal comfort and protection. The silicone tubing can dwell up to 30 days and remains flexible for optimal patient comfort during nasogastric tube use and removal.

INSERTION PROCEDURE

The procedure of nasogastric (NG) intubation, and its benefits, risks, complications, and alternatives, should be explained to the patient or the patient's relative (if the patient is not conscious). If the patient is conscious, the patency of the nostrils is checked by asking the patient to occlude one nostril and asking him to breathe through the other one. Local examination of the nostrils is done to identify any nasal septal deviation. The medical record should be checked for any possible anatomical variations due to surgery or cancer. Alternate the nostrils if the nasogastric tube is being replaced.

This will help in prevention of nasal irritation and potential ulceration. The patient may be made to raise a hand to communicate with the nurse during the procedure. This may also help to alleviate fear as the patient has some control over the procedure.

The hands are washed and an apron and gloves are worn to minimize the cross infection. The patient is placed in a semi-upright position (high Fowler's position) with the head supported in a slightly forward position. This position assists swallowing and helps prevent tracheal placement if the swallowing is compromised.

10 mL of viscous lidocaine 2% (for oral use) is instilled through the more patent nostril with the head tilted backwards. The patient is asked to sniff and swallow so that the nasal and oropharyngeal mucosa gets anesthetized. A time period of 5 to 10 minutes is required to ensure an adequate anesthetic effect.

The length of the tube to be inserted is measured as the length from the tip of the nose to the ear lobe and then from the ear lobe to the xiphoid process[3] (NEX measurement: nose, ear lobule, xiphoid process). This is believed to ensure that the distal end of the tube reaches the stomach. However, recent studies have shown that the NEX guideline is incorrect because it only approximates the nose to the gastroesophageal junction (GOJ) distance. A better approach was advocated by Taylor and coworkers to measure the distance in the opposite direction: xiphisternum to ear to nose (XEN), then add 10 cm. This ensures that the nasogastric tube is placed in the mid stomach.[4]

After measuring the desired length, the tip of the tube is inserted into the chosen nostril. The nasogastric tube is advanced gently and horizontally along the floor of the nostril; parallel to the nasal septum, into the nasopharynx, and then into the oropharynx. The patient may sneeze during the process. At this stage, the patient is reassured. If resistance is met, the nasogastric tube is withdrawn slightly and the angle of insertion is altered. If there is persistent resistance, the procedure may be abandoned and insertion should be attempted through the other nostril. To ensure a smooth insertion, it should be ensured that the natural anatomy of the nose is followed during the procedure.

If the patient is able to swallow, small sips of fluid should be taken at this stage. In an unconscious patient, a cold spoon on the tongue may stimulate the swallowing reflex. This swallowing action places the epiglottis over the trachea facilitating the entry of the tube into the esophagus. The nasogastric tube is then advanced down the esophagus with successive swallows until the proper insertion mark is seen at the nostril. In ventilated patients, the NG tube may be inserted under direct laryngoscopy. If the patient continues to cough and gag, check for coiling of the tube at the back of the throat using a tongue blade and flashlight (or a laryngoscope in intubated patients). If the nasogastric tube is coiled, it is withdrawn until it is up in the oropharynx again. After confirming the tube position, it is anchored on the nostrils or the cheeks using appropriate adhesive tapes.

CONFIRMATION OF NASOGASTRIC TUBE PLACEMENT

1. **Auscultatory method: (Air insufflation test)**. It should not be the sole method to confirm the location of the nasogastric feeding tube. "Pseudoconfirmatory gurgling" sound can be heard when feeding tubes are positioned in the tracheobronchial tree or pleural spaces as tubes inadvertently placed in the respiratory tract or esophagus can transmit a sound similar to that of air entry in the stomach.[5] However, a positive air insufflations test combined with aspiration of gastric contents is considered as a fairly reliable predictor of successful placement of nasogastric tube in the stomach.[5]

2. **pH testing:** A combination of aspirate appearance and pH testing is helpful in predicting the placement of nasogastric tube in the stomach. Around 2 ml of stomach content are aspirated using a sterile syringe and tested using CE marked pH paper.

   a. If the pH value is less than 5 it confirms a gastric placement and feeding should be initiated.[6]

   b. If the pH is between 5 and 6, the visual characteristics of the gastric aspirate are carried out. If visual characteristics indicate gastric aspirate, we can proceed to feed.

Otherwise, an x-ray is needed to confirm tube placement. The gastric secretions are grassy green in color with brown sediment. The intestinal secretions are more transparent than gastric aspirates and may appear bile stained, ranging in color from light to dark golden yellow or brownish-green, and tracheobronchial secretions consist of off-white to tan sediment.[6]

c. If pH is more than 6, it indicates an intestinal or respiratory placement of the NG tube and an X ray should be done to confirm the placement.

3. **Radiologic determination of feeding tube placement:** A request for an x-ray of the upper abdomen and chest should be made

   a. If the pH of the aspirate is between 5 and 6 and visual characteristics are not indicative of gastric or intestinal aspirate.

   b. If pH of the aspirate is >6.

   c. No aspirate is obtained.

Radiography determination of tube location is regarded as the most accurate method of checking tube placement as x-ray helps to visualize the entire course of the tube.[7]

REFERENCES

1. Stroud M, Duncan H. Guidelines for enteral feeding in adult hospital patients. *J Nightingale Gut.* 2003;52.
2. Kirby DF, Opilla M. (2005). Enteral access and infusion equipment. In: Merritt, R, ed. *The A.S.P.E.N. Nutrition Support Practice Manual. 2nd ed.* American Society of Parenteral and Enteral Nutrition, 3.1 to 3.10. [ASPEN, 2005]
3. Simons SR, Abdallah LM. Bedside assessment of enteral tube placement: Aligning practice with evidence. *Am J Nurs.* 2012;112:40-46.
4. Taylor SJ, Allan K, McWilliam H, Toher D. Nasogastric tube depth: The 'NEX' guideline is incorrect. *Br J Nurs.* 2014;23:641-644.
5. Metheny N, McSweeney M, Wehrle MA, Wiersema L. Effectiveness of the auscultatory method in predicting feeding tube location. *Nurs Res.* 1990;39(5):262-267.
6. Taylor SJ, Clemente R. Confirmation of nasogastric tube position by pH testing. *J Hum Nutr Diet.* 2005;18:371-375.
7. Lemyze M. The placement of nasogastric tubes. *Can Med Assoc J.* 2010;182:802.

45

Intraparenchymal ICP catheter insertion

NIDHI GUPTA

INTRODUCTION

Despite advances in neurocritical care, traumatic brain injury (TBI) remains a significant source of both injury-related mortality and long-term disability worldwide. Historically, monitoring intracranial pressure (ICP) and maintenance of an adequate cerebral perfusion pressure have been considered as the cornerstone of acute neurologic treatment after TBI. However, effectiveness of ICP monitoring in reducing mortality from TBI is still controversial. While several large observational studies suggest an improved outcome associated with ICP monitoring and aggressive treatment of intracranial hypertension (ICH) in severe TBI patients,[1–3] others find no difference or even an increased mortality associated with ICP monitoring.[4,5]

Results from large observational studies suggest that ICP monitoring may be more efficacious for more serious patients of TBI, who have a high probability of ICH.[6,7] These patients tend to gain the most from invasive monitoring as they often require aggressive medical therapy and cannot be effectively monitored noninvasively. A recent meta-analysis of published studies to assess the effects of ICP monitoring in patients with severe TBI suggests superior survival in patients receiving ICP monitoring.[8]

The latest Brain Trauma Foundation guidelines (4th Edition) also recommends management of severe TBI patients using information from ICP monitoring to reduce in-hospital and 2-week postinjury mortality. (Class of evidence—level II B).[9]

INTRACRANIAL PRESSURE MONITORING SYSTEMS

There are two types of transducer systems for continuous monitoring of ICP. The external strain-gauge transducers are coupled to the patient's intracranial space via a fluid-filled catheter, whereas the catheter tip transducer technologies are placed intracranially. Though external strain-gauge transducers have greater accuracy, false readings associated with obstruction, air bubbles, or movement of the patient's fluid lines are a concern. Currently, the most commonly used methods of continuous ICP monitoring includes intraventricular devices (IVDs) with pressure readings obtained either via the fluid-filled catheter attached to an external strain-gauge transducer or, by fiberoptic or strain-gauge microtransducer implanted within the tip of the ventricular catheter; and intraparenchymal devices (IPDs) with intraparenchymal catheter-tip microtransducer systems.

The ventricular catheter connected to an external strain gauge [external ventricular drain (EVD)] is considered as the most accurate, low-cost, and reliable method of monitoring ICP.[10] It also offers the ease of in vivo calibration, thus ensuring that ICP is measured correctly, while simultaneously permitting therapeutic drainage of cerebrospinal fluid (CSF) for ICH. Though considered as a "gold standard," EVDs are believed to be more frequently associated with complications than IPDs. In comparison, IPDs are extremely easy to insert and are highly accurate with consistent readings.[10–12] Intraparenchymal pressure may not be representative of the true "global ICP" because of the intraparenchymal pressure gradients that may exist after TBI.[13] This notion was, however, recently questioned by Vender and coworkers who evaluated the predictive capability of intraventricular, intraparenchymal, and fluid-coupled techniques for ICP monitoring to local, regional, and global changes in patients with severe TBI.[12] Authors found that the regional pressure measurements via the IPD did not under or overestimate global pressure changes compared to the IVD. Changes in recorded ICP began and subsided over a similar time course both in the ventricle and the parenchyma. Furthermore, when compared to the other two monitoring techniques, intraparenchymal monitoring was the only method that remained unaffected when spinal fluid was being drained. This can be helpful in providing "bridging data" that could monitor ICP and detect ICP trends while allowing uninterrupted CSF drainage as well as providing a secondary, confirmatory measure should ventricular sensor function be partially impaired. These potential advantages, along with lower infectious and hemorrhagic risks, have given the IPDs the position of the standard device for ICP monitoring in a majority of neurosurgical intensive care units (ICUs). It is, however, evident that the clinical decision making regarding the type of ICP monitor to be placed is complex and centers around determining which modality would cause maximum benefit and least harm to the patient.

To date, only a few studies have been conducted comparing outcomes in TBI patients with regards to the type of ICP monitor used.[14,15] Kasotakis and coworkers did the first study to compare the clinically relevant outcomes in TBI patients managed with either IPDs or an EVD.[14] Though device selection for ICP monitoring did not affect neurologic outcomes and mortality between the two groups; use of EVD was found to be associated with prolonged ICP monitoring and a higher device-related complication rate. The IPD group had a larger size of the midline shift, a finding reflective of the neurosurgeon's preference for IPDs in patients with lateral, space-occupying hematomas, and therefore ventricles that are likely effaced. Likewise, the incidence of intraventricular hemorrhage in the EVD-treated group was more than double that of the IPD group (37% vs. 16.3%, $P < 0.001$), reflecting the preference for EVDs that can at least partially evacuate blood from the ventricular system or simply drain CSF with nondraining, noncommunicating hydrocephalus. Contrary to the findings of the previous study, Liu and colleagues found that patients managed with EVD had a lower rate of ICH, underwent fewer craniotomies, and had higher survival rates at 1 and 6 months after injury; thereby reaffirming the therapeutic effectiveness of the EVD draining function in patients with ICH.[15]

TYPES OF INTRAPARENCHYMAL ICP MONITORING DEVICES

The IPDs are nonfluid coupled devices and can be classified into different subtypes based on their pressure transduction method; strain-gauge method [Codman® MicroSensor™ (CMS), Raumedic Neurovent-P ICP sensor, and Pressio sensor]; fiberoptic technology (Integra™ Camino® ICP monitor and Innerspace ICP monitor); or pneumatic technology (Spiegelberg ICP Monitor). The CMS and the Camino monitor are the two most known and commonly used of these devices.

Codman MicroSensor: The CMS (Johnson and Johnson, Raynham, MA, USA) ICP transducer consists of a miniature strain-gauge pressure sensor mounted in a titanium case (diameter 1.2 mm) at the tip of a 100-cm flexible nylon tube (diameter 0.7 mm) (Figure 45.1). The sensor contains a silicon microchip with diffused piezoresistive strain gauges that are connected by thin copper wires to complete a Wheatstone bridge-type circuit. When pressure is applied, the silicon diaphragm deflects a small amount in proportion to the applied pressure, thereby inducing strain in the embedded piezoresistors. This change in electrical resistance is reflected in the form of a different voltage, which is then converted into a different pressure and displayed as an ICP. The CMS

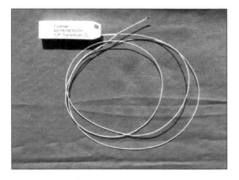

Figure 45.1 Codman MicroSensor Intracranial Pressure Transducer.

Figure 45.2 Spiegelberg parenchymal probe with small air-pouch balloon at the distal end of the catheter (black arrow).

transducer monitors ICP directly at the source—parenchymal, subdural, or intraventricular. The system can also be incorporated into a ventricular catheter, thereby allowing simultaneous drainage of CSF as well as ICP recording.

Neurovent-P ICP Monitor: Similar to the Codman system, the Neurovent-P ICP monitor (Raumedic AG, Helmbrechts, Germany) is also based on an electronic microchip strain-gauge pressor sensor. In addition to measuring ICP, the multiparameter Neurovent–PTO monitoring system also measures brain tissue oxygen partial pressure using a luminescence optical sensor fiber and brain temperature using thermistors.

Neurovent-P-tel is an implantable transdermal telemetry system for intraparenchymal ICP measurement.[16] It consists of an intraparenchymatous pressure sensor at the end of the tip and a subgaleal telemetric transducer that transfers pressure values over the closed scalp using validated radiofrequency identification principle to a reading device. The data is then captured and stored on a software for analyses. In patients with severe TBI, Neurovent-P-tel could be used for long-term ICP monitoring to exclude late complications.

Pressio® Device: The Sophysa Pressio® (Sophysa Ltd., Orsay, France) system is composed of a transducer containing a silicon microsensor with an embedded piezoresistive strain gauge for pressure measurement and micro-thermistor for temperature measurement.

Integra Camino Monitor: The Camino ICP monitor (Intergra LifeSciences Corp, NJ, USA) uses a fiber-optic catheter to direct light toward a miniature displaceable mirror placed at the catheter tip. Changes in ICP distort the mirror and the

differences in reflected light intensity are converted into an ICP value.

Spiegelberg ICP Monitor: The Spiegelberg ICP monitor (Spiegelberg GmbH & Co. KG, Hamburg, Germany) uses the pneumatic air-pouch method to measure ICP. A small air pouch balloon, containing 0.1 ml of air, is placed at the distal end of the polyurethane catheter (Figure 45.2). The ICP is transmitted across the thin pouch wall to the air volume inside the balloon. The catheter connects to an internal strain-gauge transducer that measures the internal balloon pressure changes, converting them into an electrical signal. The Spiegelberg monitor is capable of automatic zero drift correction once every hour in vivo, which avoids the problem of rezeroing and zero-drift.

PLACEMENT OF INTRAPARENCHYMAL ICP CATHETERS

Intraparenchymal ICP monitor insertions have historically been done by neurosurgeons. However, recent data show that the procedure is equally safe when performed by neurointensivists and trauma surgeons, well trained and credentialed by the neurosurgeons in the placement of these monitors.[17,18] The sensor can be inserted in any setting: under local anesthesia in the operating room or at the bedside, either in the ICU or in the emergency department; without any significant difference in the infection risk associated with the procedure.[19,20]

CODMAN MICROSENSOR ICP CATHETER INSERTION TECHNIQUE

The Codman ICP pressure-monitoring system consists of three parts: the CMS, an interface cable, and the ICP EXPRESS® unit (IEU). The IEU is a digital ICP monitor that also serves as an interface between the CMS ICP transducer and compatible external patient monitors (Figure 45.3). It provides a continuous numeric display of the mean, systolic, and diastolic ICP. As an interface unit, the IEU calibrates patient monitors, zeroes the microsensor transducer, and generates a real-time output signal for viewing the ICP waveform on external patient monitors. The cable, which is provided with the unit, is designed with an inline memory computer chip that retains the microsensors zero-reference number. Hence, the IEU can be easily interchanged or briefly disconnected without the need for calibration during patient transport.

Setting of IEU: Begin by using the "On/Off" key to turn the IEU on. If the IEU is connected to an external patient monitor, the screen on the monitor prompts to "Zero Patient Monitor." The bedside patient monitor is now zeroed according to the manufacturer's instructions. After verifying that the patient monitor displays a numeric mean ICP of zero, the IEU menu "Enter" key is pressed. The

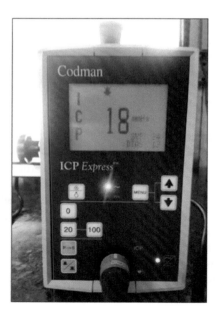

Figure 45.3 Codman intracranial pressure express unit.

patient monitor is now calibrated by pressing either the "20" or "100" key labeled "Calibrate Patient Monitor." The 20 key is used whenever the patient monitor scale is less than 100 mmHg. A 20 mmHg signal is now displayed on the patient monitor. The menu "Enter" key is pressed again when the calibration is complete. The microsensor is now connected to the IEU. Wait till the instruction "Press Zero to Zero Transducer" appears on the screen. The tip of the catheter is now submerged in 3 inches of sterile saline in the horizontal position for zeroing. The transducer is zeroed by pressing the blue "Zero" key labeled "Zero Transducer." The microsensor zero-reference number will be displayed on the IEU screen. This number is specific to the transducer that is zeroed and must be recorded in the patient's chart as well as on the microsensor connector. This number is used by the IEU to correct the zero level at implantation according to a mathematical algorithm. The menu "Enter" key is pressed again and the sensor should now show a pressure of 0 mmHg. The microsensor ICP transducer is now ready for implantation.

INTRAPARENCHYMAL CODMAN MICROSENSOR INSERTION TECHNIQUE

Traditionally, the sensor is placed through a twist drill burr hole, at Kocher's point [approximately 2 cm anterior to the coronal suture (to avoid motor strip) and 2–3 cm lateral to the midline (to avoid the sagittal sinus), in the mid-pupillary line] (Figure 45.4). The right (nondominant) side is usually preferred, unless contraindicated by the patient's pathology. The area around the incision is clipped, cleaned aseptically with povidone-iodine solution for 5 minutes and draped with sterile surgical sheets. After local anesthetic infilteration, a 5-mm parasagittal skin incision is made. The scalp is retracted to expose the skull. A small burr hole (3 mm) is made through the outer and inner tables of the skull using a twist drill bit of size 2.7 mm. Using a tunneling needle, the flexible catheter is now tunneled beneath the scalp to a separate skin puncture (about 5 cm from the surgical incision), to prevent it from being easily broken. After zeroing, the sensor tip is now introduced into the brain parenchyma to a depth of 1.5 to 2 cm through the burr hole. The incision is closed with sutures and the catheter is secured to the scalp after making a

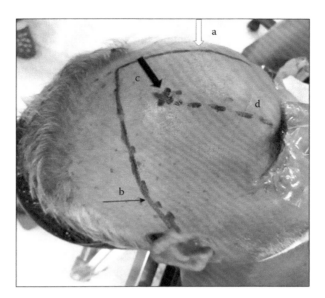

Figure 45.4 Schematic diagram of patient's head showing (a) midline, (b) coronal suture, (c) Kocher's point (approximately 2 cm anterior to the coronal suture and 2–3 cm lateral to the midline, in the midpupillary line), and (d) midpupillary line.

small loop for additional strain relief (Figure 45.5). Alternatively, the sensor can be placed at the end of the craniotomy, if ICP monitoring is planned in the immediate postoperative period. The catheter is tunneled beneath the scalp using the tunneling needle provided in the kit and calibrated according to the manufacturer's instructions. The sensor tip is inserted through the cortex into the brain, before the bone flap is secured in place. The catheter is now secured to the scalp. After the procedure, a

cerebral computed tomography scan is performed to check the position of the intraparenchymal probe tip and look for any hematoma along the catheter.

Unlike EVDs, IPDs do not require a hydrostatic zero level, as the transducer is placed intracranially on the tip of the sensor. Hence, there is no concern about the level of the transducer. Nonetheless, while inserting the sensor inside the brain parenchyma, it is of paramount importance to attain an

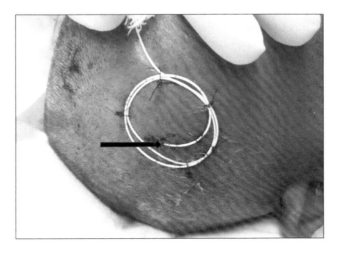

Figure 45.5 Codman microsensor transducer catheter secured to the scalp after making a small loop (black arrow represents catheter entry site beneath the scalp).

optimal implantation depth, which, under certain situations, can affect the measured ICP. Accurate pressure readings are monitored only if the patient is in a supine horizontal position with no elevation of the head. By elevating the head, a hydrostatic pressure is introduced, which depending upon the depth of the sensor tip, influences the measured ICP. Koskinen and coworkers observed a wide variation in the insertion depth of the CMS from 0 to 88 mm (mean implantation depth was 21.3 ± 11.1 mm), which should be taken into account while measuring ICP, if patients are treated with head elevation of 30°.[21] The recently introduced new CMS sensor has length markings on the catheter, which facilitates its accurate placement within the brain parenchyma.

Zero-drift: Most of the currently available IPDs (except Spiegelberg ICP monitor) are inherently susceptible to zero-drift, as the sensor tip cannot be recalibrated with atmospheric pressure while *in situ*. Hence, there is an increasing drift of zero-value with time resulting in inaccurate pressure readings, particularly when long-term ICP monitoring is contemplated. Zero-drift is calculated as the difference between the initial and final pressure measurement when the sensor is explanted, with the tip just submerged in saline.

The CMS manufacturers estimate a zero-drift of no greater than 3 mmHg per 24-hour period. Koskinen and Olivecrona evaluated the accuracy and reliability of the CMS system to measure ICP by determining the zero-drift of the device in 128 patients treated for various intracranial abnormalities.[11] In addition, they recorded the ICP simultaneously in 22 patients with an EVD and the CMS. They found very acceptable zero-drift (mean drift of 0.9 ± 0.2 mmHg) and no statistically significant correlation between the drift and duration of use of CMS. Nonetheless, there was a good correlation with the "gold standard" EVD measurements (bias, −1.2 mmHg, limits of agreement, −7.7; 5.3 mmHg). Authors thus concluded that the ICP measured by the CMS device is reliable, true, and stable, even after 1 week of use. Al-Tamimi and coworkers demonstrated a median absolute zero-drift of 2.0 mmHg (interquartile range, 1–3 mmHg), with a statistically significant positive correlation with the time that the probe was in situ.[22] However, nearly 20% of drift readings were ≥5 mmHg and 2% of the readings were ≥10 mmHg.

Astonishingly, these values had potential significant therapeutic implications in up to 50% of patients, if not accounted as inaccurate. Nevertheless, this finding underscores an important clinical dictum of critical care management of severe TBI patients that the ICP should not be treated just as a number and should be interpreted carefully in conjunction with clinical and radiological assessment of patients.

Compared to CMS, literature suggests a higher zero-drift with the Camino device.[19,23] According to the manufacturer's specifications, the Camino ICP monitor has a maximum zero-drift during the first 24 hours of 0 ± 2 mmHg and less than ±1 mmHg/day on subsequent days. Gelabert-González and coworkers observed a mean zero-drift of 7.3 ± 5.1 mmHg (range, −17 to 21 mmHg).[19] Moreover, only 12.6% of sensors were found to have no zero-drift on removal, with a mean monitoring time of 58.4 ± 8.6 hours (range 16–114 hours). Though no significant correlation was noted between zero-drift and monitoring time for global, negative, and positive drift by the authors, the data presented showed drift up to ±20 mmHg with longer periods of monitoring (>100 hours). Apparently, the accuracy of the device for longer periods of monitoring needs further evaluation.

To reduce the significance of zero-drift on the accuracy of IPDs during long-term ICP measurements, Morgalla and coworkers have suggested the use of drift index by the manufacturers of various devices.[24] In their initial laboratory testing of seven different types of ICP transducers (including Camino, Codman, and Spiegelberg ICP monitors), authors have shown that probes often do not exhibit a linear pattern of drift.[25] Instead, sometimes they seem to reveal positive and negative drift consecutively. They may also change their pressure reading quite frequently despite the actual pressure being constant. Authors later used a fixed-pressure system to assess the percentage of readings that showed drift, the maximum pressure deviation, and the mean pressure deviation in several different transducers over a 10-day monitoring period.[24] For the Camino device, the median proportion of pressure change was 1.59%, the maximum pressure change was up to 6 mmHg, the median value for the mean absolute pressure change was 2.9 mmHg, and the 10-days drift measurement was 4 mmHg.

COMPLICATIONS

Intraparenchymal ICP monitoring-related complications include infection, intracranial hemorrhage, and technical complications of the catheter.

Infection: Unlike IVDs, IPDs are usually associated with very low clinically relevant infections, even in the absence of prophylactic antibiotics.[14,15,20,26] The small size of the transducer and flexibility of the catheter allows the transducer to be tunneled beneath the scalp, thus minimizing infection. In addition, the non-CSF-derived system lowers the risk for meningitis and makes nursing of the patient much easier. Infectious complications data from recent literature have noted culture-positive monitor tips in ≤17%, with clinically relevant infection rates between 0% and 3%.[14,15,19,21,27,28] *Staphylococcus epidermidis* has been identified as the predominant organism in culture positive cases (up to 80% of cases) followed by *Escherichia coli* (10%–15% of cases).[19,20,26] Other isolated organisms include *Corynebacterium* spp., *Staphylococcus aureus*, *Haemophilus influenza*, *Klebsiella* spp., *Streptococcus* spp., *Bacillus* spp., *Serratia* spp., *Acinetobacter baumannii*, and *Pseudomona aeruginosa*.

Given the low rate of infection, the use of prophylactic antibiotics with IPDs remains controversial. The clinical practice varies widely, mostly being institution-specific, determined in terms of the antimicrobial spectrum, bio-availability, side effects, and the antibiotic cost-efficacy ratio. To date none of the study has conclusively demonstrated the beneficial role of prophylactic antibiotics in preventing IPDs-related infection. Even after comparison of the culture-positive studies, the results are either comparable or inconclusive as to the prophylactic role of intravenous antibiotics.[14,15,19,21,26,27,29] Stoikes and colleagues reported twice as many infectious complications after the administration of prophylactic antibiotics than no antibiotics prior to or during ICP monitoring along with a significant increase in the number of multidrug-resistant pathogens.[29] Martínez-Mañas and coworkers used prophylactic intravenous cephalosporins and had a 9.5% culture-positive rate with the Camino device.[27] Similarly, Kasotakis and coworkers provided prophylactic gram-positive coverage to all the patients for the duration of ICP monitoring.[14] Although infectious

complications that occurred in 2.6% of the patients managed with an EVD, no catheter-related infections were identified in the IPD group. In another prospective observational study, infections occurred in 1.7% of patients with CMS as compared to 3.2% of the patients managed with EVDs ($P = 0.448$), despite routine antibiotic prophylaxis in all subjects for the duration of ICP monitoring.[15] Studies not using prophylactic antibiotics reported 17% and 8.5% culture-positive rate, and 2.1% and 0% clinically relevant infections, respectively, for the Camino device[19,26] and an infection rate of 0.6% for the CMS.[21]

Some studies have suggested that prophylactic antibiotics may even be harmful.[19,28–30] Indiscriminate exposure to antibiotics, especially broad-spectrum antibiotics, has been reported to affect the susceptibility patterns of pathogens producing subsequent infectious complications from multidrug-resistant pathogens, anaphylactic reactions, and systemic toxicity.[29,30] May and coworkers have shown that patients who received broad-spectrum prophylaxis acquired gram-negative infections with significantly greater antibiotic resistance than patients who received narrow-spectrum or no prophylaxis at all.[28] Hence, broad-spectrum antibiotic prophylaxis of ICP monitors should be eliminated or minimized till data from randomized trials prove its efficacy.

While evaluating the risk factors and complications of the Camino device, Bekar and coworkers found no statistically significant association between duration of catheter use and infection risk.[20] Hence, in contrast to IVDs, where the risk of infection gradually increases after the fifth day, IPDs may remain for as long as monitoring is needed. Presence of rhinorrhea, wound infection, and surgical procedure for intracerebral hematoma were noted as the likely risk factors for catheter infection in this study. Considering the effect of more than one sensor placement on infection risk, no significant difference in culture results were found in patients who had >1 Camino sensor placed during their hospital course.[19,26] However, in the study evaluating the complications of CMS, all the three infected patients had two or more than two CMS inserted during the course of their treatment and had undergone major intracranial surgery for severe TBI.[21]

Morton and coworkers reported an exceptional case of a life-threatening intracerebral abscess from a Camino ICP monitor in a 35-month-old child requiring 7 days of ICP monitoring.[31] It was speculated that the reinsertion of the IPD at the same site of initial insertion and concomitant corticosteroid therapy in view of his severe airway edema may have contributed an independent risk factor for this infectious complication. Authors thus cautioned against the use of same insertion site when monitor reinsertion is required.

Hemorrhage: The catheter-induced hemorrhage is a real concern during placement of all IPDs as they are introduced blindly into the brain through a small twist drill hole. IPDs, however, have lower hemorrhagic risk than ventriculostomy catheters (1.7% vs. 4.8%), owing to the smaller size of their catheters.[15] Current literature reports a low risk (<2.5%) of hemorrhage with IPDs, with clinically significant bleeds in even less than 0.5% to 1% of insertion-related hemorrhages.[19-21]

Coagulopathic patients are considered at increased risk for complications during monitor placement, including worsening of existing injuries or a new intracranial bleed. Nonetheless, recent literature suggests IPDs as a safe option considering the risk for hemorrhage, even in patients with confirmed coagulopathy.[19,21,32] With a CMS device, nonsignificant bleeds of ≤1 ml were found in 4.4% of the patients and a hematoma of 8 ml in only one patient (0.2%), with no significant increase in hemorrhagic complications in patients who were considered coagulopathic.[21] Moreover, the initiation of anticoagulant treatment after coiling of aneurysms, sinus thrombosis, and prophylactic treatment for deep venous thrombosis did not result in hemorrhage around the sensor. Gelabert-González et al. reported an overall bleeding rate of 2.5% with the Camino fiber-optic device (including patients with and without coagulation disorders) with only six cases requiring surgical evacuation.[19]

Hemorrhagic complications are infrequent in patients with an INR of ≤1.6 and do not mandate the routine use of FFP to "normalize" INR below this threshold.[32] Prior to the placement of an ICP monitor, patients on warfarin should be reversed with vitamin K and fresh frozen plasma or prothrombin complex concentrates. Patients on antiplatelet medications should undergo prior functional assays for aspirin and P2Y12 inhibitors followed by correction of the qualitative platelet dysfunction with platelet transfusion. In the setting of severe coagulopathy (patients with grade III/IV

hepatic encephalopathy), inserting an IPD after administration of recombinant Factor VIIa (within 15 minutes to 2 hours) allows for an expeditious, reliable and apparently safe way of establishing invasive ICP monitoring without hemorrhagic or thrombotic complications.[33]

Technical complications: Device-related technical complications are up to 3 times less frequent with IPDs than with EVDs.[14] EVDs, being hollow tubes, may plug or thrombose, and may eventually require replacement, if the indication for ongoing ICP monitoring persists. On the contrary, absence of a fluid column in IPDs precludes dampening of pressure waveforms by blood clots, debris, or air bubbles. The distal location of the transducer at the tip of the sensor also eliminates the need for constant realignment of the transducer with the patient's head and repeated re-zeroing. However, IPDs are sensitive to stretch and are easily damaged when acutely bent during nursing maneuvers, during transport of the patient to the radiological unit, or by restless patients in bed.[19-21] Commonly reported technical complications include disconnection of the transducer, breakage of the catheter close to the proximal connecting part, dislocation of the fixation screw, and probe defects of unknown cause. Education of nurses and other medical staff about the proper handling of the device goes a long way in decreasing these complications.

REFERENCES

1. Farahvar A, Gerber LM, Chiu YL, Carney N, Hartl R, Ghajar J. Increased mortality in patients with severe traumatic brain injury treated without intracranial pressure monitoring. *J Neurosurg.* 2012;117:729-734.
2. Alali AS, Fowler RA, Mainprize TG et al. Intracranial pressure monitoring in severe traumatic brain injury: Results from the American College of Surgeons Trauma Quality Improvement Program. *J Neurotrauma.* 2013;30:1737-1746.
3. Talving P, Karamanos E, Teixeira PG et al. Intracranial pressure monitoring in severe head injury: Compliance with Brain Trauma Foundation guidelines and effect on outcomes: A prospective study. *J Neurosurg.* 2013;119:1248-1254.
4. Cremer OL, van Dijk GW, van Wensen E et al. Effect of intracranial pressure monitoring

and targeted intensive care on functional outcome after severe head injury. *Crit Care Med.* 2005;33:2207-2213.

5. Chesnut RM, Temkin N, Carney N et al; Global Neurotrauma Research Group: A trial of intracranial-pressure monitoring in traumatic brain injury. *N Engl J Med.* 2012;367: 2471-2481.

6. Yuan Q, Wu X, Yu J et al. Effects and clinical characteristics of intracranial pressure monitoring-targeted management for subsets of traumatic brain injury: An observational multicenter study. *Crit Care Med.* 2015;43:1405-1414.

7. Dawes AJ, Sacks GD, Cryer HG et al. Intracranial pressure monitoring and inpatient mortality in severe traumatic brain injury: A propensity score-matched analysis. *J Trauma Acute Care Surg.* 2015;78:492-501.

8. Shen L, Wang Z, Su Z et al. Effects of intracranial pressure monitoring on mortality in patients with severe traumatic brain injury: A meta-analysis. *PLoS One.* 2016;11: e0168901.

9. Carney N, Totten AM, O'Reilly C et al. Guidelines for the management of severe traumatic brain injury, 4th ed. https://www .braintrauma.org/coma/guidelines.

10. Brain Trauma Foundation, American Association of Neurological Surgeons, Congress of Neurological Surgeons et al. Guidelines for the management of severe traumatic brain injury. VII. Intracranial pressure monitoring technology. *J Neurotrauma.* 2007;24 (suppl 1):S45-S54.

11. Koskinen LO, Olivecrona M. Clinical experience with the intraparenchymal intracranial pressure monitoring Codman MicroSensor system. *Neurosurgery.* 2005;56:693-698.

12. Vender J, Waller J, Dhandapani K, McDonnell D. An evaluation and comparison of intraventricular, intraparenchymal, and fluid-coupled techniques for intracranial pressure monitoring in patients with severe traumatic brain injury. *J Clin Monit Comput.* 2011;25:231-236.

13. Sahuquillo J, Poca MA, Arribas M, Garnacho A, Rubio E. Interhemispheric supratentorial intracranial pressure gradients in head-injured patients: Are they clinically important? *J Neurosurg.* 1999;90:16-26.

14. Kasotakis G, Michailidou M, Bramos A et al. Intraparenchymal vs. extracranial ventricular drain intracranial pressure monitors in traumatic brain injury: Less is more? *J Am Coll Surg.* 2012;214:950-957.

15. Liu H, Wang W, Cheng F et al. External ventricular drains versus intraparenchymal intracranial pressure monitors in traumatic brain injury: A prospective observational study. *World Neurosurg.* 2015;83:794-800.

16. Welschehold S, Schmalhausen E, Dodier P et al. First clinical results with a new telemetric intracranial pressure-monitoring system. *Neurosurgery.* 2012;70(1 suppl operative): 44-49.

17. Sadaka F, Kasal J, Lakshmanan R, Palagiri A. Placement of intracranial pressure monitors by neurointensivists: Case series and a systematic review. *Brain Inj.* 2013;27(5):600-604.

18. Ekeh AP, Ilyas S, Saxe JM et al. Successful placement of intracranial pressure monitors by trauma surgeons. *J Trauma Acute Care Surg.* 2014;76(2):286-290; discussion 290-291.

19. Gelabert-González M, Ginesta-Galan V, Sernamito-García R, Allut AG, Bandin-Diéguez J, Rumbo RM. The Camino intracranial pressure device in clinical practice: Assessment in a 1000 cases. *Acta Neurochir (Wien).* 2006;148(4):435-441.

20. Bekar A, Doğan S, Abaş F et al. Risk factors and complications of intracranial pressure monitoring with a fiberoptic device. *J Clin Neurosci.* 2009;16:236-240.

21. Koskinen LO, Grayson D, Olivecrona M. The complications and the position of the Codman MicroSensor™ ICP device: An analysis of 549 patients and 650 Sensors. *Acta Neurochir (Wien).* 2013;155:2141-2148.

22. Al-Tamimi YZ, Helmy A, Bavetta S, Price SJ. Assessment of zero drift in the Codman intracranial pressure monitor: A study from 2 neurointensive care units. *Neurosurgery* 2009;64:94-98.

23. Czosnyka M, Czosnyka Z, Pickard JD. Laboratory testing of three intracranial pressure microtransducers: Technical report. *Neurosurgery.* 1996;38:219-224.

24. Morgalla MH, Dietz K, Deininger M, Grote EH. The problem of long-term ICP drift

assessment: Improvement by use of the ICP drift index. *Acta Neurochir (Wien)*. 2002; 144:57-60.

25. Morgalla MH, Mettenleiter H, Bitzer M, Fretschner R, Grote EH. ICP measurement control: Laboratory test of 7 types of intracranial pressure transducers. *J Med EngTechnol*. 1999;23:144-151.

26. Poca MA, Sahuquillo J, Arribas M, Báguena M, Amorós S, Rubio E. Fiberoptic intraparenchymal brain pressure monitoring with the Camino V420 monitor: Reflections on our experience in 163 severely head-injured patients. *J Neurotrauma*. 2002;19:439-448.

27. Martínez-Mañas RM, Santamarta D, de Campos JM, Ferrer E. Camino intracranial pressure monitor: Prospective study of accuracy and complications. *J Neurol Neurosurg Psychiatry*. 2000;69:82-86.

28. May AK, Fleming SB, Carpenter RO et al. Influence of broad-spectrum antibiotic prophylaxis on intracranial pressure monitor infections and subsequent infectious complications in head-injured patients. *Surg Infect (Larchmt)*. 2006;7:409-417.

29. Stoikes NF, Magnotti LJ, Hodges TM et al. Impact of intracranial pressure monitor prophylaxis on central nervous system infections and bacterial multi-drug resistance. *Surg Infect (Larchmt)*. 2008;9:503-508.

30. Prabhu VC, Kaufman HH, Voelker JL et al. Prophylactic antibiotics with intracranial pressure monitors and external ventricular drains: A review of the evidence. *Surg Neurol*. 1999; 52:226-237.

31. Morton R, Lucas TH 2nd, Ko A, Browd SR, Ellenbogen RG, Chesnut RM. Intracerebral abscess associated with the Camino intracranial pressure monitor: Case report and review of the literature. *Neurosurgery* 2012; 71:E193-E198.

32. Davis JW, Davis IC, Bennink LD et al. Placement of intracranial pressure monitors: Are "normal" coagulation parameters necessary? *J Trauma*. 2004;57:1173-1177.

33. Le TV, Rumbak MJ, Liu SS, Alsina AE, van Loveren H, Agazzi S. Insertion of intracranial pressure monitors in fulminant hepatic failure patients: Early experience using recombinant factor VII. *Neurosurgery*. 2010;66:455-458.

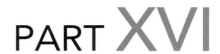
Webliography

46

Summary of Brain Trauma Foundation guidelines (2016) and scales and scores

ANKUR KHANDELWAL

BRAIN TRAUMA FOUNDATION GUIDELINES (2016)

Summary

- In 1986, Dr. Jamshid Ghajar and the Board of the Sunny von Bulow Coma and Head Trauma Research Foundation founded Brain Trauma Foundation (BTF) in order to support ongoing research on traumatic brain injury (TBI).
- Since its inception, BTF has been conducting innovative clinical research and developing evidence-based guidelines that improve outcomes for the millions of people who suffer from TBI every year.
- BTF's first, second, and third evidence-based guidelines for managing severe TBI (coma) were published in 1995, 2000, and 2007, respectively. The most recent (4th ed.) BTF guidelines were published in the year 2016 and were endorsed by the American Association of Neurological Surgeons (AANS) and the Congress of Neurological Surgeons (CNS).
- Altogether, 18 topics included in the fourth edition are organized in three categories—treatments, monitoring, and thresholds. The two new topics included in the fourth edition are decompressive craniectomy and cerebrospinal fluid drainage.

Level of recommendation

- Recommendations in this edition are designated as Level I, Level II A, Level II B, or Level III. The levels are primarily based on the quality of the body of evidence as follows:
  - Level I recommendations are based on a high-quality body of evidence.
  - Level II A recommendations are based on a moderate-quality body of evidence.
  - Level II B and III recommendations are based on a low-quality body of evidence.

In this chapter, we have summarized the BTF guidelines (2016) so as to ensure easy understanding to the readers.

Category: Treatment

1. Decompressive craniectomy (DC)
   - Level I—None (Insufficient data to support)

Level II A—Bifrontal DC is not recommended to improve outcomes as measured by the Glasgow Outcome Scale–Extended (GOS-E) score at 6 months postinjury in severe TBI patients with diffuse injury (without mass lesions), and with intracranial pressure (ICP) elevation to values >20 mmHg for more than 15 minutes within a 1-hour period that are refractory to first-tier therapies. However, this procedure has been demonstrated to reduce ICP and to minimize days in the intensive care unit (ICU).

A large frontotemporoparietal (FTP) DC (not less than 12 × 15 cm or 15 cm diameter) is recommended.
- Level II B: None
- Level III: None

2. Prophylactic hypothermia
   - Level I: None
   - Level II A: None
   - Level II B: Early (within 2.5 hours), short-term (48 hours postinjury) prophylactic hypothermia is not recommended to improve outcomes in patients with diffuse injury.
   - Level III: None

3. Hyperosmolar therapy
   - Levels I, II, III: Although hyperosmolar therapy may lower ICP, there is insufficient evidence about effects on clinical outcomes to support a specific recommendation, or to support use of any specific hyperosmolar agent, for patients with severe TBI.

4. Cerebrospinal fluid (CSF) drainage
   - Level I: None
   - Levels II A and II B: None
   - Level III: An external ventricular drainage (EVD) system zeroed at the midbrain with continuous drainage of CSF may be considered to lower ICP burden more effectively than intermittent use. Use of CSF drainage to lower ICP in patients with an initial Glasgow Coma Scale (GCS) <6 during the first 12 hours after injury may be considered.

5. Ventilation therapies
   - Levels I and II A: None
   - Level II B: Prolonged prophylactic hyperventilation with partial pressure of carbon dioxide in arterial blood ($PaCO_2$) of 25 mmHg or less is not recommended.
   - Level III: None

6. Anesthetics, analgesics, and sedatives
   - Levels I and II A: None
   - Level II B: Administration of barbiturates to induce burst suppression measured by EEG as prophylaxis against the development of intracranial hypertension is not recommended. High-dose barbiturate administration is recommended to control elevated ICP refractory to maximum standard medical and surgical treatment. Hemodynamic stability is essential before and during barbiturate therapy. Although propofol is recommended for the control of ICP, it is not recommended for improvement in mortality or 6-month outcomes. Caution is required as high-dose propofol can produce significant morbidity.
   - Level III: None

7. Steroids
   - Level I: The use of steroids is not recommended for improving outcome or reducing ICP. In patients with severe TBI, high-dose methylprednisolone is associated with increased mortality and is contraindicated.
   - Levels II and III: None

8. Nutrition
   - Level I: None
   - Level II A: Feeding patients to attain basal caloric replacement at least by the fifth day and, at most, by the seventh day postinjury is recommended to decrease mortality.
   - Level II B: Transgastric jejunal feeding is recommended to reduce the incidence of ventilator-associated pneumonia (VAP).
   - Level III: None

9. Infection prophylaxis
   - Level I: None
   - Level II A: Early tracheostomy is recommended to reduce mechanical ventilation days when the overall benefit is felt to outweigh the complications associated with such a procedure. However, there is no evidence that early tracheostomy reduces mortality or the rate of nosocomial pneumonia. The use of povidone-iodine (PI) oral care is not recommended to reduce VAP and

may cause an increased risk of acute respiratory distress syndrome.
- Level II B: None
- Level III: Antimicrobial-impregnated catheters may be considered to prevent catheter-related infections during EVD.

10. Deep-vein thrombosis (DVT) prophylaxis
- Levels I and II: None
- Level III: Low molecular weight heparin (LMWH) or low-dose unfractioned heparin may be used in combination with mechanical prophylaxis. However, there is an increased risk for expansion of intracranial hemorrhage.

11. Seizure prophylaxis
- Level I: None
- Level II A: Prophylactic use of phenytoin or valproate is not recommended for preventing late post-traumatic seizure (PTS). Phenytoin is recommended to decrease the incidence of early PTS (within 7 days of injury), when the overall benefit is felt to outweigh the complications associated with such treatment. However, early PTS has not been associated with worse outcomes.
- Levels II B and III: None

Category: Monitoring

1. ICP monitoring
- Levels I and II A: None
- Level II B: Management of severe TBI patients using information from ICP monitoring is recommended to reduce in-hospital and 2-week, postinjury mortality.
- Level III: None

2. Cerebral perfusion pressure (CPP) monitoring
- Levels I and II A: None
- Level IIB: Management of severe TBI patients using guidelines-based recommendations for CPP monitoring is recommended to decrease 2-week mortality.
- Level III: None

3. Advanced cerebral monitoring
- Levels I and II: None
- Level III: Jugular bulb monitoring of arteriovenous oxygen content difference (AVDO$_2$), as a source of information for management

decisions, may be considered to reduce mortality and improve outcomes at 3 and 6 months postinjury.

Category: Thresholds

1. Blood pressure thresholds
- Levels I and II: None
- Level III: Maintaining SBP at ≥100 mmHg for patients 50–69 years old or at ≥110 mmHg or above for patients 15–49 or over 70 years old may be considered to decrease mortality and improve outcomes.

2. ICP thresholds
- Levels I and II A: None
- Level II B: Treating ICP above 22 mmHg is recommended because values above this level are associated with increased mortality.
- Level III: A combination of ICP values and clinical and brain CT findings may be used to make management decisions.

3. CPP thresholds
- Levels I and II A: None
- Level II B: The recommended target CPP value for survival and favorable outcomes is between 60 and 70 mmHg. Whether 60 or 70 mmHg is the minimum optimal CPP threshold is unclear and may depend upon the patient's autoregulatory status.
- Level III: Avoiding aggressive attempts to maintain CPP above 70 mmHg with fluids and pressors may be considered because of the risk of adult respiratory failure.

4. Advanced cerebral monitoring thresholds
- Levels I and II: None
- Level III: Jugular venous saturation of <50% may be a threshold to avoid in order to reduce mortality and improve outcomes.

REFERENCES

Brain Trauma Foundation. https://www.braintrauma.org/.

Carney N, Totten AM, O'Reilly C et al. Guidelines for the management of severe traumatic brain injury, fourth edition. *Neurosurgery*. 2017; 80:6-15.

SCALES/SCORES USED IN NEUROANESTHESIA, NEUROINTENSIVE CARE, AND NEUROTRAUMA

Scores/Scales	Reference	Web address
Scores/Scales Used in Neuroanesthesia and Neurointensive Care		
Mallampati Score for Airway Assessment	Mallampati SR, Gatt SP, Gugino LD et al. A clinical sign to predict difficult tracheal intubation: A prospective study. *Can Anaesth Soc J*. 1985;32:429-434.	http://blogs.ubc.ca /ransonetec530b/files /2012/07/MALLAMPATI _SCORE.pdf
Cormack–Lehane Classification for Airway Assessment	Cormack RS, Lehane J. Difficult tracheal intubation in obstetrics. *Anaesthesia*. 1984;39:1105-1111.	http://www.darc-airway .com/site/images /articleofmonth /cormacklehane84.pdf
ASA Physical Status Classification System	Hurwitz EE, Simon M, Vinta SR et al. Adding examples to the ASA-physical status classification improves correct assignment to patients. *Anesthesiology*. 2017;126: 614-622.	https://www.asahq.org /resources/clinical -information/asa-physical -status-classification -system.
Modified Aldrete Recovery Score	Aldrete JA. The post-anesthesia recovery score revisited. *J Clin Anesth*. 1995;7:89-91.	http://www.sciencedirect .com/science/article/pii /095281809400001K?via %3Dihub
Modified Postanesthesia Discharge Scoring (PADS) System	Chung F, Chan VW, Ong D. A post-anesthetic discharge scoring system for home readiness after ambulatory surgery. *J Clin Anesth*. 1995;7:500-506.	http://www.sciencedirect .com/science/article/pii /095281809500130A?via %3Dihub
Ramsay Sedation Scale (RSS)	Ramsay MA, Savege TM, Simpson BR, Goodwin R. Controlled sedation with alphaxalone–alphadolone. *Br Med J*. 1974;2(5920):656-659.	https://www.ncbi.nlm.nih .gov/pmc/articles /PMC1613102/
Richmond Agitation-Sedation Scale (RASS)	Sessler CN, Gosnell MS, Grap MJ et al. The Richmond Agitation-Sedation Scale: Validity and reliability in adult intensive care unit patients. *Am J Respir Crit Care Med*. 2002; 166:1338-44. Ely EW, Truman B, Shintani A et al. Monitoring sedation status over time in ICU patients: Reliability and validity of the Richmond Agitation-Sedation Scale (RASS). *JAMA*. 2003;289:2983-2991.	http://www.acclaimhealth .ca/wp-content/uploads /2013/11/Agitation -Sedation-Scale -Richmond-RASS.pdf
Numeric Rating Scale for Pain Assessment	MacCaffery M, Beebe A. Pain: Clinical manual for nursing practice. *Mosby*; 1989.	http://www.physio-pedia .com/Numeric_Pain _Rating_Scale

(*Continued*)

Scores/Scales	Reference	Web address
Behavioral Pain Scale	Payen JF, Bru O, Bosson JL et al. Assessing pain in critically ill sedated patients by using a behavioral pain scale. *Crit Care Med.* 2001;29:2258-2263.	https://com-jax-emergency -pami.sites.medinfo.ufl .edu/files/2015/02 /behavioral-pain-scale.pdf
The Nociception Coma Scale	Schnakers C, Chatelle C, Vanhaudenhuyse A et al. The Nociception Coma Scale: A new tool to assess nociception in disorders of consciousness. *Pain.* 2010;148:215-219.	http://www.coma.ulg.ac .be/papers/vs/schnakers _pain_2009.pdf
Intensive Care Delirium Screening Checklist	Bergeron N, Dubois MJ, Dumont M, Dial S, Skrobik Y. Intensive Care Delirium Screening Checklist: Evaluation of a new screening tool. *Intensive Care Med.* 2001;27:859-864.	http://www .ubccriticalcaremedicine .ca/academic/jc_article /ICDSC%20Screening %20Tool%20Bergeron %20Int%20Car%20Med %202001%20(Apr-17-08) .pdf

Scores/Scales Used in Neurotrauma

Scores/Scales	Reference	Web address
Glasgow Coma Scale (GCS) for Consciousness Assessment	Teasdale G, Jennett B. Assessment of coma and impaired consciousness. A practical scale. *Lancet.* 1974;2:81-84.	http://www.sciencedirect .com/science/article/pii /S0140673674916390? via%3Dihub
FOUR SCORE (Full Outline of UnResponsiveness) for Consciousness Assessment	Wijdicks EF, Bamlet WR, Maramattom BV, Manno EM, McClelland RL. Validation of a new coma scale: The FOUR score. *Ann Neurol.* 2005;58:585-93.	http://rtjournalonline.com /Validation%20of%20a %20new%20coma %20scale%20-%20The %20FOUR%20score.pdf
Westmead Post-Traumatic Amnesia Scale (WPTAS)	Shores EA, Marosszeky JE, Sandanam J, Batchelor J. Preliminary validation of a clinical scale for measuring the duration of post-traumatic amnesia. *Med J Aust.* 1986; 144:569-572.	file:///C:/Users/acer /Downloads /WestmeadPTAScale (2009).pdf
Rappaport Coma/Near Coma Scale	Rappaport M, Hall KM, Hopkins K, Belleza T, Cope DN. Disability rating scale for severe head trauma: Coma to community. *Arch Phys Med Rehabil.* 1982;63:118-123.	http://www.coma.ulg.ac .be/images/cncs_e.pdf
American Spinal Injury Association (ASIA) Impairment Scale	American Spinal Injury Association. International Standards for Neurological Classifications of Spinal Cord Injury. Revised Edition, ASI Association, ed. Chicago. 2000:1-23.	http://www.ftrdergisi.com /uploads/sayilar/292 /buyuk/S25-S31y.pdf
Sub-Axial Cervical Spine Injury (SLIC) Classification	Vaccaro AR, Hulbert RJ, Patel AA et al. The subaxial cervical spine injury classification system: A novel approach to recognize the importance of morphology, neurology, and integrity of the disco-ligamentous	http://emedicine. medscape.com/article /2172534-overview

(Continued)

Scores/Scales	Reference	Web address
	complex. *Spine (Phila Pa 1976)*. 2007; 32:2365-2374.	
Botterell's Clinical Grades for Aneurysmal Sub-arachnoid Hemorrhage	Botterell EH, Lougheed WM, Scott JW, Vandewater SL. Hypothermia, and inter-ruption of carotid, or carotid and vertebral circulation, in the surgical management of intracranial aneurysms. *J Neurosurg.* 1956;13:1-42.	http://cmp-manual.wbs.cz /skaly/subarachnoid _hemorrhage_grading _scales.pdf
Modified Hunt & Hess Grading System for Aneurysmal Subarach-noid Hemorrhage	Hunt WE, Hess RM. Surgical risk as related to time of intervention in the repair of intra-cranial aneurysms. *J Neurosurg.* 1968;28:14-20.	http://cmp-manual.wbs.cz /skaly/subarachnoid _hemorrhage_grading _scales.pdf
Modified Hunt and Kosnik Grading System for Aneurysmal Subarach-noid Hemorrhage	Hunt WE, Kosnik EJ. Timing and perioperative care in intracranial aneurysm surgery. *Clin Neurosurg.* 1974;21:79-89.	http://cmp-manual.wbs.cz /skaly/subarachnoid _hemorrhage_grading _scales.pdf
World Federation of Neurological Surgeons' (WFNS) Grades for Aneurysmal Subarach-noid Hemorrhage	Teasdale GM, Drake CG, Hunt W et al. A universal subarachnoid hemorrhage scale: Report of a committee of the World Federation of Neurosurgical Societies. *J Neurol Neurosurg Psychiatry.* 1988;51:1457.	http://cmp-manual.wbs.cz /skaly/subarachnoid _hemorrhage_grading _scales.pdf
Spetzler-Martin Grading for Arteriovenous Mal-formation	Spetzler RF, Martin NA. A proposed grading system for arteriovenous malformations. *J Neurosurg.* 1986;65:476-483.	https://www.cns.org/sites /default/files/clinical _neuro/Chapter3_0.pdf

Neuroradiologic Scores/Scales in Neurotrauma

Grading of Diffuse Axonal Injury	Adams JH, Doyle D, Ford I, Gennarelli TA, Graham DI, McLellan DR. Diffuse axonal injury in head injury: Definition, diagnosis and grading. *Histopathology.* 1989;15:49-59.	http://radclass.mudr.org /content/adams -classification-diffuse -axonal-injury-dai
Blunt Carotid Arterial Injury (BCI) Grading Scale	Biffl WL, Moore EE, Offner PJ et al. Blunt carotid arterial injuries: Implications of a new grading scale. *J Trauma.* 1999; 47: 845-853.	http://www .surgicalcriticalcare.net /Guidelines/Blunt %20cerebrovascular %20injuries%202015.pdf
Fisher Scale for Aneurys-mal Subarachnoid Hemorrhage	Fisher CM, Kistler JP, Davis JM. Relation of cerebral vasospasm to subarachnoid hemor-rhage visualized by computerized tomo-graphic scanning. *Neurosurgery.* 1980; 6:1-9.	http://www.thieme.com /media/samples /pubid1181591693.pdf
Modified Fisher Scale for Aneurysmal Subarach-noid Hemorrhage	Frontera JA, Claassen J, Schmidt JM et al. Prediction of symptomatic vasospasm after subarachnoid hemorrhage: The modified fisher scale. *Neurosurgery.* 2006;59:21-27.	http://www.thieme.com /media/samples /pubid1181591693.pdf

(Continued)

Scores/Scales	Reference	Web address
Anderson-D'Alonzo Classification for Odontoid Fracture	Hsu WK, Anderson PA. Odontoid fractures: Update on management. *J Am Acad Orthop Surg.* 2010;18:383-394.	https://www.hindawi.com /journals/crior/2016 /7561682/
Anderson & Montesano Classification of Occipital Condyle Fractures	Anderson PA, Montesano PX. Morphology and treatment of occipital condyle fractures. *Spine (Phila Pa 1976).* 1988; 13:731-736.	http://www.orthobullets .com/spine/2013 /occipital-condyle -fractures
Marshall CT Classification of Traumatic Brain Injury (TBI)	Marshall LF, Marshall SB, Klauber MR et al. The diagnosis of head injury requires a classification based on computed axial tomography. *J. Neurotrauma.* 1992;9 (suppl 1): S287-S292.	http://neurocriticalcare .pbworks.com/w/page /9216463/Marshall %20CT%20Score
Rotterdam CT Score in TBI	Maas AI, Hukkelhoven CW, Marshall LF, Steyerberg EW. Prediction of outcome in traumatic brain injury with computed tomographic characteristics: A comparison between the computed tomographic classification and combinations of computed tomographic predictors. *Neurosurgery.* 2005; 57:1173-1182.	http://neurocriticalcare .pbworks.com/w/page /9216486/Rotterdam %20CT%20Score

Outcome Scores/Scales in Neurotrauma

Scores/Scales	Reference	Web address
Glasgow Outcome Scale	Jennett B, Bond M. Assessment of outcome after severe brain damage. *Lancet.* 1975;1:480-484	https://www.ncbi.nlm.nih .gov/pmc/articles /PMC3253309/
Extended Glasgow Coma Scale	Wilson JT, Pettigrew LE, Teasdale GM. Structured interviews for the Glasgow Outcome Scale and the extended Glasgow Outcome Scale: Guidelines for their use. *J Neurotrauma.* 1998;15:573-585.	https://www.ncbi.nlm.nih .gov/pmc/articles /PMC3253309/
Modified Rankin Scale	Rankin J. Cerebral vascular accidents in patients over the age of 60. II. Prognosis. *Scott Med J.* 1957;2:200-215. Farrell B, Godwin J, Richards S, Warlow C. The United Kingdom transient ischaemic attack (UK-TIA) aspirin trial: Final results. *J Neurol Neurosurg Psychiatry.* 1991.54:1044-1054.	http://www.strokecenter .org/wp-content /uploads/2011/08 /modified_rankin.pdf
Neurological Outcome Scale for Traumatic Brain Injury (NOS-TBI)	Wilde EA, McCauley SR, Kelly TM et al. The Neurological Outcome Scale for Traumatic Brain Injury (NOS-TBI): I. Construct validity. *J Neurotrauma.* 2010;27:983-989	http://www.rehabmeasures .org/Lists /RehabMeasures /DispForm.aspx?ID=1079
Barthel Index	Mahoney FI, Barthel DW. Functional evaluation: The Barthel index. *Md State Med J.* 1965;14:61-65.	http://www.strokecenter .org/wp-content/uploads /2011/08/barthel.pdf

Index

Page numbers followed by f and t indicate figures and tables, respectively.

T - #0154 - 111024 - C650 - 254/178/30 - PB - 9780367571443 - Gloss Lamination